Small Animal
Pediatrics

THE FIRST 12 MONTHS OF LIFE

Small Animal
Pediatrics

THE FIRST 12 MONTHS OF LIFE

Michael E. Peterson, DVM, MS
Staff Veterinarian
Reid Veterinary Hospital
Albany, Oregon;
Instructor
College of Veterinary Medicine
Oregon State University
Corvallis, Oregon

Michelle Anne Kutzler, DVM, PhD, DACT
Associate Professor
Companion Animal Industries
Department of Animal Science
College of Agricultural Sciences
Oregon State University
Corvallis, Oregon

with over 260 illustrations

ELSEVIER
SAUNDERS

SAUNDERS

3251 Riverport Lane
St. Louis, Missouri 63043

SMALL ANIMAL PEDIATRICS: THE FIRST 12 MONTHS   ISBN: 978-1-4160-4889-3
OF LIFE

Notices

Knowledge and best practice in this field are constantly changing. As new research and experience broaden
our understanding, changes in research methods, professional practices, or medical treatment may become
necessary.

Practitioners and researchers must always rely on their own experience and knowledge in evaluating and
using any information, methods, compounds, or experiments described herein. In using such information
or methods they should be mindful of their own safety and the safety of others, including parties for
whom they have a professional responsibility.

With respect to any drug or pharmaceutical products identified, readers are advised to check the most
current information provided (i) on procedures featured or (ii) by the manufacturer of each product to be
administered, to verify the recommended dose or formula, the method and duration of administration, and
contraindications. It is the responsibility of practitioners, relying on their own experience and knowledge
of their patients, to make diagnoses, to determine dosages and the best treatment for each individual
patient, and to take all appropriate safety precautions.

To the fullest extent of the law, neither the Publisher nor the authors, contributors, or editors, assume
any liability for any injury and/or damage to persons or property as a matter of products liability,
negligence or otherwise, or from any use or operation of any methods, products, instructions, or ideas
contained in the material herein.

Library of Congress Cataloging-in-Publication Data

Small animal pediatrics : the first 12 months of life / [edited by] Michael E. Peterson, Michelle Anne
Kutzler.—1st ed.
      p. ; cm.
    Includes bibliographical references.
    ISBN 978-1-4160-4889-3 (hardcover : alk. paper)   1. Veterinary pediatrics.   2. Puppies—
Diseases.   3. Kittens—Diseases.   I. Peterson, Michael E. (Michael Edward), 1953-   II. Kutzler, Michelle
Anne.
    [DNLM: 1. Dog Diseases.   2. Cat Diseases.   3. Cats—growth & development.   4. Dogs—growth &
development.   5. Veterinary Medicine. SF 991 S6357 2011]
    SF991.S5947 2011
636.089′892—dc22   2010011466

Vice President and Publisher: Linda Duncan
Acquisitions Editor: Heidi Pohlman
Developmental Editor: Maureen Slaten
Publishing Services Manager: Catherine Jackson
Senior Project Manager: David Stein
Design Direction: Karen Pauls

Printed in China

Last digit is the print number: 9 8 7 6 5 4 3 2 1

To my wife Kate and my children, Greyson, Rosie, Rube, and Cory. I would like to express my gratitude to Tim Reid and the staff at Reid Veterinary Hospital for their support in my academic endeavors.

Michael E. Peterson

To my husband, Sean, and to my children, Courtney, Colleen, and Connor.

Michelle Anne Kutzler

Turi K. Aarnes, DVM, MS
Clinical Instructor
Department of Veterinary Clinical Sciences
College of Veterinary Medicine
The Ohio State University
Columbus, Ohio
Pain Assessment and Management

Tomas W. Baker, MS
Supervisor
Department of Surgery and Radiological Sciences
School of Veterinary Medicine
University of California
Davis, California
Ultrasonography of the Young Patient

Karyn E. Bird, DVM, PhD
Research Assistant Professor
Department of Biomedical Sciences
College of Veterinary Medicine
Oregon State University
Corvallis, Oregon
The Hematologic and Lymphoid Systems

Linda Lou Blythe, DVM, PhD
Professor
Department of Biomedical Sciences
College of Veterinary Medicine
Oregon State University
Corvallis, Oregon
The Neurologic System

Edward B. Breitschwerdt, DVM
Professor of Medicine and Infectious Disease
Department of Clinical Sciences
College of Veterinary Medicine
North Carolina State University
Raleigh, North Carolina
Diseases Formerly Known as Rickettsial: The Rickettsioses, Ehrlichioses, Anaplasmoses, and Neorickettsial and Coxiella Infections

Gert J. Breur, DVM, PhD, DACVS
Professor
Department of Veterinary Clinical Sciences
College of Veterinary Medicine
Purdue University
West Lafayette, Indiana
The Musculoskeletal System

Barret J. Bulmer, DVM, MS, DACVIM
Staff Veterinarian
Cummings School of Veterinary Medicine
Tufts University
North Grafton, Massachusetts
The Cardiovascular System

Sharon A. Center, DVM, DACVIM
Professor
Department of Clinical Sciences
College of Veterinary Medicine
Cornell University
Ithaca, New York
The Liver, Biliary Tract, and Exocrine Pancreas

Joshua Daniels, DVM, PhD, DACVM
Assistant Professor
Department of Veterinary Clinical Sciences
College of Veterinary Medicine
The Ohio State University
Columbus, Ohio
Bacterial Infections

Craig Datz, DVM, MS, DABVP
Assistant Professor
Department of Veterinary Medicine and Surgery
College of Veterinary Medicine
University of Missouri
Columbia, Missouri
Parasitic and Protozoal Diseases

Autumn P. Davidson, DVM, MS, DACVIM
Clinical Professor
Department of Medicine and Epidemiology
School of Veterinary Medicine
University of California
Davis, California;
Staff Internist
Department of Internal Medicine
VCA Animal Care Center of Sonoma
Rohnert Park, California
Ultrasonography of the Young Patient

Emilio DeBess, DVM, MPVM
State Public Health Veterinarian
Acute and Communicable Disease Section
Oregon Department of Human Services
Portland, Oregon
Selected Zoonotic Diseases: Puppies and Kittens

James F. Evermann, MS, PhD
Professor
Department of Veterinary Clinical Sciences
Washington Animal Disease Diagnostic Laboratory
College of Veterinary Medicine
Washington State University
Pullman, Washington
Immunologic Development and Immunization
Viral Infections

Kevin T. Fitzgerald, DVM, PhD, DABVP
Staff Veterinarian
VCA Alameda East Veterinary Hospital
Denver, Colorado
Husbandry of the Neonate
Fungal Infections

Mary B. Glaze, DVM, MS, DACVO
Staff Ophthalmologist
Gulf Coast Animal Eye Clinic
Houston, Texas
The Eye

Jana M. Gordon, DVM, DACVIM
Assistant Professor
Department of Clinical Sciences
College of Veterinary Medicine
Oregon State University
Corvallis, Oregon
The Urinary System

M. Elena Gorman, DVM, MS, DACVP
Assistant Professor
Department of Biomedical Sciences
College of Veterinary Medicine
Oregon State University
Corvallis, Oregon
Clinical Chemistry of the Puppy and Kitten

Deborah S. Greco, DVM, PhD, DACVIM
Senior Research Scientist
Department of Technical Communication
Nestle Purina Petcare
St. Louis, Missouri
The Endocrine System

Diane Heider, DVM
Staff Veterinarian
Willamette Veterinary Hospital
Corvallis, Oregon
Standards of Care in Pediatrics

Melissa A. Kennedy, DVM, PhD, DACVM
Associate Professor
Department of Comparative Medicine
College of Veterinary Medicine
University of Tennessee
Knoxville, Tennessee
Viral Infections

Linda B. Kidd, DVM, PhD, DACVIM
Assistant Professor,
Department of Clinical Sciences
College of Veterinary Medicine
Western University of Health Sciences
Pomona, California
Diseases Formerly Known as Rickettsial: The Rickettsioses,
*   Ehrlichioses, Anaplasmoses, and Neorickettsial and*
*   Coxiella Infections*

Michelle Anne Kutzler, DVM, PhD, DACT
Associate Professor
Companion Animal Industries
Department of Animal Science
College of Agricultural Sciences
Oregon State University
Corvallis, Oregon
The Urinary System
The Reproductive Tract

Christiane V. Löhr, Dr. med. vet., PhD, DACVP
Associate Professor
Department of Biomedical Sciences
College of Veterinary Medicine
Oregon State University
Corvallis, Oregon
Postmortem Examination of the Puppy and Kitten

Andrew U. Luescher, Dr. med. vet., PhD, DACVB,
**   ECVBM-CA**
Director
Animal Behavior Clinic
Associate Professor
Department of Veterinary Clinical Sciences
College of Veterinary Medicine
Purdue University
West Lafayette, Indiana
Canine Behavioral Development

John Mata, PhD
Senior Research Assistant Professor
Department of Biomedical Sciences
College of Veterinary Medicine
Oregon State University
Corvallis, Oregon
Pharmacologic Considerations in the Young Patient

John S. Mattoon, DVM, DACVR
Professor
Department of Veterinary Clinical Sciences
College of Veterinary Medicine
Washington State University
Pullman, Washington
Radiographic Considerations of the Young Patient

Sean P. McDonough, DVM, PhD, DACVP
Associate Professor
Department of Biomedical Sciences
College of Veterinary Medicine
Cornell University
Ithaca, New York
The Musculoskeletal System

Maureen A. McMichael, DVM, DACVECC
Associate Professor
Department of Veterinary Clinical Medicine
College of Veterinary Medicine
University of Illinois
Urbana, Illinois
Emergency and Critical Care Issues

James B. Miller, MS, DVM, DACVIM
Professor
Department of Companion Animals
Atlantic Veterinary College
University of Prince Edward Island
Charlottetown, Prince Edward Island
Canada
Approach to the Febrile Patient

Cornelia Mosley, DVM, DACVA
Assistant Professor
Department of Veterinary Clinical Sciences
College of Veterinary Medicine
Oregon State University
Corvallis, Oregon
Anesthesia in the Pediatric Patient

Craig A.E. Mosley, DVM, MSc, DACVA
Assistant Professor
Department of Clinical Studies
College of Veterinary Medicine
Oregon State University
Corvallis, Oregon
Anesthesia in the Pediatric Patient

William W. Muir, III, DVM, PhD, DACVA, DACVECC
Chief Medical Officer
The Animal Medical Center
New York, New York
Pain Assessment and Management

Kristin L. Newquist, BS, AAS, CVT
General and Exotic Practice Technician
VCA Alameda East Veterinary Hospital
Denver, Colorado
Husbandry of the Neonate
Fungal Infections

Mark G. Papich, DVM, MS, DACVCP
Professor
Department of Molecular Biomedical Sciences
College of Veterinary Medicine
North Carolina State University
Raleigh, North Carolina
Pharmacologic Considerations in the Young Patient

Michael E. Peterson, DVM, MS
Staff Veterinarian
Reid Veterinary Hospital
Albany, Oregon;
Instructor
College of Veterinary Medicine
Oregon State University
Corvallis, Oregon
Growth
Care of the Orphaned Puppy and Kitten
Neonatal Mortality
Toxicologic Considerations in the Young Patient
The Digestive System

Jon D. Plant, DVM, DACVD
Medical Specialist in Dermatology
Central Team Support
Banfield, The Pet Hospital
Portland, Oregon
The Skin and Ear

Heather Prendergast, RVT
Practice Manager
Jornada Veterinary Clinic
Las Cruces, New Mexico
*Nutritional Requirements and Feeding of Growing Puppies
    and Kittens*
Clinical Approach to Pediatric Nutritional Conditions

Lisa Radosta, DVM, DACVB
Owner
Florida Veterinary Behavior Service
West Palm Beach, Florida
Feline Behavioral Development

Valeria Rickard, DVM
Owner and Chief of Staff
North Oatlands Animal Hospital, PC
Leesburg, Virginia
Birth and the First 24 Hours

Margaret V. Root Kustritz, DVM, PhD, DACT
Associate Professor, Vice-Chair
Department of Veterinary Clinical Sciences
Assistant Dean of Education
College of Veterinary Medicine
University of Minnesota
St. Paul, Minnesota
History and Physical Examination of the Neonate
History and Physical Examination of the Weanling and
*   Adolescent*

Craig Ruaux, BVSc, PhD, MACVSc, DACVIM
Assistant Professor
Department of Clinical Sciences
College of Veterinary Medicine
Oregon State University
Corvallis, Oregon
The Respiratory System

Bernard Séguin, DVM, MS, DACVS
Associate Professor
Department of Clinical Sciences
College of Veterinary Medicine
Oregon State University
Corvallis, Oregon
Surgical Considerations in the Young Patient

Frances O. Smith, DVM, PhD
Reproduction Specialist
Smith Veterinary Hospital
Burnsville, Minnesota
Prenatal Care of the Bitch and Queen

Erick Spencer, DVM
Assistant Professor
Department of Veterinary Clinical Sciences
College of Veterinary Medicine
Washington State University
Pullman, Washington
Bacterial Infections

Patricia A. Talcott, MS, DVM, PhD, DABVT
Associate Professor
Department of Veterinary and Comparative Anatomy,
    Pharmacology and Physiology
College of Veterinary Medicine
Washington State University
Pullman, Washington
Effective Use of a Veterinary Medical Diagnostic Laboratory

Rory J. Todhunter, BVSc, MS, PhD, DACVS
Professor
Department of Clinical Sciences
College of Veterinary Medicine
Cornell University
Ithaca, New York
The Musculoskeletal System

Andrea Van de Wetering, DVM, FAVD
Owner and Chief of Staff
Advanced Pet Dentistry
Corvallis, Oregon
Dental and Oral Cavity

Michael Weh, DVM, DACVS
Assistant Professor
Department of Small Animal Medicine and Surgery
College of Veterinary Medicine
University of Georgia
Athens, Georgia
Pediatric Fracture Management

Tamara B. Wills, DVM, MS, DACVP
Assistant Professor
Department of Veterinary Clinical Sciences
College of Veterinary Medicine
Washington State University
Pullman, Washington
Immunologic Development and Immunization

The field of veterinary neonatal and pediatric care is still in its infancy and is most advanced in the area of large animals, specifically horses. In recent years, veterinary conferences have identified feline and canine neonatology and pediatrics as areas in which practitioners are interested in additional knowledge and training. Pediatric dogs and cats are not small adults but rather have distinct anatomic and physiologic properties that must be taken into consideration.

Our purpose in developing this text is to gather into one location the current information available on puppy and kitten husbandry, normal development, internal medicine, and surgery.

The book is designed for veterinarians but can be useful for advanced breeders. All the chapters are focused on the unique considerations for the neonatal and pediatric puppy or kitten. The text is organized in four sections. The first, "General Considerations," encompasses subjects such as prenatal care of the dam or queen through birth, how to perform physical examinations, recommended husbandry, nutritional requirements, care of orphans, behavioral development, and other topics. Discussions on neonatal mortality, emergency and critical care, and immunologic development are provided.

The second section, "Common Infectious Diseases in Puppies and Kittens," includes chapters on bacterial, viral, fungal, rickettsial, and parasitic infections. The third section, "Diagnostic and Therapeutic Approaches to the Pediatric Patient," includes chapters on topics such as radiology, ultrasound, anesthesia, surgery, pharmacology, pain management, toxicology, and clinical pathology.

The fourth section "Systematic Clinical Approach to Diagnosis and Treatment of Pediatric Conditions," covers all the organ systems (e.g., cardiovascular, respiratory, dental, urinary, reproductive). Each chapter in this section is designed to approach its specific organ system with a description of normal development until that system is the same as that of the adult (this varies with the system being described) followed by descriptions of common congenital abnormalities, and finishing with common acquired conditions.

Michael E. Peterson and Michelle Anne Kutzler

ACKNOWLEDGMENTS

First and foremost I offer my profound appreciation for my wife Kate who manages to endure my literary projects and never tells me "I told you so" when roadblocks arise. She does, however, seem to have mastered the one raised eyebrow look whenever I complain. A big thanks to Maureen Slaten at Elsevier for her professionalism, dedication, and patience through the entire process. Additionally it has been a pleasure to work with David Stein and his production group.

Michael E. Peterson

My inspiration for this work is Dr. Johnny D. Hoskins for his leadership in the field of small animal pediatrics. I was also inspired by many years of questions from veterinarians and veterinary students, as well as from dog and cat breeders.

I especially appreciate my good friend and colleague Dr. Mike Peterson for being the constant driving force behind this book. Thank you, Mike. In addition, I am very grateful to each of the individual authors for sharing their time, wisdom, and passion for small animal pediatrics. They were instrumental and I am indebted to them for their contributions. Special recognition is owed to Elsevier for identifying the need and for the ongoing commitment to provide high quality information for health care professionals and support of the process. Working with the Developmental Editor Maureen Slaten was a joy. And thanks to my family, my mother who helped with the editing, and my husband and children, at whose events I could only be present in spirit.

Michelle Anne Kutzler

CONTENTS

PRENATAL CARE OF THE BITCH AND QUEEN

CHAPTER 1

Frances O. Smith

Prenatal care for bitches and queens should begin with the selection of the most desirable members of a potential breeding population. The resources of the important registration bodies and the available databases for evaluation of inherited genetic diseases should be used to select desirable traits. Information is available from the American Kennel Club (AKC), the Cat Fanciers' Association, the United Kennel Club, and many individual breed clubs. The most significant health database is the database maintained by the Orthopedic Foundation for Animals (OFA). The OFA is a private nonprofit foundation that serves as a central source of information for breeders and owners based on the standards for evaluation established by the experts in each discipline. The Canine Health Information Center (CHIC) is a joint venture of the OFA and the AKC Canine Health Foundation. The focus of CHIC is health consciousness; this focus allows breeders to manage breed-specific genetic disorders. The criteria for acceptance into the CHIC program are established by each of the parent clubs that are involved. Participation in any health database is voluntary but should be encouraged by practitioners (Box 1-1).

More than 400 genetic diseases have been recognized in the dog, and genetic diseases are responsible for 25% of all disease problems affecting dogs. With the exception of inherited renal dysplasia, all of the most commonly diagnosed inherited diseases are seen in mixed breed dogs. Designer dogs have the same prevalence of genetic disease as the purebred breeds. Responsible breeders of dogs and cats, as well as the respected breed registries, make great effort to improve the genetic health of their breeding animals and thus decrease the risk of avoidable inherited disease.

The various competitive venues available to breeders, such as conformation shows for cats and conformation shows, obedience competitions, agility competitions, hunting tests, and field trials for dogs, offer layers of selection in the choice of reproducing animals. Certainly, not every bitch or queen is worthy of reproduction and the practitioner should encourage and educate potential breeders on their responsibility to choose healthy, quality bitches and queens for their breeding programs.

Breeding dogs or cats involves tremendous commitment of time, space, knowledge, and financial resources. The practitioner should counsel prospective breeders regarding the ethical considerations involved in breeding, including the difficulty in placing puppies and kittens in permanent homes and the responsibility incurred in creating these new lives.

Bitches selected for breeding should be mature enough to have genetic clearances for their appropriate breed and young enough to produce reasonable litter size and survivability. A bitch is at her peak reproductive potential between 2 and 4 years of age. In at least one study of beagle bitches, conception failure occurred in more than 50% of bitches 5 years of age or older. Similarly, the risk of dystocia increases, neonatal mortality increases, and litter size decreases with increasing maternal age. Average litter size is known for most purebred breeds, with average neonatal losses approaching 30%.

PREBREEDING EXAMINATION

The bitch should be presented to the clinician during proestrus of the anticipated breeding cycle. A complete physical examination should include a rectal examination to evaluate the bony pelvis and a digital vaginal examination to detect any vaginal abnormalities. *Brucella canis* serology using the rapid-slide agglutination test should be done. An in-house test is available (D-Tec CB, Synbiotics; www.synbiotics.com); this test has high sensitivity and low specificity. Any positive result requires additional testing and should cause a delay in breeding during the cycle in which test results are confirmed. Regardless of previous breeding history, all bitches should be evaluated because the disease is spread orally, as well as venereally. Serologic testing for canine herpes virus should be performed on virgin bitches or in

---

BOX 1-1 **Websites of kennel clubs and health testing laboratories**

American Kennel Club: www.akc.org
United Kennel Club: www.ukcdogs.com
Orthopedic Foundation for Animals: www.offa.org
Canine Health Information Center: www.caninehealthinfo.org
Optigen: www.optigen.com
PennGen: www.vet.upenn.edu/penngen
VetGen: www.VetGen.com

BOX 1-2 **Prevention of neonatal isoerythrolysis in the feline**

1. Blood type queen and tom.
2. Breed type B queens only to B toms.
3. Foster nursing of all type A and AB kittens born to type B queens for the first 24 hours.

---

bitches with a previously negative test. If the bitch has a negative titer, she must be protected from exposure to the virus. More detailed information pertaining to herpes virus can be found in Chapter 16.

Isolation from other canids for 3 weeks before whelping to 3 weeks after whelping should prevent disease. There is no vaccine available in the United States. Vaginal cytology should be obtained and stained to assess the epithelial cells present. The bitch should either have her vaccinations brought up to date or have titers performed to assess her antibody levels. The bitch should be well protected against canine distemper and canine parvovirus to maximize maternal antibody levels.

The bitch has an endotheliochorial placenta. Puppies depend on mammary transfer of antibodies because placental transfer is minimal. With normal ingestion and absorption of colostrum, the antibody level of the puppy will approximate 95% of the dam's measured antibody level. Gut permeability to immunoglobulins begins to decline within 8 hours after birth and is no longer possible after 48 to 72 hours.

The bitch should have baseline laboratory tests performed to assess her suitability for pregnancy and lactation. A bitch with total plasma protein levels of less than 5.0 gm/dl is unlikely to whelp a litter of strong, healthy puppies. Bitches with significant renal or hepatic dysfunction are not successful brood bitches. If the bitch has a history of infertility or pregnancy loss, a vaginal culture should be performed during the first 5 days of proestrus. Although the value of vaginal cultures is controversial, most clinicians consider a pure culture in significant numbers of a known pathogen to be worthy of treatment. The vaginal culture should be interpreted within the context of patient history, physical examination findings, and vaginal cytology. Both *B. canis* and *Salmonella* sp. are always considered pathogens. *B. canis* is rarely treated in any kennel or colony situation. In kennel situations, *B. canis* is managed in a test and cull manner because it is highly contagious and nearly impossible to eradicate with therapy. Antibiotic choice and duration of treatment should be based on safety and efficacy in pregnancy. Bitches that have sustained pregnancy loss may be monitored weekly for hypoluteoidism, which is a poorly documented condition.

During normal pregnancy, progesterone reaches peak levels of 15 to 90 ng/ml. During the last trimester of pregnancy, progesterone decreases until it drops below 2 ng/ml approximately 1 day before whelping. A progesterone level above 2 ng/ml is required for the maintenance of pregnancy in the bitch. If the progesterone drops to 10 ng/ml, frequent monitoring of the progesterone levels is recommended. Progesterone values of 5 ng/ml may warrant intervention with an exogenous progestogen supplementation. Exogenous progestogen administration is an extralabel use of any of the available preparations and should always be accompanied by careful client education and a signed release form outlining the risks. Prolactin and luteinizing hormone (LH) are also luteotrophic in the bitch.

The queen should also be examined before breeding. When presented, the queen should have a complete physical examination, including baseline laboratory work, and a fecal examination should be performed. Serology for feline leukemia virus (FeLV) and feline immunodeficiency virus (FIV) should be obtained. Only queens testing negative for these two viruses should be used for breeding. Neonatal isoerythrolysis occurs in purebred cats. This condition may be avoided by blood typing the queen and breeding to a tom of an appropriate blood type (Box 1-2). The blood types of domestic felids are A, B, and AB. The breeds with the highest frequency of type B blood are the British Shorthair, the Devon Rex, and the Cornish Rex. Cats are unusual in that unlike dogs, they have naturally occurring antibodies to other blood types. The A allele (A) is dominant to the B (B) allele so only the cats with homozygous recessive condition (BB) express the type B antigen on their erythrocytes. Type A cats are either homozygous AA or heterozygous AB. The AB blood type is rare and inherited separately as a third allele recessive to A and co-dominant with B. Feline neonatal isoerythrolysis occurs when maternal anti-A alloantibody gains access to the fetal circulation after colostrum ingestion and destroys type A and type AB erythrocytes. Type A and type AB kittens from a type B queen bred to a type A or AB tom are at risk. Specifics pertaining to the clinical manifestations of the disease in neonates are discussed in Chapter 2.

In the case of breedings within catteries, the status of all cats with respect to feline coronavirus (FCOR) should be evaluated (Table 1-1). To prevent the spread of coronavirus, the tom and the queen should have the same serologic status. The *Chlamydia* status of cattery members should also be determined using serology.

<table>
<tr><td colspan="3">TABLE 1-1   Disease prevention strategies in catteries</td></tr>
</table>

Infectious agent	Cats testing negative	Cats of same serology status
FeLV	X	
FIV	X	
FCOR		X
Chlamydia		X

FeLV, Feline leukemia virus; *FIV*, feline immunodeficiency virous; *FCOR*, feline coronavirus.

<table>
<tr><td colspan="3">TABLE 1-2   Vaccination in catteries</td></tr>
</table>

Infectious agent	Vaccinate	Do not vaccinate
FeLV		X
FIV		X
FPV	X	
FHV	X	
FCV		

FeLV, Feline leukemia virus; *FIV*, feline immunodeficiency virus; *FPV*, feline panleukopenia virus; *FHV*, feline herpes virus; *FCV*, feline calicivirus.

The queen should be vaccinated for feline panleukopenia (FPL), feline herpes virus (FHV), and feline calicivirus (FCV) to prevent clinical disease within the cattery (Table 1-2). However, vaccination alone may not prevent the spread of infection. Higher levels of maternal antibody may be achieved by boostering the vaccinations just before or at the time of breeding.

The queen has an endotheliochorial placenta. Colostral antibodies are the main source of immunoglobulins in the kitten. Progesterone produced by the corpus luteum is necessary for maintenance of pregnancy in the cat since placental production of progesterone is minor. The corpora lutea remains functional throughout pregnancy and regresses after delivery. The queen typically has a progesterone level of 1.0 to 1.6 ng/ml at day 60 of pregnancy Thus pregnancy likely involves pregnancy-specific secretion of luteotrophic hormones of placental or pituitary origin. Several studies indicate that prolactin is a major luteotrophic factor in pregnant queens after implantation has occurred. Hypoluteoidism has not been reported in the queen. Progesterone therapy to prevent recurrent pregnancy loss should only be considered when infectious causes of pregnancy loss in the queen have been ruled out.

NUTRITION

Proper diet for gestation begins before the bitch becomes pregnant. The bitch should be fed a quality, name-brand diet labeled complete for all life stages by the Association of American Feed Control Officials (AAFCO) standards using feeding trials or suitable for pregnancy and lactation. There

is minimal need for increased calories during the first half of pregnancy. The bitch should be kept in fit condition, and her caloric intake should be appropriate to allow for a weight gain of approximately 36% over her normal prepregnancy weight. The diet should contain a protein level of 25% to 34% and a fat level of at least 18% with a balanced supply of n-6 and n-3 fatty acids, as well as optimum vitamins and minerals. Supplements should be avoided to prevent dietary imbalances and inadvertent toxicity.

Calcium supplementation is unnecessary and can result in decreased parathyroid hormone (PTH) stimulation of bone resorption. Eclampsia (puerperal hypocalcemia) can occur when the bitch depends on intestinal calcium absorption rather than on the PTH-stimulated bone calcium mobilization. After confirmation of pregnancy, the puppy or kitten diet is appropriate during the second half of pregnancy. Immediately after delivery, the bitch or queen should weigh approximately 5% more than her prepregnancy weight. It is nearly impossible to overfeed the bitch or queen during lactation. Recently, it has been established that nutrients may influence maternal or fetal gene expression, thereby influencing the metabolic status of an animal for life. It has been established that both prenatal and postnatal nutrition contribute to metabolic programming.

Many bitches experience a period of reduced appetite or inappetence during the second trimester of pregnancy. This period may be brief or prolonged. The bitch should be encouraged to eat by adding palatable foods to her diet (cooked meat or canned food). If inappetence persists, force feeding may be necessary.

Nutritional insufficiency of taurine may result in resorption, abortion, and stillbirth of kittens. Effects of a taurine deficient diet may persist beyond an individual lost pregnancy. This effect is unlikely to be seen in queens who are fed feline commercial diets but may be seen in situations where dog food is fed to cats. Dietary supplements are not recommended. Pregnant and nursing queens may have nutritional needs that are four times maintenance requirements. Canned foods may prove to be more palatable during pregnancy and should be offered if the queen's appetite wanes.

PARASITE CONTROL

It is possible and recommended to treat bitches to prevent transplacental and transmammary transmission of somatic *Toxocara canis* and *Ancylostoma caninum* larvae. There are no anthelmintics that are completely effective against the somatic and larval stages. The somatic larva of *T. canis* are encysted in muscle tissue but reactivated during the last trimester of pregnancy and migrate transplacentally. Transmammary transmission of *T. canis* occurs, whereas *A. caninum* is transmitted only transplacentally. The Centers for Disease Control (CDC) and the Companion Animal Parasite Council (CAPC) recommend aggressive deworming protocols of pregnant bitches, pregnant queens, and their offspring to prevent environmental contamination with parasite eggs and the potential zoonotic risk. A number of different protocols have been suggested using multiple doses of fenbendazole and ivermectin orally in bitches (Table 1-3). In both bitches and queens, topical selamectin 6 mg/kg has been shown to greatly reduce worm burdens in both puppies (98%) and kittens (100%) up to 6 and 7 weeks old.

External parasites must be controlled using products approved for pregnant bitches and queens. Frontline Plus and Revolution are approved for safety when used in pregnant animals. Products containing carbaryl should not be used because it may cause brachygnathia, taillessness, extra digits, failure of skeletal formation, and dystocia in bitches caused by uterine inertia. Heartworm preventive should be continued throughout pregnancy and has been proved to have a high margin of safety even in pregnant bitches and queens.

BIRTH DEFECTS

A birth defect is a deviation from normal morphology or function that occurs during pregnancy and is severe enough to interfere with viability or the physical well-being of the offspring. Teratology is the science of studying the etiology of birth defects. There are three critical periods in the development of the fetus. The first period is preimplantation (pregastrulation), which occurs from fertilization to implantation. The second is the embryonic period, which is when organogenesis occurs, and is an important period when birth defects develop. The third is the fetal period, which roughly encompasses the last 3 weeks of pregnancy, during which growth and maturation of organ systems occur. Serious insult during the preimplantation phase may result in an all-or-none phenomenon in which implantation does not occur or the cells survive and continue development. Most serious defects occur during the embryonic period (days 22 to 44 from the LH surge) in the dog. During the fetal stage, gross structural defects seldom occur except in structures undergoing rapid growth and maturation such as the palate, the cerebellum, and parts of the cardiovascular and urogenital system.

In humans, 60% of congenital malformations have no identifiable cause, 20% are a combination of hereditable and nonhereditable factors, and 3% are caused by chromosomal abnormalities. The remainders are caused by environmental factors or single gene mutations. Environmental factors include maternal illness and infection, pollutants, heavy metals, toxins, and drugs. Over 400 genetic diseases have been identified in canids and over 150 in felids, although most of these diseases are not associated with fetal loss (Boxes 1-3 and 1-4).

Certain breeds of dogs have increased incidence of birth defects. The English bulldog, the pug, the Boston Terrier, and the French bulldog all have increased incidence of fetal anasarca resulting in increased fetal loss and a greatly increased rate of cesarean sections. Anasarca or lethal

---

BOX 1-3 **Diseases causing pregnancy loss in the bitch**

Canine herpes virus
Canine parvovirus type 2
Canine distemper
Canine adenovirus
Campylobacter sp.
Escherichia coli
Mycoplasma sp.
Ureaplasma sp.
Salmonella sp.
Brucella canis
Canine minute virus (CPV-1)

BOX 1-4 **Diseases causing pregnancy loss in queen**

Feline leukemia virus (FeLV)
Feline herpes virus (FHV)
Feline panleukopenia virus (FPV)
Feline infectious peritonitis (FIP; feline coronavirus)
Feline immunodeficiency virus (FIV)
Toxoplasma
Chlamydia

TABLE 1-3 **Prevention of prenatal transmission of parasites**

Parasite	Drug	Dose	Dosing interval
Toxocara canis *Ancylostoma caninum*	Fenbendazole	50 mg/kg	Day 40 gestation Day 14 lactation
T. canis	Ivermectin	1 mg/kg 0.5 mg/kg	Day 20 and 42 of gestation Day 38, 41, 44, and 47 of gestation
A. caninum	Ivermectin	500 µg/kg	4-9 days before whelping *and* 1 dose 10 days later
A. caninum	Ivermectin	200 µg/kg	Weekly 3 weeks before to 3 weeks after whelping
T. canis *T. cati*	Topical selamectin	6 mg/kg	6 weeks and 2 weeks before whelping/queening *and* 2 weeks and 6 weeks after whelping/queening

congenital edema involves generalized subcutaneous edema and varying amounts of fluid in other body cavities (Figure 1-1). The condition is known to be heritable likely as a recessive trait. Many of the anasarcous puppies also are afflicted with congenital heart defects.

Cleft palates are common in all of the brachycephalic breeds (Figures 1-2 and 1-3). Cleft palates can be caused by genetic traits or by teratogenetic agents. Both griseofulvin and corticosteroids have been implicated as teratogens that can cause cleft palate. Even aspirin has been demonstrated to cause cleft palates. In general, all drugs should be avoided in the pregnant bitch or queen, including all live virus vaccines, unless they are necessary to maintain the welfare of the mother and the drug is reported to be safe during pregnancy.

Nutritional components have caused congenital defects. Excessive vitamin A between days 17 and 22 has been reported to result in cleft palates, kinked tails, and deformed auricles in kittens. Excess vitamin D has been linked with tissue calcinosis, premature closure of fontanelles, enamel hypoplasia, and supravalvular stenosis.

Congenital malformations can best be evaluated by careful necropsy of all nonsurviving puppies or kittens with the goal of eliminating the cause of such defects (see Chapter 31). There are several drugs that are contraindicated during pregnancy because they are known to cause birth defects (Box 1-5). For an explanation of the reproductive effect or for a complete list of drugs that are safe for use during pregnancy, see Chapter 27 (Table 27-4). Clinicians should obtain a good drug history, including the use of topical, herbal, and other alternative modalities (Box 1-6).

THE PREGNANCY CONFIRMATION VISIT

The bitch should have her pregnancy confirmed 25 to 30 days after her first breeding (Table 1-4). In lean relaxed bitches, it may be possible to detect discrete swellings in the uterus as early as 21 days after breeding. However, it is not possible to use palpation to differentiate uterine swellings

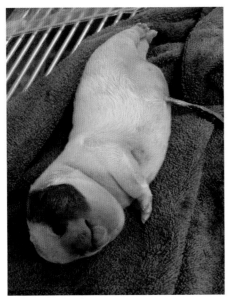

Figure 1-1 Anasarca. This miniature bulldog puppy has diffuse subcutaneous edema typically associated with anasarca.

BOX 1-5	**Drugs known to cause congenital malformations or embryotoxicity**
Altrenogest	Griseofulvin
Aspirin	Misoprostol
Ciprofloxacin	Mitotane
Corticosteroids	Oxytetracycline
Diethylstilbestrol	Pentobarbital
Doxycycline	Stanozolol
Enrofloxacin	Streptomycin
Estradiol cypionate	Testosterone
Excess vitamin A	Tetracycline
Excess vitamin D	Warfarin
Gold	

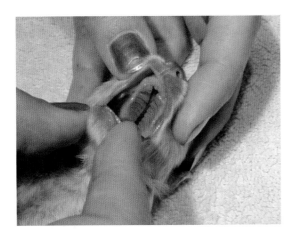

Figure 1-2 Cleft palate. Note the cleft extending the length of the palate. This 3-day-old Samoyed puppy presented with failure to gain weight and dyspnea.

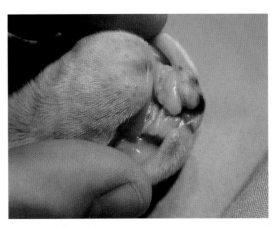

Figure 1-3 Cleft palate with harelip. Newborn Boston Terrier puppy demonstrating both a rostral cleft in the palate and a harelip defect.

BOX 1-6 Topical therapies to avoid during pregnancy

Carbaryl
Dexamethasone sodium phosphate ophthalmic
Genesis topical spray
Mometamax
Ophthalmics containing corticosteroids
Panolog cream
Pennyroyal
Rotenone
St. John's Wort
TriTop ointment

TABLE 1-4 Pregnancy diagnostics in the bitch

Diagnostic type	Appropriate/recommended time period
Abdominal palpation	• 23-30 days after breeding • 25-30 days after LH surge • Not after 30 days
Ultrasonography	• 25 days after LH surge till parturition
Radiography	• 45 days after breeding • Improved reliability closer to term
Relaxin	• Hormone level is measured by radioimmunoassay or ELISA techniques • Not as reliable as ultrasonography

LH, Luteinizing hormone; *ELISA,* enzyme-linked immunosorbent assay.

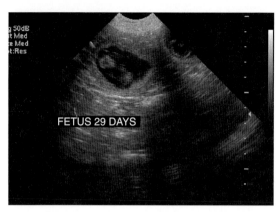

Figure 1-4 Pregnancy ultrasound shows a normal dog fetus at day 29 of gestation.

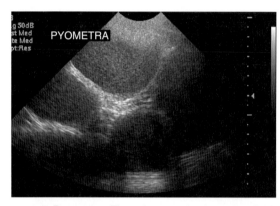

Figure 1-5 Pyometra. The ultrasound shows a fluid-filled uterus. Note the difference in echogenicity compared to the normal fetus in Figure 1-4. It is important to differentiate pathology from normal pregnancy.

associated with uterine pathology (Figures 1-4 and 1-5) from normal uterine development associated with pregnancy. After day 35, the uterine swellings enlarge, resulting in a confluence, making pregnancy palpation even more unreliable.

Real-time ultrasonography is valuable in early pregnancy diagnosis, as well as throughout the second half of gestation whenever there is a question of fetal viability or fetal loss. Ultrasonography in the bitch is accurate for pregnancy diagnosis in the hands of an experienced ultrasonographer using quality equipment as early as 19 to 21 days post-LH peak in the bitch. When the LH peak is known, pregnancy diagnosis in the bitch is very accurate after days 21 to 23. If the LH peak is unknown, ultrasonography for pregnancy detection should be performed at approximately 30 days after the last known breeding (see Figure 1-4). Fetal heartbeats are first detected 23 to 25 days after the LH peak or 16 days after the onset of cytologic diestrus. In addition to pregnancy diagnosis, ultrasonography can be used to identify fetal loss. This author has observed disparity between the sizes of gestational sacs in some pregnancies. This size disparity appears to be accompanied by low volume of embryonic fluid, cessation of fetal heart beat in the smaller sacs, shrinkage, and ultimately resorption. Ultrasound has not been proved reliable for determination of litter size. Determination of fetal age involves multiple measurements of the biparietal or trunk diameter and must take into consideration differences relative to breed and litter size.

Embryonic vesicles may be detected earlier in the queen than in the bitch (Table 1-5). Ultrasonographic pregnancy diagnosis is accurate in the queen as early as 11 to 16 days after breeding. Fetal heartbeats may be detected as early as day 16. Embryonic vesicles closest to the uterine bifurcation are detected earliest, and early examination may miss some fetuses. The ultrasound should be repeated 5 to 7 days later if no fetal vesicles are seen. Ultrasound in the queen can be used to detect fetal loss and may be used in an attempt to estimate fetal age.

Hormonal diagnosis of pregnancy varies with species. In the bitch, progesterone elevations are not different whether a bitch is or is not pregnant. Progesterone levels, however, can be used to confirm ovulation failure. In the queen, progesterone levels may be used 40 days after breeding to differentiate pseudopregnancy from pregnancy. In the pseudopregnant queen, progesterone declines to baseline levels by day 40 after breeding but remains at 1 ng/ml or above in pregnant queens. Prolactin levels increase in both the pregnant bitch and the pregnant queen; however, a commercial test is not available. Relaxin is the only reported hormone that is pregnancy-specific in carnivores and is produced by the fetoplacental unit. Relaxin is best measured by radioimmunoassay or enzyme-linked immunosorbent assay (ELISA) techniques. An in-clinic test (ReproCHEK, Synbiotics; www.synbiotics.com) has been developed but is not as reliable as ultrasonography.

At this visit, the physical examination should be repeated. The body condition of the bitch or queen should be assessed, and recommendations made for adjustments as needed. If the bitch or queen has previously been on a maintenance diet, she should be switched to a ration suitable for pregnancy and lactation. In cases where the bitch or queen is underweight and anorectic, a balanced multivitamin, such as Pet-Tabs, should be considered. There are hematologic

changes throughout pregnancy, and both the bitch and the queen will experience a gradual decline in hematocrit associated with increased plasma volume (Tables 1-6 and 1-7). Pregnancy may be accompanied by toxemia in bitches carrying large litters. Ketosis can develop in bitches not meeting the nutritional demands of pregnancy, and a negative energy balance can develop. Anorexia in late pregnancy must be corrected by force feeding or parenteral nutrition.

The owner should be questioned about any changes in behavior or appetite, increases or decreases in water consumption, extent of mammary development, and the presence of any vaginal discharge. If the bitch or queen is found to be nonpregnant at this visit, a diagnostic workup for conception failure should be discussed. This is a good time to remind the owner to avoid exposure to any infectious disease. The bitch or queen should remain in the home, kennel, or cattery environment and should not share housing or exercise areas with animals still in competition or training. This includes shared areas for exercise even if direct contact is prevented.

There are numerous viral and bacterial diseases that have potential risks for the pregnant animal. Training classes and competitive field events should be discontinued because the effect of stress on the bitch can be significant. With maternal stress, there is increased adrenaline secretion, decreased uterine and placental blood flow, decreased oxygen to the fetus, and increased fetal adrenocorticotropic hormone (ACTH).

THE PRENATAL EXAMINATION

Before term the bitch or queen should be introduced to her delivery area. This area should be safe and quiet and provide the privacy and comfort needed for the dam to become acclimated and ready for parturition. The bitch should be

TABLE 1-5	Pregnancy diagnostics in the queen
Diagnostic type	**Appropriate/recommended time period**
Abdominal palpation	• 15 days after breeding
Ultrasonography	• 11 days after breeding: embryonic vesicle
	• 16-25 days after breeding: fetal heartbeat
	• Effective till term
Radiography	• 35 days after breeding
	• Progressive increase in fetal calcification

TABLE 1-6	Effects of pregnancy on canine hematology				
Gestation	**2 weeks**	**4 weeks**	**6 weeks**	**8 weeks**	**Term**
RBC (million/µl)	8.85	7.48	6.73	6.20	4.58
PCV (%)	53	47	44	37	32
Hgb (gm/dl)	19.6	16.4	14.7	13.8	11.0
WBC (thousands/µl)	12.0	12.2	15.7	19.0	18.9

RBC, Red blood cells; *PCV,* packed cell volume; *Hgb,* hemoglobin; *WBC,* white blood cells.

TABLE 1-7	Effects of pregnancy on feline hematology					
Gestation	**1 day**	**2 weeks**	**4 weeks**	**6 weeks**	**8 weeks**	**Term**
RBC (million/µl)	8.0	7.9	7.1	6.7	6.2	6.2
PCV (%)	36.1	37.0	33.0	32.0	28.0	29.0
Hgb (gm/dl)	12.5	12.0	11.0	10.8	9.5	10.0
Reticulocytes (%, includes punctate)	9	11	9	10	20	15

RBC, Red blood cells; *PCV,* packed cell volume.

introduced to the whelping area and confined to the area where she will whelp at least 1 week before the anticipated parturition. The queen will often seek a small confined area for parturition.

The bitch or queen should have a lateral abdominal radiograph (Figure 1-6) taken 5 to 10 days before the expected delivery date to assess the number of fetuses. Radiography is an accurate method for determination of fetal numbers but can underestimate the litter size in very large litters. Radiography will also allow the assessment of the fetal skeleton for signs of fetal death (i.e., collapse of the fetal skeleton or gas within the uterus). Radiography does not truly assess the presentation of the fetus because of the mobility of the uterine horns. Ultrasonography is a better diagnostic tool for the assessment of fetal health since it allows examination of the fetal heart rate, the amount of allantoic fluid, fetal movement, and some fetal abnormalities such as abdominal wall defects (Figure 1-7). Fetal heart rates that are below 130 beats per minute indicate poor puppy viability, and the

pregnancy requires intensive monitoring. Normal fetal heart rates at term are often greater than 200 beats per minute.

During the prenatal visit, it is prudent to evaluate the dam's blood glucose and serum calcium (ionized calcium preferred) levels and packed cell volume. The physical examination should include a digital vaginal examination to detect any soft tissue obstructions (stricture or masses) and to evaluate the vaginal area for excessive edema. Any vaginal discharge warrants vaginoscopy, using either a human sigmoidoscope (Figure 1-8) or a rigid endoscope (Figure 1-9) with a video monitor to assess cervical patency and the presence of fetal membranes. The client should be given verbal and written instructions on the management of parturition and should be encouraged to inform the clinician of any change in rectal temperature (Boxes 1-7 and 1-8). The bitch's

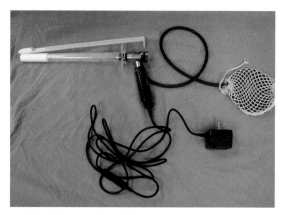

Figure 1-8 A human sigmoidoscope can be used for vaginoscopy to check the status of the cervix or if there is a puppy in the vaginal canal.

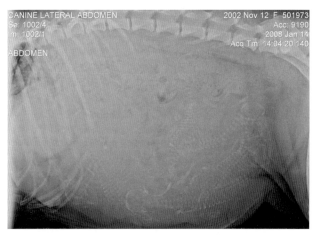

Figure 1-6 The lateral abdominal radiograph can be used to assess number of fetuses. Six puppies can be seen on this film of a Labrador retriever bitch taken 6 days before whelping.

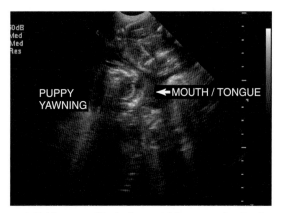

Figure 1-7 Ultrasound is the best tool for assessing fetal status and viability. It can be used to assess fetal heart beats, as well as movement of the fetus. This ultrasound captured a near-term puppy yawning.

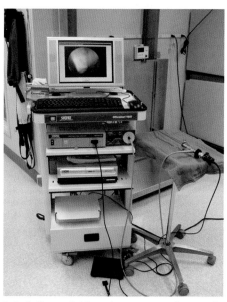

Figure 1-9 A Storz rigid endoscope can be used to examine the cervix and vagina and can also be used for transcervical insemination.

BOX 1-7   Complications of whelping

Prolonged gestation
 >71 days after breeding
 >65 days after LH peak
 >57-59 days after diestrus
 Temperature drop to 99° F (37.2° C) >24 hours
   previously
Vaginal discharge
 Mucoid—normal
 Hemorrhagic—abnormal
 Green tinged—abnormal
 Black—abnormal

Stage I labor
 Uterine inertia
 Collapse of bitch
 Vomiting
Stage II labor
 Straining continuously for 30 minutes without delivery of
   a puppy
 3 hours intermittent contractions before first puppy
 More than 3 hours between puppies

LH, Luteinizing hormone.

BOX 1-8   Normal birth in dogs (whelping)

Preparations for Whelping

Begin preparations for delivery of puppies before the female gives birth. Provide a whelping box for the mother to begin sleeping in to ensure the puppies are born in the area you have chosen. This box should be only slightly bigger than the mother, with sides 6 to 8 inches high to keep the pups from crawling out of the nest. Place the box in a secluded yet familiar area of the home, away from the family traffic, to allow the mother solitude. Newspapers make excellent bedding because they can be changed easily, are absorbent, and can be shredded by the mother as she makes her "nest." If materials such as old quilts, blankets, rugs, or towels are used, they must be washed frequently.

If you want to know precisely when delivery is near, check the rectal temperature of the mother twice daily from the 58th day of pregnancy until labor begins. Normal rectal temperature is between 100.5° F (38° C) and 102° F (38.9° C). Within 24 hours before the onset of labor, the rectal temperature drops nearly 2 degrees to 99° F (37.2° C) or below.

Labor and Delivery

Labor in the female dog (bitch) can be divided into three stages. The second and third stages are repeated with the birth of each puppy. During the first stage, the mother seems extremely restless and very nervous and often seeks seclusion. She may refuse food even if offered her favorite treats. This stage may last 6 to 24 hours. This is a good time to exercise the mother to allow her to urinate and defecate. In the second stage, uterine contractions and expulsion of the puppies begin. Usually, a small greenish sac of fluid protrudes from the vulva, followed by the puppy and its attached placenta. The normal presentation of the puppy is nose first, stomach down ("diving" position). About one-third of all puppies, however, are born hindquarters first. This presentation is considered normal in the dog. After delivery, the mother opens the sac, cleans off the pup, and severs the umbilical cord. You may have to perform these functions for the mother (see Obstetric Care). Make sure the sac is removed from the puppy immediately if it is unbroken during delivery. The third stage of labor is the resting stage, which follows delivery of each puppy. Mild contractions and delivery of the afterbirth

occur in this phase. This stage usually lasts 10 to 30 minutes, but it may range from a few seconds to an hour.

Obstetric Care

After a pup is delivered, remove all membranes covering the puppy, clean the face, and remove mucus from the mouth and nose. Rub the puppy with a clean towel to dry it and to stimulate respiration and circulation. After a few minutes of rubbing, the puppy should begin to squirm and cry loudly. The umbilical cord should be tied about an inch from the puppy's body with fine thread and then cut on the side of the knot away from the puppy. Apply a drop of Betadine to the cord end after it is cut.

Assisting with the Birth

If a puppy seems to be lodged in the birth canal and the mother cannot expel it, rapid assistance is necessary. There may not be time to call the veterinarian and drive to the hospital. Grasp the puppy with a clean towel and exert steady, firm traction. Do not jerk or pull suddenly. Traction may have to be applied for as long as 5 minutes. If you cannot remove the puppy, call the doctor.

Notify the Doctor if any of the Following Occur

- A puppy is lodged in the birth canal and cannot be removed.
- There is strong, persistent labor for 30 minutes without delivery of a pup.
- There is weak, intermittent labor for 3 hours without delivery of any puppies.
- It has been more than 3 hours since the delivery of the last pup, and it is probable that more puppies are still inside.
- There is a greenish-black vaginal discharge and no labor or puppies within 3 to 4 hours. The greenish-black color is normal, but the discharge should be followed very soon by delivery of the pups.
- The pregnancy lasts more than 65 days.
- It has been 24 hours since the drop in rectal temperature and there are no signs of labor.

temperature commonly drops to below 99°F (37.2°C) within 24 hours of initiation of parturition. The queen may experience a similar decrease in rectal temperature, although it is seldom reported by the owner. The temperature drop follows the decrease in progesterone at the end of pregnancy. During late pregnancy, the pattern of uterine electrical activity changes, which correlates with the decrease in plasma progesterone. This suggests that progesterone plays an important role in the process of parturition in the bitch. The client should be counseled to seek veterinary attention if labor is not initiated within 24 hours of the decrease in rectal temperature. The client should be given after-hours contact information if the clinician will be providing after-hours care or contact information for appropriate emergency care.

SUGGESTED READINGS

Johnson CA: Reproduction and periparturient care, *Vet Clin North Am Small Anim Pract* 16(3):417-605, 1986.

Johnston SD, Root Kustritz MV, Olson PNS: *Canine and feline theriogenology,* Philadelphia, 2001, Saunders/Elsevier.

Lee MP: *The whelping and rearing of puppies: a complete and practical guide,* Neptune City, NJ, 2003, TFH Publications.

Simpson GM, England GCW, Harvey MJ: Manual of small animal reproduction and neonatology, Gloucester, 1998, British Small Animal Veterinary Association.

BIRTH AND THE FIRST 24 HOURS

CHAPTER 2

Valeria Rickard

There are significant physiologic differences between fetuses and neonates. Puppies and kittens are born much less mature than newborns of many other domestic species and thus are more dependent on care during the first few days of life. The treatment of newborn puppies and kittens can be quite challenging to the practicing veterinarian because of the neonate's small size and immature organ function. Therefore it is very important for the veterinarian to understand the unique physiology of the neonate.

PARTURITION

To avoid a multitude of complications and to best prepare for the event, it is very important to accurately predict when the parturition will occur. There are many different ways to make this prediction, and some ways are more accurate than others (Box 2-1).

NATURAL BIRTH

Normal labor can be broken out into three distinct stages. For the descriptions of the stages of labor, the term *usually* will be used here to represent a normal range of values. It should be noted that these ranges may not be exact for every bitch or queen and for every circumstance.

Stage I usually lasts 12 to 24 hours. Clinically, bitches/queens may be restless and actively panting, scratching, and digging, whereas other bitches/queens are quiet. For the most part, on the day of delivery, they will not eat. The bitch/queen's temperature will drop to 98° F (36.7° C) and remain at that low level throughout this stage. Queens may vocalize, turn around in circles, and lick themselves constantly. Internally, cervical dilation starts. Since the cervical opening is at the level of the lumbar vertebrae in dogs, it cannot be palpated but may be visualized through a rigid cystourethroscope. Weak uterine contractions will occur during this stage

but are not visible to the human eye. These contractions can, however, be detected by the Whelp Wise service.

Stage II usually lasts 6 to 12 hours. The body temperature rises and returns to its normal level. Internally, the first fetus moves toward the pelvic canal. On entering the pelvic canal, the allantochorionic membrane of the placenta can rupture and a discharge of clear fluid may be noted. Uterine contractions will increase in force and will be outwardly visible. These uterine contractions will ultimately result in the expulsion of the fetus.

Stage III is expulsion of the placenta, usually happening immediately after the successful delivery of the fetus. Throughout the birth process, stages II and III will alternate until all fetuses have been delivered.

Dams/queens should be allowed to resuscitate their newborns. Whenever possible, the following steps should be performed by the mother:
- Licking of fetal membranes away from the mouth and nose
- Biting off the umbilical cord and eating the placenta
- Licking and nuzzling the newborn to stimulate it, encourage it to nurse, and move it closer to her to maintain its body temperature

Intervention should only happen if the dam/queen is not showing any interest in the newborn during the first 30 to 60 seconds after delivery. The action of nursing of puppies/kittens releases natural oxytocin and helps strengthen contractions and delivery of the subsequent fetuses.

Assistance in Natural Delivery

If the mother is not performing the previously mentioned duties satisfactorily, then human assistance is required. Fetal membranes should be removed by wiping the neonate with a warm towel and clearing the nose and mouth area first. A bulb syringe or a DeLee's mucus trap suctioning device can be used to suction out both nostrils and mouth. A gentle

---

BOX 2-1 **Methods for predicting delivery date**

- One timing method: Stating parturition will occur 63 days (±24 hours) from the day of ovulation (measured progesterone levels at 4 to 8 ng/ml).
- Another timing method: Stating parturition will occur 65 days from the LH surge.
- Another timing method: Stating parturition will occur 57 days from end of diestrus (confirmed by cytology).
- Measuring a drop in serum progesterone levels to <2 ng/ml, indicating parturition will occur in 12 to 24 hours.
- Measuring a temperature drop to 98° F (36.7° C), indicating parturition will occur anywhere between 8 and 24 hours.
- Using of a Whelp Wise monitoring system (www.whelpwise.com) that will pick up changes in uterine activity.
- Examining of radiographic changes that indicate a calcification of the digits; used in conjunction with ultrasonographic measurements.

LH, Luteinizing hormone.

BOX 2-2 **Clinical signs possibly associated with dystocia**

- Green/brownish-red discharge is noted, and the first puppy is not produced within 1 hour.
- Weak contractions are exhibited for more than 3 hours.
- Strong, sustained contractions without the expulsion of the fetus within 30 minutes.
- More than 3 hours elapse since the last puppy/kitten was born and more fetuses remain inside.
- The dam/queen has been in stage II labor for more than 12 hours.

---

rocking of the newborn in a head-down position (while head and neck are supported) can assist with the removal of the remaining fluid from the chest/trachea. Swinging of the newborns is no longer advocated because of potential cerebral hemorrhage from concussion.

The umbilical cord should first be clamped about ¼-inch away from the body wall, then tied off with a piece of suture, and finally dabbed with either a chlorhexidine or Betadine solution. Once the neonate is dry and breathing well, it can be put with the dam/queen. A healthy neonate should actively search for the dam's teat and should start suckling almost immediately.

Care should be taken in case the dam/queen rejects the neonate and attempts to bite it. In this situation, a light tranquilization with acepromazine (0.01 to 0.02 mg/kg) might be necessary initially and the dam/queen should not be left alone with the offspring until the problem of rejection is overcome. Sometimes, rubbing placental fluids on the neonate may help the mother to recognize it as her own. A few drops of oxytocin may be applied topically to her nostrils to assist in mothering behavior.

At times, injections (Cal-Pho-Sol 1 cc/10 lb subcutaneous [SC]) have been used to help with hypocalcemia-associated aggression. Care must be used with other SC preparations to avoid skin irritations. A dog-appeasing pheromone (DAP) diffuser or DAP collar may also be helpful in creating a calm, comfortable environment in the whelping room.

In cases of aggression it may be necessary to place puppies/kittens in a small plastic box (found at a Walmart or similar store) that has a heating supply (such as a small self-contained heating disk [e.g., Snuggle Safe]) and small round openings cut out for ventilation. Also longitudinal slits should be made in the lid so that the new mother can smell and hear her offspring, as well as see them move. It will help with the desensitization process. The offspring should be removed from the container for supervised and assisted nursing. Usually only 48 to 72 hours are needed to calm new mothers.

In normal labor, the female may show weak or infrequent contractions for up to 2 and at the most 4 hours before giving birth to the first fetus. If the female is showing strong and sustained contractions and a puppy or a kitten is not produced within 30 minutes, a possible obstruction may exist and immediate veterinary advice should be sought.

The dam/queen should be presented for veterinary examination immediately if any evidence of delivery problems is noted (Box 2-2).

Fetal viability and distress is best diagnosed with the use of ultrasound. Since the normal fetal heart rates are between 180 to 220 beats per minute (bpm), a heart rate below 180 bpm indicates fetal distress. If the fetal heart rate falls below 150 bpm, an emergency is indicated and requires an immediate cesarean section (C-section).

CESAREAN SECTION

If a C-section is deemed necessary, several aspects of this procedure should be considered to maximize success and ultimate survivability of the fetuses. The primary considerations and focus should be placed on preparation, choice of anesthesia, careful use of approved drugs, and speed of execution.

A metoclopramide injection (0.1 to 0.2 mg/kg) should be considered if there was a recent meal ingestion or if some puppies were already born and the mother has ingested placentas; in very large litters; or when there is a lot of pressure on the stomach, which can facilitate regurgitation or vomiting. Before induction, the female should receive 10 to 15 minutes of preoxygenation via a mask. Premedication with anticholinergics (atropine, glycopyrrolate) may be used to maintain a higher heart rate in the mother. An intravenous (IV) catheter needs to be inserted, and sodium chloride

(NaCl) fluids should be given at a surgical rate of 10 ml/kg/hr to maintain the proper blood pressure during the surgery. For an elective C-section in dogs, short-acting steroids (Solu-Delta Cortef) can be administered 2 to 12 hours prior to surgery at a dose of 1 mg/kg and have been shown to be beneficial in litter resuscitation. The induction itself may be performed with propofol (4 to 6 mg/kg) administered intravenously or gas induction via a mask. The use of optimal anesthetic protocols will improve neonatal survival. Certain drugs, such as ketamine, thiopental, and xylazine, should be avoided. Once induced, the anesthetic state should be maintained with an Isoflurane or Sevoflurane anesthetic gas. A local block with either a lidocaine or a bupivacaine will help with keeping the anesthesia levels lower until a centrally acting analgesic can be given. At this point, it is critical to remove all the fetuses from the uterus as expeditiously as possible so that the moderately depressed state from anesthesia will not worsen the already present distress of the fetuses, which necessitated the procedure in the first place.

After all fetuses have been removed, focus can once again return to the mother and successful completion of the procedure. It should also be noted that the sooner the procedure can be completed and the mother can be safely reunited with the newborns the better. After all puppies are removed, a standard pain control IV dose of butorphanol or buprenorphine can be given to keep the mother comfortable.

Neonatal Resuscitation after Cesarean Section

Resuscitation of neonates delivered by C-section involves mostly the same process as outlined in the section on natural birth, except that many puppies will need resuscitation simultaneously as opposed to a more evenly distributed and extended timeframe. Additionally, the fetuses that were in distress before the C-section began should be given priority and may require more extreme measures to resuscitate (see next section on more extensive resuscitation measures).

Once neonates are pink and breathing well on their own, they should be placed into a warm environment like an incubator to await their mother's recovery. At that time, all puppies/kittens should be checked for congenital defects like cleft palates, atresia ani, hydrocephalus, and so on.

EXTENSIVE RESUSCITATION MEASURES

After the initial rubbing, suctioning, and stimulating, if a newborn does not start to breathe on its own within 30 to 60 seconds, then additional and more extensive assistance is required. These more extensive measures should be employed after a quick but careful evaluation of the neonate's condition because the clinician will want to take the least invasive path possible while achieving the same result.

Thicker secretions can be removed through the use of an airway suction catheter in the mouth (DeLee aspirator). This device provides the application of controlled suction and allows inspection of the pharynx to see if meconium may have been aspirated because of in utero distress. Ventilatory support should include a constant flow of oxygen via a tightly fitted oxygen mask providing positive pressure ventilation. If this is not effective after 3 to 5 minutes or if the newborn's heart rate starts to drop, then intubation should be attempted. Although it is difficult to insert, a 2-mm endotracheal tube or a larger gauge IV catheter could be used to provide positive pressure ventilation in an attempt to inflate the lungs. Oxygen toxicity is usually not a major concern as few neonates are maintained in oxygen-rich environment for longer than the first 10 to 15 minutes.

Doxapram is thought to work via central stimulation. The effectiveness of this drug is significantly diminished if the brain is hypoxic since the action requires the central processing of the incoming signal from the periphery. Thus doxapram is unlikely to be beneficial to the apneic hypoxic neonate.

The use of Jen Chung acupuncture point GV26 has been advocated by some. A 25-gauge needle is inserted into the nasal philtrum at the base of the nostrils where it joins the haircoat and rotated clockwise when it reaches the bone.

Cardiac stimulation should follow ventilatory support through the use of direct chest compressions. If there is no improvement, epinephrine is the drug of choice for neonatal cardiac arrest. It has been shown to increase the mean arterial blood pressure and improve oxygen delivery to the heart. Suggested doses of epinephrine range from 10 µg/kg to 200 µg/kg IV. Caution should be used with higher doses because of the risks of associated hypertension. The preferred route of administration is either via IV through the umbilical vein or via an intraosseous (IO) route through the insertion of a 22- or 25-gauge needle into the humerus or femur. Endotracheal administration should be avoided because of associated vasoconstriction of the tracheal mucosa.

Since bradycardia is usually caused by hypoxemia-induced myocardial depression and not vagal mediation, the use of atropine is not recommended because it can cause a rebound tachycardia and exacerbate myocardial oxygen deficit.

The use of sodium bicarbonate is controversial but potentially could be beneficial in the treatment of neonatal acidosis in cases in which resuscitation takes longer than 20 to 30 minutes. This drug should only be administered to a patient who is well ventilated. The recommendation is to dilute it 1:1 with 5% dextrose (0.5 mEq/ml) and administer at a dose of 0.5 to 1 mEq/kg IV via the umbilical vein slowly over 2 to 3 minutes.

In the past, it was recommended that naloxone (0.1 mg/kg intramuscular [IM]) should be used in all apneic neonates. This was based on the findings that there is a surge of endorphin release during the time of parturition and especially during a stressful birth, which was associated with respiratory depression in newborns. Modern research has showed that the use of this medication is no longer effective and may be detrimental if given to a hypoxemic patient since it may worsen the existing bradycardia. It may be beneficial only in cases in which the neonate shows signs of respiratory depression and the mother received an opioid injection before or during the C-section surgery.

The clinician should examine all puppies and kittens for obvious congenital defects. If severe abnormalities are noted, humane euthanasia of the affected neonate(s) should be considered so that resuscitation efforts can be focused on the healthy ones.

RESPIRATORY SYSTEM

During intrauterine life, fetal respiration occurs through a blood-gas exchange process across the placenta. The lungs are not in use, and blood flow through them is sparse. During the last few days before birth, with the surge of adrenal activity, surfactant synthesis is stimulated by cortisol. Thus increased adrenal activity just before birth is essential for the normal lung function postnatally.

When the umbilical cord is separated at birth, the blood supply to the fetus through the placenta is suddenly disrupted. This disruption results in a state of hypoxia. Concurrently, there is an increase in vascular resistance in the peripheral vessels of the neonate. The combination of these factors creates a state of dyspnea, which leads to a reflex contraction of the chest muscles. Negative pressure occurs in the airways, which causes air suction into the lungs.

If a mammal is born alive and the pathway of normal development and maturation has been followed, the lungs will float if put in a container of water during postmortem examination. This flotation indicates the lungs have filled with air at least once. This is in contrast to the stillborn mammal, whose lungs would not float because it was never able to draw air into its lungs.

Respiratory conditions are found quite frequently in fetuses. The most common prenatal condition is hypoxia. There are many causes for hypoxia; the most common ones are overcrowding in the uterus, diseased/weakened placenta, prematurely detached placenta, and/or shock associated with conditions in the mother. Fetuses are less able to tolerate hypoxia because their brains are not as well adapted to the reduced oxygen tension and their lungs have yet to inflate to provide an oxygen reserve.

Hypoxia in the newborn is usually due to an inability to completely inflate the lungs, which can be the result of inadequate lung surfactant production (most commonly found in premature newborns) or because of an airway obstruction. Since neonates have relatively small airways, large tongues, and small nostrils, they are susceptible to hypoxia from the presence of fluid or mucus within the airways.

CARDIOVASCULAR SYSTEM

Within the fetal circulatory system, the blood is shunted past the nonfunctioning fetal lungs through the ductus arteriosus, which is located between the left pulmonary artery and the ascending aorta. When the mother severs the umbilical cord, navel circulation stops. In response to increasing oxygen tension, the ductus arteriosus narrows and the pulmonary vessels dilate. Increased left-sided pressure results in the closure of the foramen ovale between the atria. Closure of the ductus arteriosus is not immediate and normally takes place within 2 to 5 days after birth.

When those closures fail to occur completely, they result in conditions called persistent ductus arteriosus or persistent foramen ovale. This condition can be diagnosed by a characteristic heart murmur and subsequently be confirmed by an echocardiogram. After birth, the stroke volume of the right ventricle increases compared to the left ventricle. Because of this, the ratio of the right-to-left ventricular mass changes from a 1:1 ratio in the newborn to a 1:2 ratio in the adult.

Overall, in comparison to the adult, newborn puppies and kittens have a lower blood pressure, stroke volume, and peripheral vascular resistance but have a higher heart rate, cardiac output, plasma volume, and central venous pressure. The autonomic innervations of the heart and vasculature are incomplete, thus not giving neonates good baroreflex control of their blood circulation. Myocardial contractility has not fully developed, resulting in limited compensatory ability to hemorrhage, hyperthermia, and acid/base imbalances. Last, the heart rhythm of a newborn is a regular sinus rhythm, which is not associated with breathing patterns, because vagal reflexes do not develop until approximately 8 weeks of age.

THERMOREGULATION

Thermoregulation is always poor in newborns because their ability to shiver and vasoconstrict in response to decreasing temperatures is limited. Also, neonates have a large surface-area-to-body-mass ratio, little body fat, poor blood flow to the extremities, high water composition, and an inability to pant. This inability to maintain their body temperatures makes puppies and kittens sensitive to temperature fluctuations.

After the puppy or kitten is born, its body temperature will gradually decrease from the dam's body temperature to that of a neonate over the first 30 minutes of life (Table 2-1). Immediately after delivery, the mother licks the newborn to stimulate and clean it. The puppy/kitten's natural instincts should cause it to move toward the mammary glands, where

TABLE 2-1 Normal rectal temperatures for neonates

Week	Normal rectal temperature	Recommended environmental temperature
Week 1	95° to 99° F (35° to 37.2° C)	86° to 90° F (30° to 32.2° C)
Weeks 2-3	97° to 100° F (36.1° to 37.8° C)	80° to 85° F (26.7° to 29.4° C)
Week 4	99° to 101° F (37.2° to 38.3° C)	70° to 75° F (21.1° to 23.9° C)

the temperature is only slightly below that of the mother. Thus heat loss is compensated for by the mother, and the newborn's thermal balance is maintained.

Hypothermia can develop very fast if environmental temperatures are not well controlled (see Table 2-1). Another important factor is humidity, which should be maintained between 55% and 60% to avoid excessive drying of the skin and dehydration.

DIGESTIVE SYSTEM

Neonates are born with a sterile gastrointestinal (GI) system. Over the next few days, they will develop their own intestinal flora that will be influenced by the surrounding environment, diet, and their mother. As newborns start to nurse, the first milk that they ingest is called *colostrum*. This first nursing initiates the discharge of meconium, which is a very thick, sticky brown material that has collected in the bowels of the fetus. Failure to discharge meconium can be caused by a lack of suckling and mothering behavior or a congenital defect such as atresia ani or coli.

The neonate's digestive system is very fragile and is easily affected by its diet, the environment, or pathogens because the physical defense against infection is reduced in the newborn. Since the production of gastric hydrochloric acid has not yet fully developed, stomach acidity is lower in neonates than in adults. As a result of this decrease in the acid barrier, the defense against infectious agents is decreased, allowing greater survival of bacteria and increased susceptibility to GI infections. The most common infectious agents in the newborn GI tract are *Escherichia coli*, *Campylobacter* sp., *Streptococcus* sp., and *Clostridium perfringens*. The most common manifestation of GI upset is diarrhea.

NEONATAL NUTRITION/COLOSTRUM SUPPLEMENTATION GUIDELINES

Colostrum

Since only negligible amounts of maternal antibodies (<5%) are passed through the placenta to the developing fetus, an adequate ingestion of colostrum *must* occur within the first 24 hours to acquire passive immunity from the mother. Gut permeability to immunoglobulins starts to decline 8 hours after birth, and no further absorption is possible after 48 to 72 hours. It is good practice to check maternal vaccination history before breeding and measure the vaccine titers if the history is questionable.

Table 2-2 shows normal levels of immunoglobulins in canine colostrum versus canine milk.

If colostrum is not available, then maternal serum can be administered orally to a neonate less than 12 hours old via a feeding tube in the amount of 15 ml/100 gm of body weight (divided into multiple feedings).

If the ingestion of colostrum is questionable, serum levels of alkaline phosphatase (ALP) and gamma-glutamyl transferase (GGT) can be checked. If colostrum has been ingested

TABLE 2-2	Immunoglobulin comparison in canine colostrum and milk		
Source	IgG (mg/dl)	IgM (mg/dl)	IgA (mg/dl)
Canine colostrum	500-2200	70-370	150-340
Canine milk	10-30	10-54	110-620

IgG, Immunoglobulin G; *IgM*, immunoglobulin M; *IgA*, immunoglobulin A.

these serum levels should remain high during the first 2 weeks of life. Additional information pertaining to alterations in serum enzyme concentrations is available in Chapter 30. If neonates did not receive any colostrum within the first 24 hours, serum can be administered subcutaneously at a dose of 5 ml/100 gm of body weight, 3 times at 6 to 8 hour intervals. Hyperimmune canine serum preparations can be purchased through Hemo Pet (www.hemopet.org) or through other regional veterinary blood banks.

If the lack of ingestion of colostrum is due to the problems with the release of milk or amount of milk present within the mammary gland, then the dam/queen can be given low doses of oxytocin (0.2 to 2 U IM) 15 to 20 minutes before nursing in an attempt to induce milk release. Also, metoclopramide (0.1 to 0.2 mg/kg by mouth [PO] 3 times a day [TID]) or domperidone (2.2 mg/kg PO 2 times a day [BID]) have been used to help increase milk production. As a complementary treatment, acupuncture points LI4 and SI1 have also been used to promote lactation.

Weight Gain

The puppy or kitten should be weighed at birth. After that, neonates should be weighed twice a day to accurately measure weight gain. Digital scales are more accurate and gram scales work better for small and toy canine breeds and felines. Low birth weight can be correlated with poor survivability in puppies and kittens. Birth weight is not influenced by sex of the neonate and is more likely an indicator of inadequate intrauterine nutrition or congenital abnormality. It is normal for neonates to lose a little bit of weight (mostly water) in the first 24 hours. Neonates that lose more than 10% of the birth weight in the first day of life have a poor prognosis. After that, puppies/kittens should gain 5% to 10% of their birth weight daily. This equates to 1 to 3 gm/day/lb of anticipated adult weight for canines and 50 to 100 gm weekly for felines. They should double their weight by 10 days of age.

A neonate's caloric requirement during the first week of life is 133 calories/kg/day. If the mother's milk is slow to come in and neonates are not gaining weight, supplemental feedings of the puppies and kittens will be necessary. Supplementation can be provided by feeding with commercially available milk replacers such as Esbilac, Just Borne, KMR, Veta-Lac, and others. Puppies get their energy from fat during the first week of life, and kittens get their energy from protein. Lactose is not a source of energy, and if the level of lactose is too high, it can easily lead to diarrhea. When choosing a milk replacer, it is important to review the product's energy content to fluid concentration ratio. Because a neonate's stomach has a limited capacity, it is imperative that this ratio be correct to maintain proper hydration and meet the daily caloric requirement without overextending its fluid capacity.

Bottle or Tube Feeding

If a neonate is not gaining weight by itself and doing so at the rate described previously, it will need to receive nutritional supplementation either via bottle or tube feeding. When choosing a supplementation method, the strength of the neonate is the primary selection criterion. Bottle feeding might not be the best for weak neonates because their suckle reflex may be diminished and there is a possibility of aspiration into the lungs. In this case, tube feeding might be a better alternative.

Regardless of the supplementation method, prior to the feeding it is extremely important to make sure that the body temperature of the neonate is above 96° F (35.5° C). If the neonate's body temperature is too low, ileus develops and the ingested material will start to ferment instead of being digested, resulting in a bloated and distressed neonate.

For the neonate unable to be bottle-fed, tube feeding will be required. This process is not particularly difficult but needs to be done correctly. Depending on the size of the neonate, the clinician should use either a 5 Fr or 8 Fr red rubber catheter. First, measure the distance from the tip of the nose to the last rib. Then, with a permanent marker, mark 75% of that measurement on the catheter (Figure 2-1). This mark will guide the length of the tube's insertion so that it correctly reaches the stomach, avoiding kinking of the tube in the GI tract. While holding the neonate upright with its head flexed (not extended), insert the tip of the tube along the roof of the mouth, following the path of least resistance (Figure 2-2). No force is needed and most neonates will swallow the feeding tube easily. If the catheter is accidentally inserted into the trachea, the neonate might cough as a sign of the incorrect placement. Another indication of incorrect catheter placement will be that the tube will not be able to be inserted fully to the premeasured mark. Once the tube has been inserted, a syringe containing the milk replacer is attached to the end of the catheter. Correct placement of the feeding tube can also be ensured by the presence of negative pressure using the syringe on the end of the tube. Warm an appropriate amount of commercial milk replacer (based on the size and age of the neonate) and slowly feed it to the neonate. Monitor for gastric distention. Average stomach capacity in neonates is 0.7 fluid oz (4 teaspoons) per lb (40 ml/kg). After the feeding is complete, the catheter needs to be kinked before pulling it out to avoid milk dripping from the tip and being aspirated into the lungs.

Neonates being supplemented with milk replacers need to be monitored for constipation. Warm water enemas can be performed as needed if that condition occurs. After each meal, neonates need to be stimulated to urinate and defecate by rubbing the perineal and preputial areas with a cotton ball that has been soaked in warm water.

IMMUNE SYSTEM

Puppies and kittens receive virtually no antibodies through the placenta. They are born with a relatively immature immune system and are completely dependent on the passive transfer of antibodies through the colostrum. Ingestion of colostrum has to occur within the first 24 hours from birth because after that the GI tract will close and prevent absorption of antibodies. Mainly, the immunoglobulin G (IgG) and A (IgA) antibodies are absorbed since the IgM molecules are too large.

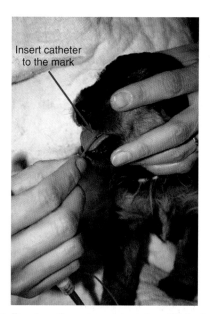

Insert catheter to the mark

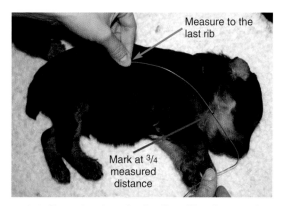

Measure to the last rib

Mark at ¾ measured distance

Figure 2-1 Preparing for tube feeding. The distance from the tip of the nose to the last rib should be measured first; then, with a permanent marker, mark 75% of that measurement on the catheter.

Figure 2-2 Passing the orogastric tube. While holding the neonate upright with its head flexed (not extended), insert the tip of the tube along the roof of the mouth, following the path of least resistance.

DRUG METABOLISM

The ability to metabolize drugs is reduced in neonates. Renal clearance is decreased as the glomerular filtration rate does not develop until the puppy/kitten nears 6 weeks of age. Hepatic clearance is also decreased, therefore any drugs metabolized by the liver and kidneys should be avoided or used with extreme caution. Additional pharmacokinetic differences between neonates and adults include increased percentage of total body water, decreased percentage of body fat, decreased albumin concentrations, and decreased binding to plasma proteins. These differences should be taken into consideration when selecting the appropriate drugs for neonates.

The volume of distribution for the water-soluble drugs is increased, so the dose used in neonates should also be increased. In contrast, the volume of distribution for the lipid soluble drugs is decreased. In this case, the dose in neonates should be decreased. Since elimination is decreased, the half-life of drugs would be longer and time between dosing intervals for the neonate should be increased as well.

EXAMINATION OF A SICK NEONATE

A methodical systemic physical examination should be performed on a neonate as it is in the adult animal as follows:
- Oral cavity should be free of congenital defects (e.g., a cleft palate or harelip).
- Hydration status should be assessed by checking mucous membranes.
- Skull needs to be examined for the presence of open fontanelles or large-size skull with domed appearance to it.
- The presence/patency of the anus should be checked.
- The ability to urinate (by stimulating the area around the urethral opening) should be verified. Color of the urine should be checked as a relative assessment of hydration status.
- Umbilicus should be dry and without any surrounding redness (Figure 2-3).
- Lungs should be clear and free of fluid on auscultation.
- Abdomen should be soft and not painful.
- Neurologic examination consists of checking the three main reflexes that are listed below. The flexor tone will predominate until days 3 to 4; thereafter, extensor tone will dominate. Presence of any weakness in the following reflexes indicates an ill neonate:
  - Righting response: Evaluating ability of the neonate to right itself from lying on the back.
  - Rooting response: Evaluating the neonate's ability to push its muzzle into circled fingers.
  - Suckle response: Make sure clinician's fingers are warm and free of smell/taste.

The recommended minimum database for further diagnostic workup includes a hematocrit, total protein, blood glucose, blood urea nitrogen, urine specific gravity, and

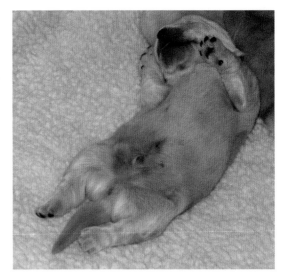

Figure 2-3 The normal neonatal umbilicus should be dry and without any redness around it.

sediment analysis. The blood sample amount collected should be no more than 1 ml/100 gm of body weight.

If septicemia is suspected in the neonate as a result of discoloration of the umbilicus or abdominal skin or because of other supportive symptoms, aggressive antibiotic therapy should be instituted immediately. Predisposing factors for this condition are a prolonged delivery or endometritis in the mother. A third-generation cephalosporin antibiotic (e.g., Naxcel) is one of the better choices because it has minimal effects on the normal GI flora of the neonate. It should be administered subcutaneously at a dose of 2.5 mg/kg twice daily and continued for 5 days.

During the first few days of life, neonates have reduced clotting capability. Vitamin K-1 may be used at a dose of 0.01 to 1.0 mg subcutaneously once because most neonates have a reduced thrombin level for the first 48 to 72 hrs.

THREE MAIN SYMPTOMS OF ILLNESS IN NEONATES

The three main symptoms of illness in neonates within the first 24 hours include hypothermia, dehydration, and hypoglycemia.

Hypothermia

Hypothermia is a very serious problem in the neonate. Gut motility slows down when the body temperature decreases, causing ileus of the intestinal tract. Previously ingested milk starts to ferment, produces gas, and leads to bloating. Subsequently, there is increased pressure on the diaphragm, which causes labored breathing and dyspnea. These factors in turn cause the neonate to swallow more air and thus worsen the bloating. Severe bloating can result in circulatory collapse and death. If hypothermic neonates are tube fed, the milk replacer is usually regurgitated and aspirated.

Neonates are considered hypothermic when their body temperature drops below 96° F (35.5° C); hypothermia should be treated promptly. Neonates should be slowly warmed but not more than 2° F (1° C) per hour. If the body temperature is raised more than 4° F (2° C) per hour, life-threatening organ failure (specifically the heart and kidneys) can result. Environmental temperatures need to be increased because higher temperatures will help neonates maintain their core temperature. Neonates should be rotated often to ensure even warming, and rectal temperatures should be checked frequently. External heat sources most commonly used are heat lamps, heating pads, and warm water bottles. The latter two need to be used with caution since weak neonates might not be able to crawl away from the heat source, resulting in burns and thermal injury. Warm IV or intraosseous (IO) fluids can also be given to raise the body temperatures, but the temperature of the fluids should not be more than 2 degrees higher than that of the body. For the reasons previously mentioned, a hypothermic neonate should never be fed.

Dehydration

Neonates are especially susceptible to dehydration as a result of the physiologic immaturity of their kidneys. Although their bodies are more than 80% water, their ability to conserve water is significantly diminished since kidneys do not fully mature until 6 to 8 weeks of age. The fluid requirement for neonates is 13 to 22 ml/100 gm of body weight per day. Low specific gravity and glucosuria are common normal findings in neonates.

To assess hydration levels in neonates, it is best to check the moistness of their mucous membranes because skin turgor of neonates is not as developed as in adults. If dehydrated, skin on the ventral abdomen and the muzzle may appear a deeper red color. For severely dehydrated patients, the shock dose of fluids can be given as quick bolus of sodium chloride solution at 30 to 40 ml/kg of body weight. Subsequently, the percentage of dehydration needed to be corrected should be estimated. Fluid deficits should be incrementally corrected over 12 to 24 hours. A maintenance fluid dose in neonates is 3 to 6 ml/kg/hr. Estimated ongoing fluid losses need to be added on top of that. Careful monitoring is essential because fluid overload is possible due to the diminished kidney function. Fluids can be given via multiple routes: IV, IO, intraperitoneal (IP), or SC. IP and SC routes are less desirable since absorption rates are slower and less predictable. IV and IO routes are the preferred ways to administer fluids to neonates. It is best to use a microdrip administration set or a syringe pump to avoid fluid overload. A saline solution of 0.45% with 5% dextrose supplementation is recommended. IV catheters are best placed in the external jugular vein (the cephalic vein can be attempted in larger patients).

If an IV catheter cannot be placed, fluids can be administered by the IO route. An 18- to 22-gauge spinal needle can be passed through the trochanteric fossa of the femur or greater tubercle of the humerus. The needle is inserted into the intramedullary canal, parallel to the long axis of the bone. The catheter needs to be placed aseptically and maintained the same as the regular IV catheter placement. Fluid is readily absorbed and rates similar to IV administration rates can be used.

Hypoglycemia

Since puppies and kittens are born with limited glycogen stores, they have minimal capacity for gluconeogenesis. Without nursing, hepatic stores will be depleted in 24 hours, and hypoglycemia will develop (serum levels dropping to less than 40 mg/dl). Clinical signs for hypoglycemia include crying, weakness, tremors, coma, and seizures. More in-depth information regarding the causes of hypoglycemia can be found in Chapter 30.

Therefore glucose supplementation is essential for sick neonates. In an emergency situation, dextrose can be given IV or IO at a dose of 0.5 to 1.0 g/kg using a 5% to 10% solution or at a dose of 2 to 4 ml/kg of 10% dextrose solution. If the neonate is not too weak, has a good circulation, and is attempting to nurse, then a 50% dextrose solution can be applied to the gums. IV or SC injections of 50% dextrose treatments should never be given because of the potential side effects of phlebitis or skin sloughing.

NEONATAL ISOERYTHROLYSIS IN CATS

Neonatal isoerythrolysis (NI) is a condition that occurs infrequently in regular domestic kittens but is one of the common causes of fading kittens in certain exotic feline breeds. It results from the immune-mediated destruction of a kitten's erythrocytes by its mother's antibodies. Kittens are born healthy, nurse, and ingest maternal IgG antibodies through the colostrum. NI occurs when kittens of blood type A or AB receive colostral anti-A alloantibodies from a type B queen. Kittens with blood type A have weak anti-B alloantibodies, whereas kittens with blood type B have strong anti-A alloantibodies. These kittens are the ones that are primarily responsible for incompatibility reactions. Affected kittens start to show clinical signs within a few hours of colostral ingestion. Some might be suddenly found dead. Others will stop nursing, become weak, and may show hemoglobinuria. These kittens may then develop jaundice, anemia, tachycardia, and tachypnea, leading to death. Kittens that survive may develop necrosis of the extremities or tip of the tail, which may later slough.

Affected kittens should be immediately removed from the mother to prevent further absorption of the antibodies. Treatment is primarily supportive. Mild cases can be fostered by the type-A queen or fed milk replacement formulas for 24 to 48 hours. Severe cases might require blood transfusion. Prevention is the key. It is best to blood-type breeding pairs of exotic breeds before breeding. B-type queens should only be mated to B-type toms. If accidental breeding of B-type queen to A-type tom has happened, newborn kittens need to be removed from the mother for 24 hours so colostrum ingestion from the B-type queen does not occur. Additional information regarding prevention can be found in Chapter 1.

SUGGESTED READINGS

Concannon PW, England GE, Verstegen J, et al (eds): *Recent advances in small animal reproduction,* Ithaca, NY, 2003, International Veterinary Information Service (www.ivis.org).

Hoskins JD: *Veterinary pediatrics: dogs and cats from birth to six months,* ed 3, Philadelphia, 2001, Saunders/Elsevier.

Johnson SD, Root Kustritz MV, Olson PNS: *Canine and feline theriogenology,* Philadelphia, 2001, Saunders/Elsevier.

Moon P, Pascoe P: Neonatal and pediatric critical care, *Proceedings of the Annual Conference for the Society for Theriogenology,* Nashville, TN, 1999.

Simpson GM, England GCW, Harvey MJ: *Manual of small animal reproduction and neonatology,* Gloucester, 1998, British Small Animal Veterinary Association.

Small Animal Neonatology Symposium: *Proceedings of the Annual Conference of the Society for Theriogenology,* Lexington, KY, 2004.

HISTORY AND PHYSICAL EXAMINATION OF THE NEONATE

CHAPTER 3

Margaret V. Root Kustritz

In this chapter, the neonatal period is defined as the period from birth through 3 weeks of age, or when the puppy or kitten is walking and capable of spontaneous urination and defecation. Box 3-1 contains a general overview of important parameters in the physical examination of neonatal dogs and cats.

COLLECTING A COMPREHENSIVE HISTORY

Although clients with a sick puppy or kitten often resent the time taken by a technician or veterinarian to ask historical questions, collection of a relevant history leads the veterinarian's physical examination and any further diagnostic testing and may alter plans for therapy. If a significant number of pediatric patients are seen in a practice, it may be beneficial to use the following history questions to create a history template that can be filled out (either as a hard copy or electronically) as puppies and kittens are admitted to the practice.

Duration of Illness

Knowledge of the duration of illness helps the veterinarian differentiate acute from chronic disease and may direct the practitioner toward a specific diagnosis. It also guides interpretation of clinical signs noted on physical examination, for example, a kitten that has been ill for days and is not dehydrated is probably less severely ill than the animal that has acutely become nonresponsive.

Clinical Signs Noted by the Owner

The owner should be asked to specifically list any clinical abnormalities noted, recognizing that some, such as diarrhea, may be difficult to assess if the bitch or queen is doing a good job of cleaning the neonate. Some clinical signs indicate an emergent situation, and any puppy or kitten exhibiting these signs should be seen immediately. Such signs include the following:

- Open-mouth breathing
- Nonresponsiveness
- Flaccid muscle tone
- Known trauma or obvious fracture or wound

Number Affected in the Litter

Infectious diseases and parasite infestations of the neonates and diseases of the bitch are more likely to affect multiple littermates, whereas trauma, congenital disorders, and abnormalities of nursing with subsequent malnutrition are more likely to affect individual puppies or kittens.

Treatments Provided

Any fluids, supplements, antibiotics, stimulants, human or veterinary drugs of other classes, or herbal therapies and any environmental changes made to allay signs of illness should be recorded. Obtaining this information may require some probing from the technician or veterinarian, since owners may be embarrassed or apprehensive about having used medications intended for humans or other animals on neonates. Knowledge of treatments used alters the interpretation of physical examination findings and may alter treatment recommendations.

History of the Dam

Questions should be asked about the birth of these offspring (e.g., were these puppies or kittens delivered vaginally or by cesarean section [C-section] and did dystocia occur at the time of parturition?); the dam's current clinical condition and behavior; history of the dam's mothering skills if she has had previous litters; and health and reproductive history of the dam, including vaccination history.

Colostrum Ingestion

Kittens may receive as much as 25% of their maternally derived antibodies through the placenta; puppies receive 5% to 10% at best. Because of this minimal antibody transfer

---

BOX 3-1 Important parameters in physical examination of neonatal dogs and cats

- Bradycardia (heart rate less than 150 bpm) in the first 4 to 5 days of life is most commonly associated with hypoxemia.
- Normal body temperature in neonates is significantly lower than that in normal adults of the same species.
- Hydration status is best assessed by examining urine color, with visible yellow color indicative of dehydration.
- Failure of the bregmatic fontanelle to close is not invariably associated with neurologic disease at the time of examination or in the neonate's future.

TABLE 3-1 Timing of significant events in pediatric development

Event	Age at occurrence
Umbilical cord dries and falls off	2-3 days
Eyelids open	5-14 days
External ear canals open	6-14 days
Extensor dominance	5 days
Capable of crawling	7-14 days
Capable of walking, urinating, and defecating spontaneously	14-21 days
Hematocrit/RBC number stabilize near that of adult	8 weeks
Renal function nears that of adult	8 weeks
Hepatic function nears that of adult	4-5 months

RBC, Red blood cell.

across the endotheliochorial placenta of bitches and queens, ingestion of colostrum is necessary for the bulk of passive transfer. Puppies and kittens should be encouraged to nurse within hours of birth. Maximal absorption of antibodies through the gastrointestinal (GI) tract occurs at about 8 hours of life, with virtually no GI uptake of antibodies by 1 day of life. In puppies, if the owner is unsure whether or not a given pup has nursed and is sure another has nursed, blood can be drawn from both and serum alkaline phosphatase (ALP) and gamma-glutamyl transpeptidase (GGT) values compared between the two. Concentrations are higher in pups that have ingested colostrum and remain high for only 1 to 2 days after ingestion. If a neonate is known not to have ingested colostrum, antibodies can be provided by administration of serum or plasma from any vaccinated adult of the same species, given orally (within the first day of life) or as subcutaneous boluses. The empirical regimen for kittens is administration of 15 ml of serum pooled from several adults (mindful of blood type to prevent neonatal isoerythrolysis), given as 3 boluses, administered at birth, and 12 and 24 hours later. The empirical regimen for puppies is administration of 10 ml/lb (22 ml/kg) of pooled adult serum; this can be given at once in large pups or split into boluses as described for kittens.

Birth Weight and Changes in Body Weight

Low birth weight is correlated with poor survivability. Normal birth weight for kittens is about 100 gm (3.5 oz). Normal birth weight for puppies varies by breed, with general averages of 120 gm (4.2 oz) for toy breed pups, 250 gm (9 oz) for medium breed pups, 490 gm (17 oz) for large breed pups, and 625 gm (22 oz) for giant breed pups. Low birth weight also may be an indicator of an abnormality of the dam, for example, hypothyroidism in bitches.

Puppies and kittens may lose a small amount of weight in the first 24 hours of life because they dehydrate slightly and defecate for the first time. Puppies and kittens should gain weight daily, doubling birth weight by 7 to 10 days of age. It has been demonstrated that those pups that lose more than 10% of their birth weight within the first 2 days of life were much less likely to survive to weaning than those that

maintain or gain weight in that time. It is recommended that all neonates be weighed at birth, at 12 and 24 hours of life, and daily thereafter, with good records maintained to document changes in body weight. Any loss of weight after 1 day of age should be a signal to have that neonate seen by a veterinarian; weight loss may precede onset of recognizable signs of disease by as much as 16 hours.

Body weight can be used to estimate age of healthy kittens. Most kittens gain weight in a fairly linear fashion so that they weigh about 1 lb at 1 month of age, about 2 lb at 2 months, and so on until reaching adult weight at about 6 months of age.

PHYSICAL EXAMINATION

The timing of significant events in pediatric development can be found in Table 3-1.

Apgar Scoring

Human neonates are scored for various viability measures at birth. The scoring system used was developed by Virginia Apgar, MD, and bears her name. A similar scoring system has been proposed for neonatal dogs and cats (Table 3-2). At present, there are no studies correlating viability scores at birth with morbidity or mortality in puppies or kittens. This system may be most useful as a way of consistently reevaluating an ill puppy or kitten during hospitalization or if they are presented repeatedly. This system provides an objective measure for the medical record for this individual and may be used to guide urgency of diagnostics or alterations in treatment by the veterinary staff.

Body Temperature

Body temperature should be measured using a rectal thermometer. It has been demonstrated that rectal thermometry is a more accurate reflection of core body temperature than any other method in adult dogs, and there is no reason to believe that this is not also true in pediatric dogs and cats.

TABLE 3-2	Neonate viability scoring*		
Parameter	**0 points**	**1 point**	**2 points**
Activity, muscle tone	Flaccid	Some tone in extremities	Active movements
Pulse, heart rate	Absent or <110 bpm	110-220 bpm	>220 bpm
Reflexes when stressed	Absent	Some movement	Crying out
Mucous membrane color	Pale or cyanotic	Slightly cyanotic	Pink
Respiratory rate	Absent	Weak, irregular	>15/minute, rhythmic

bpm, Beats per minute.

*Interpretation: Total points 0-3: weak vitality; total points 4-6: moderate vitality; total points 7-10: normal vitality.

Normal rectal body temperature in the first week of life is considerably lower than in normal adult dogs or cats. Neonatal puppies and kittens do not generate heat by movement and do not have an active shiver reflex until about 6 days of age, relying on brown fat for thermogenesis and on the environment. In the first week of life, normal body temperature is 94.5° to 97.5° F (35° to 36° C). In the second and third weeks of life, before the puppy or kitten is actively crawling and walking consistently, normal body temperature ranges from 98.6° to 100.0° F (37.0° to 38.2° C). Body temperature less than 94.0° F (34.4° C) is associated with GI stasis.

Hydration Status

Hydration status can be difficult to assess in neonatal puppies and kittens. Skin turgor or tenting is not as accurate an indicator of hydration status in pediatric animals as it is in adult animals because neonates have less subcutaneous fat. Well-hydrated puppies and kittens with light pigmentation normally have fairly deep pink coloration of the ventrum, muzzle, and oral mucous membranes (Figure 3-1). There is deepening to dark pink or red with dehydration, but this is a very subjective measure. Oral and ocular mucous membranes may be dry in dehydrated animals. Caution should be used when assessing oral mucous membranes in animals that have recently nursed; milk on the mucous membranes will make them feel slick, artifactually suggesting normal hydration. Normal urine in neonatal animals is very dilute with no discernible color. Stimulation of urination by gentle manipulation of the genitalia with a moistened cotton ball allows one to assess color of urine; any yellow color suggests dehydration is present. Packed cell volume (PCV) cannot be used as a measure of hydration in neonatal puppies and kittens because there is variation in the number of red blood cells (RBCs) passed through the placenta and umbilicus at the time of parturition and because there is a normal decline in PCV with age until it stabilizes at about 8 weeks of age.

Behavior/Mentation

Normal puppies and kittens spend the majority of the time sleeping in the first 2 to 3 weeks of life. Huddling of the pups on top of each other or near the dam is normal; healthy puppies and kittens will not lie apart from littermates or the dam until 5 to 6 weeks of age.

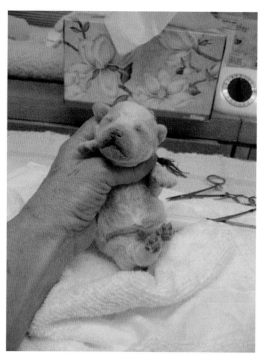

Figure 3-1 Normal 7-day-old pup with pink ventrum and muzzle.

When awake, neonatal pups should be able to respond to pain, odor, and touch. Normal pups or kittens show a strong suckle reflex that may be elicited by inserting a clean, warm finger into the neonate's mouth. Some animals will not respond because the veterinarian's finger is cold or tastes like disinfectant. Besides suckling, pups and kittens should demonstrate rooting and righting reflexes. The rooting reflex is stimulated by making a circle of the thumb and forefinger on one hand and inserting the neonate's nose into that circle (Figure 3-2). Normal pups will push against it or root. To stimulate the righting reflex, the neonate should be placed on its back on a soft, warm surface. Normal puppies and kittens should be able to right themselves fairly quickly.

Sensory Organs

Eyelids separate in most puppies and kittens from 5 to 14 days of age. There are reports of eyelid separation at birth or shortly thereafter in Abyssinian kittens. After eyelid

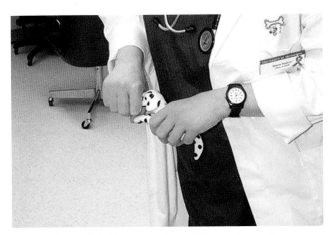

Figure 3-2 Demonstration of the rooting reflex.

separation, corneal edema may be present for 2 to 3 weeks, evidenced by slowly resolving corneal clouding. Normal iris color may not be present until after the neonatal period. Menace response and pupillary light response should be present by 10 to 21 days of age. Shirmer tear testing can be performed anytime after eyelid separation but may be difficult in pediatric animals because of their small size. Fundic examination cannot be performed consistently in the neonatal period.

The external ear canals of puppies and kittens are closed at birth, opening at about 6 to 14 days of age. Initial examination is hampered by the small size of the ear canal and presence of epithelial debris as the ear canals undergo desquamation. Otic examination and hearing testing cannot be performed consistently in the neonatal period.

Neurologic System and Calvaria

Neurologic examination cannot be performed consistently in the neonatal period. Pups should be able to respond to pain, odor, and touch. Withdrawal reflexes should be present but may be slower than in older animals. When handled, puppies and kittens exhibit flexor dominance until about 4 days of age. This means that animals held up by the scruff of the neck will curl into themselves rather than extend the spine and rear limbs; the latter is extensor dominance, which becomes prominent anywhere from 5 to 21 days of age. More advanced ancillary testing, such as brainstem auditory evoked response (BAER) hearing testing or electroencephalography (EEG), cannot be performed consistently in the neonatal period.

The skull should be palpated for assessment of closure of the bregmatic fontanelle. Open fontanelles are not invariably associated with enlargement of the ventricles of the brain nor is ventriculomegaly invariably associated with neurologic disorders. About one-third of dogs with persistently open fontanelles have no associated ventriculomegaly or neurologic disorders at any point in their life, about one-third have ventriculomegaly with no neurologic disorders at any point in their life, and about one-third have ventriculomegaly and neurologic disorders.

Cardiovascular System

Normal heart rate in puppies and kittens is about 220 beats per minute (bpm) in the first week of life and is therefore hard to assess. This rapid heart rate and the small size of the heart make auscultation difficult; use of a human pediatric stethoscope with the smallest bell and diaphragm available is encouraged.

In the first 4 to 5 days of age, puppies and kittens respond to hypoxemia with bradycardia and hypotension, with heart rate potentially falling as low as 45 bpm and systolic blood pressure potentially falling as low as 23 mm Hg. A heart rate of 150 bpm or less in a neonatal animal in the first week of life is an indication to hospitalize the animal and provide oxygen.

Sinus arrhythmia is not commonly reported in neonatal dogs and cats. Cardiac murmurs of grades I to III/VI most often are functional or innocent murmurs caused by increased flow velocity in the aorta and pulmonary artery or variations in closure of embryologic connections between chambers of the heart or between the heart and major vessels. Cardiac murmurs of grades IV to VI/VI more often are due to persistent congenital abnormalities of the heart. Other physical examination findings that may support the presence of a severe cardiac disorder include asynchrony of the femoral pulse with the heart beats, pale or cyanotic mucous membrane color, jugular venous distention, and ascites and hepatomegaly. Congenital heart disease was reported to occur in 17% of dogs and 5% of cats presented to the cardiology service of one veterinary teaching hospital in the United States. The most common congenital cardiac disorders in dogs in that study were subaortic stenosis and persistent ductus arteriosus. The most common disorders in cats were tricuspid valve dysplasia and ventricular septal defect.

Electrocardiography (ECG) is performed rarely in neonatal animals. Arrhythmias and conduction disturbances potentially could be identified using ECG in very young animals. There are no studies documenting accurate assessment of cardiac size by measurement of mean electrical axes. Assessment of cardiac function by echocardiography is difficult to perform in neonatal dogs and cats because of the lack of equipment of appropriate size and limited studies documenting normal measurements. However, appropriate ultrasonic techniques and interpretations are described in Chapters 22 and 32.

Respiratory System

Normal respiratory rate in newborns may be as low as 15 breaths per minute. By 1 day of life, respiratory rate increases to about 20 to 30 breaths per minute. Manipulation of the genitalia or umbilicus may cause an increase in respiratory rate. Respiratory rate is the same as that in adults by 4 weeks of age. Lung sounds easily can be auscultated using a stethoscope with a pediatric head. Thoracic radiography of neonates is complicated by their small size and the lack of known technique for animals of this size and body composition. Radiographs are interpreted as for adults. Transtracheal wash or other methods used to collect samples for culture or cytology may be performed as in adult animals.

Gastrointestinal Tract/Abdomen

Complete evaluation of the GI tract includes evaluation of the oral cavity, assessing which teeth have erupted, if any, and looking for any evidence of abnormal bite associated with oral trauma caused by malocclusion, cleft palate, or cleft lip. Puppies and kittens usually are born with no deciduous teeth erupted. Timing of eruption of deciduous and permanent teeth is listed in Table 35-1. Puppies and kittens most often lose deciduous teeth while eating and swallow them so these teeth rarely are found by pet owners. Dentition can be used to estimate the age of puppies and kittens by evaluating which permanent teeth have erupted (see Chapter 35).

Abdominal structures that should be palpable include the left kidney, small intestines, colon, and urinary bladder. The spleen usually is not palpable and the margins of lobes of the liver usually are not palpable beyond the ribcage; ready palpation of either of these organs is suggestive of enlargement. Abdominal effusion may be present in normal pediatric animals; the source of this fluid is undetermined. If the abdomen is distended so that no structures can be palpated as distinct entities, possible abnormalities include aerophagia caused by pain or respiratory stridor, maldigestion, or retention of feces or urine as a result of inadequate or difficult stimulation of urination and defecation.

Abdominal radiography of neonates is complicated by their small size, the lack of known technique for animals of this size and body composition, and the lack of abdominal fat to set off specific organs. Radiographs are interpreted as for adults. Abdominal ultrasonography is complicated by the animal's small size; a fluid offset may be used to ensure the focal length of the transducer is at the proper depth. Increased echogenicity may be visible in the renal cortex during the neonatal period and the kidneys are relatively large for the animal's body size, compared to adult measurements.

The GI epithelium is capable of taking up large proteins intact for the first day of life, permitting rapid absorption of antibodies from colostrum. The GI tract is sterile at birth but rapidly is colonized with multiple species of bacteria that form a stable population.

Motility of the GI tract appears to be controlled more by distention than by electrical activity before about 40 days of age. Lack of food intake and body temperature less than 94.0° F (34.4° C) are associated with GI stasis.

The neonatal kidney is immature. Nephrogenesis is not complete at birth but continues for at least the first 2 weeks of life. Glomerular filtration rate is decreased as is the rate of tubular secretion, achieving adult levels by about 8 weeks of age. Hepatic function also is decreased in neonates, with decreased protein synthesis and decreased microsomal and P450 enzyme systems until the animal nears 4 to 5 months of age. These metabolic variations must be taken into account when evaluating laboratory results from neonates or when administering drugs.

Skin and Haircoat

The umbilicus dries and falls off or is removed by the dam within days of life. Infection of the umbilicus (omphalitis) is evidenced by redness at the umbilicus, swelling, and exudation of fluid. The extremities and genitalia may be damaged if littermates suck on the neonate, contributing to skin disease. The most common dermatologic abnormalities reported in puppies and kittens are fleas and dermatophytosis. Fleas may be visible or may be evidenced by accumulation of flea excrement ("flea dirt") over the top line. Dermatophytosis usually is evidenced as areas of alopecia and crusting that may or may not be circular (see Chapter 17). Loss of hair or sloughing of the extremities or tip of the tail may indicate sepsis in either puppies or kittens or neonatal isoerythrolysis in kittens.

Musculoskeletal System

Normal neonates, although not mobile, have good muscle tone and do not feel flaccid when picked up and held. Normal puppies and kittens can lift their head from birth, will attempt to push themselves up on their forelimbs or scoot along using their hindlimbs by about 10 days of age, and will attempt walking by 14 days of age. Larger, heavier puppies often take longer to crawl and walk. Some heavy pups or pups housed on a slick surface learn to move by pushing their sternum along the ground and end up with a dorsoventrally flattened ribcage with the forelimbs or all four limbs abducted almost completely laterally to the trunk.

Radiography of the bones and joints in neonates is complicated by their small size, the lack of known technique for animals of this size, and the relative lack of mineralization of bone. General recommendations for enhancing the quality of radiographs are to decrease the kilovolt peak to one-half that used for an adult animal of the same size or to use 2 kVp for each 1 cm of soft tissue measured for up to 40 cm of thickness. Radiographs are interpreted as for adults; however, it should be remembered that the relative lack of mineralization and open physes are normal in puppies and kittens.

Reproductive Tract

The gender of kittens may be difficult to differentiate in neonates. Anogenital length is greater in males than in females, with a more obvious discontinuity between the anus and vulva. Testes of male kittens are not commonly palpable in the scrotum within the neonatal period.

Gender discrimination in puppies is not problematic. Testes are not commonly palpable in the scrotum in the neonatal period. Bitch puppies may appear to have a very recessed vulva in the neonatal period; this is normal and is not associated with disease.

SAMPLE COLLECTION

Collection of Blood

Blood volume of puppies and kittens is 25 to 40 ml/lb of body weight. The laboratory used for blood analysis should provide the absolute minimum sample size needed to ensure test accuracy. Use of in-house blood analyzers permits collection of smaller volumes of blood and faster turnaround time for results but may not be associated with rigorous quality control. Recommended tests in a minimum database for ill neonates are hematocrit, total protein, blood glucose, and blood urea nitrogen (BUN).

Venipuncture is complicated by the animal's small size and small veins, which collapse easily. In neonates, the peripheral vessels are too small for venipuncture, thus the external jugular vein is the site of choice. The puppy or kitten can be restrained as in adult animals, with the extended forelimbs drawn down over the edge of a table or counter while the head and neck are extended. Alternatively, the pup or kitten can be held in dorsal recumbency, usually within the hand of the person restraining the patient, with the animal's head and neck extended in a neutral position and the forelimbs held down against the chest and abdomen (Figure 3-3). To minimize heat loss, the area over the vein should be moistened with water not alcohol. Appropriate equipment is a 22- or 25-gauge needle attached to a 3 ml-syringe. If the syringe is seated well and the blood is drawn slowly, venous collapse and hemolysis of the sample are less likely.

Blood tubes of the smallest diameter possible should be used to ensure adequate mixing of blood with any anticoagulant present and to more readily permit aspiration of serum or plasma after clotting and centrifugation. Samples may yield more plasma than serum; if there is no artifactual change in tests requested, the use of green-topped (heparinized) tubes and submission of plasma may be preferred to the use of red-topped (clot) tubes and submission of serum.

Collection of Urine

In the neonatal period, urination can be stimulated by manipulation of the genitalia, which is preferable to cystocentesis. Minimum database for urinalysis is assessment of urine specific gravity and sediment.

INTERPRETATION OF LABORATORY RESULTS

Complete Blood Count

Normal physiologic changes reflected in complete blood count results include a decline in hematocrit in the first several weeks of life because of decreased production and shortened lifespan of RBCs and increased polychromasia, nucleated RBCs, Howell-Jolly bodies, and Heinz bodies (kittens only) (Tables 3-3 and 3-4). Hematocrit and RBC parameters remain different from those of adults throughout the neonatal period. White blood cell (WBC) differential analysis is the same as in adult animals (see Chapter 30).

Chemistry Profile

Normal physiologic changes in chemistry profile results include decreased alanine aminotransferase (ALT) and total protein, and elevated alkaline phosphatase (ALP) and phosphorus concentrations; the latter are increased during rapid bone growth (Tables 3-5 and 3-6). BUN varies readily with ingestion of food but is still a more accurate indicator of abnormalities of the kidney than measurement of creatinine in neonates. There are no good studies documenting absolute normal values for BUN or creatinine in neonatal puppies. Values may be extrapolated from work done in kittens. Blood glucose concentration is the same as the dam at birth, declines initially, and then stabilizes at about 3 days of life. ALT, total protein, ALP, and phosphorus concentrations remain different from those of adults throughout the neonatal period. Bile acid measurement is not an accurate indicator of hepatic function or disease in the neonatal period.

Urinalysis

Physiologic proteinuria may be present in the first days of life as colostral antibodies are excreted into urine. Glucosuria

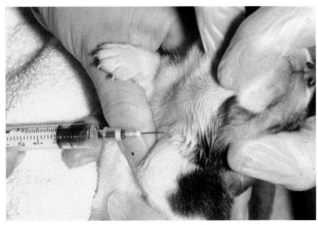

Figure 3-3 Restraint for venipuncture.

TABLE 3-3	CBC values for puppies in the neonatal period	
Age (weeks)	Hematocrit (%)	WBCs (×10³/µl)
0-2	29-53	7-23
2-4	27-37	9-26

CBC, Complete blood count; *WBCs,* white blood cells.

TABLE 3-4	CBC values for kittens in the neonatal period	
Age (weeks)	Hematocrit (%)	WBCs (×10³/µl)
0-2	34-37	9-10
2-4	26-27	14-17

CBC, Complete blood count; *WBCs,* white blood cells.

TABLE 3-5 Chemistry profile results for puppies in the neonatal period

Age (wks)	ALT (IU/L)	ALP (IU/L)	Bile acids (μmol/L)	Albumin (gm/dl)	Total protein (gm/dl)	Bilirubin (mg/dl)	Glucose (gm/dl)	BUN (mg/dl)	Creatinine (mg/dl)	Na (mEq/L)	Cl (mEq/L)	K (mEq/L)	Ca (mEq/L)	Ph (mg/dl)	Cholesterol (mg/dl)
0-2	10-34	176-560	<15	2	4	0.5	111-146	—	—	—	—	—	—	—	112-204
2-4	20-22	135-201	<15	1-2	4	0.3	86-115	—	—	—	—	—	—	—	232-344

ALT, Alanine aminotransferase; *ALP,* alkaline phosphatase; *BUN,* blood urea nitrogen; *Na,* sodium; *Cl,* chloride; *K,* potassium; *Ca,* calcium; *Ph,* phosphorus.

TABLE 3-6 Chemistry profile results for kittens in the neonatal period

Age (wks)	ALT (IU/L)	ALP (IU/L)	Bile acids (μmol/L)	Albumin (gm/dl)	Total protein (gm/dl)	Bilirubin (mg/dl)	Glucose (gm/dl)	BUN (mg/dl)	Creatinine (mg/dl)	Na (mEq/L)	Cl (mEq/L)	K (mEq/L)	Ca (mEq/L)	Ph (mg/dl)	Cholesterol (mg/dl)
0-2	11-24	68-269	—	2	4-5	0.3	76-129	<30	—	—	—	—	—	2-3	164-443
2-4	14-26	90-135	<10	2	5	0.2	99-112	<30	0.5	149-153	120-124	4-5	9-11	2-3	222-434

ALT, Alanine aminotransferase; *ALP,* alkaline phosphatase; *BUN,* blood urea nitrogen; *Na,* sodium; *Cl,* chloride; *K,* potassium; *Ca,* calcium; *Ph,* phosphorus.

also may be present during this period, which is associated with altered renal function. Urine specific gravity in pediatric patients is 1.006 to 1.017. Protein:creatinine ratio is reported to be elevated in neonatal animals. Proteinuria and glucosuria should no longer be present in normal puppies and kittens by 3 weeks of age. Decreased urine specific gravity persists throughout the neonatal period.

Coagulation Testing

In general, tests for clotting time are prolonged in neonatal animals. Prothrombin time and partial thromboplastin time normalize by 1 week of age. Antithrombin concentrations are decreased at birth but reach adult concentrations by 1 week of age.

SUGGESTED READINGS

Johnston SD, Root Kustritz MV, Olson PNS: The neonate: from birth to weaning. In Johnston SD, Root Kustritz MV, Olson PNS (eds): *Canine and feline theriogenology,* Philadelphia, 2001, Saunders/Elsevier.

Levy JK, Crawford PC, Collante WR, et al: Use of adult cat serum to correct failure of passive transfer in kittens, *J Am Vet Med Assoc* 219:1401-1405, 2001.

Little S: How I treat orphaned kittens, *Waltham Focus* 16:2-6, 2006.

MacDonald KA: Congenital heart diseases of puppies and kittens, *Vet Clin North Am Small Anim Pract* 36:503-531, 2006.

Panciera DL, Purswell BJ, Kolster KA: Effect of short-term hypothyroidism on reproduction in the bitch, *Theriogenology* 68:316-321, 2007.

Poffenbarger EM, Olson PN, Chandler ML, et al: Use of adult dog serum as a substitute for colostrum in the neonatal dog, *Am J Vet Res* 52:1221-1224, 1991.

Wilsman NJ, Van Sickle DC: Weight change patterns as a basis for predicting survival of newborn Pointer pups, *J Am Vet Med Assoc* 163:971-975, 1973.

HISTORY AND PHYSICAL EXAMINATION OF THE WEANLING AND ADOLESCENT

CHAPTER 4

Margaret V. Root Kustritz

In this chapter, the weanling period is defined as that time when the puppy or kitten is walking and capable of spontaneous urination and defecation (about 3 weeks of age) until they are weaned from the dam (about 8 weeks of age). The adolescent period is defined as that period from weaning until full adult height and normal physiology of the major organs is attained. Some may define the adolescent period as ending with puberty, defined as first estrus in females and in males, as acquisition of normal breeding behaviors and semen quality adequate to effect pregnancy. In cats, the end of the adolescent period averages 6 months of age; in dogs, it varies from 6 months of age in toy breeds to 12 to 15 months of age or older in giant breeds (Table 4-1). In most cases, once puppies and kittens attain a size allowing ready collection of blood and urine samples and performance of other diagnostic tests, rule-out lists and diagnostic and treatment plans are the same as for adults.

COLLECTING A COMPREHENSIVE HISTORY

Although clients with a sick puppy or kitten often resent the time taken by a technician or veterinarian to ask historical questions, collection of a relevant history leads the veterinarian's physical examination and diagnostic testing and may impact plans for therapy. If a significant number of pediatric patients are seen in a practice, it may be beneficial to use the following history questions to create a history template that can be filled out (either as a hard copy or electronically) as puppies and kittens are admitted to the practice.

Duration of Illness

Knowledge of the duration of illness helps the veterinarian differentiate acute from chronic disease and may direct the practitioner toward a specific diagnosis. It also guides interpretation of clinical signs noted on physical examination, for example, a kitten that has been ill for days and is not dehydrated is probably less severely ill than the animal that has acutely become nonresponsive.

Clinical Signs Noted by the Owner

The owner should be asked to specifically list any clinical abnormalities noted, recognizing that some, such as diarrhea, may be difficult to assess if the bitch or queen is doing a good job of cleaning the neonate. Some clinical signs indicate an emergent situation, and any puppy or kitten exhibiting these signs should be seen immediately. Such signs include the following:

- Open-mouth breathing
- Nonresponsiveness
- Flaccid muscle tone
- Known trauma or obvious fracture or wound

Number Affected in the Litter

Infectious diseases and parasite infestations of the neonates and diseases of the bitch are more likely to affect multiple littermates, whereas trauma, congenital disorders, and abnormalities of nursing with subsequent malnutrition are more likely to affect individual puppies or kittens.

Treatments Provided

Any fluids, supplements, antibiotics, stimulants, human or veterinary drugs of other classes, or herbal therapies and any environmental changes made to allay signs of illness should be recorded. Obtaining this information may require some probing from the technician or veterinarian, since owners may be embarrassed or apprehensive about having used medications intended for humans or other animals on neonates. Knowledge of treatments used alters the interpretation of physical examination findings and may alter treatment recommendations.

TABLE 4-1	Timing of significant events in pediatric development
Event	**Age at occurrence**
Capable of walking, urinating, and defecating spontaneously	14 to 21 days
Hematocrit/RBC number stabilize near that of adult	8 weeks
Renal function nears that of adult	8 weeks
Hepatic function nears that of adult	4 to 5 months

RBC, Red blood cell.

History of the Dam

Questions should be asked about the birth of these offspring (e.g., were these puppies or kittens delivered vaginally or by cesarean section [C-section] and did dystocia occur at the time of parturition?); the dam's current clinical condition and behavior; history of the dam's mothering skills if she has had previous litters; and health and reproductive history of the dam, including vaccination history.

Colostrum Ingestion/Immunity

Because there is minimal antibody transfer across the endotheliochorial placenta of bitches and queens, ingestion of colostrum is necessary for the bulk of passive transfer in puppies and kittens. Antibody titers fall to a nadir at 3 to 4 weeks of life, as maternal antibody concentrations decline before the animal's own immune system begins to function optimally. If there is concern that a weanling has not received maternal antibodies and needs protection against common diseases until it can respond to vaccination, antibodies can be provided by administration of serum or plasma from any vaccinated adult of the same species, given as subcutaneous boluses. The empirical regimen is administration of 15 ml of serum pooled from several adults, given as 3 boluses administered at 12-hour intervals. Adolescent animals are presumed to have sufficient immune function to permit them to respond to vaccination.

Changes in Body Weight

It is recommended that all neonates be weighed at birth, at 12 and 24 hours of life, and daily thereafter, with good records maintained to document changes in body weight. Any loss of weight after 1 day of age should be a signal to have that neonate seen by a veterinarian; weight loss may precede onset of recognizable signs of disease by as much as 16 hours. Daily weighing should continue until the puppy or kitten is weaned.

Body weight can be used to estimate age of healthy kittens. Most kittens gain weight in a fairly linear fashion so that they weigh about 1 lb at 1 month of age, about 2 lbs at 2 months, and so on until reaching adult weight at about 6 months of age.

PHYSICAL EXAMINATION

Apgar Scoring

Human neonates are scored for various viability measures at birth. The scoring system used was developed by Virginia Apgar, MD, and bears her name. A similar scoring system has been proposed for dogs and cats (see Table 3-2). This system may be most useful as a way of consistently reevaluating an ill puppy or kitten during hospitalization or if they are presented repeatedly. This system provides an objective measure for the medical record for this animal and may be used to guide urgency of diagnostics or alterations in treatment by the veterinary staff.

Body Temperature

Body temperature should be measured using a rectal thermometer. It has been demonstrated that rectal thermometry is a more accurate reflection of core body temperature than any other method in adult dogs, and there is no reason to believe that this is not also true in pediatric dogs and cats. Weanlings and adolescents have the same normal body temperature range as adult animals.

Hydration Status

Hydration status can be difficult to assess in weanlings. Skin turgor or tenting is not as accurate an indicator of hydration status in pediatric animals as it is in adult animals because neonates have less subcutaneous fat. Oral and ocular mucous membranes may be dry in dehydrated animals. Caution should be used when assessing oral mucous membranes in animals that have recently nursed; milk on the mucous membranes will make them feel slick, artifactually suggesting normal hydration. Normal urine in neonatal animals is very dilute with no discernible color. Stimulation of urination by manipulation of the genitalia is no longer possible once the weanling starts to urinate spontaneously; if the animal is large enough, collection of urine by free catch or cystocentesis may be attempted. Packed cell volume (PCV) cannot be used as a measure of hydration in weanlings because there is a normal decline in PCV with age until it stabilizes at about 8 weeks of age. PCV or change in body weight could be used as a measure of hydration status in adolescent animals, as in adults.

Behavior/Mentation

Huddling of the pups on top of each other or near the dam when sleeping is normal; healthy puppies and kittens will not lie apart from littermates or the dam until 5 to 6 weeks of age. When awake, weanling puppies spend a majority of the time exploring and playing. The suckling reflex is strong, but mouthing of other objects and attempts to eat solid food may occur as early as 4 weeks of age.

Sensory Organs

Eyelids separate in most puppies and kittens from 5 to 14 days of age. After eyelid separation, corneal edema may be present for 2 to 3 weeks, evidenced by slowly resolving corneal clouding. Normal iris color may not be present until 4 to 6 weeks of age. Menace response and pupillary light response should be present by 10 to 21 days of age, and vision is considered normal by 30 days of age. Shirmer tear testing can be performed anytime after eyelid separation but may be difficult in pediatric animals while they are small. Fundic examination can be performed after about 6 weeks of age. The tapetum may not attain full color and reflectivity until 4 to 7 months of age.

The external ear canals of puppies and kittens are open at about 6 to 14 days of age. Initial examination is hampered by the small size of the ear canal and presence of epithelial debris as the ear canals undergo desquamation; a thorough otoscopic examination should be possible by as early as 4 weeks of age. Assessment of hearing in most practice settings is difficult. Percussive hearing tests (clapping or making noise outside of the animal's field of vision and watching for a reaction) are beset with false negative (distracted animals ignoring your sounds) and false positive results (animal happening to move when noise is made or responding to air pressure changes). Brainstem auditory evoked response (BAER) testing is accurate as early as 4 to 6 weeks of age but requires specialized equipment and expertise. Partial deafness is very difficult to detect with any testing technique.

Neurologic System and Calvaria

Neurologic examination can be performed consistently once neurologic function matures at 6 to 8 weeks of age. Postural reactions (placing, hemi-walking) are fully developed by that age and generally develop in the forelimbs before the hindlimbs. Localization of neurologic deficits can be performed in young animals as it is in adults (Table 4-2).

The skull should be palpated for assessment of closure of the bregmatic fontanelle. Open fontanelles are not invariably associated with enlargement of the ventricles of the brain, nor is ventriculomegaly invariably associated with neurologic disorders. About one-third of dogs with persistently open fontanelles have no associated ventriculomegaly or neurologic disorders at any point in their life, about one-third have ventriculomegaly with no neurologic disorders at any point in their life, and about one-third have ventriculomegaly and neurologic disorders.

Cardiovascular System

Rapid heart rate and the small size of the heart may make auscultation difficult in puppies and kittens; use of a human pediatric stethoscope with the smallest bell and diaphragm available is encouraged. Sinus arrhythmia is not commonly reported in neonatal dogs and cats. Cardiac murmurs of grades I to III/VI most often are functional or innocent murmurs caused by increased flow velocity in the aorta and pulmonary artery or to variations in closure of embryologic connections between chambers of the heart or between the heart and major vessels. Cardiac murmurs of grades IV to VI/VI more often are due to persistent congenital abnormalities of the heart. Other physical examination findings that may support the presence of a severe cardiac disorder

TABLE 4-2	Localization of neurologic dysfunction
Neurologic sign or finding	**Location**
Head tilt	Vestibular
Seizures	Cerebrum
Abnormal mental status	Cerebrum
Intention tremor	Cerebellum
Ataxia	Cerebellum
Limb incoordination	Cerebellum
Gait and posture deficits—forelimbs only	Peripheral nervous system
Gait and posture deficits—all limbs, upper motor neuron all limbs	Upper cervical spine or diffuse
Gait and posture deficits—all limbs, lower motor neuron forelimbs, upper motor neuron hindlimbs	Lower cervical spine or diffuse
Gait and posture deficits—hindlimbs only, upper motor neuron	T2-L3
Gait and posture deficits—hindlimbs only, lower motor neuron	L4-S1
Gait and posture deficits—hindlimbs only plus dilated anus and/or flaccid tail	S1-S3

include asynchrony of the femoral pulse with each heart beat, pale or cyanotic mucous membrane color, jugular venous distention, and ascites and hepatomegaly. Congenital heart disease was reported to occur in 17% of dogs and 5% of cats presented to the cardiology service of one veterinary teaching hospital in the United States. The most common congenital cardiac disorders in dogs in that study were subaortic stenosis and persistent ductus arteriosus. The most common disorders in cats were tricuspid valve dysplasia and ventricular septal defect.

Electrocardiography (ECG) is performed rarely in neonatal animals. Arrhythmias and conduction disturbances potentially could be identified using ECG in very young animals. There are no studies documenting accurate assessment of cardiac size by measurement of mean electrical axes in very young animals. Echocardiography is used to assess cardiac function, although rarely performed in pediatric dogs and cats because of the lack of equipment of appropriate size and the absence of studies documenting normal measurements (see Chapters 22 and 32).

Respiratory System

Respiratory rate is the same as that in adults by 4 weeks of age. Lung sounds easily can be auscultated using a stethoscope with a pediatric head. Thoracic radiography of weanlings and adolescents is as for adults. Transtracheal wash or other methods used to collect samples for culture or cytology may be performed as in adult animals.

Gastrointestinal Tract/Abdomen

Complete evaluation of the gastrointestinal (GI) tract includes evaluation of the oral cavity, assessing which teeth have erupted, if any, and looking for any evidence of abnormal bite associated with oral trauma caused by malocclusion. Puppies and kittens usually are born with no deciduous teeth erupted. Timing of eruption of deciduous and permanent teeth is listed in Table 35-1. Puppies and kittens most often lose deciduous teeth while eating and swallow them so these teeth rarely are found by pet owners. Dentition can be used to estimate the age of puppies and kittens by evaluating which permanent teeth have erupted.

Abdominal structures that should be palpable in animals of any age include the left kidney, small intestines, colon, and urinary bladder. The spleen usually is not palpable and the margins of lobes of the liver usually are not palpable beyond the ribcage; ready palpation of either of these organs is suggestive of enlargement. Abdominal effusion may be present in normal pediatric animals; the source of this fluid is undetermined. Palpable or visible abnormalities of the abdomen, such as pain on palpation, organ enlargement, or abdominal distention, should be evaluated as in adults.

Abdominal radiography of weanlings and adolescents is generally the same as for adults (see Chapter 21). Abdominal ultrasonography (see Chapter 22) may be complicated by the animal's small size; a fluid offset may be used to ensure the focal length of the transducer is at the proper depth. The kidneys are relatively large for the animal's body size when compared to adult measurements, up to 12 weeks of age. Ultrasonographic characteristics of the liver are the same as in adults, as is liver size relative to body size.

Motility of the GI tract appears to be controlled more by distention than by electrical activity before about 40 days of age. Lack of food intake and body temperature less than 94.0° F (34.4° C) are associated with GI stasis.

The neonatal kidney is immature. Nephrogenesis is not complete at birth but continues for at least the first 2 weeks of life. Glomerular filtration rate is decreased as is rate of tubular secretion, achieving adult levels by about 8 weeks of age. Hepatic function also is decreased in neonates, with decreased protein synthesis and decreased microsomal and P450 enzyme systems until the animal nears 4 to 5 months of age. These metabolic variations must be taken into account when evaluating laboratory results from neonates or when administering drugs.

Skin and Haircoat

The extremities and genitalia may be damaged if littermates suck on the neonate, contributing to skin disease. The most common dermatologic abnormalities reported in puppies and kittens are fleas and dermatophytosis. Fleas may be visible or may be evidenced by accumulation of flea excrement ("flea dirt") over the top line. Dermatophytosis usually is evidenced as areas of alopecia and crusting that may or may not be circular (see Chapters 17 and 41).

Musculoskeletal System

Musculoskeletal examination is the same as for adults. Specific abnormalities to be assessed include laxity of joints for assessment of canine hip dysplasia, elbow dysplasia, and

TABLE 4-3 Timing of physeal closure in puppies and kittens

Anatomic area	Age at physeal closure (months)	
	Puppies	Kittens
Humerus–proximal	10-13	18-24
Humerus–distal	6-8	4-4.5
Radius–proximal	6-11	5-7
Radius–distal	8-12	14.5-22
Pelvis	4-6	–
Femur–proximal	7-11	7.5-10
Femur–distal	8-11	12.5-19
Tibia–distal	8-11	10-12

patellar luxation; abnormal angulation of the limbs, such as may be seen with asymmetry of bone growth or abnormalities of physeal closure; traumatic injury, such as anterior cruciate ligament rupture; pain as may be seen with panosteitis; proliferative bone conditions, such as craniomandibular osteopathy or hypertrophic osteodystrophy; and cartilage disorders such as osteochondritis dissecans (see Chapter 42).

Radiography of the bones and joints in neonates is complicated by their small size and the relative lack of mineralization of bone early in life. General recommendations for enhancing the quality of radiographs are to decrease the kilovolt peak to one-half that used for an adult animal of the same size or to use 2 kVp for each 1 cm of soft tissue measured for up to 40 cm of thickness. Radiographs are interpreted as for adults; however, it should be remembered that the relative lack of mineralization and open physes are normal in puppies and kittens (Table 4-3). Physeal closure also may be delayed by gonadectomy.

Reproductive Tract

Vulvar abnormalities of female cats are uncommon. The vulva of female dogs may be recessed, even to the extent that the vulvar cleft may lie horizontal to the ground. Clinical significance of this "juvenile" vulva is unknown. Testes usually are descended into the scrotum and easily palpable by 6 to 8 weeks of age. Dogs technically are not considered to have cryptorchidism until 6 months of age because that is the average age of closure of the inguinal ring (see Chapter 39).

SAMPLE COLLECTION

Collection of Blood

Collection of blood is the same for neonates in physically small animals and for adults in physically larger animals.

INTERPRETATION OF LABORATORY RESULTS

Complete Blood Count

Normal physiologic changes reflected in complete blood count results include a decline in hematocrit in the first several weeks of life because of decreased production and shortened lifespan of red blood cells (RBCs) and increased polychromasia, nucleated RBCs, Howell-Jolly bodies, and Heinz bodies (kittens only) (Tables 4-4 and 4-5). Hematocrit and RBC parameters remain different from those of adults throughout the neonatal period. White blood cell (WBC) differential analysis is the same as in adult animals (see Chapter 30).

Chemistry Profile

Normal physiologic changes in chemistry profile results include decreased alanine aminotransferase (ALT) and total protein and elevated alkaline phosphatase (ALP) and phosphorus concentrations; the latter are increased during rapid bone growth (Tables 4-6 and 4-7). Blood urea nitrogen (BUN) varies readily with ingestion of food but is still a more accurate indicator of abnormalities of the kidney than is measurement of creatinine in neonates. There are no good studies documenting absolute normal values for BUN or creatinine in neonatal puppies. Values may be extrapolated from work done in kittens. Blood glucose concentration is the same as the dam at birth, declines initially, and then stabilizes at about 3 days of life. ALT, total protein, ALP, and phosphorus concentrations remain different from those of adults throughout the neonatal period. Bile acid measurement is not an accurate indicator of hepatic function or disease in the neonatal period.

TABLE 4-4	CBC values for puppies in the weanling period	
Age (weeks)	**Hematocrit (%)**	**WBCs (×10³/µl)**
4-6	26-36	13-27
6-8	31-39	13-17

CBC, Complete blood count; WBCs, white blood cells.

TABLE 4-5	CBC values for kittens in the weanling period	
Age (weeks)	**Hematocrit (%)**	**WBCs (×10³/µl)**
4-6	26-28	16-19
6-8	29-31	16-20

CBC, Complete blood count; WBCs, white blood cells.

TABLE 4-6	Chemistry profile results for puppies in the weanling period														
Age (weeks)	**ALT (IU/L)**	**ALP (IU/L)**	**Bile acids (µmol/L)**	**Albumin (gm/dl)**	**Total protein (gm/dl)**	**Bilirubin (mg/dl)**	**Glucose (gm/dl)**	**BUN (mg/dl)**	**Creatinine (mg/dl)**	**Na (mEq/L)**	**Cl (mEq/L)**	**K (mEq/L)**	**Ca (mEq/L)**	**Ph (mg/dl)**	**Cholesterol (mg/dl)**
4-6	16-17	125-132	<15	4-5	3-4	—	125-126	9	1-4	148	105	5	11	—	—
6-8	9-24	144-177	<15	2-3	4-5	0.1	134-272	—	—	—	—	—	—	—	111-258

ALT, Alanine aminotransferase; ALP, alkaline phosphatase; BUN, blood urea nitrogen; Na, sodium; Cl, chloride; K, potassium; Ca, calcium; Ph, phosphorus.

Urinalysis

Urinalysis is the same as in adult animals. Isosthenuria is present early in life; urine specific gravity should be the same as that of adults by 9 to 10 weeks of age.

TESTING FOR HEREDITARY DISORDERS

Samples used for testing for hereditary disorders in dogs and cats include blood and cheek swabs. Cheek swabs for collection of deoxyribonucleic acid (DNA) can be purchased directly by clients from the American Kennel Club (www.akc.org) or MMI Genomics (www.mmigenomics.com). Cheek swab sampling is inaccurate in animals that are still nursing since maternal cells may be picked up along with cells from the pediatric animal.

Which tests are available and accurate vary by breed and change daily. Clients are encouraged to access their national breed club for a list of hereditary disorders of concern and tests available.

SUGGESTED READINGS

Bell JS: Testing for genetic disorders, *Proceedings of the Annual Conference for the Society for Theriogenology*, Lexington KY, 2004.

Grundy SA: Clinically relevant physiology of the neonate, *Vet Clin North Am Small Anim Pract* 36:443-459, 2006.

Johnston SD, Root Kustritz MV, Olson PNS: The neonate: from birth to weaning. In Johnston SD, Root Kustritz MV, Olson PNS: *Canine and feline theriogenology*, Philadelphia, 2001, Saunders/Elsevier.

Little S: How I treat orphaned kittens, *Waltham Focus* 16:2-6, 2006.

MacDonald KA: Congenital heart diseases of puppies and kittens, *Vet Clin North Am Small Anim Pract* 36:503-531, 2006.

Root Kustritz MV: Common disorders of the small animal neonate, *Proceedings of the Annual Conference for the Society for Theriogenology*, Lexington KY, 2004.

Root Kustritz MV: Neonatology. In Root Kustritz MV (ed): *Small animal theriogenology*, St Louis, 2003, Butterworth-Heinemann.

TABLE 4-7 **Chemistry profile results for kittens in the weanling period**

Age (weeks)	ALT (IU/L)	ALP (IU/L)	Bile acids (μmol/L)	Albumin (gm/dl)	Total protein (gm/dl)	Bilirubin (mg/dl)	Glucose (gm/dl)	BUN (mg/dl)	Creatinine (mg/dl)	Na (mEq/L)	Cl (mEq/L)	K (mEq/L)	Ca (mEq/L)	Ph (mg/dl)	Cholesterol (mg/dl)
4-6	9-41	–	–	2	4-5	–	<150	<30	0.2-1.2	151-156	119-125	5-6	10-11	6-10	125-592
6-8	23-50	–	–	2	5	0-0.1	<150	10-30	0.4-1.0	150-152	119-125	4-5	9-12	8-12	124-221

ALT, Alanine aminotransferase; *ALP,* alkaline phosphatase; *BUN,* blood urea nitrogen; *Na,* sodium; *Cl,* chloride; *K,* potassium; *Ca,* calcium; *Ph,* phosphorus.

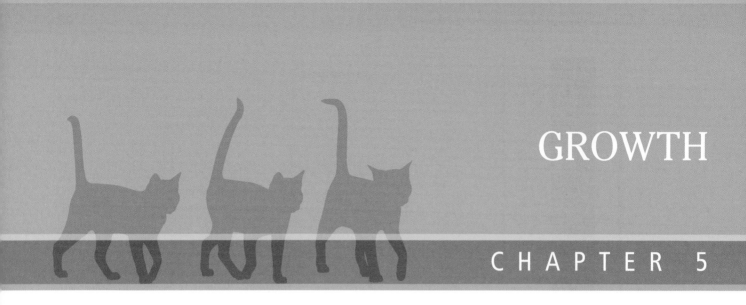

GROWTH

Michael E. Peterson

Generalizations about normal growth in puppies and kittens are difficult to make; this is particularly true in respect to dogs because of the wide variety of breeds encompassing many body shapes and sizes. Dogs are one of the few species with such a variety of size, which makes metabolic and growth rates significantly different. Normal adult dogs can vary in size from less than 5 lb to 150 lb in weight and still be healthy. This diverse morphologic range is rarely seen in any other species. Not only are there differences in the length of the exponential growth phase but also in the individual rates of growth (Figure 5-1).

Determination of appropriate growth for an individual animal can be difficult. Unless a particular animal is still with siblings or has an owner with a good understanding of not only this breed but also of this specific lineage, normal growth for a particular animal can be difficult to define. An example of this situation is manifest in the Dachshund—a breed in which miniatures (less than 11 lb) and standards (16 to 32 lb) can be whelped in the same litter. Generalizations about normal growth can be made between dog breeds that will attain approximately the same adult size (Table 5-1).

Many factors contribute to the normal development and growth of puppies and kittens. Genetics, environmental influences, endocrine and metabolic processes, nutrition, and disease are all major factors in determining growth. Growth is regulated by somatotropin (growth hormone), which triggers insulin-like growth factor-1 (IGF-1) release. When stimulated by thyroid hormone, IGF-1 is responsible for triggering cell proliferation, protein synthesis, and skeletal growth.

Growth of an animal is influenced by many factors, and it may be difficult to determine the specific contribution of each of the factors involved. These factors can include alterations in energy requirements as a result of the length of haircoat, breed temperament (compare the Jack Russell Terrier to the Clumber Spaniel), and body mass to surface area (English bulldog vs. the Whippet).

Assessment of normal stature in dogs can be difficult. Purebred breeds have written standards that include optimal size, usually height at the withers, but occasionally include weight guidelines (Table 5-2). Seasoned breeders usually have enough experience to recognize abnormal puppy growth trends. This does not mean all purebred dogs meet their standards requirement. Dogs with registration papers may or may not be "show" dogs; these "pet quality" dogs (graded as pet quality by the breeder because of a variety of faults, one of which may be size) are sold and should ideally be spayed or neutered. Unfortunately, the new pet owners may not sterilize their pets, and if the breed is particularly popular, may breed with another registered pet quality dog. Since these pet owners do not have the expertise in genetics or an understanding of the breed type, these puppies often have issues relative to their breed standards and frequently these dogs are much larger than the written standard requires. This is illustrated by the 100-lb registered Golden Retrievers (standard calls for 65- to 75-lb males) seen daily in the veterinary hospital.

Dogs that are bred, shown, and become champions have survived in the gene pool by meeting the rigors of independent judging in the show ring; by definition the dog show is designed to "exhibit" correct breeding stock. An example of this situation is the requirement for the Lakeland Terrier directed by its written parent club standard, which calls for the male to be $14\frac{1}{2}$ inches at the withers ($\pm\frac{1}{2}$ inch). Another example are the Miniature Dachshunds, which are not to exceed 11 lb. Some standards require disqualification if size requirements are breached, whereas in other breeds, deviation from the suggested size (either height or weight) is considered a significant fault in the show ring. The net effect is that purebred dog breeds do have standard sizes that a veterinarian can obtain, which is useful in determining if

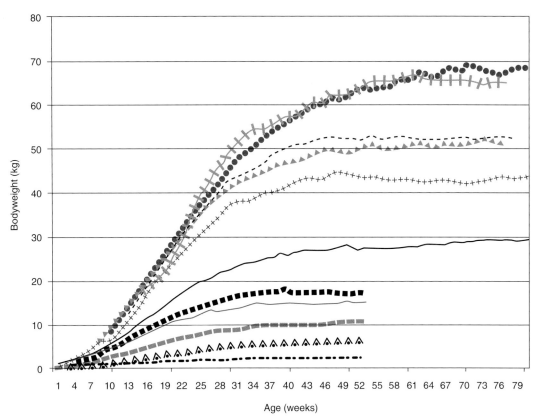

Figure 5-1 Mean growth curves for 12 breeds of dogs (SEM bars are excluded for clarity): English Mastiff (┼┼), St. Bernard (●●), Irish Wolfhound (---), Great Dane (▲), Newfoundland (+), Labrador Retriever (─), Beagle (■), English Springer Spaniel (─), Cocker Spaniel (━━), Miniature Schnauzer (▲), and Papillon (-••-). (Adapted from Hawthorne AJ, Booles D, Nugent PA, et al: Body-weight changes during growth in puppies of different breeds, *J Nutr* 134:2027S-30S, 2004.)

a particular puppy is incorrectly sized (see Table 5-2). However, it should be remembered that a puppy may be considerably sized incorrectly and still be healthy. Mongrel puppies have no known expected growth guidelines, unless the veterinarian can get some information on the parents' size. It must also be kept in mind that pregnancies that occur without human supervision may have multiple sires, thereby confounding the issue.

Breed-specific differences in growth patterns are affected by the dog's ultimate adult size, temperament, and type of hair coat. Any condition that requires an increase in energy consumption can negatively affect growth rates if nutritional adjustments are not made. A Bulldog puppy may be more languid than Parson Russell or Wire Fox Terrier puppies, which have a much higher energy demand because of their increased activity levels. Breeds with longer, denser haircoats will require less energy to keep warm in cooler climates than shorthaired or thin-coated individuals. All of these types of influences will impact energy requirements, which will permit various growth rates either faster or slower when the animal is fed any diet with a fixed caloric density.

Exponential growth rates (log-body weight increased linearly) occur in all puppies, regardless of subsequent adult stature. This exponential growth rate continues until the

puppy reaches approximately half its adult size. This period of tremendous rate of growth is prolonged with corresponding increases in adult size. English Mastiffs end this phase at about 23 weeks of age, whereas toy breeds have finished their exponential phase at 11 weeks of age. Interestingly, in one study, the fastest exponential growth rate occurred in English Springer Spaniels at 18%, whereas the slowest was in the English Mastiff at 10.8%. Growth rates, increase in percentage of body weight gain per week, are strikingly similar until half of adult size is reached. These early exponential percentage growth rates range from 13% per week in toy breeds to 17% per week in giant breeds.

The time necessary to achieve 99% of the adult body weight varies with the final adult size. Toys, small-, and medium-sized dogs achieve adult body size by 9 to 10 months of age. Giant breeds do not achieve 99% of their adult body size until 11 to 15 months of age.

There may be differences in growth rates of dogs of approximate equivalent adult size. This observance can be seen in differences between the Newfoundland, which had a lower adult body weight and a higher exponential growth rate than other giant breeds studied.

Male and female dogs have different growth patterns, with males taking longer to reach adult size. This may be a

TABLE 5-1	Growth characteristics of different dog breeds calculated by fitting a logistics equation to growth curves*						
	Dogs (No.)						
Size and breed	**Male**	**Female**	**R^2**	**a (kg)**	**1 lb (%)**	**x_0 (wk)**	**T_{99} (wk)**
Giant							
English Mastiff	2	2	0.995	66.9 ± 0.28	10.9 ± 0.24	22.9 ± 0.19	65.2 ± 0.92
St. Bernard	2	2	0.994	65.2 ± 0.27	13.2 ± 0.32	21.9 ± 0.17	56.7 ± 0.83
Irish Wolfhound	2	5	0.998	52.4 ± 0.11	15.3 ± 0.22	19.1 ± 0.09	49.1 ± 0.43
Great Dane	6	5	0.996	51.1 ± 0.14	13.5 ± 0.24	18.1 ± 0.12	52.1 ± 0.59
Newfoundland	7	8	0.997	43.3 ± 0.16	16.7 ± 0.33	18.5 ± 0.13	46.1 ± 0.55
Large							
Labrador Retriever	16	21	0.994	28.1 ± 0.12	13.7 ± 0.33	18.6 ± 0.18	52.1 ± 0.79
Medium							
Beagle	12	0	0.998	17.4 ± 0.05	17.0 ± 0.29	14.8 ± 0.08	41.9 ± 0.45
English Springer Spaniel	8	6	0.997	14.8 ± 0.07	18.3 ± 0.42	14.3 ± 0.13	39.4 ± 0.56
Small							
Cocker Spaniel	19	9	0.994	10.2 ± 0.08	15.3 ± 0.49	16.6 ± 0.22	46.6 ± 0.92
Miniature Schnauzer	11	9	0.997	7.0 ± 0.03	16.9 ± 0.36	14.1 ± 0.13	41.3 ± 0.57
Cairn Terrier	4	14	0.998	6.3 ± 0.06	16.9 ± 0.39	15.5 ± 0.17	42.9 ± 0.62
Toy							
Papillon	1	2	0.979	2.2 ± 0.01	15.0 ± 0.85	11.1 ± 0.28	41.7 ± 1.58

From Hawthorne AJ, Booles D, Nugent PA, et al: Body-weight changes during growth in puppies of different breeds, *J Nutr* 134:2027S-30S, 2004.

R^2, Fit of the equation to the curve; *a*, adult body weight; *1 lb*, exponential growth rate; x_0, time taken to reach 50% of maximum growth; T_{99}, time taken to reach 99% of adult body weight.

*Values are means ± standard error of measurement (SEM).

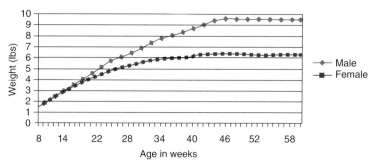

Figure 5-2 Mean growth curves for domestic cats. This graph is a relative growth time line for kittens. (Data from Harlan Sprague Dawley, Inc., July 1, 1996, catalog.)

function of sex hormones affecting growth plate closure; however, the full etiology of the difference has yet to be fully elucidated.

Domestic cats, on the other hand, with a few exceptions, such as the large Maine Coon cat, are generally fit into the same size range relative to height. There are some substantial differences in size of skeletal structure and weight. Examples would be comparing many of the heavy-boned, stout English breeds with the slender athletic Southeast Asian breeds. The Cat Fanciers of America recognizes 39 breeds, each with a written standard. Only one has actual recommendations for

ideal weight; the remaining recommendations are either generalized as small, medium, or large or do not address size at all (Table 5-3).

Kittens grow on average 100 gm/week up to 6 months of age. Average-sized kittens weigh roughly a pound per month of age up to 10 months. When reviewing the feline growth chart, male kittens are usually in the upper two-thirds, whereas females routinely fall into the lower two-thirds (Figure 5-2).

Rates of growth and subsequent energy requirements in puppies and kittens are not constant. Dietary energy

TABLE 5-2   Desired heights and weights for dogs

Breed	Height male (inches)	Height female (inches)	Weight male (pounds)	Weight female (pounds)
Affenpinscher	9-11.5	9-11.5	NA	NA
Afghan Hound	27 ± 1	25 ±1	60	50
Airedale Terrier	23	Slightly less	NA	NA
Akita	26-28 (<26*)	24-26 (<24*)	NA	NA
Alaskan Malamute	25	23	85	75
American Eskimo dog	9-19*	9-19*	NA	NA
American Foxhound	Not under 22 or over 25	Not under 21 or over 24	NA	NA
American Staffordshire Terrier	18-19	17-18	NA	NA
American Water Spaniel	15-18	15-18	30-45	25-40
Anatolian Shepherd Dog	29	27	110-150	80-120
Australian Cattle Dog	18-20	17-19	NA	NA
Australian Shepherd	20-23	18-21	NA	NA
Australian Terrier	10-11	10-11	NA	NA
Basenji	17	16	24	22
Basset Hound	14 ± 1*	14 ± 1*	NA	NA
Beagle	13	13	NA	NA
Beagle	15	15	NA	NA
Bearded Collie	21-22	20-21	NA	NA
Beauceron	25.5-27.5*	24-26.5*	NA	NA
Bedlington Terrier	16.5	15.5	17-23	17-23
Belgian Malinois	24-26*	22-24*	NA	NA
Belgian Sheepdog	24-26*	22-24*	NA	NA
Belgian Tervuren	24-26*	22-24*	NA	NA
Bernese Mountain Dog	25-27.5	23-26	NA	NA
Bichon Frise	9.5-11.5	9.5-11.5	NA	NA
Black and Tan Coonhound	25-27	23-25	NA	NA
Black Russian Terrier	27-30*	24-26.5*	NA	NA
Bloodhound	25-27	23-25	90-110	80-100
Border Collie	19-22	18-21	NA	NA
Border Terrier	NA	NA	13-15.5	11.5-14
Borzoi	28 minimum	26 minimum	75-105	60-85
Boston Terrier	NA	NA	15-25	15-25
Bouvier des Flandres	24.5-27.5	23.5-26.5	NA	NA
Boxer	22.5-25	21-23.5	NA	NA
Briard	23-27*	22-25.5*	NA	NA
Brittany	17.5-20.5*	17.5-20.5*	30-40	30-40
Brussels Griffon	NA	NA	8-10	8-10
Bull Terrier	NA	NA	NA	NA
Bulldog	NA	NA	50	40
Bullmastiff	25-27	24-26	110-130	100-120
Cairn Terrier	10	9.5	14	13
Canaan dog	20-24*	19-23*	45-55	35-45
Cardigan Welsh Corgi	10.5-12.5	10.5-12.5	30-38	25-34
Cavalier King Charles Spaniel	12-13	12-13	13-18	13-18
Chesapeake Bay Retriever	23-26	21-24	65-80	55-70
Chihuahua	NA	NA	<6†	<6†

Continued

TABLE 5-2 Desired heights and weights for dogs—cont'd

Breed	Height male (inches)	Height female (inches)	Weight male (pounds)	Weight female (pounds)
Chinese Crested	11-13	11-13	NA	NA
Chinese Shar-Pei	18-20	18-20	45-60	45-60
Chow Chow	17-20	17-20	NA	NA
Clumber Spaniel	19-20	17-18	70-85	55-70
Cocker Spaniel	15 ± 0.5*	14 ± 0.5*	NA	NA
Collie	24-26	22-24	60-75	50-65
Curly-Coated Retriever	25-27	23-25	NA	NA
Dachshund	NA	NA	Over 11	Over 11
Dachshund Miniature	NA	NA	11 or less	11 or less
Dalmatian	19-23*	19-23*	NA	NA
Dandie Dinmont Terrier	8-11	8-11	18-24	18-24
Doberman Pinscher	26-28	24-26	NA	NA
Dogue de Bordeaux	23.5-27	23-26	>110	>99
English Cocker Spaniel	16-17	15-16	28-34	26-32
English Foxhound	NA	NA	NA	NA
English Setter	Approx. 25	Approx. 24	NA	NA
English Springer Spaniel	20 ± 1	19 ± 1	50	40
English Toy Spaniel	NA	NA	8-14	8-14
Field Spaniel	18 ± 1	17 ± 1	NA	NA
Finnish Spitz	17.5-20	15.5-18	NA	NA
Flat-Coated Retriever	23-24.5	22-23.5	NA	NA
French Bulldog	NA	NA	<28†	<28†
German Pinscher	17-20	17-20	NA	NA
German Shepherd Dog	24-26	22-24	NA	NA
German Shorthaired Pointer	23-25	21-23	55-70	45-60
German Wirehaired Pointer	24-26	Smaller but not less than 22	NA	NA
Giant Schnauzer	25.5-27.5	23.5-25.5	NA	NA
Glen of Imaal Terrier	12.5-14	12.5-14	NA	NA
Golden Retriever	23-24	21.5-22.5	65-75	55-65
Gordon Setter	24-27	23-26	55-80	45-70
Great Dane	30+ (<30*)	28+ (<28*)	NA	NA
Great Pyrenees	27-32	25-29	100	85
Greater Swiss Mountain Dog	25.5-28.5	23.5-27	NA	NA
Greyhound	NA	NA	65-70	60-65
Harrier	19-21 ± 1	19-21 ± 1	NA	NA
Havanese	8.5-11.5*	8.5-11.5*	7-13	7-13
Ibizan Hound	23.5-27.5	22.5-26	50	45
Irish Red and White Setter	24.5-26	22.5-24	NA	NA
Irish Setter	27 ± 1	25 ± 1	70	60
Irish Terrier	18	18	27	25
Irish Water Spaniel	22-24	21-23	55-65	45-58
Irish Wolfhound	32 minimum	30 minimum	120	105
Italian Greyhound	13-15	13-15	NA	NA
Japanese Chin	8-11	8-11	NA	NA
Keeshound	18 ± 1	17 ± 1	NA	NA

TABLE 5-2   Desired heights and weights for dogs—cont'd

Breed	Height male (inches)	Height female (inches)	Weight male (pounds)	Weight female (pounds)
Kerry Blue Terrier	18-19.5	17.5-19	33-40	Slightly less
Komondor	27.5	25.5	100+	80+
Kuvasz	28-30 (<30*)	26-28 (<30*)	100-115	70-90
Labrador Retriever	22.5-24.5	21.5-23.5	65-80	55-70
Lakeland Terrier	14.5 ± 0.5	Not more than 1-inch less	17	Slightly less
Lhasa Apso	10-11	Slightly less	NA	NA
Löwchen	12-14	12-14	NA	NA
Maltese	<7	<7	NA	NA
Manchester Terrier Toy	NA	NA	Not more than 12	Not more than 12
Manchester Terrier	NA	NA	>12-<22†	>12-<22†
Mastiff	30 minimum	27.5 minimum	NA	NA
Miniature Bull Terrier	10-14	10-14	NA	NA
Miniature Pinscher	10-12.5*	10-12.5*	NA	NA
Miniature Schnauzer	12-14*	12-14*	NA	NA
Neapolitan Mastiff	26-31	24-29	150	110
Newfoundland	28	26	130-150	100-120
Norfolk Terrier	9-10	9-10	11-12	11-12
Norwegian Buhund	17-18.5*	16-17.5	31-40	26-35
Norwegian Elkhound	20.5	19.5	55	48
Norwich Terrier	10 or less	10 or less	12	12
Nova Scotia Duck Tolling Retriever	18-21	17-20	NA	NA
Old English Sheepdog	22+	21+	NA	NA
Otterhound	27	24	115	80
Papillon	8-11*	8-11*	NA	NA
Parson Russell Terrier	12-14*	12-14*	13-17	13-17
Pekingese	NA	NA	<14*	<14*
Pembroke Welsh Corgi	10-12	10-12	<30	<28
Petit Basset Griffon Vendéen	13-15 ± 0.5*	13-15 ± 0.5*	NA	NA
Pharaoh Hound	23-25	21-24	NA	NA
Plott	20-25	20-23	50-60	40-55
Pointer	25-28	23-26	55-75	45-65
Polish Lowland Sheepdog	18-20	17-19	NA	NA
Pomeranian	3-7	3-7	NA	NA
Poodle miniature	10-15*	10-15*	NA	NA
Poodle standard	>15*	>15*	NA	NA
Poodle Toy	<10*	<10*	NA	NA
Portuguese Water Dog	20-23	17-21	42-60	35-50
Pug	NA	NA	14-18	14-18
Puli	17	16	NA	NA
Pyrenean Shepherd	15.5-18.5*	15-18*	NA	NA
Rhodesian Ridgeback	25-27	24-26	85	70
Rottweiler	24-27	22-25	NA	NA
Saint Bernard	27.5 minimum	25.5 minimum	NA	NA
Saluki	23-28	Less than male	NA	NA
Samoyed	21-23.5	19-21	NA	NA
Schipperke	11-13	10-12	NA	NA
Scottish Deerhound	30-32	28+	85-110	75-95
Scottish Terrier	10	10	19-22	18-21

Continued

TABLE 5-2	Desired heights and weights for dogs—cont'd			
Breed	Height male (inches)	Height female (inches)	Weight male (pounds)	Weight female (pounds)
Sealyham Terrier	10.5	10.5	23-24	Slightly less
Shetland Sheepdog	13-16*	13-16	NA	NA
Shiba Inu	14.5-16.5	13.5-15.5	23	17
Shih Tzu	9-10.5	9-10.5	9-16	9-16
Siberian Husky	21-23.5	20-22	45-60	35-50
Silky Terrier	9-10	9-10	NA	NA
Skye Terrier	10	9.5	NA	NA
Smooth Fox Terrier	15.5	Slightly less	18	16
Soft Coated Wheaten Terrier	18-19	17-18	35-40	30-35
Spinone Italiano	20-26	20-26	56	56
Staffordshire Bull Terrier	14-16	14-16	28-38	24-34
Standard Schnauzer	18.5-19.5*	17.5-18.5*	NA	NA
Sussex Spaniel	13-15	13-15	35-45	35-45
Swedish Vallhund	12.5-13.5	11.5-12.5	NA	NA
Tibetan Mastiff	26	24	NA	NA
Tibetan Spaniel	10	10	9-15	9-15
Tibetan Terrier	15-16	15-16	20-24	20-24
Toy Fox Terrier	8.5-11.5*	8.5-11.5*	NA	NA
Vizsla	22-24 ±1.5*	21-23 ±1.5*	NA	NA
Weimaraner	25-27 ±1*	23-25 ±1*	NA	NA
Welsh Springer Spaniel	18-19	17-18	NA	NA
Welsh Terrier	15-15.5	Slightly less	20	20
West Highland White Terrier	11	10	NA	NA
Whippet	19-22 ±0.5*	18-21 ±0.5*	Na	NA
Wire Fox Terrier	15.5	Slightly less	18 ±1	16 ±
Wirehaired Pointing Griffon	22-24	20-22	NA	NA
Yorkshire Terrier	NA	NA	<7	<7

Data from American Kennel Club Breed Standards.
NA, Not addressed.
*Disqualification if incorrect height.
†Disqualification if incorrect weight.

requirements are three times maintenance levels at weaning. However, energy requirements are only 1.2 times maintenance as the puppy or kitten approaches adulthood.

FAILURE TO GROW*

Diagnosing a puppy or kitten with failure to grow can be challenging. As stated, the first issue is to determine the definition of normal growth for that breed. It is possible that the puppy is small but inside the normal growth curve and healthy with no underlying problems. This puppy or kitten is genetically programmed for whatever size he will become. All normal-sized dogs of a breed fit into a bell curve, with "normal" small and large individuals residing on either end of the curve.

Attaining a complete history is necessary in attempting to develop a clinical approach to defining the etiology for failure to grow. One important determination is whether the growth issue has been lifelong and the kitten or puppy has always been small, or whether the growth deficiency developed acutely. This question is the equivalent to asking the probability of the problem being congenital or acquired.

Puppy and kitten nutritional history should include the type or quality of the food, volume offered, and frequency of feedings, since dietary palatability and caloric density have a major impact on growth. Homemade diets or "fad" puppy or kitten foods may be improperly balanced or calorically insufficient. Additionally, this information is of little value if

*Adapted from Ihle SL: Failure to grow. In Ettinger SJ, Feldman EC (eds): *Textbook of veterinary internal medicine*, ed 7, St Louis, 2010, Elsevier/Saunders.

TABLE 5-3	Size recommendations for cats
Breed	**Size (lb)**
Abyssinian	NA
American Bobtail	NA
American Curl	M 7-10; F 5-8
American Shorthair	NA
American Wirehair	NA
Balinese	Medium
Birman	Medium
Bombay	Medium
British Shorthair	Med to large
Burmese	Medium
Chartreux	NA
Colorpoint Shorthair	Medium
Cornish Rex	Small to med
Devon Rex	Medium
Egyptian Mau	Medium
European Burmese	Medium
Exotic	NA
Havana Brown	Medium
Japanese Bobtail	Medium
Javanese	Medium
Korat	NA
LaPerm	Medium
Maine Coon	Med to large
Manx	NA
Norwegian Forest Cat	Large
Ocicat	Med to large
Oriental	NA
Persian	NA
RagaMuffin	Large
Ragdoll	Med to large
Russian Blue	NA
Scottish Fold	Medium
Selkirk Rex	Med to large
Siamese	Medium
Siberian	Med to large
Singapura	Small to med
Somali	Med to large
Sphynx	Medium
Tonkinese	Medium
Turkish Angora	Medium
Turkish Van	NA

Data from The Cat Fanciers' Association.
NA, Not addressed

the practitioner is not aware of the puppy's or kitten's current appetite relative to historical information. Has he always been a "picky" eater, or is this a new behavior in a dog that previously ate voraciously? Maybe the puppy is receiving an excellent diet relative to both quality and quantity and eats voraciously but fails to gain weight and grow. Answers to these questions guide the diagnostic approach.

Any history of concurrent clinical signs is important. Patients exhibiting gastrointestinal signs, such as regurgitation, vomiting, or diarrhea, can be afflicted with structural esophageal issues, systemic illness, or exocrine pancreatic insufficiency, among many other conditions. Young animals suffering with a hepatic portal caval shunt may have depressed mentation postprandially. Syncope or exercise intolerance may point to cardiovascular or hepatic structural or metabolic dysfunction. A thorough history should elucidate issues such as polyuria and polydipsia (remembering that young puppies and kittens have immature renal function).

The history should also explore what measures the owner has already employed to alleviate the growth failure, including dietary supplements and any medications or nutraceuticals. Has there been any improvement or worsening of the condition relative to the administration of these products?

Etiologies for failure to grow generally fall into one of four categories: genetic, insufficient nutrient intake, excessive caloric or nutrient loss, and abnormalities in metabolism. Genetic influences control the maximum size any animal can attain given optimal husbandry practices; however, genetic abnormalities can influence growth by inducing abnormal organ or structural development and/or metabolic dysfunctions. Examples of congenital abnormalities that would inhibit growth include megaesophagus, vascular ring abnormalities, pyloric stenosis, and portal caval shunts, among others. Genetic issues, such as chondrodystrophism caused by abnormalities in bone growth, can also be responsible for altered growth patterns.

Deficient nutrient intake may deny the body the required building blocks and energy necessary to accomplish optimal growth. The quality of commercial diets can vary widely, with some having much poorer nutritional value than others. Additionally, fad diets and homemade diets often are significantly imbalanced or lack the nutritional sophistication to adequately fuel correct growth in the puppy or kitten. Any condition that decreases appetite or impedes nutritional intake will limit growth. Conditions that cause vomiting or regurgitation or any maldigestion/malabsorptive issues will deny the growing puppy or kitten adequate nutrition. Heavy gastrointestinal parasitism will siphon nutrients from the host and decrease optimal growth.

The young animal may have adequate nutritional intake but also have conditions that increased caloric or nutrient loss. Persistent hyperthermia and protein-losing enteropathies would be examples of such conditions. Renal protein loss or urinary glucose loss as seen in diseases such as diabetes mellitus can also be a source of caloric loss, as again would be gastrointestinal parasitism.

A wide variety of abnormal metabolic conditions may precipitate inhibited growth in young animals. Hypothyroidism, insufficient growth hormone, insulin restrictive diseases, and pituitary abnormalities can all affect growth negatively. Hepatic disease can limit correct protein metabolism and decrease growth in young animals. Box 5-1 lists potential causes of growth failure in dogs and cats. Development of a structured approach to the diagnosis of the etiology of failure to grow can be found in Figure 5-3.

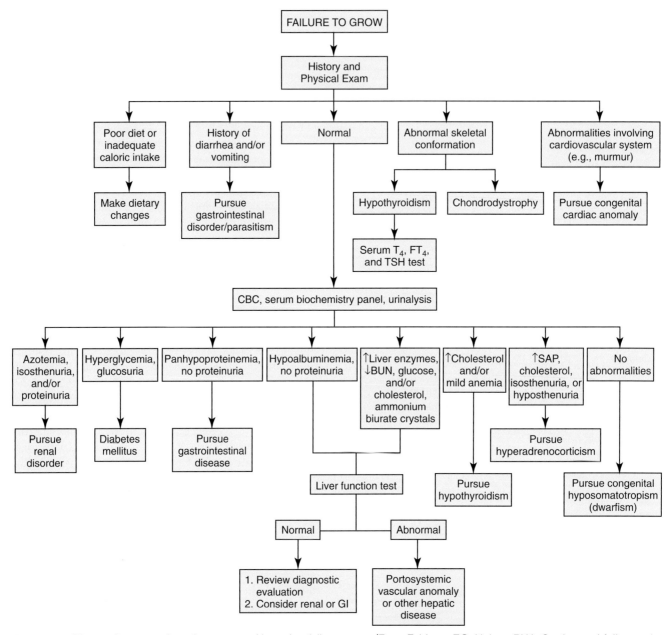

Figure 5-3 Diagnostic approach to the puppy or kitten that fails to grow. (From Feldman EC, Nelson RW: *Canine and feline endocrinology and reproduction*, ed 3, St Louis, 2004, Saunders/Elsevier.)

| BOX 5-1 | Causes of growth failure in dogs and cats |

Small Stature and Poor Body Condition
  Dietary problem
  Underfeeding
  Poor quality diet
  Cardiac disorder
  Congenital anomaly
  Endocarditis
  Hepatic dysfunction
  Portosystemic vascular anomaly
  Hepatitis
  Glycogen storage disease
  Esophageal disease
  Megaesophagus
  Vascular ring anomaly (e.g., persistent right aortic arch)
  Gastrointestinal disease
  Parasites
  Inflammatory bowel disease
  Obstruction (e.g., foreign body, intussusception)

Histoplasmosis
Exocrine pancreatic insufficiency
Renal disease
Renal failure (congenital or acquired)
Glomerular disease
Pyelonephritis
Inflammatory disease
Hormonal disease
Diabetes mellitus
Hypoadrenocorticism
Diabetes insipidus
Juvenile hyperparathyroidism (dogs)
Small Stature and Good Body Condition
  Chondrodystrophy
  Hormonal disease
  Congenital hypothyroidism
  Congenital hyposomatotropism (pituitary dwarfism)
  Hyperadrenocorticism

From Ihle SL: Failure to grow. In Ettinger SJ, Feldman EC (eds): *Textbook of veterinary internal medicine*, ed 7, St Louis, 2010, Elsevier/Saunders.

SUGGESTED READINGS

Feldman EC, Nelson RW: Disorders of growth hormone. In Feldman EC, Nelson RW: *Canine and feline endocrinology and reproduction,* ed 3, St Louis, 2004, Saunders/Elsevier.

Ihle SL: Failure to grow. In Ettinger SJ, Feldman EC (eds): *Textbook of veterinary internal medicine,* ed 7, St Louis, 2010, Saunders/Elsevier.

HUSBANDRY OF THE NEONATE

CHAPTER 6

Kevin T. Fitzgerald, Kristin L. Newquist

The word *husbandry* comes from Old English and means caretaker, manager, or provider. At no other period in an organism's lifetime is it more dependent nor does it require more care and protecting than when it is a neonate. Newborns have many unique physiologic characteristics that are in an active state of transition, as well as anatomic, nutritional, and behavioral deficiencies that distinguish them dramatically from adults. Newborn animals are complicated, but if they are approached in a uniform, systematic fashion their therapy can be extremely rewarding.

Proper neonatal husbandry must include a variety of considerations. Some sources claim birth defects in mammals approach 16%, whereas others claim a 20% fatality rate for puppies in the first 2 weeks of life. This chapter considers newborns from birth to weaning by close examination of their idiosyncrasies (Box 6-1).

THERMOREGULATION

Neonatal animals are poor regulators of their body temperature. Newborns can lose body heat because of evaporation, radiation, convection, and cooling. If newborns are wet or placed next to cold objects (cage or kennel floors), in drafts, or in outdoor enclosures, they can lose considerable amounts of heat. Orphaned newborn puppies during their first week of life require environmental temperatures of 85° to 90° F (30° to 32° C).

For puppies, newborns have lower body temperatures than adult dogs. In the first week of life rectal temperatures range from 95° to 97° F (35° to 36° C), and for the second and third weeks temperatures range from 97° to 100° F (36° to 38° C). By the time of weaning, average rectal temperatures are nearly the same as those of adults.

Reflexes, such as shivering, and vasoconstrictive mechanisms to maintain heat are not developed in the neonate. Brown adipose tissue found in newborns is the site of nonshivering thermogenesis. Wet puppies, inappetent puppies, and orphaned newborns are thus unable to successfully maintain their body temperature in cool or drafty environments. Although shivering is absent in newborn puppies, panting is present in overheated neonates.

Maintenance of normal physiologic functions is related to temperature in puppies and kittens. In puppies that become chilled, the heart rate may drop precipitously. A newborn with a rectal temperature of 96° F has a heart rate somewhere between 200 and 250 beats per minute (bpm). Once the rectal temperature reaches 70° F, the heart rate quickly drops to only 40 bpm. A decreased heart rate may result in inappetence, dehydration, and loss of suckling reflexes. In addition, nursing bitches may refuse to nurse and care for cold puppies and even push them away. When body temperature falls below 94° F, a gastrointestinal (GI) ileus develops and a chilled puppy will stop trying to nurse. If chilled puppies are not rewarmed before force feeding, regurgitation and subsequent aspiration pneumonia can result (Box 6-2).

Hypothermia in newborns can, however, have a sparing effect. The hypothermia that results in decreased cardiovascular function may conversely protect puppies from the ischemic brain injury that accompanies cardiovascular collapse. In one investigation, induction of hypothermia resulting in circulatory onset of up to 1 hour was not responsible for subsequent brain injury. If hypothermia-related circulatory arrests lasting more than an hour were induced, neuronal injury resulted. In puppies with sustained hypothermia, tissue hypoxia, metabolic acidosis, and cell death all subsequently ensue.

The ability for lymphocytes to transform and combat infection is significantly decreased when pups are chilled. The cardiovascular and GI systems depend on body temperature, and the immune system is also closely influenced by a change of only a few degrees.

Warming chilled neonates back to normal temperatures can be potentially very dangerous. Newborns must be warmed safely after cooler body temperatures are discovered.

BOX 6-1   Significant husbandry issues for the neonate

- Sick neonatal animals should always be checked for hypoglycemia. Clinical signs of hypoglycemia in neonates include lethargy, failure to suckle, depression, mental dullness, stupor, tremors, and seizures. Hypoglycemic animals may also show agitation, vocalize, be irritable, be intensely hungry, and lose consciousness.
- Diarrhea in newborns can be a result of overfeeding, hyperosmolar diets, viruses, or parasites. Body temperature is critical in neonates. At body temperatures below 94° F (34.5° C) ileus develops. This decreases their ability to suckle and nurse and increases their chances for aspiration and pneumonia.
- Both feline and canine newborns are immunologically incompetent and antibody deficient at birth. Passive immunity is acquired through the adequate ingestion and absorption of maternal colostrum during the first 24 hours after birth. Ability for antibody absorption decreases markedly after 12 hours.
- If colostrum intake is not possible or available, pooled adult serum can be administered to puppies and kittens to elevate serum immunoglobulin concentrations (22 ml/kg and 15 ml per kitten). T-cell mitogenesis and differentiation and phagocytic cell functions are not fully mature until 12 to 16 weeks of age.

- When recommending vaccine regimens for young animals, veterinary clinicians must consider a number of important criteria. These include (1) the morbidity and mortality of the specific disease, (2) the prevalence or actual incidence rate of the disease, (3) actual risk of that individual for exposure to that disease, (4) efficacy of the vaccine, (5) risks associated with the vaccine, (6) any potential for zoonotic infection by that disease, and (7) route of infection and transmission by this disease.
- Based on consideration concerning these criteria, vaccines for puppies and kittens can be regarded by either "core," "noncore," or "not recommended." However, each animal must be assessed as an individual with all the benefits and risks evaluated before any vaccine can be administered.
- Clinical signs of neonatal septicemia include weakness, failure to suckle, diarrhea, hypothermia, cyanosis, vocalization, and finally coma. Sloughing of extremities (e.g., toes, tails, ears) can be observed.
- Treatment of failing newborns involves aggressive fluid support, combating septic shock, and nutritional buttressing. Selection of a safe, efficacious antibiotic may be required.

BOX 6-2   Effects of drop in body temperature on neonates

- Heart rate drops.
- GI ileus may result.
- Chilled neonates have less ability for lymphocyte transformation.
- Mothers reject newborns with cool skin.

GI, Gastrointestinal.

Heat sources must be safe, effective, and easily monitored. Warm water bottles wrapped in towels or cloth, boiled rice heated in a sock, or warmed towels can provide adequate heat but must be judiciously scrutinized. Water should be changed and reheated as it cools, since there is the risk of chilling newborns with cold bottles and containers full of cold water. Similarly, newborns are neurologically immature and lack the ability to move away from excessive heat. Cloth coverings or pillow cases can decrease direct contact of the delicate newborn skin with hot water bottles and heat sources, but these types of heat supplements can overheat, dehydrate, and even severely burn ill, comatose, or orphaned newborns. For these reasons, heating pads, heat lamps, and electric blankets are not recommended because they are so difficult to regulate and safely manage.

Pediatric incubators are easily available and are ideal in managing sick, debilitated, or orphaned puppies and kittens. Nevertheless, these devices can also lead to problems if not rigorously attended. Environmental control for newborns must also consider humidity. Use of incubators can lead to mucous membranes that are quickly dried out. A relative humidity of 55% to 65% is considered adequate for the prevention of skin drying. In neonatal, low birth weight puppies, relative humidity of 85% to 90% is most effective in maintenance of hydration and body temperature. If high humidity is provided, care must be taken not to reach environmental temperatures greater than 90° F (32° C). Temperatures of 95° F (35° C) and greater coupled with relative humidities of over 95% lead to respiratory distress in neonatal puppies and kittens. Oxygen cages are also an excellent way to warm newborns.

The best incubators, whelping boxes, or closed environments present the newborn with a gradient of temperatures and allow the puppies and kittens to select the most comfortable zones. Nevertheless, even healthy pups and kittens initially are neurologically immature and unable to move away from excessive heat.

REGULATION OF CARBOHYDRATES

Newborns differ substantially from adults with regard to their ability to maintain normal blood glucose levels. Ill neonates must always be evaluated for hypoglycemia. Hypoglycemia in the newborn can be due to a variety of causes and can appear in conjunction with hypothermia, sepsis, starvation, toxic milk syndrome, or any combination of these things. The capacity of the newborn for the regulation of blood glucose may be directly related to the nutritional state of the dam during pregnancy. Starvation of the mother can lead to lower birth rates, lower fetal blood glucose concentrations, and increased fetal ketone levels. Starvation of the mother also reduced fetal birth weight by 23% and resulted in significantly lower fasting blood glucose levels in pups at 3 hours of age when compared to controls in one study. Furthermore, bitches fed a low-carbohydrate diet had both a higher incidence of stillbirths and a higher incidence of neonatal losses in the first 3 days after whelping.

Neonates born to healthy, well-fed mothers are better able to maintain blood glucose for even several hours after the fast. However, since the neonatal liver contains minimal glycogen stores, even slight fasts can cause hypoglycemia. The neonate is born with limited capacities for gluconeogenesis and glycogenolysis because of the immaturity of the newborn's liver. In addition, initial limited hepatic glycogen stores, small muscle mass, lack of adipose tissue, and decreased use of free fatty acids as an alternative energy source place neonates at great risk for developing hypoglycemia in the face of even the briefest fast. Impaired gluconeogenesis caused by the delayed maturation and induction of the rate-limiting gluconeogenic enzymes has been shown to result in hypoglycemia in human infants and is suspected in the same condition in kittens and puppies.

Hypoglycemia of immature (less than 6 months old) toy and miniature dog breeds is frequently reported. Just as in human infants, alanine deficiency has been implicated in this condition in young dogs. The rate of alanine release from muscle determines the rate of gluconeogenesis during starvation. These toy breeds have much smaller muscle mass, immature enzymatic machinery, and smaller muscle stores to begin with, thus hypoglycemia develops more easily.

Hypoglycemic neonates have often been under extreme stresses; they have only recently been purchased or otherwise obtained and have had a huge change in their environment, as well as their diet. GI problems, anorexia, diarrhea, and vomiting are commonly reported. These signs may also be the result of parasites. Neonates lack the feedback mechanism between hepatic gluconeogenesis and blood glucose concentrations, making regulation of blood glucose much more difficult than for adult dogs, and a variety of other factors can lead to this hypoglycemia. In addition, a host of other conditions inherited, contracted, or acquired can cause hypoglycemia in newborns. Endotoxemia, sepsis, portosystemic shunts, and glycogen storage abnormalities have all been recognized as conditions that can cause a profound decline in blood sugar concentrations.

Inherited, inborn errors in amino acid and/or carbohydrate metabolism; inadequate protein, glycogen, or carbohydrate stores; and immature, deficient, or faulty enzyme systems should be considered in neonates with repeated bouts of hypoglycemia in the absence of any identifiable contagious cause (septicemia/endotoxemia). If hypoglycemia recurs in neonates with a good diet and adequate nutrition, glycogen storage disease should be suspected. Glycogen storage disease also might be considered if neonates with recurrent hypoglycemia episodes also display acidosis, ketosis, and hepatomegaly.

TABLE 6-1	Treatment of hypoglycemia in newborn dogs
Dextrose concentration (%)	**Amount administered (ml/oz/dog)**
5%	0.25-0.6525 IV
10%	0.125 to 0.31 IV
50%	0.25 to 0.625, orally, direct to gums. Never give higher than 10% IV.

IV, Intravenous.

Normal concentrations for blood glucose in neonates are considered to be 52 to 127 mg/lb for neonatal pups between the ages of 1 to 3 days and 111 mg/lb at 4 weeks of age. The normal adult range of blood glucose concentrations has been reported at 65 to 110 mg/lb. Blood glucose less than 40 mg/lb in pups 2 to 6 weeks of age should be considered abnormal, particularly if clinical signs are present.

Clinical signs of hypoglycemia in neonates include lethargy, failure to suckle, depression, mental dullness, stupor, tremors, and seizures. Accompanying signs may include agitation, vocalization, irritability, intense hunger, and loss of consciousness.

Treatment for hypoglycemia is initiated after a diagnosis has been made. Dextrose 0.2 to 0.5 gm/lb (0.5 to 1.0 gm/kg) can be administered *slowly* (over several minutes) intravenously through the jugular veins of most pups. Solutions of 5% to 10% dextrose are recommended for intravenous (IV) administration. Higher concentrations of dextrose may be directly applied to mucous membranes but should *never* be given intravenously because of the risk of phlebitis (Table 6-1). Because of the immature metabolic mechanisms in neonatal animals concerning glucose metabolism and the potential for inherited glycogen storage diseases, blood glucose levels should be determined before more dextrose is administered to a neonate who fails to respond to therapy.

HEPATIC AND RENAL CONSIDERATIONS

Veterinarians treating neonates must come to recognize the differences between adult animals and the immature liver and kidneys of newborns. These differences are critical in terms of drug metabolism and excretion. Nephrogenesis is not completed until the third week after birth. As cortical blood flow changes and as maturation of nephrons occurs, various parts of the kidney are vulnerable to drug toxicity at various times. Protein, glucose, and amino acids are higher in the urine of neonatal pups than in adult dogs. Nevertheless, urine specific gravity is usually lower. During the first 8 weeks after whelping, the urine specific gravity ranges from 1.006 to 1.017. At or about 8 weeks, the urine specific gravity of the neonate approaches that of an adult animal. Urination begins soon after birth. The dam stimulates the vulva or prepuce of the neonate in order to get the newborn to urinate. After a few weeks, they are urinating on their own.

A variety of functions of the liver are immature or incompletely developed in the neonate enzyme system such as the P450; reduction, hydroxylation, and demethylation are not fully mature until animals are at least 5 months of age. Drugs that are metabolized and excreted by the liver should be avoided in neonates or a modified dosage scheme should be developed. However, for many drugs, no such schemes or schedules are available.

CARDIOPULMONARY COMPETENCE
(see Chapters 32 and 34)

Cutaneous stimulation and manipulation of a newborn puppy initiates a reflex respiration. This reflexive response can be seen when the bitch licks and nips the newborn or when surgery assistants rub puppies after cesarean section. Respiratory rates of adult dogs are 16 to 32 bpm. Respiratory rates of pups are 10 to 18 bpm during the first week of life, 18 to 36 bpm during the second week, and by the third week of life it becomes the same as the rate of adult dogs. Newborn pups respond to hypercapnia by reflexively increasing bronchomotor tone. However, a pulmonary response to hypoxia is either lacking or minimal. In pups, bradycardia can occur as oxygen partial pressure drops, quite unlike the tachycardia shown in response to hypoxemia by adult dogs. Veterinary clinicians must realize that hypoxemic neonatal pups may have heart rates expected for healthy adult dogs (this despite the fact that the heart rate of normal newborn pups is 200 to 250 bpm).

Baroceptors for blood pressure are operational by the fourth day of life. This causes the heart rate of pups to vary in reaction to changes in blood pressure just as occurs in adult dogs. Mean arterial blood pressure is between 30 and 70 mm Hg in 1- to 4-week-old pups, which is much lower than that found in adults. Blood pressure is affected by a multitude of factors, including body temperature and blood glucose concentration. For severely hypoglycemic pups, the mean arterial blood pressure may drop as much as 50%. After the first week, arterial blood pressure increases with age and reaches adult levels somewhere between 6 weeks and a few months of age. The electrocardiogram (ECG) of neonates is much different than that of adults. In one report, the QRS modal axis of the ECG switched from a right cranioventral direction in the first week after birth to a left caudoventral orientation 12 weeks after whelping. This significant cardiac axis change may represent the change in ratio of right ventricular to left ventricular mass. At birth, the mass of right ventricle relative to the left ventricle is 1:1 in neonates and 1:2 or 1:3 in normal, mature adult dogs. This change in mass is intimately reflected in the ECG.

NERVOUS SYSTEM (see Chapter 40)

The development, onset, and appearance of different neurologic reflexes vary tremendously in the newborn. The suckling reflex for nursing should appear within an hour of birth. Neonatal puppies and kittens can raise their heads and move by propelling themselves forward on their ventral thorax shortly after birth. Although flexion is the predominant posture of pups at birth, within the first 5 days, extensor muscles achieve dominance. Although eyes and ears do not open for almost the first 2 weeks, neonates do respond to noises and can show a slow blink to lights shined through closed eyelids.

Newborns have an immature blood-brain barrier. The gradient is permeable to lactic acid, which the body can utilize as a nutrient when starved or hypoglycemic. The immature nature of the blood-brain barrier of the neonate provides easier access for drugs into the central nervous system (CNS). Antibiotic molecules normally prevented from entering the adult brain can enter the brain of the neonatal puppy or kitten. Thus many drugs can achieve dramatic cerebrospinal fluid concentrations in the newborn. As a result, great care must be taken when drugs are administered to immature animals. Since a greater effect of the drug is possible, a greater potential for toxicity also exists. Tetracyclines, penicillins, sulfonamides, and a host of other drugs may obtain worrisome levels in the newborn CNS.

GASTROINTESTINAL SYSTEM
(see Chapter 36)

The GI tract of neonates is sterile at birth. In the first few days, the GI tract is quickly colonized by microorganisms. Diet (whether nursing or bottle fed), environment, antibiotic therapy, or bacterial, viral, or parasitic disease can affect the rate of colonization.

Puppy and kitten GI tracts are well-developed at birth and produce a yellowish, semiformed stool while nursing. Care must be taken to note the stools of neonates. They are not always observed, since mothers ingest the feces of the newborn. Orphaned pups fed formula and puppies supplemented while nursing often develop diarrhea. Diarrhea may result from bacterial overgrowth, overfeeding, hyperosmolar diets, viruses, or parasites.

Estimation of the age of pups, even when pups are orphans, becomes important after recommending appropriate vaccination schedules. Age of newborns can be estimated by identifying the eruption dates of various deciduous and permanent teeth. Somewhere between 3 and 6 weeks deciduous teeth erupt and when this occurs, the dam encourages weaning of the newborns.

IMMUNE SYSTEM (see Chapter 14)

It has long been recognized that neonatal animals have immature immune systems. Little passive immunity is acquired by developing animals in utero; the majority of passive immunity is obtained after birth from the colostrum of the mother. Colostral antibodies are received during the first 24 hours postpartum and are primarily responsible for immunity during the first several weeks of life. After the first 24 to 36 hours, little further uptake of colostral antibodies occurs across the GI tract. However, although they are no longer absorbed, colostral antibodies in the milk continue to be protective by preventing infections that initiate from the oral or intestinal mucous membranes of the neonate. These antibodies, predominantly immunoglobulins (Ig) A (IgA) and IgG, provide some level of protection. In the mouth, esophagus, and oropharynx, IgB antibodies play a major role, whereas in the stomach and intestines, IgA antibodies are at work. The protection provided by colostral antibodies drops quickly so that between 6 and 20 weeks of age they are no longer functional.

Although colostral antibodies supply the majority of neonatal immune protection, newborns are able to mount some antibody response to various antigens. This neonatal response is produced mainly by IgM. The production of antibodies by B cells depends on the activity of T-helper cells. The humoral response of pups is immature when compared to that of adults. It is not known at present whether this is due to the immaturity of B- or T lymphocyte lines.

At birth, proliferation of T cells induced by mitogens and various substances is minimal, which may explain the neonate's lack of response to early vaccination regimens and overall susceptibility to infections. Differentiation and maturation of T lymphocytes occurs in the thymus. In dogs, during the first 12 weeks postpartum, T lymphocytes increase over 200-fold.

In addition to B and T lymphocytes, other factors are necessary for a mature, operational, and fully functioning immune system. Enzymes, complement, and polymorphonuclear cells are all involved in the immune response of the young animal. In neonates, complement components can be deficient and phagocytic activity can be defective, leading to reduced killing of microorganisms, decreased phagocytosis, and defective opsonization of bacteria.

ANTIBIOTICS, DRUGS, AND NEONATAL ANIMALS (see Chapter 27)

In the husbandry and management of newborn domestic animals, veterinary clinicians must be aware of the special sensitivities of neonatal animals to certain antimicrobial drugs and only select drugs that are safe and effective. In this section, several drugs are examined that have been reported as unsafe in younger animals (Table 6-2).

Gentamicin sulfate is an aminoglycoside antibiotic. It is bactericidal and its mechanism of action is to inhibit bacterial protein synthesis by binding with the 30S ribosome. It is a broad-spectrum antibiotic, except for anaerobic bacteria and certain streptococci. Nephrotoxicity has been reported in pups and the young of several species. Animals must have adequate fluid and electrolyte balance if it is to be used. The much-described ototoxicity has not been reported in animals. It is a poor selection in animals with decreased or immature renal function.

TABLE 6-2	Antibiotic considerations in neonates
Drug	**Considerations**
Tetracycline	Known to chelate calcium. Results in abnormal teeth and bone development. Not for use in young animals.
Trimethoprim + sulfonamides	Known to cause arthropathy, anemia, skin reactions, and keratoconjunctivitis sicca. Not for use in young animals.
Gentamicin sulfate	Nephrotoxicity is the most drug-limiting toxicity. Ototoxicity and vestibulotoxicity also possible but have not been reported in animals. Not for use in animals that are dehydrated or that have compromised renal function, renal insufficiency, or renal failure. There must be adequate renal clearance present if gentamicin is to be used. Safer drugs are available for young animals.
Enrofloxacin	All of the fluoroquinolones can cause arthropathy in young animals. Dogs are most sensitive at 4-28 weeks of age. Large, rapidly growing dogs are most susceptible. High concentrations can cause CNS signs, especially in animals with renal failure. At higher dosages can cause nausea and diarrhea. Not for use in young animals.
Metronidazole	Most toxicities are dose related. Most animals showing neurotoxic signs have been receiving dosages over a prolonged period. At suggested dosages, fetal abnormalities have not been reported. However, metronidazole has been shown to be mutagenic and genotoxic in some species. As a result, it is not recommended during pregnancy.

CNS, Central nervous system.

Enrofloxacin is one of the fluoroquinolones. The antibacterial acts via inhibition of DNA gyrase in bacteria that inhibits DNA and RNA synthesis. Enrofloxacin is a broad-spectrum antibiotic and is metabolized to ciprofloxacin. Susceptible bacteria include *Staphylococcus, Escherichia coli, Proteus, Klebsiella,* and *Pasteurella.* It does not have good activity against anaerobic bacteria. All fluoroquinolones may cause arthropathy in young animals. It causes abnormal development in articular cartilage and causes destructive lesions in animals younger than 18 months of age. Rapidly growing, large, and giant breeds of dog appear most susceptible. Cats appear relatively resistant to cartilage injury. Cats at higher dosages may display retinal degeneration and subsequently develop permanent blindness. Injected solutions may be irritating to some tissues.

Tetracycline is an antibiotic whose mechanism of action is to bind to the 30S ribosomal subunit, thereby inhibiting protein synthesis. It has broad activity but is only bacteriostatic against some bacteria. It is effective against certain protozoa. Resistance is commonly seen for many bacteria when tetracycline is administered. Tetracycline chelates calcium and as a result can affect bone and teeth formation. The calcium chelation causes enamel dysplasia and tooth discoloration ("tetracycline teeth"), skeletal deformities, and inhibition of bone growth. Tetracycline is the wrong drug for use in young animals.

Trimethoprim + sulfonamide act synergistically on bacteria and have a broad spectrum of activity. The mechanism of action comes from competition with *para*-aminobenzoic acid for the enzyme that synthesizes dihydrofolic acid in bacteria. For many bacteria, it is bacteriostatic. Trimethoprim + sulfonamide combinations can cause keratoconjunctivitis sicca (KCS), skin reactions, anemia, thrombocytopenia, and allergic reactions including type II and III hypersensitivities, and arthropathies. It is not recommended in young animals and Doberman Pinschers. Dogs may be more sensitive than other species to sulfonamide reactions because they lack the ability to acetylate sulfonamides to other metabolites.

Chloramphenicol is an antimicrobial drug capable of inhibiting bacterial protein synthesis via binding to the ribosome. This antibiotic molecule can cause bone marrow suppression at high dosages or with prolonged use. Cats appear particularly sensitive to the effects of this drug. Bone marrow suppression has been seen in cats after only 14 days of treatment. Chloramphenicol should not be used in pregnant animals, neonates, or cats. It is appetite suppressive and can pose a risk of toxicity in humans. Exposure to small dosages has caused anaplastic anemia in people. There are safer, better drugs for use in neonates.

Ivermectin is an antiparasitic avermectin. These molecules are macrocyclic lactones that originally were produced from molds. These drugs are neurotoxic to parasites by potentiating glutamate-gated chloride ion channels in the parasites. Paralysis and death of parasites are caused by increased permeability to chloride ions and hyperpolarization of nerve cells. Toxicity can occur at high dosages and in breeds where ivermectin crosses the blood-brain barrier. Ivermectin should not be given to pregnant animals or those younger than 6 weeks of age. Ivermectin at doses of 400 μg/kg has produced toxicosis in kittens and doses as low as 300 μg/kg have been lethal in young cats.

All aspects of disposition of drugs by an organism, absorption, distribution, metabolism, and excretion are affected by the age and maturity of the animal. As a result, newborn patients are much more susceptible to the adverse effects of drugs, since their various physiologic pathways governing metabolism of drugs are so immature. In neonates, the permeability of the intestinal mucosa is increased

and as a result the uptake of toxic molecules is increased. Newborn animals also have decreased concentration of plasma proteins the first few weeks of life, which can lead to more unbound compound and a potentially longer plasma half-life and toxic action. Young animals have less total body water and more extracellular fluid than adults, which can lead to a longer half-life of toxic molecules. Furthermore, younger animals have decreased body fat. This results in less accumulation of lipid soluble molecules in the fat and thus persistently increased plasma levels of the drug. Because of increased skin hydration, the newborn animal has greater capacity for percutaneous absorption of molecules. As a result, the pediatric patient is at much higher risk for the significant cutaneous absorption of potentially toxic molecules. Finally, volatile gases are more rapidly absorbed from the pediatric respiratory tract than from adults. As a result, young animals are more sensitive to the potential toxic effects of inhaled gases.

Plasma protein concentration is much lower in pediatric animals, particularly glycoproteins and albumin. With less potentially toxic drug plasma-bound, the risk of toxicity increases as the concentration of free pharmacologically active compound rises. If a substance has a narrow therapeutic index and is highly protein bound, these age-related changes become significant and may make intoxication more likely to occur. Thus increased unbound toxic compounds may have longer access for free distribution to outlying tissues.

Neonates also display differences in regional organ blood supply. Differences in renal blood flow can result in wide alterations in drug or toxin excretion. Pediatric patients have proportionally greater blood supply to the heart and brain, increasing the risk of toxic effects from lower exposures to cardiac and CNS poisons. Newborns have increased permeability of the blood-brain barrier. Consequently, younger animals have increased potential for toxic exposure to CNS intoxicants. Thus, the CNS, normally more protected in adults, is at much higher risk of exposure to toxins in the neonatal animal.

Neonatal animals show incomplete hepatic metabolism and reduced renal excretion. As a result, elimination and clearance of potentially injurious molecules are reduced. Young animals show both reduced phase I (oxidative) and phase II (glucuronidation) reactions. Puppies may not show phase I activity until day 9 after whelping; this activity increases after day 25 until it reaches adult activity levels at day 135. Since hepatic drug metabolism is decreased, plasma clearance of drug is decreased, plasma half-life is increased and the compound may obtain toxic concentrations as a result. Until the liver matures, great care must be taken in prescribing drugs and prevention of toxic exposure.

Neonates demonstrate a steady increase in glomerular filtration and renal tubular function in the weeks after birth. Young animals have reduced renal excretion, decreasing clearance of renally excreted compounds and the products of hepatic phase II metabolism. In puppies, adult levels of glomerular filtration and tubular function are achieved by 10

TABLE 6-3	Drug metabolism and considerations in neonates
Drug	**Considerations**
Renally excreted antimicrobials (penicillin, ampicillin, cephalosporins, fluoroquinolones, aminoglycosides)	Caution if given to neonates
β-Lactam antibiotics	Antimicrobial drug of choice Half-life is prolonged Large therapeutic index
NSAIDs	Require hepatic metabolism Risk of renal injury from NSAIDs is greatly increased Not recommended in neonates

NSAIDs, Nonsteroidal antiinflammatory drugs.

weeks of age. Until then, water-soluble compounds have decreased clearance and extension of plasma half-life. One can anticipate even greater toxic effects in sick or dehydrated neonatal animals in which the kidneys are even further compromised (Table 6-3).

The neonate is a fragile and complex organism rapidly changing into an adult. The practicing clinician must be aware of this transition and the unique physiologic traits of young animals and make appropriate concessions to successfully treat and manage the pediatric patient.

VACCINATIONS (see Chapter 14)

In recent years, vaccination protocols and specific vaccinations have come under increased scrutiny. Duration of immunity for various vaccines and the potential deleterious effects of certain vaccines brought the whole rationale for vaccinating into question. Nevertheless, infectious diseases are still very much present that prey on the pediatric patient. Vaccinations should be administered only if the risk of an individual animal being exposed to a particular infectious agent has been rigorously considered. Furthermore, criteria, such as health risk associated with infection, actual disease incidence and severity, and vaccine efficacy, must likewise be assessed. "Core" vaccines are those immunizations that have been recommended to be administered to *every* dog and cat who is 6 months of age or younger or is not known to have had any prior vaccination. These vaccines have been deemed necessary because the diseases they prevent display significant morbidity and mortality, are widely distributed, and/or may have zoonotic potential. "Noncore" vaccines are those influenced by geographic distribution of the infectious agent, age of the patient, and lifestyle of the animal (indoor only vs. free-roaming). Noncore vaccines are those recommended against less common or less severe diseases and against those that are either self-limiting or lend themselves well to

treatment. The veterinarian has a tremendous responsibility to the animal, its caretakers, and to the American public in selecting safe and effective vaccines for young animals.

Any recommendations for vaccinations of puppies and kittens must be recognized as recommendations. Nevertheless, they are guidelines based on the most recent studies and research and the best understanding of the most current, available science concerning immunization. Certainly, there are risks inherent in vaccinating. However, vaccines represent one of the best bargains for animal health care based on their efficacy, cost, and overall safety. Vaccine selection is the responsibility of the veterinarian providing care and must be a serious decision based on determination of the animal's risk of exposure and its lifestyle and age. The decision must reflect the geographic incidence of the disease in question, its relative morbidity and mortality, the animal's overall health, and potential of the disease for transmission to human beings.

For dogs, the Task Force recommends as "core" vaccines, immunization against canine distemper virus (CDV), canine parvovirus (CPV), canine adenovirus-2 (CAV-2), and rabies. When possible, modified-live virus (MLV) vaccines are recommended over killed vaccines. Killed rabies vaccines (determined to be either 1- or 3-year vaccines) are the only types available at present within the United States and most other countries. A minimum of three doses of "core" vaccines (CDV, CPV, and CAV-2) should be given to puppies between 6 and 16 weeks of age. The final dose must be administered between 14 and 16 weeks of age. A subsequent inoculation of the core vaccines should be given 1 year after the administration of the last in the puppy series. A single rabies immunization is recommended at 16 weeks of age. This is followed up with a single injection rabies booster 1 year later.

"Noncore" vaccines for canines include *Bordetella bronchiseptica* vaccines, distemper-measles, parainfluenza virus vaccines, *Borrelia burgdorferi, Lyme borreliosis,* and *Leptospira interrogans* (all four serovars).

Nonrecommended canine pediatric vaccines include measles, coronavirus, canine adenovirus-1, and *Giardia* vaccine. Veterinarians must become familiar with recommended and nonrecommended vaccines, incidence of a particular disease in an area, frequency of administration of vaccines, type to be administered (killed vs. avirulent live), and route of administration (topical vs. parenteral).

For years the primary vaccination series in cats for core immunizations was a dose administered at 9 and 12 weeks. Currently, recommended feline guidelines are first dose of core vaccines (feline parvovirus [panleukopenia virus], herpes virus-1, and calicivirus) be administered as early as 6 weeks and then given every 3 or 4 weeks until 16 weeks of age. A booster of these components should follow in 1 year. A rabies vaccine (also considered a core immunization for cats) can be administered as early as 12 weeks of age. A rabies booster is recommended 1 year later.

At present, chlamydiosis, feline leukemia virus (FeLV) vaccine, and vaccinations for *Bordetella bronchiseptica* are not listed as feline core vaccines and should be given only if exposure risk is great. Furthermore, vaccination for feline immunodeficiency virus (FIV), feline coronavirus (FCOR) to protect against feline infectious peritonitis (FIP), and *Giardia lamblia* are generally not recommended at all.

Vaccinations are potent biologic agents created to prevent disease. As with any foreign substance administered to a living system, vaccines have the potential for adverse reactions. Vaccinations must meet United States Department of Agriculture (USDA) standards guaranteeing their safety, efficacy, potency, and purity. Nevertheless, even by requiring vaccines to meet these standards there still exists the possibility for adverse vaccine reactions. Some reactions may be seen more often with certain agents, others have increased frequency in certain breeds, and others are simply idiosyncratic and unpredictable. Clinical signs of vaccine reactions can include anorexia, pyrexia, and malaise for 1 or 2 days after the immunization. Most of the reactions are mild, self-limiting, and require little or no treatment. However, any reaction to a vaccine must be documented in the animal's legal record to protect against further incidents.

Reactions to vaccines may manifest themselves in a variety of ways. Feline injection site sarcomas or fibrosarcomas develop secondary to inflammation of the vaccination site. Certain adjuvants and other ingredients have been implicated with an increased risk of development of these tumors. Clinicians are encouraged to avoid multiple vaccines in the same site to decrease the amount of inflammation at the site and to administer only vaccines for diseases for which the animal is actually at risk. The "three-two-one" rule advocated by the Vaccine-Associated Feline Sarcoma Task Force (VAFSTF) is very helpful. It states that persistent swellings in areas of recent vaccination should be rigorously monitored. The "rule" maintains that if the swelling persists for 3 months or more, if the area is larger than 2 cm in diameter, or if the size of the swelling increases after 1 month and if any of the criteria are met, the swelling should be biopsied and samples sent out to a board-certified pathologist.

Type I hypersensitivity to vaccination is known as *anaphylaxis* or *immediate hypersensitivity* and is mediated by the IgE antibody. In this instance, the animal's immune system is reacting to adjuvants, preservatives, or the antigen contained in the vaccine. Typically, these reactions occur within 2 to 3 hours of vaccination. In dogs, most commonly seen signs are angioedema, urticaria, and pruritus, but symptoms can be worse and include respiratory collapse and full-blown anaphylaxis. For cats, the acute onset of vomiting and diarrhea, with associated hypovolemia, and respiratory and vascular collapse may be seen. Any animal showing these signs within hours of being vaccinated should be returned to the hospital immediately for thorough examination and perhaps emergency medical therapy and support. The animal's medical record should be flagged inside and out to prevent future incidents of this type and caretakers should be advised to never give this product again.

Type II hypersensitivities to vaccines (autoimmune reactions) have been reported to occur in dogs. Some reports maintain that immune-mediated hemolytic anemia and immune-mediated thrombocytopenia can develop shortly after a recent vaccination. Animals developing either condition within a month of receiving an immunization should be protected from subsequent use of that vaccine product.

Type III hypersensitivities are immune complex reactions. Anterior uveitis associated with the use of the CAV-1 vaccine and the complement-mediated rabies vaccine-induced vasculitis or dermatitis in dogs are examples of this adverse vaccine reaction.

Type IV hypersensitivity reactions are the cell-mediated responses, which can occur locally or systemically. Examples of type IV reactions include sterile granulomas at vaccine sites and polyradiculoneuritis.

Despite recent findings concerning deleterious effects of certain vaccines, vaccinations still remain one of the clinician's greatest weapons in preventing disease. Vaccines have played an incredible role in providing better health for generations of kittens and puppies. The clinician must balance the risk of disease to the animal presented against the risk of potential adverse side effects. We must also convey to the owner the comparative risks of overvaccinating vs. undervaccinating.

FADING PUPPIES (see Chapter 11)

Many neonatal losses are often ascribed to the "fading puppy syndrome." Sadly, many times any cause of death in newborns is lumped into this category. True fading puppy syndrome is believed to be caused by neonatal septicemia. Confirmation of a septic process may require histologic determination, evaluation of cultures, and identification of specific agents. Nevertheless, effective therapy for this condition must never wait for laboratory results. Aggressive therapy must be initiated early to help affected pups. Because of a neonate's minimal energy reserves, an immature immune system, and small size, neonatal septicemia can progress rapidly and quickly lead to death. Factors that can lead to neonatal septicemia include maternal infections (e.g., endometritis, metritis, mastitis), contaminated environments (puppy mills, veterinary hospitals, and boarding kennels), antimicrobial drug treatment (any drug that causes reduction in the number of anaerobic bacteria in the GI tract), feeding formulas with excessive osmolarity (the bitch's milk is best because it is high in IgA), stress (e.g., tail docking, dewclaw removal), and chilling puppies (causes reduction in transformation of lymphocytes).

Clinical signs of neonatal septicemia are found in Box 6-3. Sloughing is believed caused by hypoxia, reduced blood supply to extremities in already hypovolemic newborns, and a vasculitis directly caused by the infectious organism.

Treatment for affected puppies involves selection of an antibiotic with a wide spectrum of activity that is at the same time safe for the young animals. *Escherichia coli, Klebsiella pneumoniae, Staphylococcus intermedius,* and β-hemolytic streptococci are some of the more frequently observed microorganisms. Cephalosporins can be used safely in such

BOX 6-3	Clinical signs of neonatal septicemia

- Weakness
- Failure to suckle
- Vocalization
- Diarrhea
- Cyanosis
- Coma
- Occasional sloughing of extremities (toes, tails, ears)

puppies. Selection of safe antibiotics and safe dosages and intervals are considered elsewhere in this discussion and in Chapter 27.

NUTRITIONAL CONSIDERATIONS
(see Chapters 8 and 44)

Proper nutrition is essential for the health of the neonate. Inadequate caloric intake must be addressed promptly to prevent serious consequences. Sick pups who fail to nurse on their own may need to be bottle fed or tube fed (see Chapter 9). Newborns separated from their mothers must be kept warm. Hypothermia retards digestion and promotes GI ileus. This loss of GI motility is often present in septicemic pups.

For bottle feeding, a human infant bottle with a soft nipple is used. Healthy neonates should be bottle fed four times a day. Bottle-fed pups take longer to feed but consume more than tube-fed pups. The stomach distends gradually during bottle feeding, allowing the newborn to eat more. Since they consume more at each feeding, bottle-fed pups require fewer feedings than tube-fed counterparts. Tube feeding is done using a 5 Fr red rubber catheter for neonates under 300 gm and 8 to 10 Fr for larger neonates. Tube feeding should be done only by experienced personnel. Overdistention is easy to do and can result in regurgitation and respiration pneumonia. Improper tube placement into the trachea is easily done in neonates since no gag reflex develops until approximately 10 days of age. Overfeeding is much more likely to occur by tube feeding and it can be particularly harmful to cold puppies when ileus may be present. Tube feeding bypasses the suckle response and tube-fed pups may suckle on the vulvas, prepuces, and extremities of siblings, resulting in a moist dermatitis.

For normal neonates, less than 10% of the body weight is lost within the first 24 hours of life (loss of more than 10% greatly decreases survival rates). Healthy puppies and kittens should start to grow and double their weight by 10 days after their birth. Formula-fed neonates (via bottle or tube) grow at significantly slower rates than healthy siblings despite identical caloric intake. However, after weaning and receiving the same growth diets, normal nursing and formula-fed pups reach identical weights. In general, formula-fed pups should increase their body weight at least 10% each day during the first 3 weeks of life. Daily monitoring of the weight of newborns becomes critical and should be done on a gram scale three times daily.

SUGGESTED READINGS

Fox MW: Developmental physiology and behavior. In Fox MW (ed): *Canine pediatrics: development, neonatal, and congenital diseases*, Springfield, IL, 1966, Charles C Thomas.

Frischke H, Hunt L: Suspected ivermectin toxicity in kittens, *Can Vet J* 32:245, 1991.

Johnson SD, Root-Kustritz MV, Olson PNS: *Canine and feline theriogenology*, Philadelphia, 2001, WB Saunders.

Jones RL: Special considerations for appropriate antibiotic therapy in neonates, *Vet Clin North Am Small Anim Pract* 17:577, 1987.

Linde-Forsberg C: Abnormalities in pregnancy, parturition, and the periparturient period. In Ettinger SJ, Feldman EC (eds): *Textbook of veterinary internal medicine*, ed 7, St Louis, 2010, Saunders/Elsevier.

Miettinen EL, Kliegman RM, Tserng K-Y: Fetal and neonatal responses to extended maternal starvation. I. Circulating fuels and glucose and lactate turnover, *Pediatr Res* 17:634, 1983.

Monson WJ: Orphan rearing of puppies and kittens, *Vet Clin North Am Small Anim Pract* 17:567, 1987.

Mujsce DJ, Towfighi J, Vannucci RC: Physiologic and neuropathologic aspects of hypothermic circulatory arrest in newborn dogs, *Pediatr Res* 28:354, 1990.

Peters EL et al: The development of drug-metabolizing enzymes in young dogs, *Fed Proc Am Soc Biol* 30:560, 1971.

Poffenbarger EM et al: Canine neonatology. Part I. Physiologic differences between puppies and adults, *Compend Contin Educ Pract Vet* 12:1601, 1990.

Roth JA et al: Thymic abnormalities and growth hormone deficiency in dogs, *Am J Vet Res* 41:1256, 1980.

STANDARDS OF CARE IN PEDIATRICS

CHAPTER 7

Diane Heider

Puppies and kittens make up a large part of the private small animal practice. Developing and implementing a pediatric wellness program and standard of care are important aspects of ensuring consistent, comprehensive health care for pediatric patients, as well as promoting a long-term, client-practice bond. One of the best ways to begin this process is to establish a pediatric standard of care that is unique to your practice. A properly developed standard of care ensures that all puppies and kittens receive consistent care during their individual office visits and throughout their long-term pediatric care. According to the *New England Journal of Medicine,* standard of care is defined as a diagnostic or treatment process that a clinician should follow for a certain type of patient, illness, or clinical circumstance.

IMPORTANCE OF STANDARDS OF CARE

Having an established standard of care is an excellent reference for anyone (head technician, receptionist, new graduate, or newly hired yet experienced associate) to determine what should be done in almost any situation in a practice. This chapter focuses on the standards of care for pediatric wellness visits. These standards are not intended to be hard and fast rules but rather guidelines to follow in frequently encountered situations. These guidelines allow veterinarians to establish more consistent patient care and practice better medicine as a result of improved client understanding and compliance.

Consistent patient care will better aid clinicians in making sure every client is receiving similar information. Even clinicians within a practice have different interests and practice styles, which lead to similar cases being treated very differently within the same hospital. A written standard of care would ensure that every client, regardless of which doctor is seen, would be leaving the practice with a predictable set of information and recommendations. This is particularly important in pediatric cases because it gives each subsequent

veterinarian confidence in what information and treatments were given in the prior visits. In the pediatric wellness examinations, an important part of the veterinarian's job is to educate the client. A client who hears the same or similar recommendations from different sources within the hospital is much more likely to comply with those recommendations. For example, one veterinarian in a three-doctor practice may feel that strictly indoor cats do not require feline leukemia virus (FeLV) testing. The second veterinarian may recommend testing only in multiple cat households. The third veterinarian may recommend testing for all cats but leave it up to the client to decide. Inconsistencies create confusion with clients, as well as support staff, and the client is much less likely to follow any of the recommendations given.

A pediatric standard of care allows clinicians to practice better overall medicine. Every private small animal practice experiences busy days, juggling multiple patients simultaneously. With an established set of guidelines and protocols, there is less chance of omitting a FeLV test, failing to recommend a fecal floatation, or forgetting to discuss a particular aspect of behavior and training on those busy days. The pediatric visits are more likely to become a complete health care program, both medically and behaviorally, rather than a series of vaccines and deworming.

ESTABLISHING STANDARDS OF CARE AND PROTOCOLS

The most important aspect of establishing a standard of care is that it must be in written form. If it is not written, it does not exist. Everything must be documented within a medical chart, from recommendations (both accepted and declined) and treatments to telephone conversations with clients; thus a hospital must have written standards of care.

The first step is to schedule a doctor's meeting. Having the meeting outside of the hospital may be a good way to avoid distractions and interruptions. This is a team effort in which all doctors within the practice should contribute to create the pediatric standard of care. If everyone is able to contribute to the plan rather than having it dictated, there will be better success in following the plan that has been created. During the initial meeting, a list of areas that need standards to be developed can be generated and agreed on. The American Animal Hospital Association (AAHA), American Association of Feline Practitioners (AAFP), and Veterinary Information Network (VIN) are good resources for guidelines and can easily be tailored to fit a practice style.

Training the support staff on the newly created plan is a crucial part of the process. Each member of the staff needs to adhere to the plan to make sure the desired message is being delivered to the client at any point in their visit to your practice. Whether it is the receptionist, the veterinary assistant, or the technician delivering the message, the information given to the client should be the same. Regular staff meetings can be used to educate staff on the standards and to review and reinforce the protocols and standards of care. A list should be generated of the top 25 to 50 most frequently asked questions that are fielded by the receptionists and technicians, and the written answers to these questions can serve as a source or script for those staff members. Written protocols and standards of care guidelines aid in standardizing and enhancing the training of new staff members. A test bank of different topics from the pediatric wellness visits (or any other aspect of a practice) can be created, and staff members can be periodically tested on the information. For example, how often are vaccinations given, what are the available canine vs. feline vaccinations, or what are the common internal and external parasites of puppies and kittens? Once these tests are completed and scored, many practices will reward successful staff members. Rewards could be gift certificates, staff parties, or pay raises.

THE FIRST PEDIATRIC VISIT

The first pediatric visit generally occurs between 6 to 8 weeks of age. An adequate amount of time should be established for the first pediatric wellness visit. Creating 30- to 40-minute office visits allows doctors and technicians ample time to address all topics identified in the plan, as well as answer any questions the client may have. Some may contend that this amount of time is too much for a busy practice; however, if it ensures that the puppy is well socialized and trained, then the time will be recouped in future visits (instead of having to muzzle or deal with an unruly patient). Generally, there is too much information for the average client to digest on the first visit, especially if this is their first pet. It is recommended that information be divided into smaller sections to be discussed at each of the scheduled pediatric visits, so the client does not become overwhelmed. The pediatric visits are an opportunity to educate the clients, to make sure they understand the plan of care and recommendations, and to make sure their new puppy or kitten is going to be a good fit for their family and lifestyle.

BOX 7-1 **Suggested pediatric topics of discussion**

Supplies needed
Puppy/kitten-proofing your home
Introducing new puppy/kitten to other pets and family members
Socialization
Housetraining/litterbox training
Pet identification
Zoonoses
Parasite control
Infectious disease and vaccination
Vaccine reactions
Heartworm disease
Barking/vocalization
Biting
Chewing/digging/destructive behavior
Nail care and scratching posts
Inappropriate scratching
Training
Exercise
Nutrition
Body condition score
Spay/neuter
Declawing/tendonectomy
Pet insurance
Microchip
Grooming
Groomers/kennels
Dental care
Ear care
Emergencies

A written handout should be created for the initial and subsequent visits. There are typically 3 to 4 pediatric visits between the ages of 6 to 20 weeks (corresponding with vaccination dates), depending on the age of the pet when it is first seen. Each visit and handout should cover different selected topics. A list of suggested topics can be found in Box 7-1. Since there is a large volume of information to be given to the new puppy or kitten owner and the average client remembers about 25% of what they hear, alternative learning aids are helpful. Systematically transferring information into smaller, easier-to-digest sections in a written format for the client to take home is a significant tool in client education.

Specific website and book recommendations should be established as a source of additional information for clients. Rather than simply suggesting books or the Internet in general, find specific sites and titles that mesh with the practice's style and philosophy and supply clients with a list of those sources.

Risk Assessment

The office visit should begin with a history, followed by the physical examination and any treatments deemed necessary. The client should complete a pediatric history and a Risk

Factor Evaluation, which is an excellent method of determining the type of environment from which the new puppy or kitten came and the environment and lifestyle that it is now entering (Figures 7-1 and 7-2). Based on this information, appropriate testing, vaccination, deworming, and other parasite control recommendations can be made.

Physical Examination

After risk assessment, a complete physical examination is performed and should be emphasized not only at the first pediatric visit but also each time the pet enters the hospital. Over the years, veterinarians have excelled at promoting annual vaccinations, and as a result, clients perceive vaccination as the most important reason for their annual visit. Clients should understand that vaccinations are medical procedures that should be individualized based on history, physical examination, risk, and lifestyle of the individual animal. Placing emphasis on the physical examination at the first visit helps ensure that clients will return in the future for annual check-ups and recommended vaccinations, as opposed to returning simply for "yearly shots."

Based on the information obtained from the risk assessment, physical examination, and the geographic location, the clinician can determine the appropriate vaccinations and anthelmintics and at what interval they will be administered and assess the need for any other internal or external parasite control (e.g., heartworms, fleas, or ticks).

Vaccination and Deworming

Vaccination and internal and external parasite control protocols will all vary within a given geographic region (see Chapters 14 and 19). Using the regional incidence of disease, as well as AAHA canine vaccination guidelines, AAFP feline vaccination guidelines, and Companion Animal Parasite Control (CAPC) guidelines, appropriate standards and protocols can be established to suit the practice.

For both dogs and cats, vaccinations are generally divided into core, noncore, and not recommended categories. Core vaccines are recommended for all animals. Noncore vaccines should be administered to animals only in specific risk categories. Generally, vaccines not recommended are those that do not induce a clinically meaningful immune response or

---

Kitten History and Risk Assessment

Patient number_____

Client name _____ Pet name_____ Gender_____

Date of birth _____

1. Is this your first kitten? _____

2. Do you have other pets?_____ Are they indoors or outdoors?_____

3. Where did you acquire your kitten?_____

4. Has your kitten been tested for Feline Leukemia?_____ If so, what were the results?_____

5. Has your kitten been vaccinated?_____ If so, for what diseases, and when?_____

_____

6. Has your kitten been dewormed?_____ What product was used?_____

   When? _____

7. What are you feeding your kitten?_____

8. Is your kitten eating and drinking normally? _____

9. Has your kitten had any vomiting or diarrhea?_____

10. Has your kitten had any coughing, sneezing, runny eyes, or runny nose?_____

11. Have you seen any itching, scratching, fleas, or hair loss?_____

12. Is your kitten using the litterbox? _____

13. Will your kitten be an indoor or outdoor cat?_____

14. Will your kitten be around other cats?_____

15. Do you plan to spay/neuter or declaw your kitten?_____

Figure 7-1 Kitten history and risk assessment form.

Puppy History and Risk Assessment

Patient number _____

Client name _____ Pet name _____ Gender_____

Date of birth _____

1. Is this your first puppy? _____

2. Do you have other pets?_____ Are they indoors or outdoors?_____

3. Where did you acquire your puppy? _____

4. Has your puppy been vaccinated? _____ If so, for what diseases, and when? _____

_____

5. Has your puppy been dewormed? _____What product was used? _____

　　 When?_____

6. What are you feeding your puppy? _____

7. Is your puppy eating and drinking well?_____

8. Has your puppy had any vomiting or diarrhea? _____

9. Have you seen any itching, scratching, fleas, or hair loss? _____

10. Are you having success with potty training? _____

11. Will you be taking your puppy to dog shows? _____ Using for hunting or field trials?_____

12. Will your puppy be going to the groomers? _____

13. Will your puppy be in a fenced yard? _____ On acreage? _____

14. Will your puppy go on vacations with you? _____ Be boarded at a kennel? _____

15. Will your puppy be taken on walks?_____ Go to the park?_____

16. Do you plan to spay/neuter your puppy? _____

17. Are you planning on breeding your puppy? _____

Figure 7-2 Puppy history and risk assessment form.

have been associated with an adverse event, resulting in the risk outweighing the benefit. A list of these vaccines can be seen in Table 7-1. The initial core vaccination series is begun at the first visit, with boosters given at 3 to 4 week intervals. For example, the core puppy vaccinations (distemper-adenovirus type 2, parvovirus [DA$_2$P]) may be given at 8, 12, and 16 weeks, and core kitten vaccinations (feline viral rhinotracheitis, calicivirus, panleukopenia [FVRCP]) given at 9 and 13 weeks. State requirements may vary, so rabies vaccines may be given at the final pediatric visit or at the time of the ovariohysterectomy or castration.

Intestinal parasites common to puppies and kittens are acquired via transplacental, transmammary, or environmental routes. A list of the most common pediatric intestinal parasites and their treatments can be found in Chapter 19. Puppies and kittens should be treated early and often to prevent patent infections and potential zoonotic concerns. Generally, deworming should take place at 2, 4, 6, and 8

weeks of age. CAPC guidelines are as follows: "Puppies and kittens require more frequent anthelmintic administration than adult dogs and cats, because (1) they often are serially reinfected via nursing and from the environment, and (2) they often harbor parasite larvae in migration that later mature and commence laying eggs. Intestinal parasite infections in puppies and kittens may cause serious illness or even death before a diagnosis is possible by fecal examination. Puppies and their mothers should be treated with appropriate anthelmintics when puppies are 2, 4, 6, and 8 weeks of age, then put on a monthly preventive. Because prenatal infection does not occur in kittens, biweekly treatment can begin at 3 weeks of age, and they can be put on a monthly preventive at 8 or 9 weeks of age. Nursing bitches and queens should be treated concurrently with their offspring since they often develop patent infections along with their young."

Because geographic, seasonal, and lifestyle factors substantially affect parasite prevalence, veterinarians should

TABLE 7-1	Vaccinations
Feline Vaccinations	
Core	Panleukopenia
	Feline viral rhinotracheitis (FHV-1)
	Calicivirus
	Rabies
Noncore	Feline leukemia virus (FeLV)
	Feline immunodeficiency virus (FIV)
	Chlamydia psittaci
	Bordetella bronchiseptica
Not recommended	Feline infectious peritonitis (FIP)
	Giardia lamblia
Canine Vaccinations	
Core	Distemper
	Parvovirus
	Adenovirus
	Rabies
Noncore	Parainfluenza
	Bordetella bronchiseptica
	Lyme borreliosis
	Leptospirosis
	Leptospira canicola
	L. icterohaemorrhagiae
	L. pomona
	L. grippotyphosa
	Distemper-measles
Not recommended	Coronavirus
	Giardia lamblia
	Adenovirus-1

tailor prevention programs to fit the needs of individual patients. More complete recommendations can be found in the CAPC guidelines at www.capcvet.org.

Topics of Discussion

Once risk assessment is completed, physical examination is performed, and vaccinations and anthelmintics administered, the educational portion of the visit can be continued.

Using the handout that was created for the first pediatric visit as a guideline, the client can be guided through each topic selected for discussion (see Box 7-1). Many topics have multiple visual aids and informational materials available from distributors and drug companies for clients to see and take home in an effort to emphasize and reinforce the information you are providing. For example, both Hill's and Purina provide Body Condition Score charts for use when discussing nutrition and healthy body weight. CAPC provides many charts and diagrams illustrating parasite life cycles and life stages when discussing parasite control and zoonoses. Clinicians can use anatomical models when discussing breed-related dental or orthopedic concerns pets may encounter. People learn and process information in many different ways, so using all of the tools available to enhance the client's learning experience is recommended.

SUBSEQUENT PEDIATRIC VISITS

The remaining 2 to 3 pediatric visits take place at 3 to 4 week intervals after the first visit. These visits consist of making note of any lifestyle changes for the pet (i.e., the strictly indoor kitten becoming an indoor/outdoor cat), the physical examination, recommended vaccinations and anthelmintics, and discussion of the next set of topics as outlined in the already established client handouts. The veterinarian has an opportunity to evaluate how housetraining and behavior issues are progressing and address any questions or concerns the client may have encountered in the past few weeks. At the conclusion of each visit, the pediatric agenda should be updated, and an appointment scheduled for the next visit.

SUGGESTED READINGS

Companion Animal Parasite Control (CAPC) Guidelines: at www.capcvet.org.

Hoskins JD: *Veterinary pediatrics: dogs and cats from birth to six months,* ed 3, Philadelphia, 2001, WB Saunders.

Hoskins JD, Whitford R: *First choice medical protocols,* Lakewood, CO, 2001, American Animal Hospital Association.

NUTRITIONAL REQUIREMENTS AND FEEDING OF GROWING PUPPIES AND KITTENS

CHAPTER 8

Heather Prendergast

Nutrition during the first year of life can greatly influence the longevity and health of puppies and kittens. Inadequate protein and energy intake can decrease growth rate, inhibit neural myelination and neurotransmission, decrease brain growth, and inhibit cognitive function. Many neonatal deaths result from inadequate nutritional intake or the inability of the neonate to adequately digest and absorb nutrients as a result of the immature digestive system. At birth, the gastrointestinal (GI) tract must transition from processing amniotic fluid to digesting milk. The release of hormones and digestive enzymes and the activation of secretion, motility, and absorption are adaptations that begin shortly after birth. These changes are critical to allow the GI tract to perform required functions.

NEONATE DIGESTION

The intestinal mass of puppies increases in the first 24 hours. Pancreatic lipase production increases over the first 3 weeks as the amount of milk fat increases. The increase in lipase production increases the thickness of the GI wall and facilitates the passage of solids. Intestinal growth is decreased if milk replacer is fed in place of colostrum, possibly caused by missing hormones, fat, or other colostral components.

Neonates have decreased pancreatic digestive enzymes, which permits intestinal absorption of immunoglobulins from the colostrum. The neonatal pancreas does not begin to produce amylase until after 21 days of age. However, canine milk contains the digestive enzyme amylase, which helps digest milk sugars in the neonatal GI tract. Digestive enzymes are produced in response to consumption of solid food. Therefore consuming solid food is important to facilitate the development of normal GI tract function in the young dog and cat.

GI motility, relative to older puppies and kittens, is reduced in neonates less than 30 days old. This must be taken into consideration when a neonate requires supplemental feeding either by bottle or orogastric tube. Therefore small amounts should be fed frequently to decrease the possibility of regurgitation and aspiration.

MILK CONTENTS

Milk consists of lipids, sugars, minerals, and minor constituents. For the first 24 hours after parturition, "immature milk" is produced, which slowly matures over the next week. The immature milk, or colostrum, is rich in proteins, immunoglobulins, energy, nutrients, and growth factors that stimulate GI tract development. The energy in colostrum is 95% digestible. Species with a small body size, such as dogs and cats, produce milk higher in energy density to compensate for small gastric capacity. Puppies and kittens that do not receive colostrum are more susceptible to infection until about 35 days of age. Levels of calcium, phosphorus, and magnesium are initially high for 2 to 3 days and then decrease as the milk matures.

A healthy mother who is well-nourished should be able to provide complete nutrition for a puppy or kitten for their first 4 weeks. A healthy puppy or kitten will nurse vigorously several times a day and gain weight on a daily basis. A malnourished puppy or kitten will fail to gain weight, constantly cry, and become inactive (see Chapter 11). More neonates die from improper husbandry and nutrition than disease. Birth weight is the single most important predictor of neonate survival. Average birth weight for toy, medium, large, and giant breed dogs can be found in Box 8-1.

MILK REPLACER REQUIREMENTS

Formulated puppy and kitten milk replacer is available commercially. Both powder and liquid forms are available. Powdered formula lasts longer, since the unused powder can be

BOX 8-1   **Average birth weight for dogs**

Toy breeds: 100-200 gm
Medium breeds: 250-350 gm
Large breeds: 400-500 gm
Giant breeds: 700 gm

BOX 8-2   **Emergency milk replacer formula**

4 oz whole cow's milk
4 oz water
2 egg yolks
1 tsp vegetable oil
500 mg of calcium carbonate (Tums)
   This formula is approximately 1.2 kcal/ml. A 0.45 kg puppy would receive approximately 60 ml/day, divided over 8 feedings.

frozen for 6 months. Once powdered formula has been reconstituted, contents should be used within 48 hours, provided the unused portion is refrigerated in a glass container. Liquid milk replacer should be used within 48 hours once the can is opened, provided the unused portion is refrigerated. Formulated milk replacer is superior to homemade versions because commercial products generally provide the correct balance of protein, fat, carbohydrates, vitamins, and minerals needed for growing neonates. Ingredients and caloric density of the puppy milk replacer can vary with manufacturer. The label recommendations should be for the product being administered.

Milk replacer is made from bovine milk and is lower in protein, calories, fat, calcium, phosphorus, and carbohydrates. This may explain the decreased growth rate of orphan puppies and kittens, even though the caloric intake may be equivalent. Bovine milk is higher in lactose than either canine or feline milk, which can cause diarrhea in puppies and kittens fed milk replacer. It is advised to dilute milk replacer 25% to 50% with water or a balanced electrolyte solution for the first 2 days of feeding to minimize the occurrence of diarrhea.

If commercial milk replacer is temporarily unavailable, an emergency formula may be used (Box 8-2). This emergency formula is strictly for emergencies and should be replaced with a commercial milk formula as soon as possible.

TRANSITIONAL DIET

By the time the neonate is 3 to 4 weeks old, dry food can be mixed with water and/or formula in a 1 : 3 ratio to form a gruel. If canned food is preferred, a 2 : 1 ratio can be made. Pediatric patients receive hydration from the milk or the milk replacer, but water intake will increase once offered. Drinking water should be offered at 5 weeks. By 6 weeks of age, 50% of the pediatric patient's diet should be from unmixed puppy or kitten food. Puppies and kittens can be totally weaned from the dams' milk at approximately 6 to 8 weeks. Early weaning (defined as completely removed from their mother) is discouraged, since it can lead to malnutrition, stress-related diseases, diminished social skills, and behavioral problems. However, nutritional weaning can start as early as $4\frac{1}{2}$ weeks of age. The advantages of this earlier nutritional weaning in the opinion of some are preventing debilitation of the dam nursing a large litter and allowing the transitioning process of the GI tract to solid food while still under the protection of colostral antibodies. From the time of weaning until 6 months old (9 months in large-breed dogs), it is advised to feed juveniles three times a day and more frequently for smaller and toy breeds. Thereafter dogs and cats should be fed twice daily on a regular schedule.

AMERICAN FEED CONTROL OFFICIALS

The Association of American Feed Control Officials (AAFCO) was established in response to the increasing number of pet food diets available on the market, some of which did not meet the specific nutritional needs of animals. The AAFCO is made up of a variety of individuals and is not regulated or managed by any pet food manufacturer. Any foods that are recommended by veterinarians should meet the expectations and testing of AAFCO. A label that reads "complete and balanced" must either meet a nutrient profile or pass a feeding trial. To be classified as "safe," the food must meet all nutrient minimum and maximum ranges that have been established by the AAFCO as being safe.

To compare diets, food must be looked at on a "dry matter (DM) basis." The AAFCO's definition of DM basis is the level of nutrients contained in a food. A "guaranteed analysis," or "as fed basis," must be converted to DM to effectively compare diets. For example, a canned diet contains approximately 75% moisture, whereas a dry diet contains approximately 10% moisture. To effectively compare the two products, the moisture content must be removed. Ingredients are listed on the label by weight and can include moisture. Therefore some products may list chicken as their main ingredient, but it may only weigh more than the corn or wheat products that follow because of its moisture content.

The most commonly used unit of measurement is the kilocalorie (kcal), defined as the amount of heat necessary to raise the temperature of 1 kilogram (kg) of water by 1 degree Celsius. Calories are used to maintain physical activity, digestion, growth, and basal metabolism. Most foods are recommended in kilocalorie/8 oz cup of dry food or kilocalorie/can. Puppies and kittens require a larger amount of energy early in life, which decreases as they age. It is important to follow the feeding recommendations established by the pet food manufacturer, since diets vary by company, as well as within a specific product line. The AAFCO nutrient requirements for puppies and kittens are listed in Tables 8-1 and 8-2, respectively.

TABLE 8-1	AAFCO dog food nutrient profiles*			
Nutrient	**Units DM basis**	**Growth and reproduction minimum**	**Adult maintenance minimum**	**Maximum**
Protein	%	22.0	18.0	–
Arginine	%	0.62	0.51	–
Histidine	%	0.22	0.18	–
Isoleucine	%	0.45	0.37	–
Leucine	%	0.72	0.59	–
Lysine	%	0.77	0.63	–
Methionine-cystine	%	0.53	0.43	–
Phenylalanine-tyrosine	%	0.89	0.73	–
Threonine	%	0.58	0.48	–
Tryptophan	%	0.20	0.16	–
Valine	%	0.48	0.39	–
Fat[†]	%	8	5	–
Linoleic acid	%	1.0	1.0	
Minerals				
Calcium (Ca)	%	1.0	0.6	2.5
Phosphorus (P)	%	0.8	0.5	1.6
Ca:P ratio		1:1	1:1	2:1
Potassium	%	0.6	0.6	–
Sodium	%	0.3	0.06	–
Chloride	%	0.45	0.09	–
Magnesium	%	0.04	0.04	0.3
Iron[‡]	mg/kg	80	80	3000
Copper[§]	mg/kg	7.3	7.3	250
Manganese	mg/kg	5.0	5.0	–
Zinc	mg/kg	120	120	1000
Iodine	mg/kg	1.5	1.5	50
Selenium	mg/kg	0.11	0.11	2.0
Vitamins				
Vitamin A	IU/kg	5000	5000	250,000.0
Vitamin D	IU/kg	500	500	5000
Vitamin E	IU/kg	50	50	1000
Thiamine[¶]	mg/kg	1.0	1.0	–
Riboflavin	mg/kg	2.2	2.2	–
Pantothenic acid	mg/kg	10	10	–
Niacin	mg/kg	11.4	11.4	–
Pyridoxine	mg/kg	1.0	1.0	–
Folic acid	mg/kg	0.18	0.18	–
Vitamin B_{12}	mg/kg	0.022	0.022	–
Choline	mg/kg	1200	1200	–

From Association of American Feed Control Officials (AAFCO).

DM, Dry matter.

*Presumes an energy density of 3.5 kcal ME/gm DM, based on the "modified Atwater" values of 3.5, 8.5, and 3.5 kcal/gm for protein, fat, and carbohydrate (nitrogen-free extract [NFE]), respectively. Rations greater than 4.0 kcal/gm should be corrected for energy density. Rations less than 3.5 kcal/gm should not be corrected for energy.

[†]Although a true requirement for fat per se has not been established, the minimum level was based on recognition of fat as a source of essential fatty acids, as a carrier of fat-soluble vitamins, to enhance palatability, and to supply an adequate caloric density.

[‡]Because of very poor bioavailability, iron from carbonate or oxide sources that are added to the diet should not be considered as components in meeting the minimum nutrient level.

[§]Because of very poor bioavailability, copper from oxide sources that are added to the diet should not be considered as components in meeting the minimum nutrient level.

[¶]Because processing may destroy up to 90% of the thiamine in the diet, allowance in formulation should be made to ensure the minimum nutrient level is met after processing.

TABLE 8-2 **AAFCO cat food nutrient profiles***

Nutrient	Units DM basis	Growth and reproduction minimum	Adult maintenance minimum	Maximum
Protein	%	30	26	–
Arginine	%	1.25	1.04	–
Histidine	%	0.31	0.31	–
Isoleucine	%	0.52	0.52	–
Leucine	%	1.25	1.25	–
Lysine	%	1.20	0.83	–
Methionine-cystine	%	1.10	1.10	–
Methionine	%	0.62	0.62	1.50
Phenylalanine-tyrosine	%	0.88	0.88	–
Phenylalanine	%	0.42	0.42	–
Threonine	%	0.73	0.73	–
Tryptophan	%	0.25	0.16	–
Valine	%	0.62	0.62	–
Fat[†]	%	9	9	–
Linoleic acid	%	0.5	0.5	–
Arachidonic acid	%	0.02	0.02	–
Minerals				
Calcium	%	1.0	0.6	–
Phosphorus	%	0.8	0.5	–
Potassium	%	0.6	0.6	–
Sodium	%	0.2	0.2	–
Chloride	%	0.3	0.3	–
Magnesium[‡]	%	0.08	0.04	–
Iron[§]	mg/kg	80	80	–
Copper (extruded)[¶]	mg/kg	15	5	–
Copper (canned)[¶]	mg/kg	5	5	–
Manganese	mg/kg	7.5	7.5	–
Zinc	mg/kg	75	75	2000
Iodine	mg/kg	0.35	0.35	–
Selenium	mg/kg	0.1	0.1	–
Vitamins				
Vitamin A	IU/kg	9000	5000	750,000
Vitamin D	IU/kg	750	500	10,000
Vitamin E[¶]	IU/kg	30	30	–
Vitamin K**	mg/kg	0.1	0.1	–
Thiamine[††]	mg/kg	5	5	–
Riboflavin	mg/kg	4	4	–
Pantothenic acid	mg/kg	5	5	–
Niacin	mg/kg	60	60	–
Pyridoxine	mg/kg	4	4	–
Folic acid	mg/kg	0.8	0.8	–
Biotin[‡‡]	mg/kg	0.07	0.07	–
Vitamin B12	mg/kg	0.02	0.02	–
Choline[§§]	mg/kg	2400	2400	–
Taurine (extruded)	%	0.10	0.10	–
Taurine (canned)	%	0.20	0.20	–

From Association of American Feed Control Officials (AAFCO).

DM, Dry matter.

*Presumes an energy density of 4.0 kcal/gm ME, based on the "modified Atwater" values of 3.5, 8.5, and 3.5 kcal/g for protein, fat, and carbohydrate (nitrogen-free extract [NFE]), respectively. Rations greater than 4.5 kcal/gm should be corrected for energy density; rations less than 4.0 kcal/gm should *not* be corrected for energy.

[†]Although a true requirement for fat per se has not been established, the minimum level was based on recognition of fat as a source of essential fatty acids, as a carrier of fat-soluble vitamins, to enhance palatability, and to supply an adequate caloric density.

[‡]If the mean urine pH of cats fed ad libitum is not below 6.4, the risk of struvite urolithiasis increases as the magnesium content of the diet increases.

[§]Because of very poor bioavailability, iron from carbonate or oxide sources that are added to the diet should not be considered as components in meeting the minimum nutrient level.

[¶]Because of very poor bioavailability, copper from oxide sources that is added to the diet should not be considered as components in meeting the minimum nutrient level.

[¶]Add 10 IU vitamin E above minimum level per gram of fish oil per kilogram of diet.

**Vitamin K does not need to be added unless diet contains greater than 25% fish on a DM basis.

[††]Because processing may destroy up to 90% of the thiamine in the diet, allowance in formulation should be made to ensure the minimum nutrient level is met after processing.

[‡‡]Biotin does not need to be added unless diet contains antimicrobial or antivitamin compounds.

[§§]Methionine may be substituted for choline as methyl donor at a rate of 3.75 parts for 1 part choline by weight when methionine exceeds 0.62%.

SPECIFIC NUTRIENTS

Nutrients are required for basic bodily function, including acting as structural components, enhancing chemical reactions, transporting substances throughout the body, maintaining temperature, and providing energy. Nutrients are divided into six categories as shown in Box 8-3.

As diseases associated with nutrient deficiencies became more prominent, minimum level requirements were established for protein, fat, carbohydrate, and essential amino acids. Maximum level requirements were established for calcium, phosphorus, magnesium, fat, water-soluble vitamins, and trace minerals to prevent nutrient excess. Nutritional excess has become a larger problem than nutrient deficiencies with pet foods currently available. Maximum levels for methionine and zinc, as well as vitamins A and D, have been established for adult cat foods, reflecting current studies available on the toxic effect of these nutrients. Taurine levels have been established for both canned and dry cat food because the bioavailability of taurine in canned food is decreased.

Homemade diets are generally incomplete and therefore not recommended. When preparing meals at home, owners may omit ingredients because of expense or inability to find a product or may substitute an ingredient as the result of the owner's personal preference. Many homemade canine diets contain excessive protein but may be deficient in calories, calcium, vitamins, and microminerals. Often, homemade diets have an inverse calcium to phosphorus ratio. Home-prepared

---

BOX 8-3   **Nutrient categories and functions**

Water
Water is the most important nutrient and has several functions. It helps regulate temperature, provides shape and resilience to the body, enhances chemical reactions, and transports substances through the body.

Carbohydrates
Carbohydrates include sugars, starches, and fiber and function primarily to provide energy.

Protein
Protein is composed of various amino acids and provides energy. Protein is the principal structural component of body tissues and organs.

Fat
Fats supply energy and essential fatty acids that the body cannot produce.

Minerals
Minerals comprise all inorganic elements in food. Minerals play a large role in enzyme and hormone systems.

Vitamins
Both water-soluble and fat-soluble vitamins are co-factors in enzyme reactions and play a role in DNA synthesis.

---

feline diets tend to be deficient in fat, energy, and micronutrients. Uncooked recipes (e.g., raw diets) contain high levels of pathogenic bacteria that not only pose harm to the pet receiving the diet but also to the owner preparing the meal as well.

All commercial foods must be categorized as either growth and lactation or maintenance. Foods labeled "For all life stages" must meet the most stringent requirements for both categories. For the purpose of this chapter, foods recommended should fall into the growth and lactation category. Canine growth and lactation nutrient requirements have higher levels of zinc, iron, and fat and decreased levels of calcium, phosphorus, and sodium.

Omega-3 and omega-6 fatty acids are important for development. Decreased levels of docosahexaenoic acid (DHA) can lead to abnormal neurodevelopment, as well as decreased visceral and psychomotor development. Researchers have found that fatty acids improve the trainability of puppies, which suggests a beneficial effect on neurodevelopment. Omega-3 fatty acids can come from a variety of sources, including flaxseed oil and fish meal. Flaxseed oil has an abundant amount of alpha-linoleic acid (ALA) but little DHA. Cold water fish contain DHA and eicosapentaenoic acid (EPA), which is more beneficial to the puppy or kitten.

DIETARY EXCESSES

Choosing the correct diet for a puppy or kitten requires evaluation of the breed, age, activity level, and environmental conditions. Some breeds are less active than others, and a house-bound dog will likely use less energy than a farm dog. Many breeds are predisposed to obesity. Fat has a higher caloric density than protein or carbohydrates. Excess dietary fat may be a primary contributor to excess energy intake. Extra energy is stored as fat once the maximum growth rate has been achieved. Puppies and kittens that develop a large number of adipose cells during growth may also be predisposed to obesity as adults. Clients should be educated in how to prevent obesity by body-condition scoring their pets, which minimizes the number of diseases related to obesity the pet will face in its senior years.

Excess dietary energy and caloric intake may support a growth rate that is too fast for appropriate skeletal development and result in a higher incidence of skeletal abnormalities. Large breed puppies require fewer calories per unit of body weight and mature more slowly than small breed puppies. Rapid growth occurs in the first few months in all breeds but occurs over a longer period of time in large breeds. Large breed dogs need diets that support a slower growth rate to help decrease skeletal abnormalities. It is important to take into consideration the age, breed, gender, body condition, genetics, and environmental components when designing an adequate nutritional program that decreases the risk of developing skeletal disease.

Excess protein is also detrimental to large breed puppies. However, decreased protein will also affect the skeletal system. Therefore a diet should contain >25% protein in dry matter. Excess calcium affects the skeletal system by increasing the severity of osteochondrosis. The absolute value of calcium appears to be more significant than the calcium to phosphorus ratio. Subsequently, it is contraindicated to supplement large breed puppies with calcium when they are fed a complete and balanced commercial diet. The AAFCO has demonstrated the safety and efficacy of a 1.1% calcium DM diet for large breed puppies.

A proper balance of vitamins A, C, and D and trace minerals (e.g., copper and zinc) is very important to skeletal development. Vitamin D metabolites regulate the uptake of calcium and phosphorus from the GI tract. Commercial diets contain between 2 to 10 times the amount of AAFCO-recommended vitamin D, therefore supplementation is absolutely discouraged. Studies evaluating excess amounts of vitamin A and C, copper, and zinc in the diet and the relationship to skeletal abnormalities are lacking. Specific diseases resulting from nutritional excess or deficiency can be found in Chapter 44.

CONTROLLING INTAKE

Feeding methods can help control excess nutrient intake. Methods of feeding include free-choice feeding, time-restricted feeding, and food-restricted feeding. Free-choice feeding allows the pet to eat ad libitum, thereby increasing the risk for excess nutrient intake. Time-restricted feeding allows the owner to feed 2 to 3 times per day for a set period of time, which may encourage the pet to eat ravenously, past the normal satiety mechanism. Food-restricted feedings allow the owner to control caloric intake and maintain optimum growth rate and body condition. Determining a daily energy requirement (DER) allows the owner to feed the correct amount of food, which can be changed as the puppy increases in size and age. The formula for calculating the DER can be found in Box 8-4.

The body condition should be evaluated every 2 weeks. Food can be adjusted as needed to decrease excess fat, which will decrease the growth rate. Puppies and kittens should be scored on a 9-point body-condition scale (Figures 8-1 and 8-2). The ideal body condition is an hourglass shape when viewed from above, with a definitive waist behind the ribs.

Environment, genetics, and nutrient composition play key roles in skeletal development. We can minimize the

---

BOX 8-4	**Calculating daily energy requirement (DER)**

DER can be calculated by multiplying the appropriate growth factor and the resting energy requirement (RER). RER is calculated by the following formula:

RER (kcal/day) = 30 (weight in kg) + 70.

Appropriate Growth Factor	**Calculated DER**
Weaning to 16 weeks	DER = 3 × RER
16 weeks to 1 year	DER = 2 × RER
1 year	DER = 1.6 × RER

---

effects of skeletal disease in large breed puppies by regulating nutrient and caloric intake. The goal is to regulate growth rate not maximize it. Feeding an AAFCO-approved commercial diet is recommended to help achieve this goal.

EXPECTED WEIGHT GAIN

Neonates that die after 48 hours old have most likely succumbed from starvation rather than infectious disease. Inadequate nutrition leads to dehydration and muscular weakness. In general, growing puppies need twice as much energy as adults for growth, activity, and body maintenance. Low birth weight produces poor performance, increases morbidity and mortality, and can be caused by congenital cardiac and pulmonary defects. Newborns that are less than 25% of the average birth weight are at a higher risk of developing hypoglycemia, hypothermia, and pneumonia. Hypothermia decreases GI motility, further slowing the digestion of nutrients. Body weight should be monitored daily to ensure normal weight gain. Neonates not gaining weight require supplementation. Additional information pertaining to monitoring neonatal growth can be found in Chapter 5.

The required caloric intake for puppies changes weekly and should be adjusted with weight gain (see Box 8-4). An approximate feeding guide of volume to feed based on neonatal weight per day is also summarized in Box 8-4. The total daily feeding for orphan puppies should be divided into eight feedings per day the first week of life, then decreased to five feedings per day thereafter. Smaller and toy breeds require more frequent feedings to prevent hypoglycemia. The frequency of feedings can slowly be decreased as the amount being fed increases. Puppies should gain 5% to 10% each day or 2 gm/kg of their expected adult weight. For example, a 13.5 kg adult should gain 30 to 60 gm/day during the first 5 months.

If one puppy is not gaining weight while the rest of the litter is, a physical examination should be performed. Providing the underfed puppy time alone with the mother may be beneficial. The litter may be pulled away from the mother for 5 to 10 minutes, 3 or 4 times a day to give the underweight neonate an opportunity to increase milk intake. Successful hand rearing of orphans can depend on several factors, including appropriate feeding schedule, selection of milk replacer, meeting caloric needs of the neonate, and proper feeding methods.

Orphan newborns should be fed every 3 hours for the first week. Once the neonate has doubled its birth weight, feeding can be decreased to 4-hour intervals. Doubling of birth weight can take up to 14 days for a puppy receiving milk replacer (see Chapter 9).

Kittens require the most energy (20 kcal/100 gm/day) their first 2 weeks of life. The normal birth weight of healthy kittens is between 90 to 110 gm. Kittens should gain 10 to 15 gm/day, and double their birth weight by day 10. Thereafter kittens should gain an average of 0.45 kg/month of age until 4 months. Formula-fed kittens grow slower, only being able to double their body weight at 14 days, regardless of

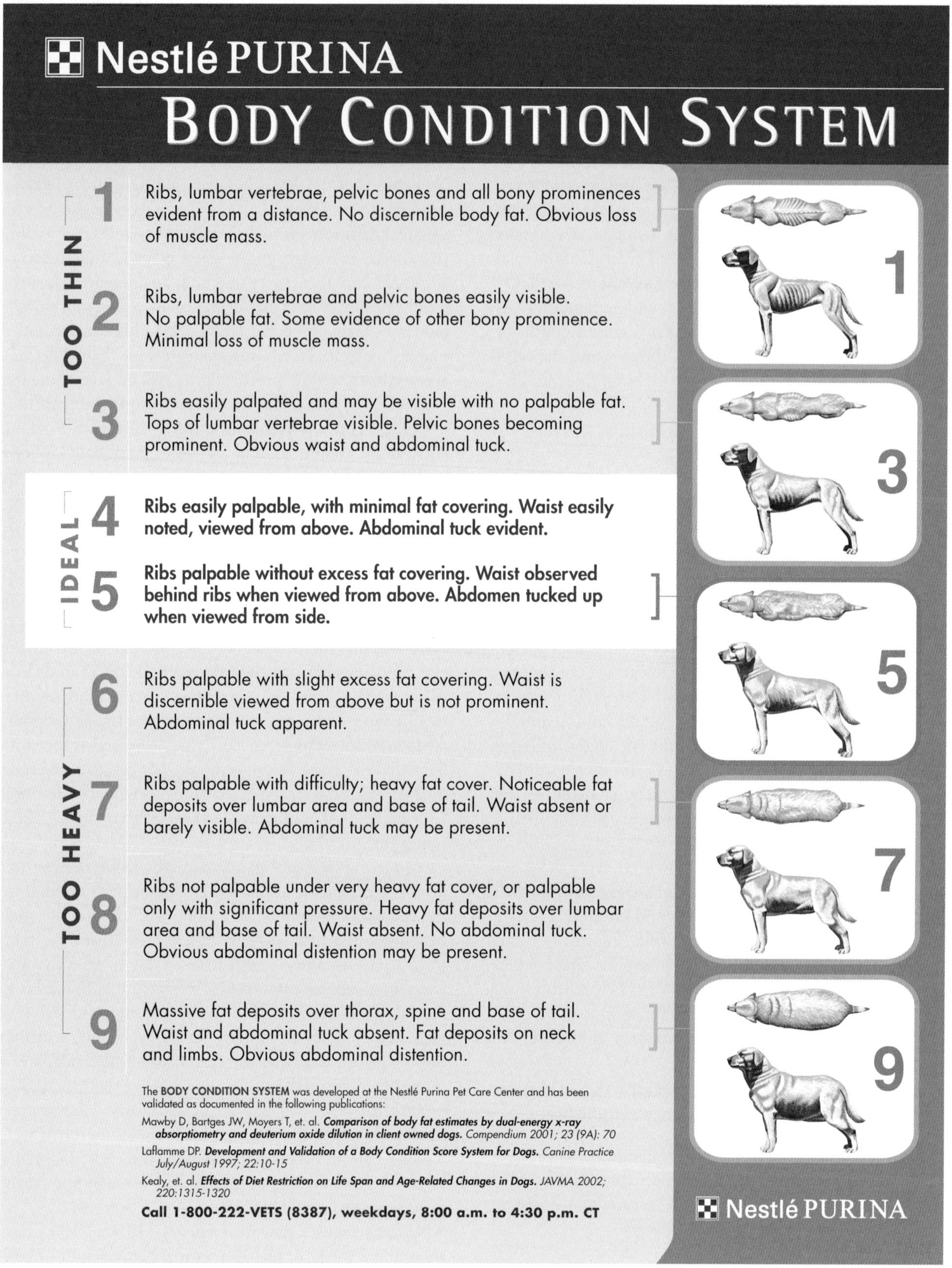

Nestlé PURINA

BODY CONDITION SYSTEM

TOO THIN

1 Ribs, lumbar vertebrae, pelvic bones and all bony prominences evident from a distance. No discernible body fat. Obvious loss of muscle mass.

2 Ribs, lumbar vertebrae and pelvic bones easily visible. No palpable fat. Some evidence of other bony prominence. Minimal loss of muscle mass.

3 Ribs easily palpated and may be visible with no palpable fat. Tops of lumbar vertebrae visible. Pelvic bones becoming prominent. Obvious waist and abdominal tuck.

IDEAL

4 Ribs easily palpable, with minimal fat covering. Waist easily noted, viewed from above. Abdominal tuck evident.

5 Ribs palpable without excess fat covering. Waist observed behind ribs when viewed from above. Abdomen tucked up when viewed from side.

TOO HEAVY

6 Ribs palpable with slight excess fat covering. Waist is discernible viewed from above but is not prominent. Abdominal tuck apparent.

7 Ribs palpable with difficulty; heavy fat cover. Noticeable fat deposits over lumbar area and base of tail. Waist absent or barely visible. Abdominal tuck may be present.

8 Ribs not palpable under very heavy fat cover, or palpable only with significant pressure. Heavy fat deposits over lumbar area and base of tail. Waist absent. No abdominal tuck. Obvious abdominal distention may be present.

9 Massive fat deposits over thorax, spine and base of tail. Waist and abdominal tuck absent. Fat deposits on neck and limbs. Obvious abdominal distention.

The **BODY CONDITION SYSTEM** was developed at the Nestlé Purina Pet Care Center and has been validated as documented in the following publications:

Mawby D, Bartges JW, Moyers T, et. al. **Comparison of body fat estimates by dual-energy x-ray absorptiometry and deuterium oxide dilution in client owned dogs.** Compendium 2001; 23 (9A): 70

Laflamme DP. **Development and Validation of a Body Condition Score System for Dogs.** Canine Practice July/August 1997; 22:10-15

Kealy, et. al. **Effects of Diet Restriction on Life Span and Age-Related Changes in Dogs.** JAVMA 2002; 220:1315-1320

Call 1-800-222-VETS (8387), weekdays, 8:00 a.m. to 4:30 p.m. CT

Nestlé PURINA

Figure 8-1 Nine-point body-condition scale for dogs. (Reprinted with permission of Nestlé Purina Co, St Louis.)

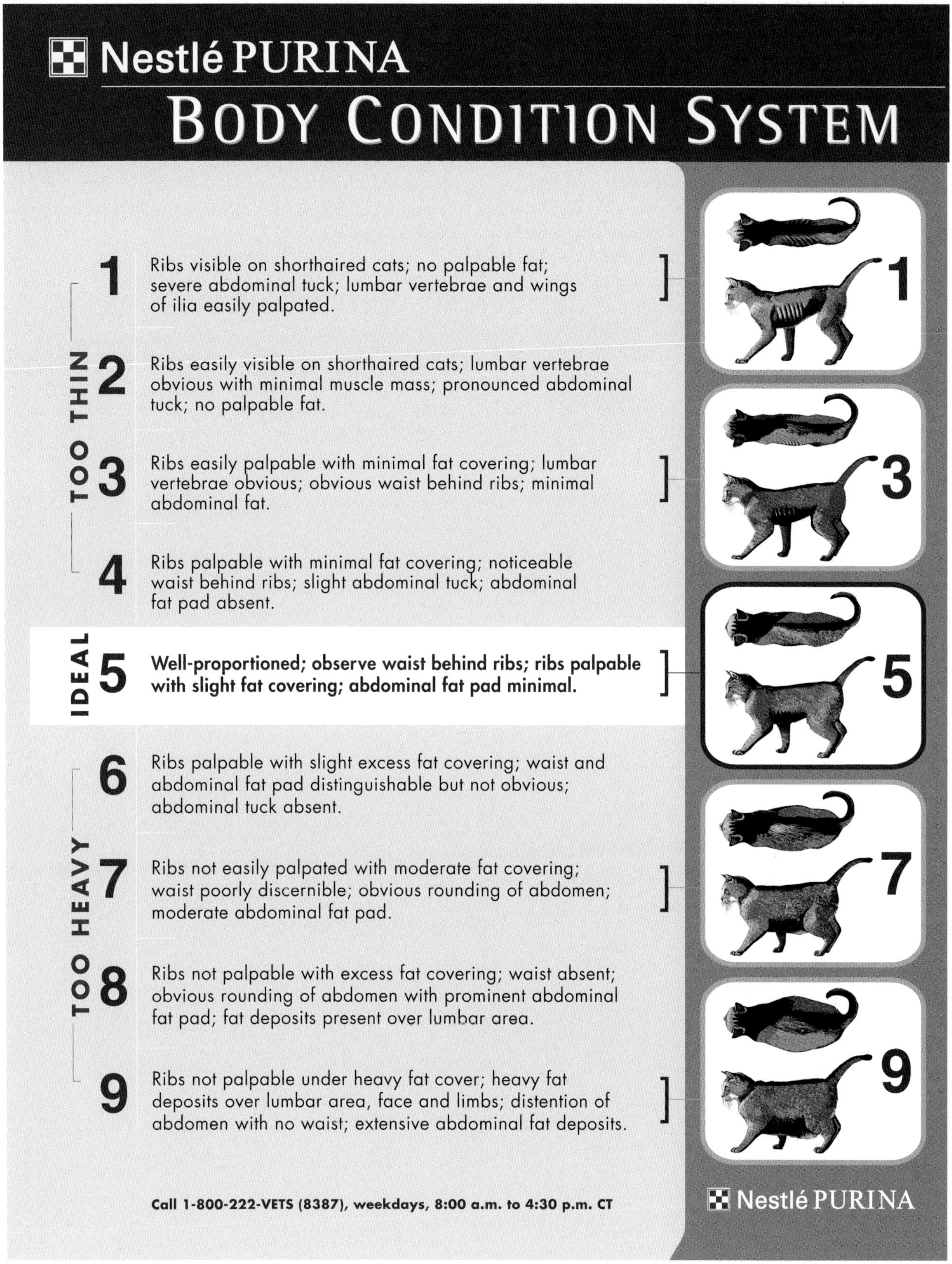

▦ Nestlé PURINA
BODY CONDITION SYSTEM

1 Ribs visible on shorthaired cats; no palpable fat; severe abdominal tuck; lumbar vertebrae and wings of ilia easily palpated.

TOO THIN

2 Ribs easily visible on shorthaired cats; lumbar vertebrae obvious with minimal muscle mass; pronounced abdominal tuck; no palpable fat.

3 Ribs easily palpable with minimal fat covering; lumbar vertebrae obvious; obvious waist behind ribs; minimal abdominal fat.

4 Ribs palpable with minimal fat covering; noticeable waist behind ribs; slight abdominal tuck; abdominal fat pad absent.

IDEAL

5 **Well-proportioned; observe waist behind ribs; ribs palpable with slight fat covering; abdominal fat pad minimal.**

6 Ribs palpable with slight excess fat covering; waist and abdominal fat pad distinguishable but not obvious; abdominal tuck absent.

TOO HEAVY

7 Ribs not easily palpated with moderate fat covering; waist poorly discernible; obvious rounding of abdomen; moderate abdominal fat pad.

8 Ribs not palpable with excess fat covering; waist absent; obvious rounding of abdomen with prominent abdominal fat pad; fat deposits present over lumbar area.

9 Ribs not palpable under heavy fat cover; heavy fat deposits over lumbar area, face and limbs; distention of abdomen with no waist; extensive abdominal fat deposits.

Call 1-800-222-VETS (8387), weekdays, 8:00 a.m. to 4:30 p.m. CT

▦ Nestlé PURINA

Figure 8-2 Nine-point body-condition scale for cats. (Reprinted with permission of Nestlé Purina Co, St Louis.)

appropriate caloric intake. At about 3 to 4 weeks of age, orphan kittens can be fed a gruel consisting of dry kitten food mixed with formula and/or water (2 : 1) and fed in a saucer. They will increase consumption over the next 2 weeks, during which the amount of water and/or formula added to the kitten food can be decreased, eventually weaning them onto kitten food. Generally, kittens can be totally weaned at 6 to 8 weeks. Early total weaning is not advised, since separation from littermates can result in behavioral changes and declined social skills. However, kittens can be nutritionally weaned starting at $4\frac{1}{4}$ weeks. Advantages and disadvantages to earlier nutritional weaning are controversial.

Kittens should be fed 3 times daily for 6 months, then twice daily for life. The label on each food the kitten is eating should be read to determine the correct amount to feed. If the kitten is eating both canned and dry, the total caloric intake needs to be considered. As kittens mature, the energy requirements become less. At 10 weeks of age, the average DER is 200 kcal/kg. By 10 months of age, the DER has decreased to 80 kcal/day.

Kittens can become obese, leading to a variety of diseases later in life. Some cats will limit themselves and simply "graze" all day, whereas others will simply eat until they have a distended abdomen. The same rules apply for kittens and cats that apply to puppies and dogs: owners should be well-educated on body scoring their pets for obesity. The ribs and spine should easily be palpable, with an hourglass shape from above, and a trim waistline behind the ribs. Figure 8-2 demonstrates the appropriate technique to determine the body-condition score of cats.

SUGGESTED READINGS

AAFCO Guidelines: www.fda.gov/cvm/petfood.htm.

Hand M, Thatcher C, Remillard R et al: *Small animal clinical nutrition,* Topeka, KS, 2000, Mark Morris Institute.

Kirk R: *Current veterinary therapy X,* Philadelphia, 1989, WB Saunders.

Nestle Purina Research Report, volume 9, issue 2, St Louis, 2005, The Nestle Company.

CARE OF THE ORPHANED PUPPY AND KITTEN

CHAPTER 9

Michael E. Peterson

Puppies and kittens may require hand rearing for a variety of reasons; the most obvious is death of the mother. However, some mothers are agalactic, have mastitis, have an underlying disease, or are so debilitated that they cannot care for the litter. Occasionally, litters are so large the dam is incapable of supplying adequate nutrition to the offspring. Some neonates are much smaller or weaker than their siblings and have difficulty competing, thus necessitating hand rearing to improve their chances of survival.

A common assumption is that most neonatal orphans die from infectious disease. However, the majority of orphan puppy and kitten deaths are due to caregiver error by either a delay in identifying a problem or inadequate husbandry knowledge or technical capability to correctly respond. Normal puppies and kittens should eat or sleep for 90% of the day for the first 2 weeks of their lives; if not, all efforts should immediately be directed at identifying the source of their discontent.

Orphans are at higher risk of infection because of a variety of factors, including but not limited to a decreased immune response secondary to stress and not receiving local antibodies from their mothers' milk. Visits from individuals outside the home should be limited. Handling of the litter should be primarily restricted to the caregiver; and everyone should wash their hands before handling the neonates.

Orphaned puppies and kittens along with their mothers and littermates should receive complete physical examinations to ascertain the possible cause of the abandonment. Often, abandoned neonates have significant medical problems, including hypothermia, hypoglycemia, dehydration, and a variety of congenital malformations that need to be addressed. Dams that are preeclamptic secondary to low calcium levels often are nervous and poor mothers and may savage their young.

FOSTERING

Fostering is an excellent approach for managing abandoned or orphaned puppies and kittens. Fostering, if successful, allows issues of proper nutrition, stimulation to eliminate, and temperature control to be managed by the surrogate mother. This approach is not without risk as some bitches or queens may neglect or attack and kill the adoptive puppies and kittens. Successful foster mothers usually accept and nurse orphan neonates immediately. Often, caregivers try to put some odor from the natural offspring onto the adoptive neonates to aid in the process. This is not always necessary; however, care should be taken to monitor the interaction between the new foster mother, her offspring, and the orphan neonates, particularly early in the adoptive process.

HAND REARING

The basic precepts of raising orphaned kittens and puppies involve providing the proper environment (e.g., temperature and bedding), nutrition, stimulation to eliminate, and socialization.

Environmental Control

Control of the physical environment is very important. Orphans need a dry, warm, draft-free, and comfortable nesting box. The nesting box should have sides that are tall enough so the neonates cannot climb out when unattended and get chilled. The nesting box should be easy to clean. However, there are risks with materials that are easier to clean, since they can often be a tremendous heat sink; for example, stainless steel cleans easily, but any neonate coming into contact with this material will rapidly chill.

Plastic sweater boxes work very well as nesting boxes; heating pads can be set on low under a portion of the box.

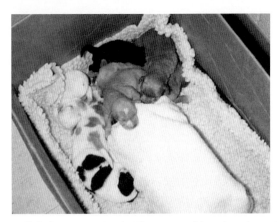

Figure 9-1 A warm water bottle wrapped in a towel provides an adequate external heat source for neonatal puppies; the water must be changed when it cools. (From Poffenbarger EM, Olson PN, Ralston SL, et al: Canine neonatology. Part II: Disorders of the neonate, *Compend Contin Educ Pract Vet*, 13:25-37, 1991.)

TABLE 9-1	Environmental temperatures for neonates	
Age in days	Nesting box temperature	Normal neonatal body temperature
0-7	85° F (29° C)	96-98° F (35.5° C-36.5° C)
8-28	80° F (26.5° C)	99° F (37° C)
29-35	75° F (24° C)	100.5° F (38° C)
35+	70° F (21° C)	100.5° F (38° C)

This will limit the risk of moisture conducting heat from the electric heating pad, inducing significant burns of the neonates. One drawback of plastic or glass containers is that they are not absorbent, so care should be taken to deal with any fluids that may end up in the box. Some caregivers advocate locating the nesting box at table height, since neonates receive closer attention if caregivers do not have to bend over (Figure 9-1). Nesting boxes should not be placed near heating vents or air conditioning ducts.

Once puppies reach 4½ to 5 weeks of age and are much more ambulatory, the use of a child's plastic swimming pool works well as a housing solution. These pools are inexpensive and easily cleaned. Additionally, standard-sized folding exercise pens will fit firmly around the pool, keeping the puppies contained. Rubber-backed floor mats with close cloth nap work well as bedding, providing excellent footing and warmth. These are easily removed and cleaned, and when used as a pair, can be rotated so while one is in use the other is being cleaned and dried.

Bedding material should be soft, absorbent, nonabrasive, and easily cleaned and should comfortably insulate the neonate from heat loss. Bedding should provide good footing and be incapable of bunching up and trapping the neonate. Many breeders like newspaper (some purchase unprinted newspaper from local newspaper publishers) because it is easily obtained, absorbent, and inexpensive. Other caregivers (including this author) prefer fabric because it tends to provide better footing; however, material should be selected that does not allow the neonates nails to snag. Poor bedding will retain moisture, dissipating the heat away from the puppies and allowing increased bacterial growth. Regardless of how appropriate the bedding material employed, it must be kept clean or changed frequently.

Environmental temperature control is important for a variety of reasons. Normal rectal body temperature in the first week of life is considerably lower than in adult dogs or cats. Neonatal puppies and kittens do not generate heat by movement and do not have an active shiver reflex until about 6 days of age, relying on the environment and brown fat for thermogenesis. In the first week of life, normal body temperature is 95° to 97.5° F (35° to 36° C). In the second and third weeks of life, before the puppy or kitten is actively crawling and walking consistently, normal body temperature ranges from 98.6° to 100.0° F (36° to 38° C).

Puppies and kittens rely on environmental temperatures to keep warm, particularly early in life. Room temperature during the first few weeks of life should be no less than 72° F. Remember that floor temperatures are significantly lower than thermostat height (heat rises).

Requirements for strict temperature control are particularly needed when there is a single orphan. When there are multiple neonates, they will huddle together to preserve their heat. Neonates in the first week of life need an incubator-like environment with temperatures approximately 85° to 90° F (29° to 32° C). The nesting box temperature can then be dropped to 80° F (26.5° C) for the next 3 to 4 weeks (Table 9-1).

A variety of heat sources are available; however, radiant heat is preferred. Hot water bottles wrapped in towels are effective but can be frustrating since they are labor intensive and necessitate frequent monitoring and reheating. The use of heat lamps is common; however, drawbacks include poorer humidity control and increased risk of burning down the house, kennel, or cattery. Another disadvantage of the heat lamps are that many kittens dislike the open bed required for their use. Heating pads are avoided by some as they can generate inconsistent temperatures (the low setting on one pad can be significantly different from another pad) and are much more likely to induce thermal burns (or scalding) if moisture soaks through from the neonate to the electric pad. Heating pads set on low with some moisture barrier between the pad and the neonates is the most common heat source employed. Very young neonates do not respond well to high environmental temperature and cannot be relied on to crawl away if overheated.

Correct humidity should be 55% to 65%; less humidity is dehydrating and more increases the chances for bacterial growth and subsequent infection. The risk of dehydration is high in the newborn, since 82% of their weight is water. Glomerular filtration rates are 21% of those of the adult at birth but increase in function to 53% by 8 weeks of age.

Minimizing stressful situations is important, allowing the neonates to sleep, eat, and grow. Orphaned neonates are already stressed as they try to cope with a new environment and life without the calming effects of their mothers. Areas with lots of foot traffic and noise increase the stress level. Overhandling, particularly by children, significantly increases stress levels and should be avoided until the neonates are at least 3 to 4 weeks old. High stress levels decrease the immune system, increasing the risk of infection, and can have potentially detrimental effects on future socialization. Some kennels and catteries use pheromone dispensers in the nursery area (Feliway for cats from Veterinary Products Laboratories, Phoenix, AZ, and Dog Appeasing Pheromone for dogs from CEVA Animal Health Inc., Manchester, MO) in an attempt to minimize neonatal stress levels.

Proper hygiene is vital because puppies and kittens have a variety of structural, metabolic, and immune conditions that, although normal for their age, make them more susceptible to infectious disease. Orphans are at greater risk for infectious disease, and the owner should be meticulous about cleanliness of bedding and feeding supplies. The number of individuals handling the orphans should be kept at a minimum, and everyone should frequently wash their hands.

Cleaning and disinfecting should not be considered as synonymous because few disinfectants work well in the face of organic debris; therefore proper cleaning should occur before disinfecting the area. Proper cleaning consists of mild soap, warm water, and elbow grease. This activity along with frequent removal and washing of bedding material needs to be accomplished before any disinfecting activity.

Proper selection of disinfectants is important and care should be taken to keep these from becoming environmental toxins. Neonates have very thin skin and transdermally absorb toxins more readily than adults. Additionally many disinfectants are significant respiratory irritants at higher concentrations. The owner should be particularly careful with cleaning agents such as pine oils and phenols. Overuse of bleach or other disinfectants or employing high concentrations of these products put the neonates at risk.

Feeding

The most common questions regarding feeding of orphans are what to feed, how to feed, how much to feed, and how frequently. Proper hygiene is paramount when feeding neonates. All bottles, nipples, tubes, and any other equipment must be kept clean. Caregivers should carefully wash all feeding equipment, mixing only enough formula to last for 24 to 48 hours and refrigerating any unused quantities in a glass container.

Picking up and handling each neonate for feeding can often alert the caregiver to problems. The neonates should be vigorous, squirmy, and fat. Orphaned puppies and kittens should be weighed twice daily, and the caregiver should acquire an adequate scale for this task (Figure 9-2). Weight loss or failure to gain is one of the earliest indicators of health problems, which should provoke an immediate investigation into the cause.

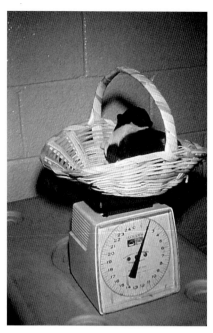

Figure 9-2 A food scale used to weigh a neonatal pup. (From Johnston SD, Root Kustritz MV, Olsen PNS (eds): *Canine and feline theriogenology*, St Louis, 2001, Saunders/Elsevier.)

BOX 9-1	Homemade milk replacer for puppies

120 ml cow's or goat's milk
120 ml water
2 to 4 egg yolks
1 to 2 tsp vegetable oil
1000 mg calcium carbonate

Adapted from Hoskins JD (ed): *Veterinary pediatrics: dogs and cats from birth to six months*, ed 3, St. Louis, 2001, Saunders/Elsevier.

BOX 9-2	Homemade milk replacer for kittens

90 ml condensed milk
90 ml water
120 ml plain yogurt (not low fat)
3 large or 4 small egg yolks

Adapted from Hoskins JD: Nutrition and nutritional problems. In Hoskins JD (ed): *Veterinary pediatrics: dogs and cats from birth to six months*, ed 3, St. Louis, 2001, Saunders/Elsevier.

Weaning usually begins at 4 to 4½ weeks of age and is discussed in detail later in this chapter. Until weaning age, it is necessary to provide proper nutrition to the orphans. This can be accomplished by feeding an appropriate milk replacement diet. Administering improper replacement diets, such as cow's milk, leads to poor nutrition with inadequate rates of growth and is usually accompanied by the onset of diarrhea. Commercial replacement diets are generally used because they come with a balanced nutritional content. Homemade diets can be made; sample recipes are included in this chapter (Boxes 9-1 and 9-2). However, formulating a nutritionally balanced homemade milk-replacer is difficult. Some owners would prefer homemade diets over commercial diets; however, several problems need to be overcome. Preparing homemade diets has some significant drawbacks, including acquiring quality ingredients, increased risk of bacterial contamination, and difficulty replicating the dam's normal milk constituents. Bitch's milk contains high amounts of fat, low amounts of lactose, and moderate amounts of protein. Cow's milk and goat's milk are high in lactose, lower in protein and fat, and have less caloric density than bitch's milk. Although supplements can be added to cow's milk and goat's milk to make them more closely approximate bitch's milk, they are too high in lactose, which increases the risk of diarrhea. Studies have demonstrated that homemade diet recipes, even when administered in larger volumes and more frequently, still resulted in slower growth rates than commercial formulas. Cottage cheese should never be used in diets for neonatal puppies and kittens as it congeals in the stomach and can obstruct the neonate. Homemade diets should only be used in an emergency situation until a commercial diet can be acquired. The primary problems with powdered commercial milk formula revolve around mixing errors. Improperly mixed milk formula may be too concentrated, leading to vomiting, bloating, and diarrhea; conversely, formula that is too diluted diminishes the caloric density of each milliliter fed, necessitating more feedings.

There are many commercial formulas on the market for milk replacement in puppies and kittens. One new commercial diet (Gastromate with IgY from PRN Pharmacal, Pensacola, FL) has further simulated mother's milk by adding immunoglobulins (avian IgY) against common canine and feline neonatal gastrointestinal (GI) pathogens. According to the company, these antibodies support local digestive tract immunity and bridge the "blank" period between natural local immunity and immunization. Some commercial diets have added bovine colostrum, which is not as effective as canine or feline colostrum.

Feeding can be accomplished by either bottle or tube feeding with an appropriate milk replacement diet. Bottle feeding works well for vigorous puppies and kittens with a strong suckle reflex because they will suckle until they are full. Weaker or sick neonates are often not able to sustain suckling long enough to receive adequate quantities of formula. If the neonate cannot suck satisfactorily, tube feeding becomes necessary.

Bottle feeding can be accomplished after selecting a properly sized nipple; larger puppies can use human baby bottles and nipples, whereas smaller puppies and kittens require specific neonatal commercial bottles with much smaller nipples (Figure 9-3). Nipples on the commercially purchased bottles usually do not have a premade opening. A proper hole can be made with a hot needle (to melt the hole open). The nipple opening should be just large enough for milk to slowly drip out if the bottle is held upside down; any less and the neonate has to work too hard for the formula, and any larger and the formula flows rapidly, increasing the risk of aspiration. Formula should always be sucked and never squeezed from the bottle.

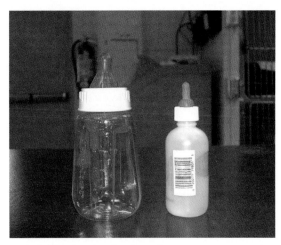

Figure 9-3 Nursing bottle sizes for puppy compared to toy puppy or kitten.

Feeding position is important. Sternal recumbency is the proper position for feeding with a bottle, the neonate should be able to push off with its front legs (as it would with its mother) and the nipple should be aligned straight into the mouth. Nipple placement is important, since the nursing neonate rolls its tongue around the nipple and creates a seal when nursing. If the nipple is placed at an angle in which this seal cannot be accomplished, the neonate sucks in air and develops colic. The neonate should not overextend its head during feeding because this position increases the risk of aspiration.

If proper technique can be learned, tube feeding has some advantages over bottle feeding, including better approximation of quantity of formula administered, faster administration (important if multiple orphans are to be fed), and increased efficiency. The disadvantages to tube feeding include a learning curve to develop proper tubing technique and increased risk of instillation of formula into the neonates' lungs. The equipment necessary for tube feeding includes a syringe and a flexible rubber or plastic feeding tube. The tube size should be large enough to have some stiffness so it will not flex back on itself, usually between 7 and 8 Fr and occasionally smaller, depending on the neonate's size. The tube should be measured from the neonate's last rib to the end of the nose with the head extended. The tube should be marked at this point. Inserting the tube to this mark will ensure the end of the tube is in the stomach and not in the esophagus or in the lungs. Multiple tube-feeding demonstration videos performed by veterinarians are available on Internet websites. The tube should be placed into the warm milk replacer and the formula pulled up into the syringe in such a way as to keep the tube full of milk so it will not introduce air into the stomach. The neonate should be upright with its head flexed (not extended) and the tip of the tube inserted along the roof of the mouth, following the path of least resistance. No force is needed and most neonates will swallow the feeding tube easily. The tube should be held in place as the milk is slowly infused into the neonate's stomach. Instill the formula slowly because rapid feeding by stomach tube can cause vomiting or bloating. Infuse the milk over 1 to 2 minutes. Once the feeding is finished, the catheter should be kinked, then slowly removed to avoid milk dripping from the tip and risking aspiration.

With tube feeding, the caregiver determines the volume of formula the neonate receives, as opposed to bottle-feeding in which the neonate decides when it is full. The average stomach capacity in neonates is 0.7 fl oz (4 tsp) per lb (40 ml/kg). The proper amount of formula gives the neonate a rounded belly appearance, but care should be taken to keep from overextending the stomach. Some caregivers advocate "burping" neonates after feeding, although this is not a necessary procedure unless air has been introduced into the stomach.

Most kitten and puppies need about 100 kJ of daily energy per 100 gm of body weight. Milk replacers usually have recommended feeding amounts printed on the label. Most commercial milk formulas provide approximately 5 kJ of metabolizable energy in each milliliter (Table 9-2). The total calculated volume of milk should be divided into multiple feedings. The frequency of feedings is controlled by the size of the recipient's stomach or by the neonate crying for more food.

Avoid overfeeding at any one meal because this can lead to diarrhea, vomiting, or even aspiration. If the neonate is not gaining adequate weight, increase the frequency of feedings to increase the total daily caloric input. This is easier than dealing with the vomiting, diarrhea, or aspiration that results from overfeeding.

Normal puppies and kittens need about 60 to 100 ml of water per lb of body weight per day. Water should be given until 90 ml/lb body weight has been given. Correct hydration is important, and intake should be calculated since the formula may not supply adequate water at the recommended dilution.

Feeding frequency depends on several factors, including age of the orphan, volume of each feeding, and caloric density of the food. Newborns should be fed 6 to 8 times daily or about every 2 to 3 hours. Once the neonates are a couple of weeks old, the feeding intervals can be increased.

Hungry kittens and puppies are restless and will cry until fed. Food must be warmed before feeding and should be at maternal body temperature (101.5° F) (38.6° C); the milk's temperature can be tested on the back of the clinician's hand before feeding to make sure the temperature is slightly warmer than skin. Cold food can stimulate vomiting, induce hypothermia, and inhibit absorption by slowing peristalsis. Food that is too hot can burn the neonate's mouth, esophagus, and stomach. The first few feedings with milk replacer should be diluted (if using canned) or made (if using powder) with a balanced electrolyte fluid to diminish the risk of osmotic diarrhea (Table 9-3).

Puppies and kittens need to be stimulated to urinate and defecate for the first 3 weeks of life. A warm, wet cotton ball can be used to gently wipe the urinary and anal openings. Many caregivers stimulate elimination just before each feeding. Usually, elimination is quickly stimulated, and puppies and kittens have a couple of moderately yellowish stools daily, although neonates may not defecate with every stimulatory session.

Monitoring Growth

Hand-reared neonates may not grow as fast as maternally nursing puppies and kittens. However, once weaned, they usually quickly catch up to their littermates. As a general rule, puppies and kittens double their weight in the first week and then gain 1 to 2 gm/lb of anticipated adult weight each day. Therefore a German Shorthair puppy expected to weigh 50 lb as an adult should gain approximately 50 to 100 gm/day as a puppy.

TABLE 9-2   Volume to feed

Week of life	Daily caloric requirements per ounce of body weight
Puppies	
1	3.75 cal/oz
2	4.50 cal/oz
3	5.00 cal/oz
4	5.50 cal/oz
Kittens	
1-2	6.00 cal/oz
3-4	8.00 cal/oz

Milk substitutes roughly contain about 1 cal/ml. Read milk replacer label for actual calories per milliliter. Use puppy milk replacer for puppies and kitten milk replacer for kittens.

TABLE 9-3   Common causes of feeding-related problems

Problem	Clinical manifestation	Corrective action
Poor feeding positioning	Increased risk for aspiration	The neonate should be sternal with head in relatively flexed position
Incorrect formula temperature	Hypothermia, poor digestion, burns	Food should be mother's body temperature when feeding
Feeding too rapidly	Vomiting, colic, bloating	Infuse the milk over 1-2 minutes
Incorrectly mixing the milk replacer	Diarrhea, bloating, poor nutrition	Mix formula according to directions, first few feedings mix or dilute with balanced saline solution
Poor hygiene	Diarrhea, vomiting, infection	Wash all feeding equipment, mix only enough formula to last for 24 hours; keep refrigerated

Neonates should be weighed at the same time twice daily for at least the first 2 weeks. After the initial 24 hours, in which a slight weight loss is expected (10% or greater weight loss in the first 24 hours is evidence of a very poor prognosis for survival), steady growth should occur. After that, monitoring growth every few days should be sufficient. A poor growth rate indicates that there is a problem. It is possible that the entire litter could have some infectious or management issue (e.g., temperature, stress) that could cause failure to thrive (see Chapter 11). If other management issues seem to be in order and all the neonates are losing weight, then strong suspicion arises with the quality of the milk replacer, the amount being fed, the method of feeding, or the frequency of feeding. If the majority of the litter is growing except for a single neonate, then suspicion turns to some underlying problem with the individual puppy or kitten.

Weaning or Introducing Solid Food

Weaning generally begins at about 4 to 4½ weeks of age. Smaller puppies and kittens wean at about 5 weeks of age. Weaning is a stressful event for the neonate. The GI system will be exposed to new protein, carbohydrate, and fat sources. Additionally, the change in texture and bulk of the ingesta is significant. Alterations in GI microbial populations occur. Rapid introduction of solid foods can precipitate constipation. The weaning puppies and kittens not only have to adjust to solid food but also significantly increase their water consumption to maintain hydration. Fresh water should be readily available at all times for weaning puppies and kittens.

Solid food soaked in the milk formula the puppies and kittens are currently receiving can be made into a warm gruel and offered to the neonates. Some readily take to the food, and once one does, the others mimic and begin eating. The initial meal quantities should be limited to smaller portions until the GI tract has had time to adequately adjust (usually a few days). Some kitten and toy breed caregivers use human baby foods as initial diets (no garlic or onions). Any warmed food releases more odors and can stimulate the neonate to taste. Smearing some of the gruel onto the kittens' or puppies' lips can often induce them to lick the food away and get their first taste of solid food. After a couple of days the qualities of food can be increased and often the amount of fluid added can be decreased. The author's Lakeland Terrier puppies are often eating dry food with their mothers at 5 weeks of age; these puppies weigh less than 3 lb.

A note of caution: water dishes should have low sides since puppies have been known to drown in buckets.

Socialization

Proper social development is important for any puppy or kitten since the expectation is that they will become healthy, well-adjusted pets as adults. Key developmental stages and proper socialization techniques to maximize them are beyond the scope of this chapter. Raising orphan puppies and kittens to adulthood with unacceptable social behaviors defeats the goal of the initial intervention, which should be the development of pets with balanced temperaments for their eventual owners. Why rescue them as orphans just to see them euthanized for significant behavioral issues later?

A kitten reared in total isolation from other cats is at risk of developing psychological abnormalities, including nervousness, aggression, and a reduced ability to cope with strange surroundings, people, or animals (see Chapter 12).

Dogs are highly social animals and are significantly affected by interacting with other dogs, people, and the environment. Several important developmental stages in their lives mold their future temperament and ability to interact acceptably as adults (see Chapter 13).

Passive Transfer Failure

A major question with very young orphaned neonates is whether they received colostrum. Obviously, when the mother dies at parturition, colostrum ingestion has not occurred. Kittens may receive as much as 25% of their maternally derived antibodies through the placenta, whereas puppies receive 5% to 10% at best. Ingestion of colostrum is necessary for significant passive transfer of maternal antibodies. Maximal absorption of antibodies through the GI tract occurs at about 8 hours of life, with virtually no GI uptake of antibodies after 1 day of life. If the clinician is unsure if a neonate has ingested colostrum and is sure another has, then blood can be drawn from both and serum alkaline phosphatase (ALP) and gamma-glutamyl transpeptidase (GGT) levels compared. The enzyme concentrations are dramatically higher (often in the thousands) in neonates that have ingested colostrum and remain high for up to 10 days after consumption.

In those neonates who have not ingested colostrum, antibodies can be provided by administration of serum or plasma from any vaccinated adult of the same species, given orally if the neonate is less than 24 hours old or as subcutaneous boluses in older puppies and kittens. Generally, kittens are administered 15 ml of serum pooled from several adults, given as 3 boluses (oral or subcutaneously), which are administered at birth, 12 hours, and 24 hours later. There is concern about the possibility for isoerythrolysis, and serum should be crossmatched before it is administered. The empirical regimen for puppies is administration of 10 ml/lb (22 ml/kg) of pooled adult serum; this can be given at once in large pups or split into boluses as described for kittens.

SUGGESTED READINGS

Abrams-Ogg A: Hand-rearing newborn puppies and kittens. In Mathews K (ed): *Veterinary emergency and critical care manual*, ed 2, Guelph, Ontario, 2006, Lifelearn.

Hoskins JD: Nutrition and nutritional problems. In Hoskins JD (ed): *Veterinary pediatrics: dogs and cats from birth to six months*, ed 3, St. Louis, 2001, Saunders/Elsevier.

Johnston SD, Root Kustritz MV, Olsen PNS: The neonate: from birth to weaning. In Johnston SD, Root Kustritz MV, Olsen PNS (eds): *Canine and feline theriogenology*, St Louis, 2001, Saunders/Elsevier.

EMERGENCY AND CRITICAL CARE ISSUES

CHAPTER 10

Maureen A. McMichael

In human medicine, neonatology and pediatrics are distinct specialties because of the unique physiologic systems of neonatal and pediatric patients. It is essential that veterinarians be familiar with normal neonatal biochemical, hematologic, radiographic, and physical examination values to recognize the compromised patient. Pediatric and neonatal patients are afflicted with some of the same disease processes as adults; however, because of their unique physiologic systems, they differ significantly in several key areas of diagnosis, monitoring, and treatment. Hemodynamic parameters, drug dosages, laboratory data, and diagnostic imaging differ significantly compared to adults of the same species, making interpretation a challenge. This chapter briefly reviews normal findings in the neonate and pediatric patient and then discusses several emergency presentations in detail.

INITIAL EXAMINATION AND CATHETERIZATION

Essentials to evaluate in all neonates are the presence or absence of a strong suckle reflex and whether they are nursing and sleeping. Constant crying occurs if they are prevented from nursing or do not ingest enough milk. Generally, pups and kittens sleep after nursing if a sufficient amount was ingested. Nutrition is crucial to neonatal health and should be addressed early (see Chapter 8).

Normal body temperature in puppies is 96° F (35.5° C) to 97° F (36° C) for the first 1 to 2 weeks of life and should increase to 100° F (37.8° C) by the end of the first month. Normal body temperature in kittens is 98° F (36.7° C) at birth and increases to 100°F (37.8° C) by the end of the first week.

Physical examination of all neonates includes an oral examination to check for a cleft palate, abdominal palpation to check for an umbilical hernia, skull palpation to check for an open fontanelle, and verification of the presence of patent urogenital openings. Pain sensation is present at birth and analgesia is essential for all procedures that are anticipated to be painful. Normal heart rate (200 bpm) and respiratory rate (15 to 35 bpm) are higher in neonates than adults, which becomes very important when addressing shock states (see section on Hypovolemia).

When venous access is required, the intravenous (IV) route is preferred and should be attempted first. Neonates often require very small gauge catheters (i.e., 24 g), which can burr easily when being driven through the skin. A small skin puncture with a 20 g needle (while the skin is kept elevated) can be made and then the catheter can be fed through the skin hole, which can prevent burring. If attempts at IV catheter placement fail, an intraosseous (IO) catheter should be placed. An IO catheter can be inserted in the proximal femur or humerus using an 18- to 22-g spinal needle or an 18- to 25-g hypodermic needle. An IO catheter can be used for fluid and blood administration. The area must be prepared in a sterile manner, and the needle is inserted into the bone parallel to the long axis of the bone (Figure 10-1). The IO catheter is gently aspirated to assure patency and then secured with a sterile bandage. Neonates, who have a large portion of "red" marrow compared with adults who have more "yellow" marrow consisting of fat, are ideal candidates for IO catheters. IV access must be established as soon as possible, ideally within 2 hours, and the IO catheter should be removed to minimize IO infection. IO catheter complications correlate with duration of use in humans.

FLUID REQUIREMENTS

Fluid requirements are much higher in neonates than adults because of a higher percentage of total body water, a greater surface area to body weight ratio, a higher metabolic rate, a decreased renal concentrating ability, and decreased body fat. Although dehydration is common, overhydration is also a serious concern because the kidneys cannot dilute urine to

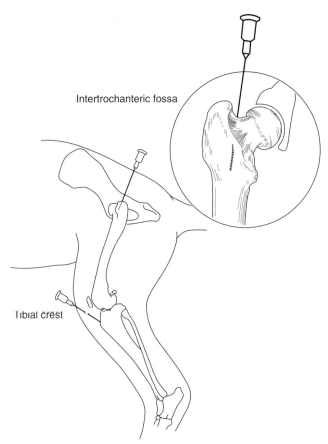

Figure 10-1 Anatomic locations for intraosseous (IO) access. (From Bateman SW, Buffington CA, Holloway C: Emergency and critical care techniques and nutrition. In Birchard SJ, Sherding RG (eds): *Saunders manual of small animal practice*, ed 3, St Louis, 2006, Saunders/Elsevier.)

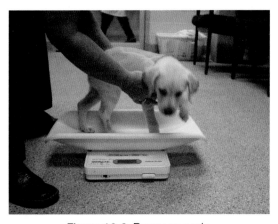

Figure 10-2 Puppy on scale.

rid the body of excess water. The best way to monitor for underhydration or overhydration is to have an accurate pediatric gram scale and weigh the patient frequently (ideally 3 to 4 times per day) (Figure 10-2). If possible, baseline thoracic radiographs are helpful. It can be difficult to diagnose fluid overload because the neonatal heart takes up so much of the thoracic cavity and normal neonate lungs have more interstitial fluid than adults. Baseline radiographs can be very

helpful in serially monitoring for fluid overload. Other ways to monitor fluid therapy include checking hematocrit (HCT) and total solids. The HCT decreases in normal neonates from days 1 to 28, and total solids are lower than adults.

A fluid bolus of 30 to 40 ml/kg is recommended in moderately dehydrated neonates followed by a constant rate infusion of 80 to 100 ml/kg/day of warm crystalloids. A liter of fluids warmed to 104° F (40° C) cools down to room temperature (70° F; 21° C) within approximately 10 minutes. A fluid warmer placed in the line is a good option to keep the fluids warmed. Lactated Ringer's solution may be ideal, since lactate is the preferred metabolic fuel in the neonate during times of hypoglycemia.

LABORATORY VALUES (See Chapter 30)

Young puppies and kittens have a lower HCT than adults (Boxes 10-1 and 10-2). The HCT decreases from 47.5% at birth to 29.9% by day 28 in puppies. This decrease is normal and is thought to be the result of the change from a relatively hypoxic environment to an oxygen-rich environment. The HCT will start to increase by the end of the first month of life in healthy neonates. Kittens also have a HCT nadir at 4 to 6 weeks of 27%. Knowledge of this normal decrease in HCT is essential during treatment of any neonate, and during this time period, a rise in the HCT is usually indicative of significant dehydration.

If at all possible, surgical procedures should be delayed until after the first week of life because of low concentrations of clotting factors and antithrombin. These values increase to normal by the end of the first week. Prothrombin time

(PT) is increased to ≈1.3 times adult values and normalizes by 7 days. Partial thromboplastin time (PTT) is also increased (1.8 times adult values) but decreases to 1.6 times adult values on day 7.

Knowledge of the slight increases in bilirubin (0.5 mg/dl; normal adult range 0 to 0.4) and dramatic increases in liver enzymes at birth in puppies is essential when creating a differential diagnoses list (Boxes 10-3 and 10-4). In puppies, serum alkaline phosphatase (ALP; 3845 IU/L, normal adult range 4 to 107) and gamma-glutamyl transferase (GGT; 1111 IU/L, normal adult range 0 to 7) are over 20 times greater than adult values. In kittens, the ALP (123 IU/L, normal adult range 9 to 42) is 3 times that seen in adults. Serum blood urea nitrogen (BUN), creatinine, albumin, cholesterol, and total protein are lower in neonates than adults. Lower creatinine is thought to be due to decreased muscle mass, and lower BUN and cholesterol are due to immature liver function. Knowledge of these values is crucial to prevent a misdiagnosis of liver disease in the neonate (elevated liver enzymes and low levels of BUN, cholesterol, and albumin can all mimic liver dysfunction).

Bone growth causes elevations in calcium and phosphorus in the young. Urine is isosthenuric in neonates because the capacity to concentrate and dilute urine is limited in this age group. Knowledge of this limitation becomes crucial when deciding on fluid resuscitation rates, since overhydration is just as much a concern as underhydration.

Blood pressure has been shown to be significantly lower in puppies, and central venous pressure (CVP) has been shown to be higher. Mean arterial pressure (MAP) is lower (49 mm Hg at 1 month of age in puppies) and normalizes (94 mm Hg) by 9 months of age. CVP is higher (8 cm H_2O) at 1 month of age in puppies but decreases (2 cm H_2O) by 9 months of age.

Radiographic interpretation can be challenging in pediatric patients if the veterinarian is not familiar with the normal anatomic differences in the young (see Chapter 21). The thymus can mimic a mediastinal mass or lung consolidation on thoracic radiographs. The heart can falsely appear enlarged and the lung parenchyma appears more opaque in neonates (because of higher water content). The liver appears to protrude further from under the rib cage than expected as a result of the absence of costochondral mineralization (making a misdiagnosis of hepatomegaly more likely). There is loss of abdominal detail because of the lack of fat and a small amount of abdominal effusion and this can be misdiagnosed as pathologic peritoneal effusion.

Although there are several significant differences in neonatal and pediatric pharmacology (see Chapter 27), cardiovascular drugs are the focus of this discussion. Cardiovascular drugs (e.g., epinephrine, dopamine, dobutamine, and so on) can be quite difficult to dose in neonates because of the individual variations in maturity of the autonomic nervous system. The autonomic nervous system is not mature until up to 8 weeks in neonates, and maturity occurs at different rates in individuals. Response to treatment and continuous monitoring of hemodynamic variables is essential when using these drugs. Elevations in heart rate after administration of dopamine, dobutamine, or isoproterenol cannot be predicted until 9 to 10 weeks of age, and the response to atropine or lidocaine is decreased in the neonate.

A normal neonate's respiratory rate is about 2 to 3 times higher than an adult's because of higher airway resistance and higher oxygen demand (Box 10-5). Drugs that depress respiration should be avoided in neonates. Neonates have a lower percentage of contractile fibers in their myocardium than adults and do not have the ability to increase cardiac output by increasing contractility (i.e., stroke volume). Since cardiac output is equal to stroke volume multiplied by heart rate, the neonate's heart rate must be increased to increase cardiac output. Since the neonatal heart depends on a high heart rate to increase cardiac output, drugs that depress heart rate should be avoided. Although opioids are very good for analgesia because of their reversibility, the animal must be monitored closely, since these drugs have a propensity to depress heart and respiratory rates.

BOX 10-3 Biochemistry profiles: pediatric canine*

Bilirubin: 0.5 mg/dl (range: 0.2-1.0, normal adult range: 0-0.4)

Alkaline phosphatase (ALP): 3845 IU/L (range: 618-8760, normal adult range: 4-107)

Gamma-glutamyl transferase (GGT): 1111 IU/L (range: 163-3558, normal adult range: 0-7)

Total protein: 4.1 gm/dl (range: 3.4-5.2, normal adult range: 5.4-7.4)

Albumin: 1.8 gm/dl at 2-4 weeks (range: 1.7-2.0, normal adult range: 2.1-2.3)

Glucose: 88 mg/dl (range: 52-127, normal adult range: 65-100)

From Silverstein DC, Hopper K (eds): *Small animal critical care medicine,* St Louis, 2008, Saunders/Elsevier.
*At birth, except otherwise specified.

BOX 10-4 Biochemistry profiles: pediatric feline*

Bilirubin: 0.3 mg/dl (range: 0.1-1.0, normal adult range: 0-0.2)

Alkaline phosphatase: 123 IU/L (range: 68-269, normal adult range: 9-42)

Gamma-glutamyl transferase: 1 IU/L (range: 0-3, normal adult range: 0-4)

Total protein: 4.4 gm/dl (range: 4.0-5.2, normal adult range: 5.8-8.0)

Albumin: 2.1 gm/dl (range: 2.0-2.4, normal adult range: 2.3-3.0)

Glucose: 117 mg/dl (range: 76-129, normal adult range: 63-144)

From Silverstein DC, Hopper K (eds): *Small animal critical care medicine,* St Louis, 2008, Saunders/Elsevier.
*At birth, except where specified.

BOX 10-5	Clinical values for pediatric canine and feline

Heart rate: 200 bpm (puppy) and 250 bpm (kitten)
Respiratory rate: 15 bpm (birth) and 30 bpm (by 1-3 hours after birth)
Temperature: 95°-98.6° F at birth and normalizes to adult values at 4 weeks
Mean arterial pressure: 49 mm Hg at 1 month of age, 94 mm Hg at 9 months (puppies)
Central venous pressure: 8 cm H_2O at 1 month of age, 2 cm H_2O at 9 months (puppies)

From Silverstein DC, Hopper K (eds): *Small animal critical care medicine*, St Louis, 2008, Saunders/Elsevier.

HYPOVOLEMIA AND DEHYDRATION

Hypovolemia results in decreased perfusion and subsequent decreases in oxygen delivery to tissues. The most common syndromes associated with hypovolemia in neonates are diarrhea, vomiting, or decreased fluid intake. In adults, hypovolemia is compensated or partially compensated for by increasing the heart rate, concentrating the urine, and decreasing urine output. In neonates, compensatory mechanisms may be inadequate or even nonexistent. Contractile elements make up a smaller portion of the fetal myocardium (30%) compared to the adult myocardium (60%), making it difficult for the fetus to increase cardiac contractility in response to hypovolemia. Neonates also have immature sympathetic nerve fibers in the myocardium and cannot maximally increase heart rate in response to hypovolemia. Complete maturation of the autonomic nervous system does not occur until after 8 weeks of age in puppies.

MAP is lower (49 mm Hg) in normal neonates at 2 months of age and normalizes (94 mm Hg) by 9 months of age. This difference appears to be due to the immaturity of the muscular component of the arterial wall at birth. In adults, the kidneys autoregulate blood pressure over a wide range of systemic arterial pressures, but neonatal kidneys are unable to accomplish this. The neonate's glomerular filtration rate (GFR) decreases as the systemic blood pressure decreases, making restoration of fluid volume critical in neonates.

Immature kidneys are incapable of concentrating urine in response to hypovolemia. Appropriate concentration and dilution of urine is not seen until approximately 10 weeks of age. The capacity to concentrate urine increases almost linearly with age during the first year of life in humans. Inefficient countercurrent mechanisms, decreased sodium resorption in the thick ascending loop of Henle, relatively short loops of Henle, and decreased urea concentration are thought to be causative. Simultaneously, BUN and creatinine are lower in neonates than adults, making monitoring of azotemia in this group very challenging.

The skin of a neonate has an increased fat and decreased water content compared to adults; therefore skin turgor cannot be used to assess dehydration. Mucous membranes remain moist in the face of severe dehydration in neonates and cannot be used to adequately assess it.

Because neonatal fluid requirements (higher than adults) and increased losses (decreased renal concentrating ability, higher respiratory rate, and higher metabolic rate), dehydration can rapidly progress to hypovolemia and shock if not adequately treated. The most common causes of hypovolemia in neonates are gastrointestinal (GI) disturbances (e.g., vomiting, anorexia, and diarrhea) and inadequate feeding. The most common cause of diarrhea in neonatal puppies and kittens is owner overfeeding with formula.

Because it can be so difficult to adequately assess hypovolemia in neonates, some assumptions should be made. One should assume that all neonates with severe diarrhea, inadequate intake, or severe vomiting are dehydrated, and potentially hypovolemic and aggressive treatment should be started immediately. Treatment of hypovolemia includes rapid replacement fluid therapy, monitoring of electrolyte and glucose status, and nutritional support. The patient should be weighed at least every 12 hours, preferably every 8 hours. Dehydration is likely when the urine specific gravity reaches 1.020, and this should be monitored as an indicator of rehydration. An initial bolus of 45 ml/kg of warm isotonic fluids in severely dehydrated or hypovolemic animals is given as fast as possible and followed by a constant rate infusion of maintenance fluids (80 ml/kg/day), as well as estimated fluid losses. Losses can be estimated (i.e., 2 tbsp of diarrhea is equal to 30 ml of fluid). If the neonate is hypoglycemic or unable to eat, dextrose is added to the IV fluids at the lowest amount that will maintain normoglycemia (i.e., start with 1.25% dextrose).

HYPOGLYCEMIA

There are several reasons that meticulous monitoring of glucose is essential in neonates. Inefficient hepatic gluconeogenesis, decreased liver glycogen stores, and loss of glucose in the urine all increase the potential of a hypoglycemic episode. Urinary glucose reabsorption does not normalize until approximately 3 weeks in puppies. The brain requires glucose for energy in the neonate, and brain damage can occur with prolonged hypoglycemia. The fetal and neonatal myocardia use carbohydrate (glucose) for energy rather than the long chain fatty acids used by the adult myocardium. The neonate therefore has an increased demand for, an increased loss of, and a decreased ability to synthesize glucose compared to adults.

Clinical signs of hypoglycemia can be a challenge to recognize because of the inefficient counterregulatory hormone release during hypoglycemia in neonates. In adults, the counterregulatory hormones are released (i.e., cortisol, growth hormone, glucagon, and epinephrine) in response to low blood glucose. These hormones facilitate euglycemia by increasing gluconeogenesis and antagonizing insulin. Clinical signs of hypoglycemia, if seen, may include lethargy and anorexia. Vomiting, diarrhea, infection, and decreased intake all contribute to hypoglycemia in neonates. Infusions of

1.0 ml/kg of 12.5% dextrose (i.e., dilute 50% dextrose 1 : 3) followed by a continuous rate infusion (CRI) of isotonic fluids supplemented with 1.25% to 5.0% dextrose are required to treat this condition. It is important to remember that any bolus of dextrose should be immediately followed by a CRI that is supplemented or there is a risk of rebound hypoglycemia. In rare cases, neonates may have refractory hypoglycemia and may only respond to hourly boluses of dextrose in addition to a CRI of crystalloid with supplemental dextrose. Carnitine supplementation should be considered in these cases, since in some studies in human babies, carnitine supplementation facilitated treatment of refractory hypoglycemia.

HEAD TRAUMA

Human children have a higher percentage of diffuse brain injury during trauma to the head compared to adults, and this is thought to be the result of their greater head-to-torso ratio. The neonatal brain also has greater water content, lacks complete axonal myelinization, and may be more susceptible to hypoxia and hypotension than adults. There may also be a greater susceptibility to apoptosis and delayed cell death during head trauma in children compared with adults. With all head trauma cases, the goals are to improve oxygen delivery, decrease intracranial pressure (ICP), and maximize cerebral perfusion pressure (CPP). Children have a lower ICP, as well as a lower MAP compared to adults. Puppies also have a lower MAP, although the author is unaware of ICP values in normal puppies.

To optimize treatment the MAP must be kept as close to normal as possible. Since CPP is equal to the MAP minus the ICP, it can be seen that MAP must be kept high, and ICP kept low to maximize CPP. Appropriate fluid therapy to keep the systolic blood pressure above 90 mm Hg is suggested in adult head trauma and has been associated with improved survival. However, this figure is based on normal adult systolic blood pressure. Since neonates have a lower MAP than adults, a lower value should be the target goal. In puppies younger than 2 months of age, MAP of 50 mm Hg may be acceptable. The author is unaware of data on normal MAP in puppies between 2 and 9 months of age.

Since CPP depends on adequate cardiac output and adequate ventilation, these should be optimized in head trauma patients. Both hyperventilation and hypoventilation should be avoided in favor of a normal ventilation rate. Hyperventilation to reduce the $PaCO_2$ to less than 35 mm Hg may be helpful as a temporary bridge (usually to surgery to remove a subdural hemorrhage) in an emergency patient with impending signs of brain herniation. The resulting vasoconstriction caused by the hyperventilation can decrease the CPP in the healthy brain (as a result of intact autoregulation), leading to decreased oxygen delivery and hypoxia. Once volume has been addressed (i.e., fluid therapy), vasopressors may be administered in humans if MAP is still low.

Mannitol (at 0.5 to 1.0 gm/kg IV over 20 minutes) can be used if neurologic status is declining or the patient shows evidence of increased ICP that is not responsive to fluid therapy. It is contraindicated if the serum osmolality is greater than 330 mOsm/L or the patient is hypotensive. Alternatively, hypertonic saline 3% (at 4 ml/kg IV over 20 minutes) can be used if the patient is not hypernatremic and the serum osmolality is not greater than 330 mOsm/L.

In human children, seizures are more frequent after head trauma than in adults and can occur with minimal brain damage. Elevation of the head to 30 degrees has been suggested, but this must be done without compressing the jugular veins (i.e., using a tilt table or a foam wedge). Placing a rolled-up towel under the neck to elevate the head is potentially dangerous, since compression of the jugular veins has been shown to increase ICP. Jugular catheters or neck bandages should not be placed in head trauma patients. Any blood needed should be drawn from a peripheral vein or a long saphenous catheter.

In humans, measurement of ICP can be made directly, but this is impractical in most veterinary situations. In adult dogs, the Cushing reflex can be helpful to gauge increasing ICP. When ICP increases, the systemic blood pressure rises, and in response, the heart rate decreases. A bradycardic, hypertensive head trauma animal is highly suggestive of increased ICP. Unfortunately, this has not been evaluated in neonatal and pediatric patients. Since the autonomic nervous system does not mature until after 8 weeks of age, there is reason to believe that the Cushing reflex may be unreliable in this age group.

In summary, the magnitude of head trauma can be difficult to assess in neonatal and pediatric patients. Treatment involves optimizing systemic blood pressure using fluids and vasopressors as needed, raising the head 30 degrees without compression of the jugular veins, and optimizing oxygenation and ventilation.

SEPSIS

Most often, neonatal sepsis is secondary to wounds, such as tail docking and umbilical cord ligation, or respiratory and GI infections. Clinical signs, as in hypovolemia, are often subtle, and sepsis can be difficult to detect in this population. Some clinical signs that may be associated with sepsis include crying and reluctance to nurse, decreased urine output, increased lactate, and cold extremities. In humans, three serial C-reactive protein (CRP) levels had a negative predictive value of 99% in neonatal sepsis. Neonates with a suspicion of sepsis had CRP levels evaluated on initial presentation and then 24 and 48 hours later. However, the positive predictive value of elevated CRP levels is low. Lactate is an excellent indicator of hypoperfusion in adults and has been shown to be higher in normal neonatal puppies. Four-day-old puppies had a mean venous blood lactate of 3.83 mmol/L compared to adult values of 1.80 mmol/L. In puppies from 10 to 28 days of age, mean lactate concentration was 2.70 mmol/L.

Aggressive fluid resuscitation is associated with decreased mortality in children with sepsis and in several animal models of sepsis. Large volumes of fluid are often needed in septic patients because of increased capillary permeability (increased losses) and vasodilation. It is suggested to start with a bolus of 45 ml/kg of warm isotonic fluids and monitor serial checks of perfusion via mucous membrane color (should be less pale), pulse quality (should get stronger), extremity temperature (should go up), lactate levels (should go down), and mentation. A CRI of fresh or fresh frozen plasma from a well-vaccinated adult dog has been suggested to attempt to augment "immunity," and some have advocated giving serum from a vaccinated adult subcutaneously. In kittens, both intraperitoneal and subcutaneous administration of adult cat serum in three 5 ml increments (at birth, at 12 hours, and at 24 hours) resulted in immunoglobulin G (IgG) concentrations equivalent to those seen in kittens that suckled normally in one study. Frequent electrolyte and blood glucose checks are essential with supplementation as needed. Warmth and nutrition are addressed as well.

Septic neonates that have been adequately fluid resuscitated and continue to be hypoperfused (i.e., cold extremities, high lactate levels, low urine output, dull mentation, and slightly concentrated urine specific gravity) may benefit from inotropic support. Because of variations in the maturity of the autonomic nervous system, all inotropic drugs need to be individually tailored to each animal. Acceptable endpoints of perfusion include increases in extremity temperature, decreases in lactate levels, increased urine production, and improved attitude.

Ideally, a culture and susceptibility of the area of concern will be submitted before beginning antibiotics. Broad-spectrum antibiotics may be required if the source of infection cannot be identified (see Chapter 27).

Oxygen therapy should be kept at or below a FiO_2 of 0.4 (i.e., 40% inspired oxygen concentration) to avoid oxygen toxicity, which is even more of a concern in neonates than in adults. Excess oxygen supplementation in neonates can cause retrolental fibroplasia, which can lead to permanent blindness in addition to primary pulmonary damage.

Sepsis can be very difficult to detect in neonates. An index of suspicion should be maintained for all neonates with risk factors and treatment should be instituted rapidly and should be aggressive. In humans, the incidence of pediatric sepsis is highest in premature newborns. Respiratory infections and primary bacteremia are the most common infections seen in human neonates.

RESPIRATORY DISTRESS OF THE NEWBORN

According to the most recent guidelines on neonatal resuscitation, "ventilation of the lungs is the single most effective step in cardiopulmonary resuscitation of the compromised infant." If respiratory distress is encountered at birth (Figure 10-3), it may indicate pulmonary hypertension, decreased surfactant levels (prematurity), aspiration of meconium, or excess fluid in the airways. Congenital defects may cause persistent pulmonary hypertension and respiratory distress that is refractory to treatment.

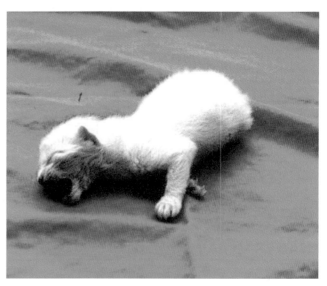

Figure 10-3 Kitten in respiratory distress.

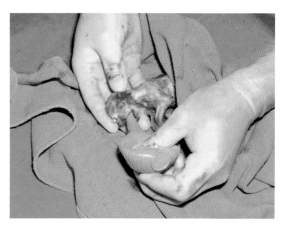

Figure 10-4 Bulb syringe to clear airway.

Emergency treatment of a newborn in respiratory distress starts with reversal of any drugs that were used during anesthesia (if a cesarean section was performed). Airways can be suctioned with a bulb syringe to help clear out any accumulated fluid (Figure 10-4). Aggressive suctioning of the airways (i.e., with a suctioning device) should be avoided as this can cause a vagal response or laryngospasm. Gentle rubbing of the neonate all over can also help stimulate respirations. Shaking or hitting the newborn is contraindicated and can cause loss of surfactant among other complications. Doxapram hydrochloride can be given under the tongue to stimulate respirations in a newborn with no respiratory drive.

Before birth, pulmonary arteries in the fetus have a higher percentage of smooth muscle than do those in adults. The elevated pulmonary vascular resistance that results causes shunting of blood from the pulmonary trunk through the patent ductus arteriosus to the aorta into the systemic circulation. Blood also reaches the systemic circulation via the foramen ovale. At birth, physical expansion of the lungs causes release of prostacyclin, which increases pulmonary blood flow through pulmonary vasodilation. Nitric oxide contributes to pulmonary vasodilation and is thought to be released in response to oxygenation at birth.

Surfactant reduces the tension of the air-fluid interface of the alveoli and prevents collapse. It is essential to improve compliance (i.e., reduce stiffness) and therefore decrease the work of breathing. Surfactant is released at birth in response to lung inflation. Dramatic decreases in pulmonary vascular resistance and adequate surfactant synthesis and release are essential to neonatal survival at birth. The two most important interventions for respiratory distress at birth are oxygenation and lung expansion. These will maximize the release of prostacyclin and nitric oxide and surfactant release.

Oxygen should be supplied via facemask or endotracheal tube, as adequate lung expansion is crucial for pulmonary blood flow. Intubation with an endotracheal (ET) tube is optimal but can be very difficult and frustrating in a newborn. A brief attempt (1 minute or less) should be made to intubate the newborn. If intubation is unsuccessful a tight fitting face mask may be tried. It is often easier than intubation of a newborn and can be lifesaving. Although adequate lung expansion is essential for survival, overexpansion can cause damage so it is essential to use the minimal amount of pressure for ventilation. Use of an ambubag designed for pediatric patients with a pressure gauge attached can minimize damage to the lungs. The neonate should be ventilated at 40 to 60 bpm; this should be done for ≈30 seconds before cardiac compressions are started, if required. If the chest is not expanding check the seal on the face mask or the ET tube placement, re-suction the airway, or consider opening the mouth slightly in animals with small or stenotic nares (e.g., Bulldog pups).

CARDIOPULMONARY CEREBRAL RESUSCITATION

New guidelines for neonatal, pediatric, and adult cardiopulmonary cerebral resuscitation (CPCR) were published in the December 2005 issue of *Circulation*. Veterinary recommendations have adopted some of these guidelines that are particularly pertinent to animals (see Suggested Readings). Important changes include a focus on continual compressions (rather than interrupting them frequently to check other parameters), a more diligent approach to avoiding overventilation (it is associated with higher mortality in animal studies and humans), and immediate resumption of cardiac compressions for 2 minutes after each defibrillation attempt. Resumption of compressions after a defibrillation attempt is associated with a better chance of converting to sinus rhythm (increased perfusion to the heart), and the new guidelines suggest not assessing the rhythm until after 2 minutes of compressions.

Oxygen should be supplied via ET intubation (see section on Respiratory Distress of the Newborn for specific details), and after the initial 40 to 60 bpm during the first 30 seconds, the ventilatory rate should be decreased to 12 to 20 bpm.

In adults, cardiac compressions are only done when the heart is not beating. But cardiac compressions are

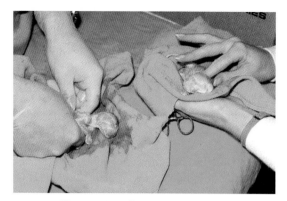

Figure 10-5 Puppy resuscitation.

recommended in human babies when the heart rate remains below 60 bpm after 30 seconds of effective ventilation. Compressions in animals are done with the thumb and forefinger on either side of the thorax with approximately 100 to 120 compressions per minute (Figure 10-5). In a piglet model of cardiac arrest, it was shown that thoracic compressions actually cause cardiac compression (vs. generalized thoracic compression seen in larger animals). IV access is ideal for delivery of drugs for resuscitation, but IO routes also work well. When an IO catheter is placed, it is essential to remove it as soon as possible. In humans, complications of IO catheters are kept to a minimum by removing them within 2 hours. The goal is to use the IO catheter as a bridge to increase volume and make placement of an IV catheter possible.

Epinephrine has both alpha- and beta-adrenergic activity and is the first-line drug during cardiopulmonary arrest. It is started after 30 seconds of chest compressions while the animal is effectively ventilated. The first dose is 0.01 mg/kg and then 0.1 mg/kg for subsequent doses. In humans with cardiopulmonary arrest from asystole, vasopressin has been shown to be slightly superior to epinephrine in one clinical trial. In a pediatric porcine CPCR model, vasopressin combined with epinephrine was superior for resuscitation than either drug alone. Vasopressin is an accepted treatment for children with vasodilatory shock after cardiac surgery and for neonatal congestive heart failure. It was also successful in a case series as a rescue therapy for children after prolonged cardiac arrest. The suggested dosage of vasopressin for CPCR is 0.8 units/kg body weight intravenously. Medications to be administered via the intratracheal (IT) route should be diluted in 5 to 10 ml of sterile water, which is absorbed better than 0.9% NaCl. If sterile water is not available, 0.9% NaCl should be utilized. The dosage should be increased 2 to 2.5 times the IV dosage for IT administration, with the exception of epinephrine, which should be increased by 3 to 10 times the IV dosage (0.03 to 0.1 mg/kg). In human and animal studies, lower dose epinephrine administered via the IT route caused hypotension and decreased cerebral perfusion pressure, due to transient beta-adrenergic effects.

Acidosis caused by decreased perfusion (i.e., lactic acidosis) and decreased ventilation (i.e., respiratory acidosis) is common during cardiopulmonary arrest and ideally should be addressed by treating the primary problems (i.e., increasing perfusion and ventilation). Severe acidosis can decrease myocardial contractility, which could be critical in neonates who have a lower percentage of myocardial contractile fibers than adults. It can also blunt responses to catecholamines, which again is critical in neonates who have a lower percentage of sympathetic fibers in their myocardia compared to adults. The use of buffers (e.g., sodium bicarbonate) is controversial because they increase sodium levels, cause hyperosmolality, can cause paradoxic central nervous system (CNS) and intracellular acidosis, and increase carbon dioxide. The guidelines from the American Heart Association Manual on Neonatal Advanced Life Support in humans do not recommend bicarbonate as front-line therapy because of lack of evidence for its efficacy.

Glucose is the main energy substrate of the neonatal brain and myocardium and should be monitored frequently during an arrest and supplemented as needed. Ionized calcium has been shown to be low in human neonates. Neonates also have an increased requirement for calcium for contractility compared to adults. Calcium has not been shown to be beneficial in adult CPCR and is not recommended for cardiopulmonary arrest in humans. Future trials may suggest a beneficial effect in neonatal CPCR, but no information is available currently.

Arrhythmias

Although rhythm analysis is important and ECG assessment should occur early in CPA, it should be done as briefly as possible to avoid impeding chest compressions. The four rhythms of concern during pulseless cardiac arrest are asystole, ventricular tachycardia, ventricular fibrillation, and pulseless electrical activity (PEA).

Asystole and Pulseless Electrical Activity

In adult dogs and cats, asystole is the most common arrest rhythm and the author is not aware of data on arrest rhythms in pediatric companion animals. Asystole can result from disease processes, trauma, and increased vagal tone. Resuscitation efforts should be directed at performing high-quality CPCR with minimal interruptions and to identify and treat reversible causes or complicating factors. No medications have proved effective in the treatment of asystole in neonatal and pediatric patients.

Pulseless electrical activity (PEA; previously called electrical mechanical dissociation) is the condition in which there is absence of myocardial contractility despite a normal heart rate and rhythm on an ECG. Under the new guidelines, asystole is combined with PEA, as well as several other rhythms, including idioventricular rhythms and ventricular escape rhythms. No medications have proven effective in the treatment of PEA (i.e., defibrillation is not beneficial), and resuscitation should focus on performing high-quality CPCR and treatment of reversible causes or complicating factors.

Ventricular Tachycardia

Ventricular tachycardia, caused by repetitive firing of an ectopic focus or foci in the ventricular myocardium or Purkinje system, is dangerous and can precipitate ventricular fibrillation. There are multiple causes of ventricular tachycardia, including hypoxia, pain, ischemia, sepsis, electrolyte changes, trauma, and primary cardiac disease. Treatment of the underlying cause should be attempted first and all abnormalities addressed before instituting specific antiarrhythmic treatment.

Ventricular Fibrillation

Ventricular fibrillation is unorganized ventricular excitation resulting in poorly synchronized and inadequate myocardial contractions that causes cardiac pump failure. Sudden loss of cardiac output leads to global tissue ischemia, with the brain and myocardium being the most susceptible. Defibrillation is an electrophysiologic event that occurs several milliseconds after the delivery of a defibrillatory shock. Ventricular fibrillation is more responsive early and should be identified as soon as possible.

Chest compressions should be performed while the defibrillator is being connected and charged. With a manual defibrillator, the defibrillator operator selects the shock energy (in joules); however, it is the amplitude of current flow (in amperes) that causes depolarization of the myocardium and results in defibrillation. Alcohol, ultrasound gel, or other nonconductive gels should not be used on electrode paddles. Conductive paste should be applied liberally to the paddles or self-adhesive pads should be used. The largest electrode paddles or pad that will fit on the patient's chest should be used because small electrodes may cause myocardial necrosis. The patient should be placed in dorsal recumbency, and then the paddles are placed with pressure on opposite sides of the chest.

When the defibrillator is charged, "clear" should be shouted to warn personnel to cease contact with the patient and anything connected to the patient, and then one shock should be administered as quickly as possible. The person administering the shock must avoid contact with the patient and everything connected to the patient. The initial countershock energy for external defibrillation is 2 to 5 J/kg. The energy of the countershock for internal defibrillation is $\frac{1}{10}$ of the dose for external defibrillation (0.2 to 0.5 J/kg).

To minimize the interruption in chest compressions, one shock should be administered, rather than the three successive shocks previously recommended. Chest compressions should immediately be resumed for 2 minutes before reassessing the cardiac rhythm and administration of an additional shock.

CONCLUSION

The unique anatomic and physiologic characteristics of neonatal and pediatric patients make diagnosis, monitoring, and treatment very challenging. Adult parameters cannot be used in these patients, and an awareness of the specific differences is essential for any practitioner with a neonatal and pediatric patient base. In addition, many laboratory and pharmacologic data differ dramatically in neonates compared to adults of the same species. New CPCR guidelines are significantly different, and familiarity with the variations in treatment of CPCR and other illnesses, such as hypovolemia, shock, head trauma, and sepsis, is essential to assure maximum chances of success in this age group.

SUGGESTED READINGS

McMichael M: Critically ill pediatric patients. In Silverstein DC, Hopper K (eds): *Small animal critical care medicine,* St. Louis, 2008, Saunders/Elsevier.

McMichael M: Pediatric emergencies, *Vet Clin Small Anim* 35(2):421, 2005.

Plunkett S, McMichael M. Cardiopulmonary resuscitation in small animal medicine: an update, *J Vet Intern Med* 22:9, 2008.

NEONATAL MORTALITY

CHAPTER 11

Michael E. Peterson

Owners frequently present a dead puppy or kitten to the veterinarian, seeking the cause of death. The veterinarian should always remember that the dead neonate is the end result of a process that may have been mediated by problems with the owner, stud, dam, environment, or the neonate itself. This stark fact dictates that a systematic, methodical approach be employed in pursuing a diagnosis for puppy and kitten losses. Even then, there are many deaths whose etiology escapes discovery.

The primary chronologic benchmarks for neonatal survival generally are birth, the first 24 hours, the first week, and weaning. The neonatal mortality rate for each of these benchmarks decreases as the neonate progresses along the timeline; 75% of puppy deaths occur in the first 3 weeks of life, 50% of neonatal deaths happen in the first 3 days, and 65% in the first week. In some studies, stillbirth accounts for 50% of the losses (Table 11-1).

The vast majority of these early losses are due to neonatal hypoxia, malnutrition, and hypothermia. Mortality can be caused by dystocia, physiologic abnormalities, environmental problems, genetic issues, infections, and behavior abnormalities. Some dams historically have increased rates of fading puppies and kittens.

The majority of the factors responsible for early mortality are centered on poor management and suboptimal husbandry. Certain breeds are known for increased neonatal mortality such as the brachiocephalic breeds in both dogs and cats. Some breeds are known anecdotally for early whelping with an increased number of weak puppies, for example, the Cavalier King Charles Spaniel. Likewise, the Norwich/Norfolk Terriers and the Schipperke have reputations among breeders for delayed onset of puppy deaths (fading puppies), beginning at 2 and 3 weeks of age.

The veterinarian may be presented with a dead neonate by a wide variety of owners. Sometimes, the breeder has significant financial interest in the litter and is seeking a specific diagnosis as a long-term herd health business solution. Other times, a new owner wants to know why the neonate has died; those cases in which a newly purchased pet is involved can carry an increased risk of litigation between the owner and breeder (the classic financial interest and who is paying for this scenario). Occasionally, owners let their dog/cat have one litter to show their children the miracle of life and were ill prepared for the miracle of death and desperately looking for a cause of death to answer their children's questions. The extent that each of these owners is willing to pursue a diagnosis varies. Often, no answer is found. The local diagnostic laboratory can provide guidelines on sample preparation before submission; following guidelines can increase the probability of obtaining a specific diagnosis (see Chapter 29).

The key to enhancing the probability of finding the etiology for neonatal puppy and kitten deaths is to obtain a quality history through encompassing questions regarding the owner, stud, dam, and environment. Physical examination of a dead neonate is usually insufficient to determine the cause of death. Use of a quality diagnostic laboratory for a complete necropsy and special studies, if indicated, is usually required. A full physical examination of the mother and living siblings can be extremely informative and should be performed.

The diagnostic approach to neonatal death is dictated by several factors. The loss of a single puppy or kitten often offers a different problem set than multiple deaths in a litter. Is a single death strictly an individual problem or is it the first in a series of multiple deaths? Is the body in good condition and weight or is it emaciated? Was the dead offspring the largest, fastest-growing littermate or was it always the smallest, weakest "runt"? These and many other questions need to be answered.

TABLE 11-1 Summary of 421 puppy deaths	
Age	Number (%)
Parturition (stillbirth)	126 (29.9)
Days 0-3 (live birth)	209 (49)
Days 4-28	71 (16.9)
Days 29-42	5 (1.2)
Days 42-45 (postweaning)	10 (2.4)

From Lawler DF: Neonatal and pediatric care of the puppy and kitten, *Theriogenology* 70(3):384-392, 2008.

BOX 11-1   Owner-related questions

- How experienced is the owner at breeding dogs/cats?
- How experienced is the owner with this breed?
- Was this a planned litter? Inbreeding coefficient?
- How experienced is the owner with managing litters?
- How experienced is the owner at helping deliver newborns?
- Did the owner physically have to help with the delivery of the litter?
- Were airways suctioned and umbilical cords disinfected?

OWNER ISSUES

A thorough history includes information on the experience and management approach of the owner. It is important to know if this was a planned breeding and if the owners have any pedigree information, since matings with high inbreeding coefficients have smaller litter sizes and increased neonatal mortality. Was the owner present at the whelping or queening? Is there a mortality history of previous litters managed by the owner? Was this a planned breeding? Was the breeding timed so a known birthing date was available? Did the owner try to treat the dam or offspring; if so, with what medication or nutraceutical? How closely are the newborns monitored, are they out in the garage or is the owner sleeping next to the whelping box in the family room? A wide variety of questions about owners and their involvement in the breeding, delivery, and postbirthing management of the newborns can elicit important data in determining the cause of neonatal mortality. Box 11-1 lists common, relevant questions for owners.

STUD ISSUES

The impact of the stud is not generally considered by owners as a possible cause of neonatal mortality. However, owners often acquire a stud with no previous health or reproductive history. Additionally, they may use a male from some other facility, with a minimum of testing for preexisting diseases, which may affect his fertility and/or the health of the dam and offspring. The stud's age, size, and health all contribute to neonatal losses. Questions that should be pursued relative to the stud are listed in Box 11-2.

BOX 11-2   Stud-related questions

- How old is the stud?
- How long has the owner had the stud?
- Where was the stud acquired?
- Is the stud previously proven?
- How often has this stud been used?
- What is his reproductive history (i.e., average litter size)?
- Is there any mortality data on his previous litters?
- What was the stud's health before breeding?
- Is the stud currently healthy?
- Was the stud tested for communicable diseases before breeding?
- Is the stud significantly larger or smaller than the dam?
- What is the tom's blood type?

BOX 11-3   Environmental causes of neonatal mortality

- Low ambient temperature/draft
- High ambient temperature
- Poor whelping box design
- Poor bedding material
- Improper hygiene
- Stressful location

ENVIRONMENTAL ISSUES

Early, preweaning neonatal vulnerability is influenced most by the dam and the environment into which the neonates are born (Box 11-3).

Incorrect environmental temperatures can have devastating impacts on neonates. Puppies and kittens are unable to shiver or generate much heat by movement in the first 6 days of life. When temperatures are low, their immunity and metabolism are significantly decreased. If the neonate's temperature is less than 94° F (34.4° C), intestinal ileus develops, shutting down the digestive process. Hyperthermic environments can stress the dam, and she may be resistant to lying close to her puppies or kittens. Additionally, hyperthermia can also lead to neonatal dehydration.

Poor whelping or nesting box design can be a major source of neonatal mortality. If the box is too large, the chances for a neonate to get separated from the mother are increased. If the box is too small, the chances of neonates being stepped on or laid on is increased. Whelping or nesting boxes without "hog rails" (Figure 11-1) increase the probability of neonates being crushed against the wall by their mother. Additionally, the whelping box should be made of materials that are easily cleaned and disinfected and do not retain moisture.

Improper placement of the whelping box can heighten the mother's stress level, particularly if the area is loud, with lots of human and/or animal traffic. Stressful locations or environments have the potential to increase neonatal

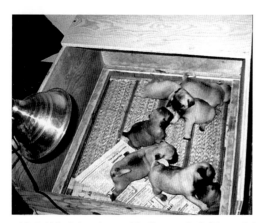

Figure 11-1 Whelping box with "hog rails." (From Johnston SD, Root Kustritz MV, Olsen PNS: *Canine and feline theriogenology*, St Louis, 2001, Saunders/Elsevier.)

TABLE 11-2	Disinfectants*
Disinfectant	**Effective spectrum of activity**
Phenolics	Most bacteria except spore formers, possibly some viruses
Alkalis	Most bacteria, some spore formers, some viruses
Chlorine	Wide bacterial spectrum, viruses and protozoa, little activity vs. spore formers†
Chloramine	Most bacteria
Quaternary ammonium	Most bacteria, some viruses†
Chlorhexidine	Most bacteria and fungi, poor on spore formers or viruses†
Hydrogen peroxide	Most bacteria, spore formers and virus

*Use at manufacturer's recommended concentration.
†Significantly decreased activity in organic material.

BOX 11-4	Environmental questions

- Where were the neonates born?
- Do they have a proper whelping or nesting box?
- Does the nesting box have "hog rails"?
- Are the neonates kept in a warm area?
- How is the temperature regulated?
- Is the area free of drafts?
- Is the bedding appropriate?
- What schedule is used for changing bedding?
- What schedule is used for cleaning?
- What schedule is used for disinfecting?
- What cleaning agents are used (concentrations)?
- What disinfectant agents are used (concentrations)?
- What strategies are employed to minimize stress?
- How quiet is the area where the neonates are kept?
- How closely are the newborns monitored?
- Are there lots of visitors?
- Are there children in the home? What are their ages and do they have access to the newborns?
- How much handling are the newborns exposed to?

mortality. Stress elevates the anxiety of the dam, which can promote poor mothering and decrease milk let-down. Anxious mothers do not quietly lie with their offspring, instead, they are up and down and very restless, which means the young are at increased risk of being stepped on and cannot settle in for quality nursing. Poor whelping box placement can also allow drafts from open doors or windows in other locations in the building.

Improper bedding materials can allow neonates to become buried or lost and unable to find their mothers and therefore are unable to nurse, becoming both hypoglycemic and hypothermic. Poor bedding retains moisture and dissipates the heat away from the puppies, allowing increased bacterial growth. Regardless of how appropriate the bedding material is, it must be kept cleaned or changed frequently or it can contribute to higher neonatal death rates.

Proper environmental hygiene is paramount, since puppies and kittens have a variety of structural, metabolic, and immune conditions that although normal for their age, makes them more susceptible to infectious disease. Proper selection of disinfectants is important; however, care should be taken to keep these from becoming environmental toxins (Table 11-2). Neonates have very thin skin and transdermally absorb toxins more readily than adults. The owner should be particularly careful with cleaning agents such as pine oils and phenols. Overuse of bleach or other disinfectants or employing high concentrations of these products puts the neonates at risk. Few disinfectants work well in the face of organic debris, therefore proper cleaning should occur before disinfecting the area (Box 11-4).

Kennels that seem to have elevated neonatal losses may benefit from a site visit. The veterinarian should develop a systematic checklist to aid in the kennel inspection. Box 11-5 lists some relevant issues for site visits.

NUTRITIONAL ISSUES

Neonates have minimal body fat, and this places them at great risk for hypoglycemia when coupled with a diminished capacity to metabolically generate glucose. Glycogen stores are quickly depleted in the newborn; therefore it is imperative that they nurse relatively soon after birth. Hypoglycemia can develop in these patients from a variety of etiologies, including endotoxemia, septicemia, portosystemic hepatic shunts, and glycogen storage problems.

The risk of dehydration is high in newborns. Since 82% of their weight is water, glomerular filtration rates (GFRs) are 21% those of the adult at birth, but GFRs increase in function to 53% by 8 weeks of age.

Puppies and kittens are particularly at risk at the time of weaning. This is very stressful to the neonate, depressing its immune system at a time that its gastrointestinal (GI) tract is responding to a new nutrient substrate.

BOX 11-5	Site visit checklist

- General kennel hygiene
- Where are the pregnant dams housed?
- Where does birthing occur?
- Nesting (whelping) box
  - Location
  - Drafts
  - Construction material
  - Traffic: human and animal
  - Stressors
  - Bedding: type and changing schedule
- Heat source: type and location
- How are mothers kept confined with newborns?
- Cleaners: type and schedule
- Disinfectants: type, concentration, and schedule
- Ventilation

BOX 11-6	Maternal causes of neonatal mortality

Agalactia
Mastitis
Crazy bitch
Eclampsia
Poor mothering skills
Diabetes mellitus in bitch
Uterine inflammations
Obesity
Dystocia
Premature delivery
No or poor-quality colostrum

BOX 11-7	Dam-related questions

- How long has owner had dam?
- Where did the owner acquire the dam? How long ago?
- Was she purchased pregnant?
- How old is the dam?
- What breed is the dam? What breed is the stud?
- Did dam survive delivery of newborns?
- How many previous litters?
- What are normal litter sizes?
- Mortality history of previous litters?
- Was this a planned breeding?
- Is this the dam's first litter? First heat cycle?
- Was or is the dam receiving any medication?
- Was delivery on time (early or late)?
- What is the dam's general health?
- What is the dam's vaccine and worming history?
- What is the dam's medical history, any underlying disease?
- Was the dam tested for communicable diseases before breeding?
- What is the dam's general body condition? Is it appropriate to litter size?
- Was it a natural or surgical delivery?
- What was the dam's diet when pregnant?
- What is the dam's diet after delivery?
- Did the dam have good colostrum volume?
- Did/does the dam have good milk supply?
- Does the dam show good mothering skills?
- Is there any evidence of eclampsia or preeclamptic activity?
- What is the queen's blood type?

MATERNAL ISSUES

A wide variety of maternal issues can affect neonatal mortality (Box 11-6). Fetal death can be due to poor uterine health, which can interfere with proper placental and/or fetal blood flow with subsequent hypoxia or nutritional interference. Any issue that impacts normal birthing directly affects mortality rates. These are the classic dystocia issues, including a narrow birth canal, abnormal pelvic shape, vaginal canal malformation, primary or secondary uterine inertia, abnormal fetal presentation, and uterine torsion. Additionally, conditions that may initiate early parturition and delivery of premature offspring can be a significant cause of mortality. If the condition is slower in onset and stresses the fetus, it is possible for surfactant production to be induced. These puppies and kittens are born with low birth weights and are usually weaker than term neonates.

The highest mortality rates occur with the first litter and are lowest with the fifth litter in dogs. The highest feline mortality rate is in single kitten litters, and loss rates are lowest in five-kitten litters. Additionally, older bitches or queens have decreased litter sizes and increased neonatal death rates.

The dam should be presented for a full veterinary examination, along with the dead neonate and its siblings. Many clues can be obtained from the physical examination and complete history relative to the dam. Pertinent information can be obtained from the guidelines for questions relative to the dam's history presented in Box 11-7.

Maternal obesity decreases litter size, and overweight bitches and queens have a higher neonatal mortality rate. Another maternal nutritional issue is eclampsia caused by imbalances in maternal calcium metabolism (particularly in small dogs). The early signs of eclampsia are often restlessness and irritability, which can be a significant contributor to poor mothering. Restless mothers and "crazy bitches" who attack their offspring (these are often medium, small [Terrier-sized] dogs) are on the verge of the muscle cramping and seizing of full-onset eclampsia. These dogs may have serum calcium levels in the normal range; however, they seem to be calcium responsive and often lay quietly with their offspring shortly after oral calcium administration.

Some bitches and queens are inexperienced or poor mothers and accidentally step or lay on their young. Some dams will try to cull specific neonates from the litter. It is possible that they can detect some underlying problem in the neonate; however, some of these offspring can be rehabilitated back on to the dam.

Mothers with poor nutritional status give birth to weak offspring with higher mortality incidents. Poor nutritional and vaccine status can contribute to insufficient quality colostrum, leading to failure of passive transfer of immunity to the puppies and kittens.

Progesterone levels during pregnancy interfere with the action of insulin and can induce maternal diabetes mellitus. Maternal diabetes mellitus can result in larger neonates, thereby increasing the risk of dystocia. Hypothyroid mothers have smaller, weaker puppies and a higher neonatal death rate.

Mammary issues can also contribute to neonatal mortality. Mastitis can occur at any time, causing offspring to stop nursing or to develop gastroenteritis. Puppies and kittens with erupted canine teeth can cause trauma to the mammary gland and induce mastitis in their dams. Agalactia may occur transiently in very stressed dams; however, some mothers fail to produce milk. Agalactia would seem to be an easy condition to evaluate; however, it is often overlooked in the diagnostic workup. Every mother should have her mammary glands examined daily and more frequently when offspring are restless and crying.

NEONATAL ISSUES

The most dominant neonatal prognostic factors related to mortality are low birth weight and failure to thrive (slow growth rates). In one study of 477 kittens, 60% of those with low birth weight failed to survive to weaning. Primary neonatal problems in puppies and kittens are usually caused by hypoxia, hypoglycemia, hypothermia, poor hydration, infection, and improper nutrition (Box 11-8).

Large litters are difficult for mothers to manage, with a resultant increase in neonatal losses. Dams accidentally sit on or step on neonates in these large litters. Stronger neonates dominate nipples and grow faster than their smaller siblings, who then fail to thrive and grow because of restricted nutrition. If owners are not vigilant, these weaker individuals are at higher risk of early death. Any neonate who is constantly crying indicates that they are either cold or hungry; occasionally, they are sick, but in any event they need immediate attention.

Owners should be queried about birth weights of the neonates. Even if the owner does not have actual weights, they may be able to subjectively describe the newborns as fat and vigorous or thin and weak. Box 11-9 lists neonatal-relevant questions.

Anoxia may occur as the result of low surfactant levels, atelectasis, pulmonary air leaks, meconium aspiration, fluid aspiration, anemia, and pulmonary hemorrhage. Pulmonary hemorrhage can be caused by a variety of factors such as trauma or coagulopathies. Weak contractions of the intercostal muscles or diaphragm can inhibit proper pulmonary function.

Some puppies and kittens fail to thrive, which can be induced by several factors such as congenital malformations, thymic insufficiency, hypocalcemia, and various metabolic disorders. Toy dog breeds have exhibited a fatty liver syndrome at 4 to 16 weeks of age that can be fatal.

Puppies and kittens who fail to ingest or absorb colostrum within the first 12 to 24 hours are at high risk for

---

BOX 11-8   **Neonatal causes of mortality**

Failure of passive immunity
Low birth weight
Hypoglycemia
Neonatal isoerythrolysis (kittens)
Dehydration (feeding errors)
Hypothermia
Meconium aspiration
Persistent pulmonary hypertension of newborn
Atelectasis
Traumatic birth injuries
Bleeding disorders
Congenital anatomic defects
Thymic insufficiency
Respiratory distress
Air leaks
Disorders of cardiovascular system
Hepatic disorders
Hypocalcemia
Metabolic disorders (inborn errors)

BOX 11-9   **Neonate-related questions**

- What was the litter size
- Was the delivery early or late?
- Is the neonate nursing?
- What was the neonate's general condition when born?
- What was the birth weight?
- Was there a size disparity within the litter?
- Was it an easy or difficult birth?
- What was the method of birth (natural vs. surgical)?
- If surgical delivery, what type of anesthesia was used and were any postoperative medications used?
- Who did umbilical separation (owner or dam)? Was it disinfected?
- Was there one puppy death or were there multiple puppy deaths?
- Were the puppies robust or weak, and then started dying?
- Was colostrum ingested?
- Has the owner noticed evidence of trauma?
- Has the owner noticed any evidence of medical issues (milk out nose, increased respiratory rate, and so on)?
- How long has the neonate been sick or was the neonate unthrifty before death?
- What is the age when deaths started occurring?
- Did the owner provide any medication?

infection as the result of failure of passive transfer. Testing neonates' blood levels of hepatic enzymes, alkaline phosphatase (ALP) and gamma-glutamyl-transpeptidase (GGT), can show if colostrum has been ingested. Often, the enzyme levels after colostrum ingestion in these individuals are many times higher than normal adult levels (see Chapter 30).

Congenital problems that are severe enough to cause death are estimated to occur at a rate of 1% to 2% in pedigree puppies. These congenital defects can be either genetic or nongenetic. Nongenetic defects can be induced with drugs, toxin exposures, or nutritional issues such as ingesting high levels of vitamin A. There are many common congenital conditions, as well as a tremendous number of uncommon congenital conditions. The most common would include swimmer puppy syndrome, water puppy syndrome, cleft palate, hepatic vascular shunt, cardiac vascular abnormalities (e.g., patent ductus arteriosus, persistent right aortic arch), and spinal dysraphism.

Traumatic injuries, such as birth injuries, maternal trauma, or littermate-induced trauma (from sucking on each other), can be a major source of early mortality.

Neonatal isoerythrolysis can be a cause of death in kittens (usually purebred kittens). This condition occurs when kittens with group A blood type receive colostrum from queens with group A alloantibodies. These kittens are born healthy but develop a hemolytic crisis several hours after colostrum ingestion. Neonatal isoerythrolysis can occur in blood type A kittens born to blood type B queens who were bred to toms with blood type A. The blood of these kittens is attacked by the antibodies received from the queen's colostrum. Siamese cats and those related breeds, such as Tonkinese, Oriental Shorthair, Burmese, and American Shorthair, only have group A blood type.

INFECTIOUS ISSUES

Owners usually suspect the cause of early mortality to be infectious disease. However, the results of postmortem examination by the pathology laboratory often fail to find an infectious etiology for the demise of the patient. Additionally, infectious disease may be the cause of death, but poor husbandry or other factors may be the primary issue that allows the infection to occur initially. Umbilical infections are often the initial cause of septicemia, and owners should be asked if the cords were disinfected at birth.

Boxes 11-10 and 11-11 list some common causes of infectious diseases involved in neonatal and pediatric deaths (see Chapters 15, 16, 17, and 18).

Many breeders are aggressive in requiring dams to be tested for communicable diseases, such as *Brucella canis*, but dam owners do not seem to have the same rigorous requirement of studs servicing their queens or bitches. Additionally, some kennels and catteries may bring in new animals to their

---

BOX 11-10 Common infectious causes of canine neonatal mortality

Herpesvirus
Parvovirus
Infectious canine hepatitis
Canine distemper
Septicemia

BOX 11-11 Common infectious causes of feline neonatal mortality

Upper respiratory infection
Panleukopenia (parvovirus)
Feline leukemia virus
Feline infectious peritonitis
Bartonella sp.
Bacterial or viral septicemia

---

facilities while the dams are pregnant or after litters are born. These new animals may be carriers of diseases that will put the newborns at risk. Many owners do a poor job of quarantining these new animals and do not immediately see the possible connection with neonatal losses.

Parasitic infections and/or infestations can be a major cause of puppy and kitten mortality. Internal parasites can be passed in utero to the fetus, and infestations of other internal parasites can occur when animals are born into contaminated environments. Package inserts should always be read because some medications used for external or internal parasite control for the mother can be passed in the milk to the neonate at levels capable of inducing toxicity (see Chapter 19).

Puppies and kittens are born with a higher red blood cell count (most likely from living in a relatively hypoxic environment); as they age, their hematocrit decreases to a nadir at about 7 weeks (approximate packed cell volume of 20%). This is the reason they are so susceptible to fatal flea infestation anemia at this age.

SUGGESTED READINGS

Abrams-Ogg A: Fading neonatal puppy and kitten. In Mathews KA (ed): *Veterinary emergency critical care manual,* ed 2, Guelph, Ontario, 2006, Lifelearn.

Hoskins JD: Puppy and kitten losses. In Hoskins JD (ed): *Veterinary pediatrics: dogs and cats from birth to six months,* ed 3, Philadelphia, 2001, Saunders/Elsevier.

Johnston SD, Root Kustritz MV, Olsen PNS: *Canine and feline theriogenology,* St Louis, 2001, Saunders/Elsevier.

Rickard V: Neonatal losses. In Cote E (ed): *Clinical veterinary advisor: dogs and cats,* St Louis, 2007, Mosby/Elsevier.

FELINE BEHAVIORAL DEVELOPMENT

CHAPTER 12

Lisa Radosta

Feline behavioral development mirrors the kitten's neurologic and musculoskeletal development. As the kitten gains the ability to perceive objects visually, investigative behavior increases. Likewise, as the kitten gains motor skills, play develops. Weaning precipitates many changes in the kitten's development such as predatory behavior. Soon, the kitten develops voluntary elimination and an elimination substrate preference is not far behind. From gestation onward, any interruption in nutrition, care, or exposure to necessary stimuli can result in behavioral abnormalities later in life. This chapter examines the behavioral development of kittens and the common behavioral disorders that may arise as a result of abnormal development and lack of proper exposure.

PRENATAL FACTORS

The factors that affect a kitten's behavioral development and subsequent behavior as an adult begin in utero. Kittens from undernourished mothers not only exhibit abnormal physical development but also abnormal behavioral development. When queens were fed one-half of their ad libitum intake during the second half of gestation and the first 6 weeks of nursing, serious behavioral changes were seen in the kittens when compared with queens who had adequate nourishment. Even after being fed a nutritionally appropriate diet for 10 weeks, kittens were more prone to accidents when playing and performed poorly on certain behavioral tests. In addition, male kittens showed increased aggressive social play and females showed less climbing behavior and more random running. Multiple factors have been shown to cause behavioral changes in kittens from undernourished mothers, including abnormal development of the cerebrum, cerebellum, and brainstem, fewer queen/kitten interactions, and increased irritability/aggression of the queen toward the kittens. If queens are nutritionally restricted to one-half of their ad libitum food intake during the entire gestation period, kittens show delayed posturing, crawling, suckling, eye opening, running, playing, climbing, and predatory and exploratory behavior. In addition, these kittens have difficulty learning new tasks and exhibit fear, aggression, antisocial behavior, and increased reactivity toward stimuli. Unfortunately, many kittens are adopted from litters of feral queens who had a poor plane of nutrition, leaving them predisposed to behavior problems. Kittens of queens subjected to severe nutritional restriction have suppressed play, whereas kittens from queens who had a less restricted but less than adequate diet show increased contact play. Although developmental changes may be obvious early in life, behavioral changes may not be brought to the veterinarian's attention until adulthood when a behavior problem has become chronic or unbearable for the owner. Although it can be challenging to obtain an accurate history of a chronic behavior problem, it is critical that an extensive history be taken with all behavior appointments, regardless of the age of the animal, so that early life experiences can be taken into account. This allows the clinician to educate the owner on the factors that have caused the final, intolerable behavior and construct an accurate diagnosis list and treatment plan.

Another factor shown to increase reactivity in rats that most likely occurs in other mammals, including cats, is the degree of physiologic and psychological stress of the mother during gestation and nursing. In general, when gestating mammalian mothers are chronically stressed, anxious, or fearful, the offspring exhibit increased reactivity to stimuli, increased emotionality, and decreased learning. As the brain of the fetus develops, it is subjected to the hormones that are secreted by the mother. The brains of neonates and nursing animals whose mothers are under stress are organized differently than the brains of those whose mothers are not. Animals subjected to stress release endogenous glucocorticoids as part of the normal physiologic stress response. When the animal is a gestating mother, those glucocorticoids are passed on to the neonate. It is postulated that the increase in endogenous glucocorticoids chronically causes an impairment of the negative feedback mechanism of the hypothalamic-pituitary-adrenal (HPA) axis in the offspring. This in turn causes the offspring of stressed mothers to respond with increased reactivity when placed in situations in which they are under stress. Depending on when the physiologic or psychological stress occurs in gestation, the changes in the HPA axis of the offspring can be permanent. This "up-regulation" of the HPA axis is suspected to underlie many behavioral problems in animals that involve impulsivity and aggression. Typical feline behavioral disorders of this type include fear-related aggression, conflict-related aggression, predatory aggression, and redirected aggression to people or other animals.

Clinical Implications: Stressed/ Undernourished Queen

Some potential cat owners search out a breeder when they are thinking of adopting a kitten, whereas most find kittens born to stray/feral queens or adopt kittens from a humane shelter, rescue organization, or veterinary office. Subsequently, many kittens that are adopted are born to queens who have a poor plane of nutrition and/or who are anxious or frightened during gestation and nursing. If possible, these kittens should be adopted into a household in which the owners are aware of potential problems such as increased reactivity, fear, and aggressive play. Kittens of this type should be socialized as soon as possible, and socialization should continue past 9 weeks of age (see section on Socialization). In addition, each member of the household should be consistent and structured in their interactions with the kitten. The kitten should have a very enriched environment. Many toys and multiple resting and hiding spaces should be offered so that the kitten does not learn inappropriate behavior.

EARLY DEVELOPMENT

The early behavioral development of the kitten is guided by the extent to which other body systems and senses have developed. In addition, other factors, such as the variability of the kitten's environment, handling, genetics, age of the queen, mothering style of the queen, weaning, sex of the kitten, and exposure to stimuli, all influence the kitten's development. Kittens are altricial, which means that they are born relatively helpless with eyes and ears closed; however, tactile sensitivity is present. Until the kitten is 2 weeks old, tactile, thermal, and olfactory senses guide its behavior (Table 12-1). The kitten's development is divided into stages: neonatal, transitional, socialization, juvenile, and adulthood. The neonatal stage lasts from 0 to 9 days of age. For the most part, the kitten is completely dependent on the mother at this stage and spends most of its time nursing and sleeping. The transitional stage is the stage between complete reliance on the mother and the beginning of independence for the kitten. It lasts from 10 to 14 days of age. The eyes open during this stage, and the kitten begins to orient to sounds. The socialization period lasts from the second to the seventh

TABLE 12-1	Feline behavioral development (birth to 23 weeks)
Age	**Behavior**
0 days	Moves toward warmth
2 days	Purring starts
5 days	Responds to sounds
10 days	Conditioned responses to sounds
2 weeks	Orients to sound
2-3 weeks	Oral grooming emerges
2-7 weeks	Sensitive period for socialization
0-3 weeks	Orients to nest using olfactory/thermal
3 weeks	Visual orienting and following objects
	Olfactory system fully developed
	Weaning begins
	Rudimentary walking emerges
	Orientation to nest visual
	Play 4×/day
3-4 weeks	Social play emerges
3-5 weeks	Voluntary elimination
4 weeks	Adult-like orienting
	Weaning begins
	Queen brings live prey to the nest
	Solitary play begins to decline
	Group play is common
4-5 weeks	Visual orienting/obstacle avoidance
	Learn tasks with visual cues alone
5 weeks	Running emerges
	Starts to kill prey
5-6 weeks	Hides while playing
	Elimination substrate preference begins to develop
6 weeks	Mild piloerection to cat silhouette
6-8 weeks	Adult-like response to threatening visual and olfactory stimuli
7 weeks	Weaning complete
	Gape is fully expressed
7-8 weeks	Adult sleep patterns
	Object/locomotor play emerges
8 weeks	Paired play is most common
9 weeks	Play for 1 hr/day (4 bouts)
12-14 weeks	Social play declines
4 months	Solitary play declines
19 weeks	Males show sexual behavior
23 weeks	Females show sexual behavior

week of age. This period is filled with exploration, development of locomotor function, formation of social relationships, development of predatory behavior, and increased motor skills. The juvenile stage starts at the end of the socialization stage and extends to sexual maturity (7 to 12 months of age) when adulthood begins.

By 5 days of age, kittens respond to sounds; by 10 days of age, they have the ability to exhibit conditioned responses to sounds (Box 12-1); and by 2 weeks of age, they orient to

BOX 12-1   Conditioning 101

The laws of conditioning are in play as long as the cat is awake and interacting with someone or the environment.

Classical Conditioning
A neutral stimulus is paired with an event that causes an unconditioned response until the neutral stimulus becomes the trigger for the unconditioned response.
- Example: The sound of a can opener (i.e., neutral stimulus) is paired with food (i.e., positive event), which causes an unconditioned response (i.e., salivation). Eventually, the can opener will cause the cat to salivate, regardless of whether food is presented each time or not.

Operant Conditioning
A neutral stimulus is paired with a conditioned response followed by a consequence.
- Example: The cat is told to sit (i.e., neutral stimulus) while being lured into a sit position (i.e., eventual conditioned response). When he is sitting, he is given a cat treat (i.e., consequence).
- Operant conditioning depends on the type of reinforcement used.

Positive Reinforcement
- Something rewarding is added to the behavior to increase the likelihood that the behavior will occur in the future.
- Example: The owner calls the cat's name → the cat comes to the owner → the owner gives the cat canned food. The cat is more likely to come to the owner when she calls in the future.

Negative Reinforcement
- An aversive (something that the cat does not like) is removed to increase the likelihood that the behavior will increase in the future.
- Example: The cat is restrained for vaccinations at the veterinary hospital → during restraint, the cat hisses and struggles → he is let up. The cat is more likely to hiss and struggle at the next veterinary examination.

Positive Punishment
- An aversive (something that the cat does not like) is added to the situation to decrease the likelihood that a behavior will occur.
- Example: The cat jumps on the counter → the owner squirts him with water. The cat is less likely to jump on the counter in the presence of the owner in the future.

Negative Punishment
- Something rewarding to the cat is removed to decrease the likelihood that a behavior will occur.
- Example: During play, the cat bites the owner → the owner gets up and walks away, ignoring the cat. The cat is less likely to bite the owner during play in the future.
- Regarding classical or operant conditioning, the neutral stimulus can be paired with a positive or negative event/consequence.

natural sounds. On average, kittens open their eyes 7 to 10 days after birth. One study found four factors that affect when a kitten will open its eyes. They include light exposure, sex of the kitten, age of the mother, and paternity. Of the factors studied, paternity was found to have the strongest influence on how early kittens opened their eyes. Additionally, dark-reared kittens opened their eyes earlier than light-reared kittens; female kittens opened their eyes earlier than male kittens; and kittens from young mothers opened their eyes earlier than kittens from older mothers.

By 3 weeks of age, many sensory systems are developing rapidly, with some having already developed to their adult state (see Table 12-1). The olfactory system reaches full development, but vision takes the lead in guiding the kitten's behavior. During this time, kittens move from paddling to rudimentary walking and oral self-grooming emerges. Between 15 and 25 days, kittens gain the ability to visually orient toward and follow objects, including the queen. One influential change in kitten development at this time is a decrease in initiation of nursing bouts by the queen in preparation for weaning (see section on Weaning). At 4 weeks, the visual and auditory systems have developed further as evidenced by more adult-like hearing and vision, as well as better coordination and motor skills. Behavioral development reflects these physical changes as the kitten begins to show play and hunting skills. At this age, the kittens orient to sounds as an adult cat would and begin to stray farther from the nest. Also, during this period (between 25 and 35 days), kittens can learn tasks with visual cues alone and their heart rate can be classically conditioned to respond to a neutral event paired with an aversive event (see Box 12-1). Additionally, at 4 weeks weaning (see section on Weaning) is typically underway. By the fifth week of life, kittens have developed the motor skills to run. They are becoming more adept hunters, and some will kill the prey that the queen brings to the nest (see section on Predatory Behavior).

Between 6 and 7 weeks, kittens show more adult responses to stimuli (see Table 12-1). They are capable of all of the gaits exhibited by adults. This new-found mobility and coordination allows kittens to engage in the complex interactions that make up typical kitten play (see section on Play). Another adult response that emerges with adult-like frequency by 7 weeks of age is the *gape*, which may imply that the vomeronasal organ is developed more completely. The gape (also called a *grimace*) is a variation of the flehmen response seen in horses and cattle. It is typically demonstrated by cats who encounter another cat's urine or a novel smell. It allows the cat to pull odors, such as pheromones, into the vomeronasal organ. Pheromones are present in urine and facial secretions, making the expression of the gape an important part of sexual and social behavior. At 6 weeks of age, kittens will orient toward a silhouette of a cat in a socially threatening position, and by 8 weeks of age, kittens display adult responses, including piloerection to a silhouette and to cat urine. By 10 to 11 weeks of age, kittens are starting to exhibit the complex motor abilities needed when climbing, walking, and turning along thin tree branches.

NURSING

Suckling is an innate reflex for young kittens. Kittens who are bottle-raised or fed intragastrically for up to 3 weeks will still initiate nursing on a queen. The olfactory system is well developed at birth and plays an important role in proper suckling. Kittens begin to suckle soon after birth (1 to 2 hours). Although exactly how kittens find the nipple has not been determined, they most likely use a combination of tactile and olfactory cues. Kittens may follow their own scent trail or the scent trail of other kittens to find the queen for subsequent nursing bouts. To properly nurse, kittens must have perception in the mouth (to find nipple) and the tongue (to suckle). Most kittens develop a nipple preference 1 to 3 days after birth, although the largest kitten does not always win the most productive teat. Kittens initiate suckling by pulling their head back and then moving it quickly forward. In addition, they massage the area around the teat with their forepaws to stimulate milk let-down. Some cats retain suckling and massaging behaviors well into adulthood (see sections on Clinical Implications: Nonproductive Sucking and Clinical Implications: Kneading). Even before the eyes open, the kitten is subject to the laws of learning. Kittens can be conditioned to prefer a nipple with bumps over a nipple with ridges when the former is paired with positive reinforcement (milk).

Clinical Implications: Kneading

Some kittens retain the juvenile behavior of kneading or "mixing" when they are about to lie down with the owner or on a soft surface. It can be accompanied by purring and extension of the front claws with each tread. The front claws may catch on fabrics or the owner's skin, making this an undesirable behavior. Kneading is considered within normal limits for a kitten and unless annoying to the owner, should be ignored. If the owner finds this behavior untoward, there are multiple treatment options available. If the kitten is kneading primarily on the owner, they should be advised to stand up, letting the kitten gently fall off their lap or place the kitten on the floor the moment that the behavior begins so that the kitten never experiences reward from the owner for this behavior. When the kitten stops kneading (after being placed on the floor), the owner should pick the kitten up and put him back on their lap. This will require many repetitions, and the owner should be advised to be patient. If the kitten is kneading on other pieces of furniture regardless of where the owner is, withdrawal of attention by the owner is not likely to be effective as the behavior is not dependent on owner attention for reinforcement. Instead, the owner should designate appropriate places for the kitten to knead, such as cat trees and pet beds, and differentially reward the kitten with food treats or catnip (if it does not cause aggression) when he kneads in appropriate places. In addition, remote devices such as the Spray Sentry (Premier,

Midlothian, VA) motion-activated, compressed air spray can be used to repel the kitten from inappropriate surfaces. Kittens should not be physically punished (e.g., flicking in the face, slapping) for kneading because it can lead to conflict behaviors owing to the fact that it fails to show the kitten what to do instead of kneading in inappropriate locations. Without proper direction as to where the kitten can perform this behavior, anxiety can increase and other conflict behavior patterns can develop that are likely to be much more annoying to the owner than kneading.

Clinical Implications: Nonproductive Sucking

Nonproductive sucking is another behavior "left-over" from the suckling behavior of nursing. Kittens who exhibit this behavior may suck on the owner's hands, arms, or clothing, as well as other substrates not associated with the owner. Most often, this type of behavior is first exhibited before the kitten is 1 year old. Although it is typically a benign behavior, it can cause destruction of the owner's belongings, danger to the kitten from ingestion, and injury to the owner. Often, young-onset, nonproductive sucking resolves on its own by the time the kitten is 6 to 12 months old; however, through reinforcement or if fueled by anxiety or genetic predisposition, nonproductive sucking may evolve into a displacement behavior or a compulsive behavior. Other factors aside from reinforcement, which can affect the likelihood that nonproductive sucking will evolve into a displacement or compulsive behavior, are early weaning, anxiety, breed (oriental breeds are predisposed), and heredity. Kittens who perform this behavior should have a highly enriched environment, including many items to suck or chew on such as rawhides (soak them first in water), cat grass, beef jerky, food stuffed toys, and chewy food, as well as dry food. In addition, if the kitten prefers a certain substrate but also sucks on the owner's skin or clothing, the owner can differentially reward him when he sucks only on an appropriate substrate. For example, if the cat prefers cotton, an old towel can be given to him so that he will have an item with his scent that is appropriate to suck on. When the kitten sucks on the owner or the owner's clothing, the owner should place the kitten on the floor, a pet bed, or a cat tree and give the kitten something acceptable to suck on or redirect the kitten to a completely different behavior. The kitten should not be physically punished because this behavior can be anxiety based and physical punishment will increase conflict, leading to much more undesirable behaviors. In addition, it should not be encouraged with petting or positive reinforcement.

WEANING

Age at weaning plays an important role in many aspects of the kitten's behavioral development. In natural situations, weaning begins at 4 weeks and is usually complete by 7 weeks of age. Kittens weaned at 2 weeks of age engage in increased random activity and do not adapt well to the presentation of novel stimuli. They also perform poorly in operant conditioning tests (see Box 12-1) and in situations in which they must compete with other cats for food.

Clinical Implications: Early Weaning/ Hand-Raising

Orphan kittens are not uncommon in the United States. Litters are often the result of a feral or stray mating. Once captured, the litter may be separated to ease with fostering or only one kitten may be able to be captured because of the feral state of the litter. Hand-raised, orphan kittens can develop a plethora of problems such as impulsive behavior, increased reactivity to stimuli, inappropriate play behavior characterized by a lack of inhibition, and play-related aggression. Early weaned kittens, on the other hand, show predatory behavior and object play earlier than normally weaned kittens. One reason that hand-raised kittens exhibit different behaviors than kittens raised with the litter is that hand-raised kittens are not exposed to other cats during the time when they would typically be learning appropriate play and predatory behavior.

When kittens are weaned by the queen, she does so gradually while offering them another outlet (hunting) in which to direct their behavior. The queen begins to limit the length of nursing bouts from 3 weeks of age by walking away from the kittens. Generally, 1 week later, she also begins to bring prey to them. She encourages the kittens to interact with the prey in addition to watching her kill it. These lessons teach them where predatory behavior should be directed, encourage a prey preference, and teach them how much force with which they should bite. Other important lessons learned during this time are independence from the queen (their only source of nurturing and food up until this time) and how to deal with minor stressors and frustration. In this way, kittens learn how to be independent and deal with stressful situations. Hand-raised kittens lack the types of interactions that encourage independence and exert a manageable amount of stress on them daily. Instead of encouraging independence as the queen does, human caretakers typically encourage reliance on the caretaker. As a result, the orphan kitten may become very closely bonded to the caretaker, as well as lacking appropriate bite inhibition, prey preference, and ability to deal with stressors on a daily basis. It is postulated that the inability to deal with stress and learn independence are factors in the impulsive and often aggressive behavior of the typical orphan kitten toward people.

To avoid the deleterious effects of hand-rearing singleton kittens, kittens should be kept with their siblings or cross-fostered onto another queen. If the litter must be broken up, kittens should at least be kept in pairs. The presence of littermates, the queen, or even an older cat can help to modulate the kitten's play behavior so that it is more appropriate. If neither of these options are available, at 4 weeks, kittens should be exposed to older, healthy cats or kittens who are not overly aggressive but will appropriately correct hard bites and rough play so that they have a higher likelihood of learning appropriate, species-typical behavior. Also, at this time, owners should begin interacting with the kitten in a structured way. They should encourage independence from them during the weaning process. Play should focus on toys that distance the owner from the kitten and stimulate predatory behavior. In addition, they should never use their hands or feet as playthings. If the kitten places his mouth or claws on the owner, even if by accident, the owner should make a sharp sound (as a crying kitten would) and immediately withdraw, ending the game of play. This acts as negative punishment, which can be a very effective training tool. If the kitten pursues the owner, they can calmly pick the kitten up and place him in a separate, kitten-proof area for 2 to 3 minutes. After that time, they can open the door and let the kitten out. Although the kitten is not likely to associate the "time out" in another room with the act of biting or scratching the owner, it will give the kitten time to calm down.

When the kitten bites or scratches the owner in play, it is challenging for even the most diligent owner to act as quickly and with just the right amount of force to stop inappropriate behavior as another kitten or the queen would. Because of this, the kitten should not be physically corrected as this may cause him to be frightened of the owner. In addition, the kitten may interpret this as play behavior escalating the level of play. As with most cat behavior problems, kittens exhibiting predatory behavior or play-related aggression toward the owners should have a highly enriched environment so that they are occupied regardless of the owner's presence.

PLAY

In the fourth week, as the kitten gains the ability to orient toward objects visually, follow objects visually, and walk more efficiently, social play arises. Between 5 and 6 weeks of age, kittens hide when moving toward another kitten. At this age, it would not be uncommon to observe three or more kittens playing in a group. By the time that kittens are 8 weeks old, group play will have decreased and pair-wise play will have become more common. Social play typically continues to increase until 11 to 14 weeks of age when it starts to decline. However, as many cat owners know, social play may continue throughout a cat's life. By 9 weeks of age, kittens typically play for 1 hour per day spread into 4 bouts.

A specific play signal has not been identified in cats as it has in dogs (i.e., play bow). While body language can vary, in general, an arched tail and back and "bouncy" movements are consistent with play. In addition, rolling, pawing, pouncing, rearing, batting, leaping, belly-up, side-step, horizontal leap, face-off, and chasing are all typical elements of play. In kittens 6 to 12 weeks of age, the pounce, belly-up, side-step, and standing up are very effective in soliciting play from other kittens. By 12 weeks, the vertical stance becomes more effective in soliciting play while the side-step becomes less important. Kittens who are adopted into homes where there are no other cats will often play with other species such as humans, dogs, and ferrets. Interspecies play can be very interesting to observe because each animal is able to interpret the other species' play signals despite the fact that they are very different. A dog may offer a play bow to a kitten while the kitten may rear up to bat at the dog's face. It is possible in this situation that there are subtle signs that each species uses to understand the play of the other such as a bouncy, soft body posture. Another possibility is that one species learns about the other and which body postures solicit play through trial and error learning. Certain postures are reinforced by the other animal's willingness to engage in play (see section on Clinical Implications: Interspecies Play).

Kittens engage in solitary play as well. Although it declines starting at 4 months of age, many adult cats will continue to engage in solitary play to some extent. As would be expected, object and locomotor play increase between 7 to 8 weeks when the kitten gains better locomotor skills. While there are elements of predatory behavior in social and object play (e.g., pouncing, hiding, batting), the development of these two types of behavior is via separate pathways. Unlike dogs where sexual postures may be included in play behavior, this type of interaction has not been identified in cats. Sex of the kitten, however, does influence the type of play engaged in by kittens. Male kittens engage in twice the amount of object play as female kittens at 7 weeks and this difference continues to some extent through the age of 8 to 12 weeks. Females which have male littermates show increased object play when compared to female kittens without male littermates. Interestingly, there are no differences between the sexes with regard to social play in weeks 4 through 12. After 12 weeks, males emerge as the more socially playful of the two sexes with increased frequency of social play from weeks 12 to 16. Much like object play, females who play consistently with male littermates show increased male-like social play behavior. By 12 to 16 weeks of age, a difference in aggressive play is detectable between all-male and all-female litters with the all-male litters showing more aggressive play than all-female litters. In litters of mixed sex, the difference is less apparent.

Clinical Implications: Interspecies Play

Interspecies play can be an excellent way to enrich an animal's environment and avoid behavior problems associated with decreased outlets for energy release and frustration; however, interspecies play can also result in serious behavior problems and a decrease in the quality of life of one or both animals if early interactions are not monitored closely. As with most species, a kitten's behavior is constantly being shaped by its interactions with social group members and its environment. If inappropriate interactions, including play, are permitted, the kitten could learn the wrong lessons, which could lead to aggressive play, fearful behavior, hiding, and increased anxiety, putting the kitten at greater risk of developing inappropriate elimination, as well as other anxiety-related behavior problems. It is recommended that owners observe the interactions between a new kitten and existing pets or people in the household to ensure that proper lessons are learned. Consider the case of a kitten that is fearful of the dog in her new home. The dog is interested

in the kitten and is not at all aggressive to her. The dog attempts to solicit play appropriately as he would with another dog and the kitten returns the play with species-typical behavior of her own. The dog begins to bounce forward barking (i.e., appropriate play behavior), and the kitten becomes frightened and runs to hide. The dog chases the kitten (i.e., a rewarding game for the dog). In that instant, the paradigm will have changed to a chase game that is rewarding for the dog and frightening for the cat. In many cases, the dog will continue to chase the cat in other situations (because the behavior is consistently rewarded) and will likely start to chase her earlier in the interaction because of the positive reinforcement associated with the chase. On the other hand, the kitten will most likely begin to run from the dog earlier in the interaction because the dog is paired with a fear response, causing a vicious cycle. This same type of fear-reinforcement interaction can occur when playing with a person as well.

To make sure that the kitten learns the correct way to play, interspecies play should be closely monitored. The kitten should be separated from other animals initially when the owners are not home. The dog's behavior should be observed and controlled if he starts to chase or frighten the kitten. Rough play should be discontinued by calling the dog to the owner. The kitten should have multiple cat-friendly places, such as low hiding spaces and high perching spaces, where it can escape from the dog.

Regarding play with humans, the same rules apply. Rough play should be avoided. Play sessions at the owner's convenience should be scheduled daily so that the kitten learns to play when the owner has time and the owner averts the inevitable stalking and pouncing of an energetic kitten. The owner should provide many types of toys and rotate the toys so that the kitten is never bored. Play should involve toys that distance the kitten from the owner and never involve the hands or feet.

SOCIAL DEVELOPMENT

In the average pet home, social behaviors influence the interactions between the kitten and the owner (possibly the only social interactions that the kitten has), as well as the other animals in the household. Inappropriate social behavior and fear of other cats are also common problems that occur in multi-cat households. Social behaviors are very important because cats are social animals. Free-ranging cats form matrilineal colonies when there are adequate resources to do so. In addition, they engage in cross-suckling of each other's kittens. Genetics, health of the queen, health of the kitten, interactions of the kitten with the littermates and the queen, environment, socialization, and ongoing learning all affect the kitten's behavioral growth and its final behavior as an adult. Again, the paternity of the kittens has been shown to be of great significance when measuring friendliness toward people. As mentioned previously, for proper social development, kittens should have adequate time with the queen and ideally the littermates. Kittens removed from the queen at 2 weeks of age and hand-raised are more fearful and aggressive toward cats and people; have increased random, locomotor activity; are slow to form attachments with other kittens; and exhibit poor learning ability. Also, kittens raised without the interactions of a queen or littermates are slower to learn social skills than naturally raised kittens. Kittens will also follow the lead of other kittens within their litter, facilitating prey behavior and social learning. Unfortunately, often "rescued" kittens are removed from the queen as soon as possible, setting the stage for future behavioral issues. The queen also influences the food preferences and prey preferences of the kittens. Kittens are more likely to try new foods when the queen is present as opposed to when she is not.

SOCIALIZATION

Socialization is another important factor in developing "friendly" kittens. Socialization is the process by which an animal learns to relate to and form relationships with the stimuli within its environment, including people, cats, and other species. Early handling and exposure to novel stimuli while a kitten is young is vitally important for shaping a friendly, social adult cat. Many animals have defined sensitive periods for socialization and the cat is no different. A sensitive period is a defined time period in an animal's development in which a small amount of interaction has a large impact. Unfortunately, the reverse is also true. No interaction with or exposure to particular stimuli during this period can produce profound fear of those stimuli. Often, it is very difficult to overcome this type of fear later in life, even with proper exposure. Although the sensitive period for each species has a defined beginning and end, it is commonly accepted that there is individual variation among individuals. In addition, the potential of each sensitive period declines rapidly when the period expires, but the window of socialization is not completely closed at midnight on the day that the sensitive period ends. The sensitive period in kittens is 2 to 7 weeks. Unfortunately, kittens are typically adopted after the sensitive period has ended. While the kitten's behavior can be altered after 7 weeks, it is more difficult than if exposure was completed during the sensitive period (see section on Clinical Implications: Sensitive Period).

Kittens raised in isolation from birth to 4 weeks will be wary of approaching people even if the queen and tom were friendly cats. As with other social species, isolation from cats or other species when young can have detrimental effects. Isolation until 7 months of age causes kittens to accept other cats more slowly. Handling young kittens is a valuable way to decrease fear of humans and other stimuli. The amount of handling necessary to shape a friendly kitten varies, depending on which study is examined. One study showed that handling for 5 minutes a day between birth to 45 days of life decreased fearfulness of humans and novel toys. In another study, kittens handled for 15 minutes a day from 2 to 6 weeks of age were friendlier than kittens that were not. Handling kittens from birth to 12 to 14 weeks of age for 15 minutes a day, shaped friendlier kittens as measured by increased time interacting with the handler. In another study, kittens who were handled early in life, opened their eyes earlier, developed characteristic Siamese coat colors earlier, and showed a more bold nature when compared with unhandled kittens. Part of effective handling is varying the handler. Kittens between 5½ and 9½ weeks of age handled by 5 people were more affectionate, less fearful, and more playful with people than kittens handled by only one person or not handled at all. Kittens handled for 15 minutes per day from 3 to 14 weeks of age stayed with the handler longer and approached the handler in less time than the kittens who were handled from 7 to 14 weeks of age and the kittens who were not handled. When the handling time was increased to 40 minutes per day, both sets of handled kittens (3 to 14 weeks, 7 to 14 weeks) allowed restraint for longer periods of time compared with when they were handled for 15 minutes per day. Kittens handled for longer periods of time who are reared in a more varied environment appear more adaptable and able to relax in new places. Kittens should be socialized to other species early as well. If kittens are exposed to dogs from 4 to 12 weeks of age, they are not afraid of them.

Clinical Implications: Sensitive Period

Kittens should be handled by as many people as possible for a minimum of 5 minutes a day, from 2 to 7 weeks of age. However, handling should not stop at 7 weeks. There is some benefit to handling kittens up to 14 weeks of age. The type of handling that kittens get should also be monitored. Rough play (e.g., rubbing a kitten's abdomen as he rakes his back feet on the owner's hand) can cause serious behavior problems later in life. Kittens should be held, touched in all areas of the body in a gentle way, picked up frequently, and sometimes gently restrained as they would be during a veterinary examination. During this time, kittens should also be exposed to as many stimuli as possible. Cat carriers, syringes, veterinary offices, dogs, birds, small mammals, and babies are just some of the stimuli that should be a part of proper socialization. It does not appear that kittens can be handled too much or by too many people as long as the handling is gentle. Kittens should enter kitten kindergarten at 7 to 8 weeks of age. Topics covered in an average 4 to 6 week course include cat carrier training, basic obedience training, handling, socialization, and acceptance of restraint.

PREDATORY BEHAVIOR

Predatory behavior in kittens is influenced by many factors. Similar to other aspects of the kitten's development, the queen's behavior has great influence on the kitten's behavior, although being taught how to hunt by the queen is not necessary for a kitten to develop into a good hunter as an adult. Kittens are good observational learners, with the mother's influence generally being greater than the littermates regarding predatory behavior. They are more likely to be drawn to and hunt prey that their mother exposed them to when they were young. In addition, they generally will not hunt prey with which they were communally raised from birth such as a specific breed of rat. Queens begin to bring live or dead prey to their kittens between 4 and 5 weeks of age. The queen will attract kittens to the prey and then attack and eat it. As the kittens get older, the queen will bring the prey to the nest and let the kittens "play" with it to stimulate predatory behavior. When necessary, the queen will demonstrate how to interact with the prey. Although kittens show predatory behavior as early as 4 weeks of age and will kill prey as early as 5 weeks of age, their interest increases notably at 8 weeks of age. At this age, kittens often prefer to hunt and kill prey over playing with littermates.

While there are elements of predatory behavior in play behavior, they are not dependent on each other for proper development. Kittens raised without opportunities to play will still hunt prey-like objects if given the opportunity. The development of predatory behavior is altered by the age at which the kitten is weaned. Early-weaned kittens (4 weeks of age) develop predatory behavior sooner than late-weaned kittens (9 weeks of age) and are more likely to become effective mouse killers. Killing and eating prey are not dependent on each other and are controlled by different parts of the brain. This can be seen in the behavior of many pet cats who will hunt diligently and then kill the prey but never eat it. Although satiated cats will still spend a significant amount of time hunting each day, hunting behavior may be suppressed by keeping the cat well-fed. The reverse is also true. Hungry cats are more likely to hunt.

Clinical Implications: Predatory Aggression

Kittens have a natural drive to hunt. If left without an outlet for predatory behavior, negative behavior, such as predatory aggression toward the owner or other animals in the house, can develop. To avoid this, owners should concentrate on enriching the kitten's environment with predatory toys. Ideally, the toys would have lifelike sounds and preylike movements to stimulate predatory behavior. Toys should be rotated so that the kitten maintains interest in each individual toy. Also, the owners should set aside designated play time for the kitten each day so that he has guidance as to where predatory behavior should be directed. Owners should never use their hands or feet as playthings. Kittens have no way of discerning when it is appropriate to bite and swat at the owner's feet and when it is not.

Clinical Implications: Hunting

Some owners become upset when their cat kills rodents and small animals. It is important for owners to recognize that hunting is a normal part of the cat's behavioral repertoire. If this behavior is not permitted to some extent, cats can become aggressive toward the owners or other pets and destructive in the home at windows and doorways where they can see prey. For owners who would not like their kitten to hunt, the easiest thing to do is keep it inside. If the kitten hunts inside the home or on a screened enclosure, they can wear a belled collar. Owners can make an outside enclosure for their cat, put metal rings around trees so the

kitten cannot climb, use commercial cat repellents or animal repellents for the yard, or use a Cat Bib (Cat Goods, Inc, Springfield, OR). If the kitten is kept inside and is already showing signs of redirected aggression or frustration at not being able to hunt, the owners should be advised to enrich the environment with predatory toys, including food toys and to hide food treats around the house so that the cat has to hunt all day for its food, satisfying much of its predatory drive.

ELIMINATION

Before 3 to 5 weeks of age, kittens are stimulated to eliminate by the queen. Kittens begin to eliminate in open areas in which there is a well-drained substrate by 3 to 5 weeks of age. By 5 to 6 weeks of age, kittens will begin to voluntarily eliminate in an appropriate substrate with adult patterns, including digging a hole and covering. It appears to be within normal limits for some kittens and subsequently some adult cats to leave feces uncovered. This may be an attempt to mark territory with feces (i.e., middening). The behavior pattern regarding covering urine and feces develops by the time most kittens are 7 weeks of age. Kittens can develop a preference for a substrate at this age as well.

Clinical Implications: Inappropriate Elimination

Owners should be warned that kittens develop preferences for elimination substrates at a young age. When a kitten is initially adopted, the owner should use the same litter that had been used previously. Changes to the litter should be made slowly, over 7 days so that a substrate aversion is not formed, causing elimination outside of the litter box. Owners can either put out multiple boxes, some with the new litter and some with the old litter or they can gradually mix the new litter with the old litter over 7 days. In addition, the box should be accessible to the kitten; unable to be blocked by other animals; in a quiet, well-lighted place; and large enough for the kitten to posture normally for elimination. The box should grow as the kitten grows. Most adult-sized cats need a box that is roughly 20 × 30 inches. If there are other cats in the household, additional boxes should be added in different areas so that the kitten cannot be intimidated away from the elimination area, causing an inappropriate elimination problem.

SEXUAL BEHAVIOR

Sexual behavior, such as mounting and neck grasping, can be seen in male kittens as early as 4½ months of age, and many are capable of spermatogenesis at 5 months of age. Males do not reach sexual maturity, demonstrating the ability to copulate, until 9 to 12 months of age. Females reach sexual maturity between 7 and 12 months of age, although heat cycles can be seen as early as 4 months of age. Females generally attempt to repel male kittens who engage in sexual behavior at a young age. Sexual maturity should not be confused with social maturity, which occurs typically between 2½ to 4 years of age.

Clinical Implications: Sexual Behavior

Mounting is considered normal behavior in unneutered male kittens over the age of 4½ months. After neutering, it should subside in most kittens. Neutering is generally most effective in stopping this behavior in kittens who have never had sexual experience. If it persists into adulthood, it is often very distasteful to owners. Multiple factors can contribute to the persistence of mounting in a neutered cat, including lack of socialization, lack of environmental stimulation, unpredictable interactions with other cats in the household, and sexual frustration. The owner should be advised to redirect the kitten to an appropriate outlet for its energy such as a large toy it can mount or an energetic game of play. Mounting of inappropriate objects, animals, and people can be discouraged by using aversive devices. When the kitten is repelled from a certain area, he should be directed to an appropriate outlet for his energy. In this way, he will learn appropriate behaviors and which items are appropriate for mounting. The owner should keep a log of when and who the kitten mounts. Often, these types of behaviors occur at a certain time of day or to a certain victim. If this is the case, the owner can preemptively keep the kitten busy with another activity during that time.

LEARNING

Cats participate in observational learning, which is the ability to learn from observing another animal's behavior. In the case of kittens, what they learn is greatly influenced by the queen. Kittens are more likely to try a novel food if their queen is present and are more likely to learn an operantly conditioned response (see Box 12-1) when they have watched the queen perform the behavior when compared to other cats.

SUGGESTED READINGS

Bowen J, Heath S: *Behavior problems in small animals,* London, 2005, Saunders Ltd.
Horwitz D, Mills DS, Heath S: *BSAVA Manual of canine and feline behavioural medicine,* Gloucester, 2002, British Small Animal Veterinary Association.
Landsberg G, Hunthausen W, Ackerman L: *Handbook of behavior problems of the dog and cat,* ed 2, London, 2004, Saunders Ltd.

CANINE BEHAVIORAL DEVELOPMENT

CHAPTER 13

Andrew U. Luescher

Experiences during development have a long-lasting effect on temperament and adult behavior, therefore it is important to understand normal and abnormal development to prevent and resolve behavior problems.

COMPLEXITY OF EARLY ENVIRONMENT

An animal's central nervous system only develops its genetically predetermined functions if exposed to appropriate environmental stimulation, especially early in life. A restricted environment early in life results in an animal with abnormal sensory perception. The animal may not be able to perceive stimuli to which it was not exposed during development. An animal reared in a restrictive environment will also be emotionally unstable. A restricted early environment also may result in reduced learning ability and trainability, thus an interesting, stimulating early environment must be provided. It is also important that the early environment be predictable and consistent. If not, the animal will not only be frustrated and under stress, but it will also learn that its behavior has no impact on what is happening around it. Such animals will be in a state of learned helplessness and are exceedingly hard to train later.

EFFECT OF NEONATAL STRESS

Some degree of stress (e.g., handling or cold temperature) in a dog's neonatal period may accelerate growth, reduce emotionality later in life, increase social status, and promote resistance to some diseases. Handling sessions from the first days of a puppy's life are recommended because they not only expose the puppy to a mild stress but also facilitate socialization when the puppy gets older. In addition to handling sessions, puppies may be removed from the nest (best while someone else walks the mother) and placed singly on a cool vinyl floor for a brief time (30 seconds) before being put back into the warm nest. Flashing lights, noises, and motions have also been used as mild stress. The Army's super-dog program used slow, refrigerated centrifuges to apply a mild stress. If done in the first few (3) days after birth when the hypothalamic-pituitary-adrenal (HPA) axis develops, the expected result is reduced behavioral and physiologic reaction to chronic stress, an increased physiologic reaction to acute stress, and reduced emotionality of the adult dog. Chronic stress is caused by unavoidable and long-lasting aversive conditions. Since they are unavoidable, the stress reaction does not result in coping and drains the animal's resources. In humans, such chronic stress causes stomach ulcers and other health impairments. A strong reaction to acute stress, however, is desirable. If an animal is exposed to a sudden, intense, and potentially damaging stimulus, it may save its life to mobilize all its resources to escape. Thus a reduced reaction to chronic stress and an increased reaction to acute stress are both beneficial.

Mild early stress also results in increased resistance to some diseases, a more stable and less emotional temperament, and increased learning ability and trainability.

SENSITIVE PERIODS OF DEVELOPMENT

It is well documented that there are "sensitive periods" in the behavioral development of the dog. These are periods of development during which certain experiences are needed to achieve normal development. Lack of these experiences during these sensitive periods may have lifelong irreversible effects. For example, between 4 and 12 weeks of age, a puppy learns how a social partner looks. During this time, the brain develops a sort of filter system in the visual cortex, which becomes sensitized to the shapes of the social partners of the puppy. In the wolf, these would be adult wolves and other pups; in the dog, they include humans and other pets. This filter system ensures that certain neurons in the visual brain are only activated when the puppy sees a social partner. After 12 weeks, it is difficult to further modify this system so that

TABLE 13-1 Periods of development in puppies

Period	Age
Fetal period	up to birth
Neonatal period	0 days to 10 days
Transition period	11 days to 21 days
Socialization period	3 to 12 (or 14) weeks
Fear period	Around 8 to 10 weeks
Juvenile period	3 months to puberty
Second fear period(s)?	3 weeks duration between 4 and 11 months?
Adolescent period	Puberty to social maturity

BOX 13-1 Fetal period: up to birth

During the fetal period, the male brain is defeminized and masculinized. This process determines gender differences in behavior.

BOX 13-2 Neonatal period: days 0 to 10

The puppy is blind and deaf and completely dependent on mother for thermoregulation, food, and elimination.

The senses of balance, touch, smell, and taste and sensitivity to temperature are already developed.

Mild stress of the neonatal dog, such as induced by handling or placing the puppy on a cool surface, increases the puppy's ability to cope with stress later in life.

the puppy will not learn (or only learn with difficulty) to accept previously unknown species as social partners.

The recognition of critical periods in canine behavioral development may be one of the most important discoveries about dogs. By controlling the puppy's environment during its early life, we can influence the emotionality, temperament, sociability, confidence, and learning ability of the dog. Early and appropriate intervention can result in the dog being more adaptable, easier to train, and physically and emotionally healthier.

The exact time course of development varies between authors (and probably between dogs to some degree!), since the sensitive periods do not start and end abruptly, but rather, they phase in and out gradually. The development of puppies has been divided into the periods seen in Table 13-1.

Fetal Period (Up to Birth)

Shortly before parturition, the male fetus produces a burst of testosterone, which has an organizational effect on the brain of the male fetus: it masculinizes and defeminizes the brain (Box 13-1). Masculinization results in the organization of typical male behavior such as roaming, urine marking, inter-male aggression, and male sexual behavior. Castration is usually successful in reducing these behaviors but does not entirely eliminate them. The effectiveness of castration in altering these behaviors is individually very variable. Defeminization results in the destruction of the mechanism that results in cyclical sexual behavior in females (intact male dogs do not have an estrus cycle and are always ready to breed) and eliminates the predisposition to show female sexual behavior. A male dog castrated after birth when given estrogen will show male and not female sexual and social behavior.

The priming of the fetal male brain is irreversible and affects all behavior that is gender-dimorphic, including various types of aggression, even in the castrated dog. Therefore a castrated male dog is still very much male; a spayed female dog is still very much female.

Neonatal Period (0 Days to 10 Days)

A puppy is born both blind and deaf but is capable of whining to attract attention from its mother (Box 13-2). It is born with the senses of balance, taste, smell, touch, and temperature. Until 3 weeks of age, the puppy is not able to urinate and defecate spontaneously and depends on stimulation (licking) by the mother to fulfill these functions. Its nervous system is poorly developed: for the first 3 days of age it has "flexor dominance" (i.e., it curls up when you pick it up by the head) and from day 4 to day 21, it has "extensor dominance" (i.e., it stretches when you pick it up). Although puppies depend on the mother for thermoregulation, they are born with a sense of temperature and will root against a warm object. Newborn puppies will also move against the grain of the hair of their mother so they will get closer to the udder and also turn or move toward the side they are touched on. From about 2 to 3 days of age, a puppy is able to crawl by throwing its head from side to side, using its nose as a sensory touch and temperature probe. All of the puppy's behaviors are designed to get it back into the heap of littermates and to the udder.

Already during this early stage, human contact and handling are important as environmental enrichment and for inducing a mild stress. As mentioned, a mild stress can also be imposed by removing the puppy from the nest for a brief period (30 seconds) and placing it on a cool surface such as a vinyl floor. This may allow the animal to better cope with stress, be more trainable, and be more emotionally stable later in life.

Puppies may vocalize when hurt, cold, or uncomfortable or when they lose contact with the littermates or the mother. However, most bitches will not react to these vocalizations. Learning with positive reinforcement is already possible, although the puppies' responses are very limited. Conditioned aversion has also been achieved in very young puppies.

Transition Period (11 Days to 21 Days)

Puppies are born in a very early stage of development. Such animals are called "altricial." In the transitional period, a

---

BOX 13-3   Transition period: days 11 to 21

During this time, the puppy begins to develop its senses of vision and of hearing. Therefore a complex environment should be provided to allow optimal development of the nervous system. From 3 weeks on, the puppy can already be desensitized to potentially frightening sights and sounds.

BOX 13-4   Socialization period: weeks 4 to 12 or 14

Socialization to dogs and to people has to occur during this time. If this opportunity is missed, the puppy will most likely always be fearful of dogs and/or humans.

During the socialization period, the puppy should also be exposed to all situations that it is likely to encounter during its life. The best prevention of behavior problems is to take the puppy to puppy classes during that time.

During the socialization period, the puppy can already learn some commands. It should learn a biting inhibition and start to learn to fit into a social group.

---

puppy catches up with those animals that are born in a much more developed state, such as foals or calves, which are examples of "precocial" animals. The puppy begins to develop its senses, gains control over thermoregulation, and at the end of the transitional period, becomes able to eliminate spontaneously (and the mother stops eating its stool) (Box 13-3). From this point on, the puppies should have the possibility to leave the nest site to eliminate. Puppies thwarted from doing so may become almost impossible to house train.

The development of vision and hearing makes the puppy more reactive to environmental stimuli. Since the puppy is also able to habituate to stimuli and still profits from environmental complexity for normal neurological development, the provision of sensory, visual, and auditory stimuli is very important. This can be done through handling; placing the puppies for short periods into a playpen with toys, platforms, tunnels, and so on (under supervision!); and playing commercially available recordings of various noises. Puppies will also begin to play-fight and are better able to learn, especially with positive reinforcement.

At around 3 weeks of age, the mother and/or father may start to regurgitate food for the puppies. However, probably as a result of domestication, not all dogs will do that. The puppies will solicit food regurgitation by pushing their noses into the corners of the parents' mouths, a behavior that later develops into appeasement behavior. At this time, it is appropriate to begin feeding solid food to puppies.

Socialization Period (4 to 12 or 14 Weeks)

The socialization period has been subdivided into a period of primary socialization, normally to conspecifics (earlier on in the socialization period), and secondary socialization to other species (later in the socialization period) (Box 13-4). Social play is the most prominent behavioral aspect of this period. During the primary socialization period, a puppy learns to interact appropriately with other puppies, to read canine body language, about bite inhibition, and to fit into a social group. During secondary socialization, the puppy learns to predict actions of members of other species and to interact with them successfully.

A puppy taken early from the litter and raised by hand will form its paramount relationships with people. If this isolation from its own species continues until after twelve weeks, the dog may become fearful of and aggressive toward other dogs. On the other hand, if the puppy is not socialized

to humans during the socialization period, it will most likely always be fearful of and possibly become aggressive toward people.

Although weaning may occur from 4 to 6 weeks of age, a puppy should never be adopted before 7.5 to 8 weeks of age and best not before 10 weeks of age. Although this has not been studied well in dogs, clinical observations indicate that the interaction occurring within the litter at that time and the effect of the mother are too critical to a puppy's development, and early removal from the litter may result in emotional instability.

During the socialization period, every effort should be made to fully socialize the puppy and expose it to a wide range of different sights, sounds, and other sensory experiences. Environmental complexity is still very important in assuring normal neurological and emotional development. A puppy park that contains all kinds of objects and stimuli and where the puppies spend time under supervision is a helpful tool to provide complex sensory experience. A puppy park may contain unusual footing, objects that make noise, a water bath, objects hanging overhead, and so on.

The puppy can now learn more easily from positive experiences and, particularly from 8 weeks of age, also from negative experiences. The puppy should be trained with positive training techniques, so it learns that its behavior can operate on the environment (learning to learn). Training done at this stage is easily retained and probably enhances later trainability. Many of the exercises that are useful for problem prevention (e.g., teaching the off command, food bowl safety, bite inhibition, and so on) are done most easily during this period. Puppy classes can provide this and more in a structured and systematic way.

Fear Period (8 to 10 or More Weeks)

The fear period lies within the socialization period and is included in that period by many authors. It starts at about 8 weeks of age, but the age of onset seems to vary considerably between breeds and individuals. If 5-week-old Beagle puppies were punished (e.g., with an electric shock for approaching a person), they showed fear, but approached that person again when retested later. If the puppies were

BOX 13-5	Fear period: weeks 8 to 10

Within the socialization period lies the fear period. A traumatic experience during this time may render the puppy a globally fearful, neurotic dog. This should be considered when arrangements for shipping a puppy are made.

BOX 13-6	Juvenile period: approximately months 3 to 6

The juvenile period is a time of rapid physical development and increased independence. This is a particularly difficult time to train the young dog, if a basis has not been established early on.

between 8 and 9 weeks of age, they retained the fear of that person. Puppies older than 12 weeks are less influenced by a mild shock and may approach the person in spite of the shock. Because of the increased fearfulness and the enhanced learning from bad experiences during the fear period, it is not recommended to ship a puppy at that time (Box 13-5). Any aversive experience during that time is to be avoided, since it may have lifelong effects on emotionality, anxiety, fear hyperactivity and reactivity, and aggressiveness. Dogs that have been affected by adverse experiences during the fear period often cannot be rehabilitated. Some dogs that are genetically predisposed to fearfulness may start to show fear during the fear period and remain fearful even in the absence of any trauma.

Juvenile Period (3 Months to Puberty)

The juvenile period is one of rapid physical growth and increasing activity, excitability, and independence. This is a difficult stage to go through (for the owner), in particular if the puppy has not yet been trained at all (Box 13-6). Early training pays off during this developmental stage.

Many owners of young puppies do not see the need to take their dog to puppy class. They say their puppy is so well behaved and follows them everywhere voluntarily, and it is the "best dog in the world" without any training. Once the puppy gets around 4 months of age, they are often greatly disappointed. Their once so voluntarily obedient puppy suddenly does not seem to care much about them anymore, and it becomes a chore to keep the puppy under control. This is a reason why many dogs are relinquished around 5 to 6 months of age.

A dominance order is now beginning to develop among the puppies. Compared to wolves that have a highly structured social order, the social order among dogs of most breeds always remains one resembling that among wolf puppies. Depending on neotenization of the breed, this social order may be loose and flexible, or it may be more rigid and linear. In a few breeds, social status may depend on gender, with all males being dominant over all females, such as was found to be the case in Terriers and Basenjis, two breeds that are less neotenized than most.

The juvenile period ends with sexual maturity around 5 to 14 months of age, depending on individual and breed. However, attainment of sexual maturity does not imply social maturity.

Further Fear Periods (3-Week Duration, Between 4 and 11 Months)

During the juvenile period, dogs may go through one or several more fear periods, lasting around 2 to 3 weeks each, during which the dog is much more easily scared and learns particularly well from adverse experiences. These additional fear periods have not been scientifically documented. However, many breeders have made the observation that juvenile or adolescent dogs go through stages during which they become much more easily frightened even by familiar things. For example, a dog that encountered garbage cans twice a week on his daily walk may be suddenly frightened by and not dare go near them and raise the hackles and bark. This behavior should not worry owners too much, since it just needs to be waited out in most cases. Counter-conditioning (making the situation pleasant by offering food or playing with the dog), response substitution (teaching an alternate behavior in that situation and rewarding it), and in severe cases, systematic desensitization (gradually exposing an animal to something and rewarding relaxation) can be used to help the animal to get through this. A normal dog will outgrow this and revert back to being confident very quickly. Aversive training techniques, punishment, and other traumatic experiences could have a long-lasting effect on fearfulness, aggressiveness, and emotionality and should be avoided.

Adolescent Period

The adolescent period starts with puberty and ends with attainment of social maturity relative to the breed. When compared to wolves, dogs remain puppyish into adulthood and never become socially mature. The degree of social maturity attained varies between breeds, with herd-guarding dogs remaining very puppyish, followed by retrievers and spaniels, then pointers and stalkers, with heelers and Terriers becoming relatively most mature. Breeds that remain socially immature are among other things less predatory, more playful, and enjoy physical contact more; they therefore may have more desirable pet qualities than breeds that become more mature.

PROBLEM PREVENTION

Complex Early Environment

As discussed previously, providing a complex early environment is important in preventing behavior problems. Also, handling and exposing puppies to a mild stress in the first few days of life should be beneficial. Exposure to variable environments during the socialization period is important to reduce fear and aggression. Puppies should be taken on car rides and to other people's homes, ideally before they are taken away from the litter, and certainly once they are with their new owner.

Socialization

Puppy classes that allow for puppy play can provide a safe way of exposing a puppy to other puppies. Under the supervision of an expert, a puppy can learn to interact appropriately with other puppies with minimal risk.

Since dogs are part of human society, socialization to humans is of paramount importance. This includes socialization to people of both genders and all races; those with physical disabilities, using crutches or being wheelchair-bound; and most of all to children. Especially puppy owners who plan on having children should plan ahead and expose the puppy in a safe way to babies (or at least the smell and sounds of babies), toddlers, and children of all ages because dogs do not appear to generalize from one age group to another. Obviously, all interactions should be pleasant and safe. In any case in which a puppy shows fear, giving it a treat immediately will tilt the balance toward a more positive experience.

Children also need to be educated in how to appropriately interact with a puppy and need to be supervised around the dog at all times. They need to be taught how to pet a dog and especially how to play with a dog. Dogs cannot be expected to put up with everything a child wants to impose on them, and many dogs can be expected to resort to aggression if a child bothers them or excites them too much.

Managing for Success

Problem prevention includes managing the puppy for success (arranging the environment so that the puppy cannot do the wrong thing and automatically chooses to do the right thing). If appropriate behaviors are successful from the puppy's point of view from the beginning, it will repeat these and not try other behaviors (and if we have set the environment up correctly, if it ever tries other behaviors, these are not successful). This includes puppy-proofing the house and appropriate confinement and supervision.

For example, a puppy will chew on any object it finds. It is therefore important to remove all objects it should not chew on (and make the ones that cannot be removed unattractive by applying an unsavory taste) and provide enough interesting chew toys. To keep the toys interesting, they can be exchanged with others every day. Toys that are filled with food are attractive to the puppy at any time. The same principle is utilized for house training a puppy (see later section).

Crate Training

Crate training is another tool for preventing behavior problems, including aggression. Lots of dogs become aggressive or anxious when confined in a crate. Teaching the puppy that the crate is a wonderful place to be can easily prevent these problems. A puppy will like its crate if it finds a hidden treat each time it enters and/or has a toy in the cage, especially one that contains some food and if the puppy gets fed in the cage. Giving a treat through the door after closing the cage door and giving a treat when approaching the cage can also prevent aggression in these situations.

Crate training is also important because a dog will need to be crate-confined at some time in its life, whether for transportation, after surgery, or for house training.

House Training

Where to eliminate is one of the most important things for a puppy to learn, since many young dogs are relinquished because they are not house trained. House training is usually easily achieved if from the beginning, the puppy is taken outside at times when elimination is most likely (i.e., after rest, feeding and drinking, or exercise and play) and frequently enough in-between. The puppy should always be taken to the same area outside and be rewarded once it has eliminated. The puppy should be observed at all times for signs of impending elimination. If it shows any sign of being about to eliminate, it should be distracted and immediately taken outside. The owner needs to stay outside with the puppy until it has eliminated, then reward the puppy immediately before taking it back into the house. At times when the puppy cannot be supervised, it should be confined (see section on Crate Training). The cage should just be big enough for the puppy to stand and lie comfortably. Cages with a movable partition are especially useful for house training. Long confinement should be avoided. A 3-month-old puppy may be able to wait for up to 4 hours, a 4-month-old for about 5 hours; however, such long times of confinement should be the exception. If a puppy does eliminate in the cage and is forced to lie in the excrements, it may lose all ability to be house trained.

Exercise

Exercise off the property will satisfy the puppy's innate motivation to explore new things, help with exposure and desensitization to stimuli, and facilitate socialization. Exercise off the property also decreases arousal and reactivity and reduces anxiety and the risk of owner-directed aggression. This necessitates training the puppy to walk on leash and to come when called.

Environment Enrichment

Interactive toys and games, food-dispensing toys, rotating the toys so they maintain novelty, and appropriate play serve to enrich the environment and provide mental stimulation. Obedience training has a similar effect. Furthermore, humane obedience training (lure training, clicker training) provides predictable, consistent, and stress-free interaction and an opportunity for the dog to act on the environment with predictable outcome. If we are consistent in training, the dog has a lot of control over the situation (i.e., over our behavior and the rewards). In clicker training, they literally can make us click. Predictability and controllability of the environment will make dogs feel more secure and relaxed, reduce anxiety, and decrease the chance for owner-directed aggression.

Consistent Rules

We do not have to dominate our puppies because our relationship with puppies is unlikely one of dominance and submissiveness. However, it is necessary to control the contingencies on the dog's behavior, which means to ensure that behaviors we desire pay off for the dog and those that are undesirable do not pay off. The establishment and strict enforcement of rules is extremely important. If rules are not consistent, the puppy can never figure them out and cannot function within them to achieve success. This situation would be similar to visiting with friends who play a card game that you do not know. They ask you to participate and explain the rules to you. You go along with it and after some time, think you have the winning hand, put your cards down, and claim that you have won. Then, of course, your friends add another rule. After two or three times of this, you become frustrated and angry (aggression as a conflict behavior!) and refuse to participate any longer. This is how dogs must feel if we have no rules or constantly change them. They may compensate for this either by developing survival behaviors that yield short-term predictable consequences (such as aggression) or by developing learned helplessness (i.e., they learn that their behavior has no effect on what happens around them). Enforcing strict rules therefore has nothing to do with dominance but rather with giving the dog a chance to operate successfully within his environment and achieving predictable outcomes. A highly trainable dog is especially keen on operating on his environment and will be in a state of compromised welfare if a consistent rule structure is not maintained.

Desirable behavior should be consistently rewarded (once a behavior is well trained, an intermittent reinforcement schedule can be used). Undesirable behavior should be ignored (a behavior that is not rewarded [i.e., not successful] will go into extinction). Of course, a behavior that is self-rewarding, such as going through the trash or ripping up a kitchen towel, does not go into extinction when ignored. Such behavior needs to be prevented by setting up the environment accordingly or by supervising and by engaging the puppy in an alternative, appropriate behavior (such as chewing on a chew toy).

Training to Control

In addition to providing consistent interaction, training to basic commands, such as come, sit, down, go to your bed, and so on, also provides the owner with the possibility to control the dog and to diffuse potentially dangerous situations (such as the dog showing aggression to visiting children or chasing a car). For example, if a dog is on the couch and growls when the owner approaches and the owner can send the dog to his bed on command, the growling is hardly a problem for the owner. Furthermore, the dog learns a behavior that gets him out of the situation without harm and to avoid the need to defend himself.

Leash Training

An important thing to teach a puppy is to walk on leash without pulling. Since dogs that do not walk properly on leash are often not exercised at all, not walking on leash contributes to anxiety and thus to behavior problems. There are many ways to teach a puppy to walk on leash, and they do not need to include aversive techniques. One easy way is to simply stop every time the puppy pulls.

Preventing Jumping Up on People

To stop a puppy from jumping up on people, people can simply take a step back each time the puppy attempts to jump up, so it lands on its feet again (a behavior that is not successful is not maintained). If the puppy knows the sit command, it can then be told to sit and be rewarded. If the puppy goes up to a person and spontaneously sits, it needs to get attention; when it jumps up, it needs to be ignored.

The "Off" Command (Leave-It and Drop-It)

Another useful command to prevent aggression over items is the "off" command (or the leave-it and drop-it commands), which teaches the puppy to let go or step back from something (many trainers use two commands, "leave-it" and "drop-it"; however, this author prefers the use of one command to simplify it for the dog and to possibly achieve better generalization). The "off" command is easily taught by holding a treat in your hand, letting the puppy sniff and nuzzle, waiting until the puppy backs off, and then immediately giving the puppy a treat from the other hand. Once the puppy reliably just touches the hand and then backs off, the "off" command can be issued just before the puppy backs off. This command easily generalizes to other situations such as scratching at the door, jumping up at a person, having a forbidden or potentially harmful object in the mouth, and so on. It teaches the puppy to happily give up an object since that behavior reliably pays off and eliminates the motivation to defend an object.

Bite Inhibition

Puppies may play very rough. Normally, they learn to inhibit their bite from playing with their littermates. If a puppy plays too rough, its playmate will no longer play along. However, many puppies are removed from their litters before learning this lesson, so puppies need to be taught to inhibit their bite to prevent bite injuries later. This is done by abruptly stopping play and ignoring the puppy for awhile. Most authors recommend yelping first. However, in our experience, this is unnecessary and in some cases may further excite the puppy. Gradually, the humans become more and more sensitive, until they stop play whenever the puppy touches their skin with its teeth. Note that no aversive treatment is necessary or advisable in teaching bite inhibition.

Desensitization and Counter-Conditioning

Since fear may be closely associated with aggression, fear should be prevented by desensitizing the puppy to all frightening things, especially to being picked up, being restrained, having the feet handled and the toe nails clipped, and so on. Some frightening situations can instead simply be paired with a pleasant experience. In fact, every time a puppy shows fear, a treat should be placed in its mouth.

This latter suggestion may seem counterintuitive, since one might think that giving a food treat when a puppy is fearful might reinforce fear. Think for a moment of being trapped in a stalled elevator. You are getting more and more frightened since no help arrives for some time. Now another person in the elevator brings out a box of donuts and offers one to everybody. How would that affect your fear? What in fact happens is that classical conditioning, being a more primitive type of learning, takes precedence over operant conditioning. You associate being in the elevator with the pleasant experience of getting a donut (rather than your fear being reinforced with a donut) and your fear diminishes.

A fear response is designed to solicit group support or find shelter from the danger. Physical contact or picking the dog up and so on is therefore likely to reinforce a fear reaction and should be avoided.

If a puppy gets a treat every time it is grabbed by the collar, it will quickly learn to enjoy being grabbed by the collar and not be fearful. If a puppy learns that each time you reach all the way into its mouth you deposit peanut butter there, it will happily let you pill it, which is a procedure that lots of dogs will not allow. Similarly, if you sit beside the puppy's food bowl and add food or treats to the bowl while the puppy eats, the puppy will love having you near the food bowl. These simple procedures go a long way to prevent aggression in situations in which dogs commonly are aggressive.

Alone Training: Preventing Separation Anxiety

A puppy can also be desensitized to being alone by placing it into its cage for increasingly longer times (with a toy that contains treats). Initially, this is done while the owner remains in the home. Then the exercise is repeated, starting again at very short times, with the owner actually leaving. Another aspect of preventing separation anxiety is to ignore the puppy for some time before leaving, so the puppy is not motivated to interact with the owner at these times and thus is less frustrated when the owner leaves.

Aversive Techniques

No aversive techniques or punishments are to be used when teaching puppies, since puppies will learn first and foremost to associate the situation with the unpleasant experience (classical conditioning takes precedence over operant conditioning). Thus the puppy will easily learn to associate their owner or another person with an aversive experience. Owners would also only rarely be able to administer punishment consistently (each time, within $\frac{1}{2}$ second of the behavior, and at the right intensity) and thus to the puppy the aversive stimulus occurs randomly and unpredictably. Inconsistent and inappropriate attempts at punishment teach the puppy that it cannot control or avoid aversive stimuli through correct behavior and increase anxiety and often aggression.

Puppy Tests

Puppy tests are of little value to determine if a puppy is at risk for becoming aggressive later in life.

SUGGESTED READINGS

Fox MW: *Canine behavior,* Springfield, IL, 1965, Charles C Thomas.
Lindsay SR: *Handbook of applied dog behavior and training: adaptation and learning,* Ames, IA, 2000, Blackwell.
Scott JP, Fuller JL: *Dog behavior, the genetic basis,* Chicago and London, 1965, The University of Chicago Press.
Serpell J, Jagoe JA: Early experience and the development of behavior. In Serpell J (ed): *The domestic dog, its evolution, behavior and interactions with people,* Cambridge, 1995, Cambridge University Press.
Van Dam P, Bleicher S: *The ultimate puppy toolkit,* Toronto, 2005, Urban Puppy Inc.

IMMUNOLOGIC DEVELOPMENT AND IMMUNIZATION

CHAPTER 14

James F. Evermann, Tamara B. Wills

The immune response is essential for survival from the wide array of infectious microorganisms to which the puppy and kitten are exposed. The immune responses of neonates are inferior to those of mature dogs and cats, not because components of the immune system are lacking, but because the soluble mediators are present in suboptimal concentration and cellular elements are in a naive state.

OVERVIEW OF IMMUNITY OF THE PUPPY AND KITTEN

The transition from a protected environment in the uterus to an environment containing a variety of potential infectious agents requires a rapid response by the immune system to protect the neonate from infections. Many factors play a role in the newborn's survival, including its innate immune system, acquired immune system, and passive transfer of maternal antibodies. Other factors, such as the dam or queen's health, nutrition status, immunization status, parasitic control, breeding management, and environment, also have an impact on health, sickness, or survival of the neonate. Understanding immunologic development of the newborn is necessary to recognize the role of immune protection from birth to 12 months, the role of maternal antibody in early immune protection, as well as the response and effect of vaccination at an early age.

In general, innate immunity is a rapid, nonspecific first line of defense. Neutrophils, macrophages, and natural killer lymphocytes are the first responders, whereas cellular products such as complement and cytokines also play a role in innate immunity. Barriers, such as skin and mucosa, and normal bacterial flora are other components of innate immunity. Acquired immunity is a slower, but a specific second line of defense involving B lymphocytes, T-helper (Th) lymphocytes (CD4+ cells), and T cytotoxic lymphocytes (CD8+ cells). Acquired immunity is further broken down into humoral immunity (e.g., Th2 immunity) and cell-mediated immunity (e.g., Th1 immunity). Humoral immunity is typically directed against antigens that survive extracellularly, such as bacteria, protozoa, or fungal organisms, and relies on interactions between B lymphocytes and a subset of T helper lymphocytes, resulting in antibody secretion. Secreted antibody binds antigens, flagging them for destruction. The second part of acquired immunity is cell-mediated immunity, which involves activation of macrophages, natural killer cells, and antigen-specific T cytotoxic lymphocytes, which are the primary effector cell. The function of cell-mediated immunity is to destroy obligate intracellular organisms such as viruses, some protozoa, and bacteria. If neonatal puppies and kittens ingest colostrum, passive immunity, consisting of maternal immunoglobulins, will also aid in early immune protection. Puppy and kitten immunity depends on all parts of the immune system, although the function of each system varies with age and colostrum ingestion.

Puppies

Development and function of complement pathways, antigen-presenting cells (APCs), phagocytic cells, and other pathways of the innate immune system have not been well characterized in puppies. However, one study observed increased phagocytic activity of neutrophils and macrophages in neonatal puppies compared to young adult dogs, suggesting there may be adequate function of phagocytic cells in puppies to help with the first line of defense against potential pathogens. In humans and mice, APCs have reduced ligand expression, which is necessary for stimulating specific immune responses, compared to adults. Although this has not been specifically evaluated in dogs, APCs may not be mature in neonatal puppies.

Immunologic development of the lymphoid system is incremental in all species. As a generality, the shorter the gestation, the less developed the immune system is at birth.

104

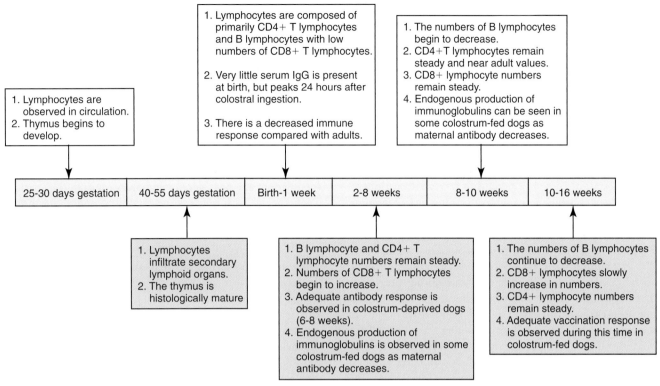

Figure 14-1 Immunologic development of the dog.

In puppies, immunologic development is an early event, beginning in midgestation with lymphocytes present in circulation at 25 days of gestation (Figure 14-1). Thymic development begins on day 27 of gestation, followed by lymphoid infiltration into secondary lymphoid organs, including spleen and lymph nodes, on days 45 to 52 of gestation. Thymic development appears histologically normal by day 45 of gestation. In contrast, splenic and lymph node architecture is not completely developed in the fetus and lacks germinal centers and B cell follicles until shortly after birth.

At birth the numbers of peripheral lymphocytes increase and are initially composed of primarily B cells and CD4+ T cells with lower numbers of CD8+ T cytotoxic lymphocytes. The majority of T cells, almost 90%, are naive at birth compared to only 40% at 4 months of age, indicating progressive maturation of the T cell population during this time. The number of B lymphocytes in neonates is much higher than adults, but after the initial increase, B cell lymphocyte numbers decline until 16 weeks of age. The high proportion of B lymphocytes in newborns likely represents early B cell stimulation and maturation in response to new antigens. T cytotoxic lymphocytes are important in cell-mediated immunity and are low at birth. This finding may lend support to human and mouse studies showing downregulation of cell-mediated immunity in neonates. Because T cytotoxic lymphocytes are important for detecting and inactivating intracellular pathogens, the low numbers of T cytotoxic lymphocytes at birth may predispose a newborn to intracellular viral or bacterial infections. T cytotoxic lymphocytes increase

steadily with age, whereas CD4+ T lymphocytes maintain at relatively steady numbers from birth to adulthood.

Knowledge of the distribution of peripheral lymphocytes is important to help determine if there are areas of immune deficiency in the neonate; however, function is another defining characteristic. Functional lymphocytes have been observed in the fetus, which is able to respond to antigens after lymphoid tissue develops in the last third of gestation. However, the antibody responses are variable and not as pronounced when compared to adults. Functional and specific lymphocyte responses are also present at birth, but similar to the fetus, antibody responses are often only a portion of the adult antibody response. One study observed adequate antibody response in day-old puppies immunized with a modified live canine parvovirus strain, suggesting some antigens may elicit an adequate antibody response, or some puppies have a higher level of immune development. In general, it is recognized that domestic animals are immunocompetent at birth; however, complete maturation of the immune system occurs postnatally.

Kittens

Development of the kitten's first line of defense, the innate immune system, including complement pathways, APCs, and other pathways of the innate immune system has not been well described. Neutrophil function has been evaluated, and phagocytic function is present at birth to help combat initial potential pathogens but is only a portion of adult response. The observed phagocytic response is independent of colostrum ingestion and matures to an adult response by 8 weeks of age. Based on human and mouse studies, it is speculated that APCs may also have reduced function in kittens; however, this hypothesis requires further evaluation.

Unlike the dog, there are only a few studies published discussing lymphoid development from the fetus to six months of age in kittens. Similar to the dog, lymphocytes have been detected in fetal circulation at approximately 25 days of gestation. Lymphocytes have also been detected in the thymus, spleen, and liver at between 28 to 52 days of gestation supporting fetal development of lymphoid tissue. In late gestation, there is a significant increase in peripheral T lymphocytes, which remain elevated after birth becoming the primary circulating lymphocyte in the adult. CD4+ T lymphocytes are present in higher numbers than CD8+ T lymphocytes, resulting in a high CD4:CD8 ratio at birth. The low numbers of CD8+ T lymphocytes at birth may be an effect of the queen's immune status during pregnancy downregulating cell-mediated immunity, although this has not been evaluated in cats. CD8+ T lymphocytes begin to increase through 8 weeks of age, lowering the CD4+:CD8+ ratio. B cell numbers increase right after birth until 4 weeks of age, likely representative of maturation of the humoral immune response, then steadily decrease to adult values. The timeline for reaching adult distribution of lymphocyte subsets has not been definitively established but is thought to occur before 12 months of age. Similar to the puppy, kittens are immunocompetent at birth but appear to have restricted immune responses compared to adults. Antigenic stimulation of the fetus has not been documented in kittens so conclusions about fetal response to antigens are unknown.

CONCEPTS OF MATERNAL IMMUNITY AND TEMPORARY PREGNANCY-ASSOCIATED IMMUNE SUPPRESSION

The areas of maternal immunity pertaining to pregnancy, fetal survival, and postpartum periods have been the subject of active investigation. In its broadest context, the immune response of the pregnant dam and queen becomes compromised as the fetus matures. Although this immunodeficient state is transitory, it is now considered to extend through the postpartum period for up to 4 weeks.

The cellular mechanisms responsible for the pregnancy and postpartum immunosuppression are considered to revolve around two key cell populations. These involve the shift of T-helper cells from a Th1 to a Th2 response and a decrease in neutrophil functions. The T cell populations are affected by progesterone, prostaglandin $F_{2\alpha}$, and α-fetoprotein. The Th1 cells are important effectors of the cell-mediated immune (CMI) response and interact with T cytotoxic lymphocytes. As mentioned earlier, the T cytotoxic lymphocytes are the main defense against intracellular pathogens. With the onset of pregnancy, the hormonal factors cause macrophages to release predominantly Th2-stimulating cytokines that contribute to the overall domi-nance of humoral immunity during pregnancy and immediately postpartum. This phenomenon of the Th cell populations is referred to as the "Th1-Th2 shift of pregnancy" and is generally regarded as a contributing factor to maternal tolerance of the fetus by suppressing the antifetal CMI response.

The second key cell population affected during pregnancy and in the postpartum period is the neutrophil. The point of maximum immunosuppression occurs in the latter stages of pregnancy when there is an acute elevation in glucocorticoids. Neutrophil dysfunction and the effects on the Th cell population are considered temporary during this period. Nonetheless, with impaired neutrophil response, the animal is now vulnerable to increased bacterial infections caused by the compromised bactericidal functions.

The outcomes of the temporary immunodeficiency states allow for fetal survival but may also result in an increased susceptibility to environmental infections by bacteria and fungi. Intracellular infections, such as viruses and protozoans, which may have been acquired during postnatal development, may become exacerbated during pregnancy because of the suppressive effects on the Th1 cells. This suppression results in a decreased CMI response. The CMI effector cells, the T cytotoxic lymphocytes, function normally to control virtually all the viral infections such as canine herpesvirus. Intracellular bacterial infections, such as *Brucella canis*, become more pathogenic during pregnancy. In addition to the aforementioned effects on T cell function, macrophage function is also compromised, allowing opportunistic bacteria, which are usually confined to external mucosal surfaces of the body, to become systemic. Concurrent with the immunosuppression that accompanies pregnancy, there is an increased shedding of infectious microorganisms. This is considered to be an extension of impaired T cytotoxic lymphocyte function. Although the pregnant animal may appear clinically normal, her altered immune response results in an increased shedding of gastrointestinal viruses, such as canine coronavirus and canine rotavirus, and bacteria, such as *Escherichia coli*, usually during the periparturient period. This increase in shedding of infectious microorganisms is an important factor when addressing the issues of management of animals through this period of time (Figure 14-2). The suppression of neutrophil functions during later stages of pregnancy and immediately postpartum are the subject of active investigation.

Although the immunosuppressive periods during pregnancy and up to 4 weeks postpartum is well recognized, our understanding of this process is still somewhat rudimentary. However, we can proceed with control measures that accomplish two primary goals: to maximize reproductive performance and to assure successful neonatal survival. Over the years, we have emphasized the importance of effective vaccination programs prebreeding, clean birthing areas, and good hygiene for the lactating animal. In conjunction with good colostral management, these measures allow us to compensate for the temporary immunosuppressive states encountered during pregnancy and immediately thereafter.

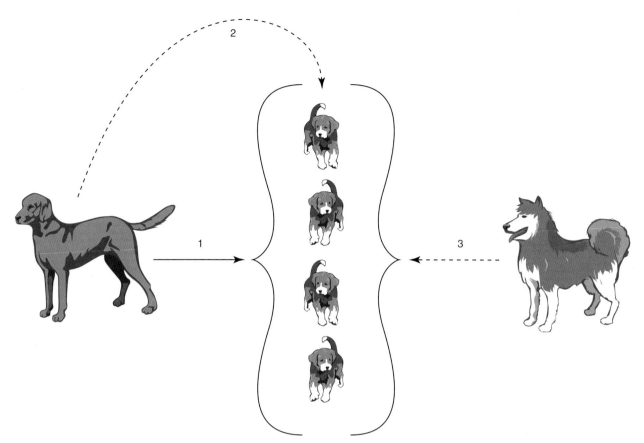

Figure 14-2 Diagram depicts the three possible ways that neonatal puppies can be naturally infected. The dam infects the puppies before whelping or shortly thereafter *(1)*; the dam acquires infection after whelping and infects the puppies *(2)*; and the puppies are infected from an external source such as another dog *(3)*.

MONITORING MATERNAL PASSIVE IMMUNITY

Puppies

Passive immunity from maternal antibodies is a vital component of immune protection to help prevent disease in neonates. In comparison to humans in which a significant amount of immunoglobulins are transferred transplacentally, dogs have an endotheliochorial placenta with four layers separating fetal and maternal blood. This type of placentation results in very little maternal immunoglobulin transfer to the fetus, with reported transplacental immunoglobulin transfer ranging from 5% to 10%. Colostrum is important for early antibody protection in puppies. In puppies, only small amounts of immunoglobulin G (IgG) are detected before colostrum ingestion and immunoglobulin A (IgA) is undetectable until after colostrum intake, supporting poor transplacental transfer. In mammals, intestinal permeability for immunoglobulin absorption is highest right after birth and decreases by 6 hours to a very low level of absorption 24 hours after birth. A low level of intestinal absorption of immunoglobulins continues while the puppy is nursing. Specific receptors in the intestine bind the immunoglobulin, which is then taken up by epithelial cells, transferred into

lacteals, and into the circulation. Immunity from colostrum depends on the vaccination and immune status of the dam, as well as the quantity of colostrum ingested. The amount of colostral antibody can be quite variable between littermates, depending on the amount of colostrum ingested, the time ingested, and the size of the litter.

Colostrum is composed of immunoglobulins, and in some species, such as cows, there are also numerous lymphocytes and proteins. Little information has been published about leukocytes or other proteins in canine colostrum, but some cellular material is transferred from the dam to the puppy. In dogs, IgG predominates in colostrum with slightly less IgA and very little immunoglobulin M (IgM). The peak immunoglobulin concentration in puppies ingesting colostrum is 12 to 24 hours after birth. Once colostrum transitions to milk, the concentrations of immunoglobulin significantly decrease in milk. The predominance of IgG in colostrum switches to a predominance of IgA in milk with only low levels of IgM and IgG detected at 6 weeks of lactation. This form of passive immunity is referred to as *lactogenic immunity*. The IgA has been shown to inhibit adherence of infectious agents to mucosal surfaces, neutralizing potential intestinal mucosal pathogens. Maternal antibody helps protect the neonate puppy but will also cause a refractory period to vaccination until maternal antibody declines.

TABLE 14-1	Half-life of maternally derived immunoglobulins in neonatal dogs and cats	
Disease	Half-life (days)	Usual duration of protection against disease (weeks)
Canine distemper	8.4	9-12
Canine parvovirus	9.7	10-14
Infectious canine hepatitis	8.4	9-12
Feline panleukopenia	9.5	8-14
Feline leukemia	15.0	6-8
Feline rhinotracheitis	18.5	6-8
Feline calicivirus infection	15.0	10-14
Feline coronavirus infection	7.0	4-6

From Greene CE, Schultz RD: Immunoprophylaxis. In Greene CE (ed): *Infectious diseases of the dog and cat*, ed 3, St Louis, 2006, Saunders/Elsevier, p 1072.

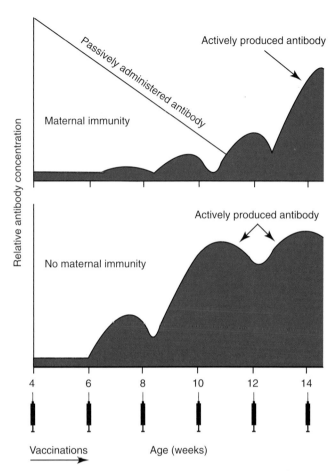

Figure 14-3 Comparison of response to sequential (2-week interval) vaccination in neonates with *(top)* and without *(bottom)* maternal antibody protection. The presence of maternal antibody delays the neonates' ability to produce successful active immunization. (From Greene CE, Schultz RD: Immunoprophylaxis. In Greene CE (ed): *Infectious diseases of the dog and cat*, ed 3, St Louis, 2006, Saunders/Elsevier.)

Endogenous immunoglobulin secretion will only be stimulated when maternal antibody decreases to a low level. Between 6 and 16 weeks, maternal antibody declines to undetectable limits and depends on the half-life of maternal canine immunoglobulin, which is approximately 8.4 days (Table 14-1). Loss of immunoglobulins is also dependent on antibody class with IgA degraded first, followed by IgM, and then IgG. Rapidly growing breeds have also been shown to break down maternally derived immunoglobulin at a faster rate. As maternal antibody decreases, endogenous immunoglobulin secretion steadily increases. The immunoglobulins tend to increase in order from IgM to IgG followed by IgA. These immunoglobulins reach adult levels at 2 to 3 months, 6 to 9 months, and 12 months, respectively.

Although maternal antibody is necessary for early protection in the neonate, it can be problematic as the puppy gets older by interfering with vaccine-induced immunity and the ability to respond to new antigens. As maternal antibody is decreasing, there is a window in which maternal immunoglobulin may decrease below protective levels but persist at high enough levels to interfere with vaccination and protective immune responses. This dangerous window is one reason that multiple vaccines are given close together in puppies less than 16 weeks of age to stimulate the immune system at the earliest time possible before exposure of antigen. It is important to know if the puppy has received colostrum because vaccination guidelines will differ, depending on whether colostrum was ingested. Puppies not receiving colostrum can elicit an adequate antibody response much sooner than puppies with maternal passive immunity (Figure 14-3).

In general, puppies begin life with a competent but immature immune system that matures over the first 6 to 12 months of life. The time frame of complete immuno-competence and adequate response to vaccination or natural antigens depends on the concentration of colostral immunoglobulin ingested, as well as progressive development of the immune system.

Kittens

Passive immunity is also important in the kitten for early immune protection. Like the dog, placentation is endotheliochorial, which means very little immunoglobulin is transferred from the queen to the fetus during pregnancy. The concentration of immunoprotective immunoglobulins in colostrum depends on the queen's immune and vaccination status, as well as the amount and timing of colostral ingestion. Similar to dogs, there can be variation of immunoglobulin ingestion within the same litter and between different litters from the same queen.

At parturition, kittens have no IgG and little to no IgA before colostrum ingestion. Feline colostral IgG is very concentrated, almost 4.5 times the concentration of the queen's serum levels, and colostral IgA is present in much lower concentrations than IgG. Absorption of immunoglobulins in the intestine is similar in all mammals with the highest permeability occurring right after birth and very little immunoglobulin absorption by 24 hours after birth. Peak serum concentration of immunoglobulin occurs 1 to 2 days after parturition with low levels of immunoglobulin absorbed during the nursing period. As colostrum transitions to milk, there is a rapid decline of IgG concentration through day 7, which then remains the same for approximately 6 weeks. IgA levels remained steady throughout lactation. In contrast to dogs, feline milk is dominated by IgG rather than IgA.

Similar to all species, maternal antibody suppresses endogenous secretion of immunoglobulin until it decreases to low concentrations. Maternal immunoglobulin has an approximate half-life of 4.4 days, and maternal antibody can be undetectable in some kittens by 4 to 5 weeks, although the range varies from 4 to 14 weeks (see Table 14-1). Endogenous IgG production starts at approximately 5 to 6 weeks of age in kittens with colostrum ingestion, whereas production of IgA begins a short time later. IgM slowly increases until approximately 8 weeks of age and then concentrations remain steady. Colostrum-deficient or -deprived kittens have significantly lower IgG than colostrum-fed kittens until 4 weeks of age and then have a higher level of endogenous IgG than colostrum-fed kittens by 8 weeks of age.

Maternal antibody creates the same vaccination challenges for cats as described in dogs. Colostrum-fed kittens have a window between 4 to 14 weeks, in which maternal antibody drops to nonprotective levels; however, it is still high enough to interfere with vaccination and the kitten's response to foreign antigens. Predicting when this window will occur and the precise time to vaccinate will be different in each individual animal, complicating vaccination in kittens. It is also important to know if the animal has received colostrum because vaccination guidelines will differ, depending on colostrum ingestion as the result of differences in immunologic development.

AGE-APPROPRIATE VACCINATION FOR PUPPIES AND KITTENS

Vaccination for the infectious microorganisms that can affect puppy and kitten survival and well-being and for public health concerns has been of vital importance for disease control. The major problem with vaccination protocols is determining the appropriate time to administer the vaccine to achieve optimal immunization. There are three main obstacles to consider when vaccinating puppies and kittens, including the immature immune system, possible bias toward humoral immunity, and presence of maternal antibodies. Although in-depth research has not been performed specifically in cats and dogs, comparative studies done in humans and mice have observed reduced expression of ligands on APCs and lymphocytes in neonates, resulting in decreased interaction between these cells. The APC and lymphocyte interaction is necessary to stimulate a specific T cell response. Another difference in neonates compared to adults is the late

development of splenic architecture with APCs, such as macrophages and B cells, developing later than T cells. Additionally B cells, which are also APCs, have decreased expression of receptors and ligands, leading to less crosstalk between B lymphocytes and T lymphocytes compared to the adult, resulting in a blunted antibody response. Some of these factors are contributors to a shift toward the humoral-mediated immune response, as well as a blunted immune response. In addition to the immaturity of the immune system, maternal antibody interferes with endogenous production of immunoglobulins, as well as response to vaccine antigens until 6 to 16 weeks of age.

The immune response of puppies and kittens will always be variable due to differences in immune development, maternal antibody, antigen load, or route of vaccination. Taking into account differences in the immune system of the neonatal puppy or kitten will help determine future vaccination guidelines. Further characterization of the predominant immune system in neonates may be beneficial for developing new vaccinations to promote a balanced immune response. A balanced immune response will stimulate both the cell-mediated and humoral immune–mediated responses to help prevent pathologic inflammation or hypersensitivity that can occur when only one side of the immune system is stimulated.

Since the duration of protection provided to puppies by maternal antibodies varies 5 weeks for canine coronavirus (CCV) to 20 weeks for canine distemper virus (CDV), it is recommended that puppies be vaccinated until active immunization occurs. Newer vaccines have proven to be effective in overcoming maternal antibodies and effectively stimulating the immune response as early as 12 weeks of age. Table 14-2 provides a list of immunogens and a time frame for administration. Once the puppy series has been completed, a booster at 1 year of age is recommended. Subsequent boosters can be administered at annual, biannual, or triennial periods, depending on the risk of subsequent infection.

Kittens become susceptible to infectious disease once they begin to lose passive protection provided by the queen's colostrum. The length of this protection varies from 3 weeks for feline coronavirus (FCoV) to 15 weeks for feline panleukopenia (FPL) virus. Table 14-3 presents a list of immunogens and time for administration for kittens. The initial vaccination is given at 8 to 10 weeks of age and a booster at 14 to 16 weeks of age. A booster is recommended at 1 year of age. Subsequent boosters on an annual, biannual, or triennial basis are given according to the risk.

There has been increased emphasis on maternal vaccination for protection of puppies and kittens from infectious diseases. Box 14-1 lists the reasons to maintain an active immunization program. The latter three points pertain specifically to the beneficial effects of maternal vaccination. These include those already mentioned (stimulation of high levels of protective immunoglobulins in the colostrum and early milk), fetal protection from congenital infection, and decreased shedding of infectious microorganisms from subclinical carriers.

TABLE 14-2	Vaccination guidelines for puppies
Age	**Vaccine**
6-7 weeks	Canine distemper virus (C)
	Canine adenovirus-2 (C)
	Canine parvovirus-2 (C)
	Canine parainfluenza (NC)
	Canine coronavirus (NC)
	Leptospirosis (4-way, NC)
	Bordetella (NC)
	Borreliosis (NC)
9-10 weeks	Same
12-13 weeks	Same + rabies (C)
16-17 weeks	Rabies booster (C)
Annual, biannual, and triennial, according to environmental risks	

C, Core; *NC*, noncore (does not mean nonessential).
Data from Hosgood G: Preventative care. In Hosgood G, Hoskins JD, Davidson JR, et al (eds): *Small animal paediatric medicine and surgery,* Boston, 1998, Butterworth-Heinemann; Davis-Wurzler GM: Current vaccination strategies in puppies and kittens, *Vet Clin Small Anim* 36:607, 2006; and Paul MA (Chair): *The 2006 AAHA canine vaccine guidelines. American Animal Hosp Assoc.* www.aahanet.org/publicdocuments/vaccine guidelines06revised.pdf

TABLE 14-3	Vaccination guidelines for kittens
Age	**Vaccine**
8-9 weeks	Feline herpesvirus (C)
	Feline calicivirus (C)
	Feline panleukopenia (C)
	Feline leukemia (NC)
	Chlamydia (NC)
	Bordetella (NC)
12-13 weeks	Same + rabies (C)
16 weeks	Rabies booster (C)
Annual, biannual, and triennial, according to environmental risks	

C, Core; *NC*, noncore (does not mean nonessential).
Data from Hosgood G: Preventative care. In Hosgood G, Hoskins JD, Davidson JR, et al (eds): *Small animal paediatric medicine and surgery,* Boston, 1998, Butterworth-Heinemann; Davis-Wurzler GM:Current vaccination strategies in puppies and kittens, *Vet Clin Small Anim* 36:607, 2006; and Richards JR (Chair): The 2006 American Association of Feline Practitioners Feline Vaccine Advisory Panel Report, *JAVMA* 229:1405, 2006.

This latter point is worth further explanation. It is known that there are subclinical carriers in the dog and cat populations that are immune from disease but still capable of shedding infectious microorganisms consistently or intermittently such as canine parainfluenza in aerosols and canine parvovirus (CPV)and FCoV in feces (Figure 14-4). Shedding animals are sources of infections for susceptible animals in the population. These include pregnant animals, young puppies and kittens (<6 months old), and immunocompro-

BOX 14-1	Reasons to maintain an active immunization program

1. Protect individual dog and cat from disease.
2. Protect the majority of animals in the population from disease (kennel/cattery "herd" immunity).
3. Serve as an immune barrier for zoonotic and emerging infectious diseases.
4. Protect fetus from infection (congenital infections; abortions; stillbirths; and so on).
5. Decreased shedding of infectious agents from subclinical carriers to susceptible animals.
6. Protect puppies and kittens from disease by colostral immunity and lactogenic (early milk) immunity.

mised animals (immunosuppressive medications, susceptible breeds, concurrent viral or bacterial infections, and nutritional stress).

ADVERSE REACTIONS ASSOCIATED WITH VACCINATION

Over the past decade, there has been a concerted effort to increase the duration of protective immunity while decreasing the adverse effects associated with certain vaccines. The use of vaccines is highest during the first year of life for puppies and kittens. The benefits of vaccine use are listed in Box 14-1. There are also vaccine reactions that may occur after vaccination.

Adverse reactions must always be considered when vaccinating a neonate or adult dog or cat; fortunately the most common side effect is protection against an infectious disease that could cause morbidity or mortality. Numerous vaccinations are given without consequence, but it is important to remember that vaccines are biologic agents and adverse reactions can occur even after undergoing strict testing for safety, efficacy, and purity. Vaccine reactions can occur locally at the injection site or systemically. Systemic effects can range from generalized malaise to hypersensitivity reactions or sometimes neoplasia. The most common side effects include local inflammation at the site of injection and generalized malaise lasting for 1 to 2 days after immunization. However, some localized inflammation can persist for weeks to months.

The type of vaccine, breed, administration guidelines, and immune status can all play roles in whether an animal will have a vaccine reaction. For example, modified live-virus vaccines elicit a stronger antigenic response in the host than killed vaccines and are often very effective. However, in immunocompromised patients or young kittens and puppies, there may be a heightened risk of adverse reactions with these types of vaccines. There are also breed predispositions to vaccine reactions, such as the Akita, Great Dane, American cocker spaniel, dachshund, poodle, Old English sheepdogs, among others, and these predispositions should be considered with immunization.

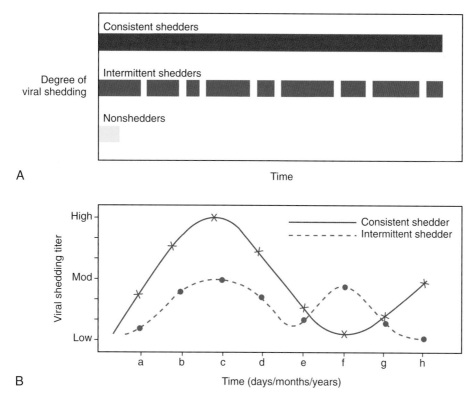

Figure 14-4 Schematic depicting the variation in viral shedding over time. **A**, Panel indicates the types of viral shedders in the animal population. **B**, Panel indicates the variability in viral shedding amount (titer) between consistent and intermittent shedders.

Systemic vaccine reactions are often the result of hypersensitivity reactions. Hypersensitivity reactions can include immediate reactions occurring within minutes to hours to more delayed reactions that occur 24 to 72 hours or even 7 to 45 days after vaccination. Hypersensitivity reactions can result from a type I hypersensitivity reaction mediated by IgE resulting in anaphylaxis. Anaphylactic reactions occur within minutes to a few hours after vaccine administration and clinical signs can include edema and pruritus, often seen in the dog, or vomiting and diarrhea in cats. More significant sequelae can occur, including respiratory distress, hypovolemia, and shock. Type II hypersensitivity, which is an autoimmune reaction, is also thought to occur after vaccination in some dogs. This has not been definitively proved; however, immune-mediated thrombocytopenia and anemia have been reported in conjunction with recent immunization. Type III hypersensitivity, or immune complex disease, is another type of reaction that can be seen with some vaccines. A specific example in the dog includes anterior uveitis, which occurs approximately 10 to 21 days after canine adenovirus-1 (CAV-1) vaccination as a result of antibody-antigen complex deposition. The last type of hypersensitivity is type IV hypersensitivity, which is a delayed response resulting in granuloma formation at the site of vaccination. Granulomas can resolve within weeks to months in some animals and are typically seen with adjuvant vaccines. In cats, inflammation can persist sometimes, transitioning from chronic inflammation to a neoplastic process resulting in an injection site sarcoma.

In human medicine, there is a lot of attention given to suspected associations between vaccination and autoimmunity. Although not scientifically proved, these concerns should persist until evidence proves otherwise. A possible mechanism of vaccine-associated autoimmunity is epitope mimicry, in which an antigen in a vaccine is similar to a self–antigen, causing the immune response to be directed at an antigen on a population of the animal's cells. Certain types of adjuvant can stimulate different pathways of the immune response and some vaccines may stimulate differentiation of pathogenic lymphocytes that recognize self–antigens. It has been shown that all adult humans have some B and T cell lymphocytes that recognize self–antigens; however, these cells are typically quiescent. With some vaccinations, these cells could become reactive or overreactive, resulting in autoimmunity. Because neonates often have a reduced immune response, it is thought they may be more protected from autoimmune reactions. Further studies need to be performed to confirm vaccine-associated autoimmune reactions and potential consequences in the neonate.

MONITORING THE IMMUNE RESPONSE WITH ANTIBODY TITERS

The practice of measuring an immune response to determine infection by using acute and convalescent serology, by IgM serology, or by enzyme-linked immunosorbent assay (ELISA) has been accepted for diagnostic purposes and for assessing vaccine challenge studies for a number of years. With the increased concerns about adverse effects of vaccination, there has been a trend to use antibody titers to specific viral antigens to assess immune competence and in some cases, provide information on protective levels of antibody. This practice has gained acceptance for those breeds of dogs and cats that have adverse effects after vaccination but usually applies to animals over 1 year of age. Antibody titer evaluation has been used more within the first year of life to determine if puppies and kittens are receiving adequate levels of maternal antibody and if they would benefit from a booster at 6 months of age. Antibody (IgG) levels of 1:100 or greater to CDV and CPV are generally regarded as protective against disease.

It is important to recognize that a protective antibody titer does not mean that the dog is not infected or that it is not a subclinical carrier-intermittent shedder. Cats with FPL IgG antibody titers of 1:100 or greater are regarded as protected against disease but that does not mean that the cat is not a subclinical carrier.

Immune assessment antibody profiles are available through most veterinary diagnostic laboratories. Assays that measure the CMI response/T cell responsiveness are currently being developed and will utilize measures to monitor T cell–specific cytokines.

SUGGESTED READINGS

Clinkenbeard KD, Cowell RL, Meinkoth JH, et al: The hematopoietic and lymphoid systems. In Hoskins JD (ed): *Veterinary pediatrics: dogs and cats from birth to six months,* ed 3, Philadelphia, 2001, Saunders.

Davis-Wurzler GM: Current vaccination strategies in puppies and kittens, *Vet Clin Small Anim* 36:607, 2006.

Day MJ: *Clinical immunology of the dog and cat,* ed 2, London, 2008, Manson Publishing Ltd.

Day MJ: Immune system development in the dog and cat, *J Comp Pathol* 137:S10, 2007.

Furth MA, Shewen PE, Hodgins DC: Passive and active components of neonatal innate immune defenses, *Anim Health Res Rev* 6:143, 2005.

Tizard IR: *Veterinary immunology: an introduction,* ed 8, St Louis, 2009, Saunders/Elsevier.

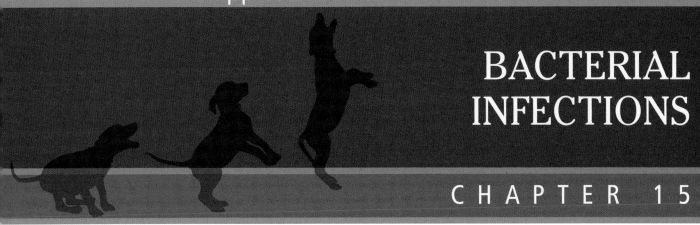

BACTERIAL INFECTIONS

CHAPTER 15

Joshua Daniels, Erick Spencer

ROLE OF BACTERIA IN JUVENILE SMALL ANIMAL DISEASE

There are relatively few bacterial diseases to which juvenile animals are inherently more predisposed in comparison to adults. This starkly contrasts with their vulnerability to viral infections (see Chapter 16). This chapter covers the most common syndromes in which bacteria act as primary pathogens in juveniles, as well as some practical considerations in obtaining definitive diagnoses in working with a diagnostic laboratory.

Classification of Bacteria

Bacteria are most commonly classified by their cell wall type and their ability to grow in the presence or absence of oxygen (aerobic/anaerobic). The majority of pathogens can be classified according to cell wall type with a Gram stain; however, some microbial genera, such as *Mycoplasma* and *Chlamydophila*, stain poorly. Other staining agents help to identify agents more specifically such as the Ziehl-Neelsen acid-fast stain for mycobacteria. Knowledge of predilections of bacterial families to colonize particular body sites is useful in empirical selection of antimicrobial agent(s) for initial therapy (Table 15-1).

Working with a Diagnostic Microbiologist

Frequently, it is desirable to obtain a definitive bacteriologic diagnosis (e.g., when empiric therapy is failing, infections are recurrent, and specific knowledge of an infectious agent is required for prognostication and/or duration of treatment). Despite the fact that culture and identification from animal specimens can be performed by human microbiology laboratories, it is in the best interest of practitioners and their clients to work with a veterinary laboratory diagnostician; doing so will save time, money, and frustration and yield better clinical outcomes. The veterinary microbiologist is able to guide the laboratory bacterial workup so that the bacteriologic differential diagnoses are covered efficiently and that isolates selected for antimicrobial susceptibility testing are appropriate. Moreover, state and university veterinary diagnostic laboratories make available consultant microbiologists via telephone at no charge.

SYSTEMIC INFECTIONS

General Neonatal Septicemia and Bacteremia

Septicemia is a major cause of mortality in puppies and kittens during the first 3 weeks of life. At parturition, puppies and kittens are in an immunocompromised state; they are susceptible to infection by bacteria that are regarded as "commensal" (i.e., normal microbial colonizers of the mucosal surfaces and skin). Despite some transplacental passage of immunoglobulins in dogs and cats, to successfully defend themselves against infection, neonates depend on passive immunity via colostrum imbibed in the first 1 to 2 days of life. Also important is the innate immune mechanism, which is afforded in large part by maintaining healthy mucosal surfaces. Puppies and kittens must be assured unfettered nursing access and kept in a room with proper ambient temperature so energy can be spent growing rather than trying to thermoregulate. In the first week of life, ambient temperature should be 85° to 90° F (29° to 32° C) and approximately 80° F (26.5° C) for the second through fourth weeks of life.

Puppies are most susceptible to septicemia during the first week of life. Septicemia is also a common sequela to viral enteritis, which occurs most commonly from 8 to 16 weeks of age. The most common organisms implicated in these infections belong to the family Enterobacteriaceae, notably *Escherichia coli*, *Klebsiella* spp., and *Proteus* spp. To a lesser extent, other gram-negative pathogens, such as *Pseudomonas* spp., may be associated with sepsis. Of the gram-positive bacteria, β-streptococci (usually group G or B) have

TABLE 15-1	Examples of common expected normal flora by body site			
Oral mucosa	**Epidermis**	**Conjunctival mucosa**	**Genital mucosa**
Gram-positive			
α-, γ-Streptococcus spp. *Corynebacterium* spp. *Peptostreptococcus* spp. *Propionibacterium* spp.	*Staphylococcus* spp. *Corynebacterium* spp. *Propionibacterium* spp.	*α-, γ-Streptococcus* spp. *Corynebacterium* spp.	*α-, γ-Streptococcus* spp.
Gram-negative			
Prevotella spp. *Bacteroides* spp. *Fusobacterium* spp. *Pasteurella* spp. *Mycoplasma* spp. (Occasional)	*Pseudomonas* spp. *Proteus* spp. No	*Moraxella* spp. *Pseudomonas* spp. Yes	Enterobacteriaceae Yes

the potential to cause systemic infection during this time frame. These organisms are normal colonizers of mucosal surfaces of the dam, particularly the vagina and anus.

E. coli is the most frequent agent involved; they are numerically dominant in feces (among the facultative organisms), and many *E. coli* serotypes that comprise the normal commensal microflora have intrinsic complement resistance caused by long lipopolysaccharide residues (O-antigens). These organisms typically gain access to the bloodstream via translocation across the intestinal mucosa and/or by a compromised umbilicus.

Kittens are also susceptible to neonatal sepsis by commensal Enterobacteriaceae during the first few weeks of life; however, bacteremic *Pasteurella multocida* infection is also common in the feline neonate. More common than in puppies, kittens are particularly at risk for systemic group G streptococcal infection. This agent is a ubiquitous inhabitant of the vaginal mucosa of queens.

Because these diseases progress rapidly in neonates and sudden death often occurs, the problem is frequently diagnosed postmortem. Typical histopathologic findings include bacterial emboli in multiple organs, and if culture is performed on fresh tissues, one bacterial species typically dominates as a pure culture in high numbers. Expired animals submitted for histopathology should be refrigerated (not frozen) and sent to the diagnostic laboratory intact within 1 day. If animals are too large to send in their entirety, they should be necropsied as soon as possible with fresh and fixed tissues collected for histopathologic examination and ancillary testing (Table 15-2).

History and physical examination findings are the basis for the clinical suspicion of systemic bacterial infections. Sepsis should be a differential diagnosis for a puppy or kitten with any of the following general signs: inappetence, inactivity, excessive crying, hypothermia, failure to thrive, and diarrhea. Any seizure activity also merits sepsis on the differential diagnosis list. Clinicopathologic results are generally nonspecific, although they may reveal failure of a specific organ.

TABLE 15-2	Samples for postmortem diagnosis of the acutely dead neonate
Fixed tissues for histopathology (10% buffered formalin)	**Fresh tissues for bacteriology, virology, serology**
Heart (LV, RV, septum), lung, kidney, adrenal glands, stomach, duodenum, jejunum, ileum, colon, urinary bladder, spleen, cerebrum, thyroid gland, cerebellum, brainstem, trachea, tongue	As tissue pool: liver, kidney, spleen, brain Separate bag: feces Separate bag: lung Serum from dam (if canine herpesvirus is suspected).

LV, Left ventricle; *RV,* right ventricle.

The leukogram may reflect evidence of inflammation such as a neutrophilia with a left shift or a normocytic, normochromic anemia. Hypoglycemia is a common finding on the chemistry profile of patients with bacteremia, although it is not pathognomonic for systemic bacterial infections. Immediate empiric antimicrobial therapy and supportive care should be instituted in these patients rather than seeking an etiologic diagnosis; these are emergencies.

If obtaining cultures does not significantly delay initiation of empiric antimicrobial therapy, the following is recommended:

1. Blood culture using a pediatric culture system, such as the BACTEC Pediatric (Becton Dickinson, Short Hills, NJ) or the Isolator system (Wampole Laboratories, Cranbury, NJ). A clinical microbiology laboratory will recommend a specific collection/transport system to use because of downstream processing.
2. Urine culture.

Identification of the organism(s) and their susceptibility data will guide the antimicrobial regime in the patient. If littermates are also affected, obtaining clinical microbiologic data on each patient is recommended, since the bacteria involved in each puppy or kitten may be different.

Methods to prevent neonatal septicemia include the use of pooled adult serum administered to colostrum-deprived puppies and kittens to attempt to increase serum immunoglobulin concentrations. In the puppy, 22 ml/kg of pooled adult dog serum can be administered subcutaneously. Approximately 15 ml/kitten of pooled cat serum can be administered subcutaneously or intraperitoneally to kittens to correct a suspected immunoglobulin deficiency.

Prevention of some infections can be achieved by administering antimicrobial agents to queens in the peripartum period (Table 15-3), if there is a known or suspected genital colonization by β-hemolytic streptococci. Proper sanitation of the birthing area is also essential in the prevention of both umbilical infections and neonatal septicemia. Antiseptic solutions, such as povidone-iodine, should also be applied to the umbilicus of the neonate to help prevent umbilical infections.

Treatment of neonatal systemic infections involves antimicrobial agents and supportive care. Balanced electrolyte solutions, such as lactated Ringer's solution or Normosol R, should be used for fluid therapy. Some patients may require dextrose or potassium chloride supplementation as part of their fluid therapy. Patients that are profoundly hypoglycemic should receive a bolus (1 to 2 ml/kg) of 50% dextrose that should be diluted to make a 10% to 25% solution. Thermal support, oxygen supplementation, and nutrition are also important elements of supportive therapy for the bacteremic patient (see chapter 10).

Oral drug absorption is unreliable in neonates and decreased perfusion of peripheral capillaries in septic shock renders subcutaneous administration of antimicrobial agents of little value, especially in dehydrated patients. Therefore antimicrobials should be administered either intravenously or intraosseously. Second- and third-generation cephalosporins, such as cefoxitin (30 mg/kg intravenous [IV] every 8 hours [q8h]) and cefotaxime (25 to 50 mg/kg IV q8h), respectively, are good initial empiric therapies because they provide broad-spectrum antimicrobial coverage against gram-positive, gram-negative, and anaerobic bacteria. If there is concurrent renal compromise, try to use a cephalosporin that is not renally cleared; however, if renally cleared cephalosporins are all that are available, use the following formula:

$$\text{Normal interval} \times \text{serum creatinine (if} > 1)$$

Respiratory Infections: Puppies

Bordetella bronchiseptica

Infectious canine tracheobronchitis (ITB) or "kennel cough" is a clinical syndrome and is associated with infection with one or more of several viral and/or bacterial agents (although to many practitioners, the term has become synonymous with *Bordetella bronchiseptica* infection in particular). Canine parainfluenza-2, adenovirus-2, and *Mycoplasma* sp. infections play roles in this syndrome and are addressed as individual agents in Chapter 16. Although *Bordetella* infection is often present as a coinfection with viral agents, it is capable of causing disease by itself.

ITB usually presents as an acute honking cough, which is classically elicited on tracheal palpation. Oculonasal discharges may accompany this cough, especially when multiple-agent infections occur. Dogs may also be febrile and lethargic. Usually, infection is self-limiting, but in a small proportion of cases (<5%), in which puppies are disproportionately overrepresented, pneumonia may develop. *B. bronchiseptica* causes specific damage to respiratory epithelium, which impacts mucociliary clearance. This damage permits superinfections with resident commensal bacteria, such as *Streptococcus* spp., *Mycoplasma* spp., and *Pasteurella* spp., that may worsen the prognosis and complicate antimicrobial therapy. Brachycephalic breeds appear to be at increased risk for the development of pneumonia, perhaps because of the combination of a short upper airway and frequently turbulent inspiratory effort (or snorting).

Agents of ITB are spread via aerosolization or by fomites such as feeding bowls. Incubation postexposure ranges from 3 to 10 days. It is important to note that viral and *Bordetella* vaccines do not prevent infection; they decrease clinical signs and shedding associated with infection. Postrecovery, dogs may shed *Bordetella* for several months, although naturally acquired mucosal immunity to the infecting strain will prevent clinical signs for 6 months or more. Bactericidal cleansers (including 20:1 water:bleach for 10 minutes of

TABLE 15-3	Prophylaxis of β-streptococcal infections in cats at parturition				
Drug	Age	Dose*	Route	Interval (hours)	Duration (days)
Ampicillin	Neonate	25 mg/kg	SC	8	5-7
Amoxicillin	Neonate	25 mg/kg	PO	8	5-7
Procaine and benzathine penicillin	Neonate	6,250 IU†	SC	48-72	3-5‡
	Queen	150,000 IU†	SC	48-72	3-5‡

Modified from Greene CE: *Infectious diseases of the dog and cat*, ed 3, St Louis, 2006, Saunders/Elsevier.

SC, Subcutaneous; *PO*, by mouth.

*Dose per administration at specified interval.

†Total dose needed for each drug in a fixed combination, based on a 2 to 3 kg cat. This drug is associated with injection site sarcomas.

‡Only one or two doses are given during this treatment regimen.

contact) are effective at killing *B. bronchiseptica,* which can be stable in the environment for days to weeks.

The etiologic agent(s) responsible for ITB are rarely identified, since most infections are self-limiting and resolve with empiric therapy. However, in animals that do not improve within 2 weeks of initial presentation, reevaluation is advised to determine if pneumonia or additional systemic problems are present. In cases involving multiple affected animals a specific diagnosis could aid future prevention efforts. If pneumonic, aspiration of tracheal fluid for cytology and culture is recommended to guide antimicrobial therapy. It is of little use to submit nasal or pharyngeal swabs, as overwhelming overgrowth of commensal bacteria will almost invariably hinder the growth of *Bordetella* (if present). It is also advisable to rule in the possibility of canine distemper infection with immunofluorescent antibody testing on buffy coat and tracheal aspirates (if cellular) and serology.

Respiratory and Ocular Infections: Kittens

The agents that cause upper respiratory disease in cats frequently cause ocular disease (primarily conjunctivitis), so they are discussed together.

Infections with feline calicivirus and/or feline herpesvirus are primarily responsible for the majority of upper respiratory disease in cats and kittens. *Chlamydophila felis* may complicate viral respiratory infections but has the ability to cause disease as a solitary agent in experimental infections. Clinically, its presence should be suspected in the most severe cases of respiratory disease and is a frequent cause of primary bronchopneumonia in kittens. The precise role of *Mycoplasma felis* as a cause of feline upper respiratory and ocular disease is not known. It is a commensal organism of the feline nasopharynx and conjunctiva and may be isolated from healthy cats, as well as those experiencing respiratory/ocular signs. Interestingly, in shelter cats, *M. felis* may play a more important role in causing respiratory disease than in the general cat population. *M. felis* has been implicated as an important cause of pneumonia in kittens and is also associated with infectious polyarthritis, which usually presents initially as a fever of unknown origin.

B. bronchiseptica in cats is a relatively uncommon cause of upper respiratory disease and is most aptly described as a commensal organism that can act as an opportunist. In a recent study of seven California animal shelters, *B. bronchiseptica* had a low prevalence relative to other upper respiratory infection (URI) pathogens and more importantly was not significantly associated with URI signs.

Prevention is primarily based on infection control (limited contact with infected patients), but appropriate vaccination, adequate ventilation, good sanitation, balanced nutrition, and routine parasite control are also important factors in limiting the transmission of these agents.

Outpatient treatment is recommended for patients with URIs; however, some patients may require hospitalization for supportive measures such as nebulization, humidification of inspired air, and/or removal of oculonasal discharge. Doxycycline 5 to 10 mg/kg PO q12h should be used in kittens, since *Chlamydophila* may be a common cause of upper respiratory disease.

Puppies and kittens suspected to have infectious tracheobronchitis should be isolated from other animals and maintained in a minimal-stress environment. Infectious tracheobronchitis is generally self-limiting, but treatment is recommended for patients with clinical signs that do not resolve within 14 days because of the potential of bronchopneumonia as a sequela. Initial treatment choices should be effective against both *B. bronchiseptica* and *Mycoplasma* sp. Doxycycline (5 to 10 mg/kg by mouth [PO] q12h), chloramphenicol (dog: 50 mg/kg PO, IV, intramuscular [IM], subcutaneously [SC] q8h; cat: 25 to 50 mg/kg PO, IV, IM, SC q12h), or amoxicillin/clavulanate (13 to 22 mg/kg PO q12h) can be used effectively in both cats and dogs for both microorganisms. Antitussives are contraindicated, since suppression of the cough reflex increases the potential for bacteria to colonize the lower airways.

If bronchopneumonia is present radiographically, it is strongly recommended that a transtracheal wash be performed to obtain material for aerobic culture and sensitivity to guide antimicrobial therapy. While waiting for clinical microbiologic data (48 to 72 hours for sensitivity), empiric therapy must be initiated. Broad-spectrum coverage using IV antimicrobial agents is recommended—ideally a β-lactam plus an aminoglycoside such as gentamicin.

With specific culture and sensitivity data, antimicrobial therapy can be modified and continued for at least 2 weeks after resolution of clinical signs and radiographic cure. Patients with bronchopneumonia also benefit from supportive therapy such as fluid administration, humidification of inspired air, nebulization, and coupage.

Bacterial Urogenital Infections

The juvenile small animal patient presents a unique challenge to the practitioner when presented by a client who assumes (and complains) that the animal has a urinary tract infection (UTI). Frequently, the animal in question is presented because it is urinating in an undesirable location, so the perceived medical problem may actually be a behavioral one. A careful history will assist the clinician in ranking behaviorally inappropriate urination in the differential diagnosis. A thorough history should be obtained, including information pertaining to frequency and volume of urination and whether the patient is posturing to urinate. In addition, the presence or lack of clinical signs associated with lower urinary tract disease, such as stranguria, pollakiuria, and hematuria, should be obtained from the caretaker. Urinalysis with culture will allow you to rule in or rule out the presence of infection and/or inflammation.

Bacterial cystitis in puppies is usually due to a primary anatomic problem. In puppies, vaginal strictures, juvenile vulvar conformation, and ectopic ureter in females and hypospadias in males permit excessive urethral ascension of bacteria, which leads to colonization of the bladder. Patent urachus in either sex may also lead to bacterial colonization of the bladder.

Like the dog, uncomplicated UTIs are also uncommon in the cat. Moreover, congenital anatomic defects that predispose the urinary tract to infection are also extremely uncommon in cats. However, idiopathic feline lower urinary tract disease (FLUTD) is a common syndrome characterized by stranguria and hematuria and is associated with sterile inflammation of the bladder. The onset of FLUTD can occur in cats less than 1 year of age. Fewer than 5% of cats with FLUTD signs have positive urine cultures.

In both puppies and kittens, assessment of the urinalysis for patients younger than 6 to 8 weeks of age can be difficult because the renal tubules have not fully matured. The presence of glucosuria, proteinuria, and a low specific gravity are normal in the immature kidney. However, the constellation of supportive clinical signs and urinalysis findings of proteinuria, hematuria, and pyuria are supportive of a urinary tract inflammation. These findings are highly suggestive for a UTI but a positive culture result is required to definitively diagnose a bacterial UTI.

Urine culture can be attempted to aid in the diagnosis. Three methods of sampling may be utilized when obtaining a urine sample: cystocentesis, catheterization, or free-catch sample. Cystocentesis permits the clearest interpretation of culture results because when performed with good aseptic technique, any bacterial growth is diagnostically meaningful. However, extremely sparse growth on culture media (<10 colonies) should be interpreted skeptically, especially if the urine does not contain an active sediment. When catheterization or midstream free-catch sampling is performed, quantification of bacteria in urine is required to aid interpretation of culture results. A result of less than 10,000 CFU bacteria/milliliter in urine should be eyed skeptically, since the distal urethra is amply colonized by bacteria.

If infections are recurrent or there is no abatement of signs in the face of appropriate antimicrobial therapy, underlying functional, structural, or neurologic abnormalities should be ruled out. Therefore it may be necessary to pursue abdominal radiographs, contrast radiography, abdominal ultrasound, urethrocystoscopy, or biopsy with histopathology of the tissues of the urinary tract.

β-Lactam antimicrobials are the preferred treatment in the neonate because they are effective against the majority of urinary bacterial pathogens, achieve high urine concentrations, and have a wide therapeutic margin. The dose or frequency of administration may need to be altered when treating with antimicrobials that are renally metabolized or excreted as they may have a prolonged half-life in the neonate. Length of antimicrobial therapy should be based on resolution of clinical signs, as well as improvement in urinalysis and urine culture. Urine culture may be performed 72 hours after the initiation of therapy to detect resistant organisms in cases where urinary signs are not abating.

Bacterial Infections of the Gastrointestinal Tract

In pediatric patients, viruses and parasites cause the majority of infectious gastrointestinal (GI) disease. However, a few bacterial species occasionally act as primary pathogens in this animal population and are discussed briefly in this section.

Many cats and dogs with enteric bacterial infections are asymptomatic, particularly when concurrent pathogens are absent. They may, however, have nonspecific clinical signs such as inappetence, vomiting, and diarrhea. The diarrhea may be small intestinal, large intestinal, or diffuse in origin. Hematemesis, melena, or hematochezia may also be noted in patients with enteric bacterial infections. The presence of blood is not pathognomonic for bacterial infection because other disease processes, such as GI foreign bodies, hemorrhagic gastroenteritis, and hypoadrenocorticism, can result in a similar clinical picture in the pediatric patient.

Salmonella enterica

Salmonella are gram-negative, facultatively intracellular bacteria that have the ability to cause enterocolitis and sepsis in rare cases. There are thousands of *Salmonella* serovars, but disease is most often associated with a small subset of the nontyphoidal serovars in mammals, especially Typhimurium, Enteritidis, and Newport. Pet owners present the greatest risk of exposing their animals to *Salmonella* through the feeding of raw diets and permitting predatory behavior (especially on songbirds). *Salmonella* may be isolated from the feces of healthy animals, and it is unclear precisely what host factors are necessary for *Salmonella* to transform from transient intestinal colonizer to pathogen, but lowered immune status and concurrent antimicrobial therapy (which lowers host colonization resistance) are believed to be important factors.

Campylobacter jejuni

Campylobacter jejuni is a gram-negative microaerophilic bacterium that may cause enterocolitis in puppies and kittens. Ingestion of raw poultry is the primary risk factor for *C. jejuni* infection, but beef may also be contaminated, thus feeding raw diets should be strongly discouraged. Like *Salmonella*, this agent may be found in the feces of healthy animals, and it is unclear what factors are required for it to act as a pathogen.

Clostridium perfringens

Clostridium perfringens is a normal inhabitant of the GI tract of dogs and cats and its role in enteric disease is controversial. However, Clostridia have an important role as preformed-toxin producers in dogs experiencing acute gastroenteritis after garbage eating. *Staphylococcus aureus* also produces toxins that are ingested preformed in garbage.

Diagnostic Approach to Diarrhea

Practitioners should initially focus on ruling in viral and parasitic causes of diarrhea with in-house parvovirus ELISA and fecal floatation/smears.

A combination of culture and examination of specially stained fecal smears is recommended for establishing a

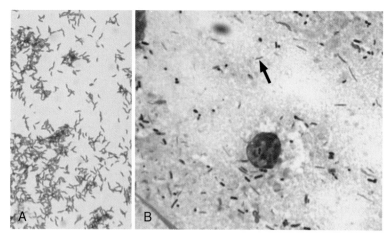

Figure 15-1   Victoria Blue stain of *Campylobacter jejuni* (100×). **A,** Pure culture growing on blood agar. **B,** Impression smear from small intestine of a puppy at necropsy. *Arrow* denotes classic "seagull" appearance of organism.

bacterial etiology. Costly anaerobic fecal cultures are discouraged, since *Clostridium perfringens* is virtually ubiquitous in the intestines of all mammals. Gram-stained fecal smears may reveal higher than normal clostridial forms relative to other bacterial morphologies, which merits a role for this agent as a participant in the clinical picture but not necessarily as the primary etiology. Classically, the presence of sporulating Clostridia ("safety pin forms") on fecal cytology has been used as a diagnostic feature of clostridial diarrhea. Newer methods, including immunodetection of clostridial enterotoxin and polymerase chain reaction (PCR), are also available, but their low specificity renders them of questionable value diagnostically.

The Victoria Blue stain is useful in establishing a diagnosis of *Campylobacter* enteritis. Because *Campylobacter* is commonly shed by healthy cats and dogs, positive culture alone is of limited diagnostic value; moreover, it is relatively expensive to perform. However, if curved rods or "seagull forms" are observed easily in fecal smears using the Victoria Blue stain, a presumptive diagnosis is reasonable (Figure 15-1) and culture for *Campylobacter* is then warranted. Aerobic fecal culture is recommended for determining if *Salmonella* is present. The presence of fecal leukocytes is always an indication to perform *Salmonella* and *Campylobacter* cultures.

Specific antimicrobial therapy should be based on the underlying cause of the GI signs. Moreover, all neonates that present with vomiting and/or diarrhea should be treated supportively. Supportive therapy at a minimum should address dehydration. Dietary modification, antiemetic agents, antidiarrheal agents, laxatives, and gastric protectants should be used as necessary.

Treatment of *Salmonella* gastroenteritis is not recommended unless there is clinical evidence of septicemia, such as neutropenia, a left shift, or hypoglycemia. If sepsis is present, then antimicrobial therapy must be based on susceptibility results because multiple antimicrobial resistance among the most common strains of *Salmonella* is expected.

It is not known whether treatment with antimicrobials effectively alters the outcome of patients with *Campylobacter*-associated diarrhea. Treatment of cats and dogs with *Campylobacter*-associated diarrhea with erythromycin has resulted in elimination of the organism, based on negative fecal cultures, and clinical improvement. Mixed results have been obtained when treating *Campylobacter*-associated diarrhea with chloramphenicol. β-Lactam antibiotics are generally ineffective against *Campylobacter* because many strains are β-lactamase producers. *Campylobacter* spp. may also develop resistance to tetracycline and fluoroquinolone antimicrobials. Some clinical veterinary microbiology laboratories have the ability to run antimicrobial susceptibility tests against *Campylobacter* spp.

Antimicrobials that have efficacy in the treatment of *Clostridium perfringens*–associated diarrhea include metronidazole, ampicillin, tylosin, erythromycin, and tetracycline.

SUGGESTED READINGS

Davidson AP: *Vet Clin North Am Small Anim Pract* 36:443, 2006.
Greene CE: *Infectious diseases of the dog and cat*, ed 3, St. Louis, 2006, Saunders/Elsevier.
Gyles CL: *Pathogenesis of bacterial infections in animals*, ed 3, Ames, IA, 2004, Blackwell.
Murray PR, Baron EJ: *Manual of clinical microbiology*, ed 9, Washington, DC, 2007, ASM Press.

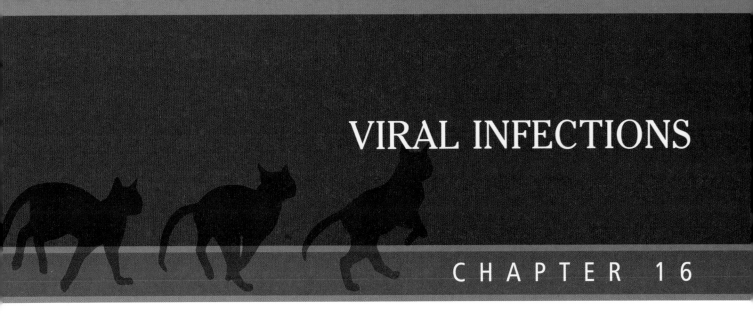

VIRAL INFECTIONS

CHAPTER 16

James F. Evermann, Melissa A. Kennedy

Neonatal and puppy-kitten mortality rates (animals dying before 1 year of age) are often used as clinical indicators of the general level of health in the community, including the level of vaccination that is used in the area (Table 16-1). Infectious diseases are a major threat to the health of neonatal animals and may contribute to the mortality rate. Neonatal puppies and kittens depend in large part on the presence of sufficient maternal immunity, which provides short-term, passive immunity to protect them against microbial pathogens in the neonates' environment. The severity of clinical symptoms (disease) in puppies and kittens that may result from infectious microorganisms depends on several key factors (Box 16-1). In addition to current maternal passive immunity, they include preexisting maternal infection status, maternal and neonatal nutrition, neonatal thermoregulation, concurrent neonatal infections and parasitism, and hereditary defects of the immune system.

Viral pathogens in particular can be life threatening for the neonate because for most infections, no specific antiviral therapy is available. Spread within a litter can be rapid as a result of the contagious nature of these pathogens. Adults with subclinical infections, including the dam, can be an important source of infection. Although some viruses, such as the feline retroviruses, are relatively labile outside the carrier host, others such as feline calicivirus and canine parvovirus are extremely hardy and can persist for months in contaminated environments. Transmission from dam to offspring can occur in utero or during birth of the neonate, whereas others are transmitted via nursing or grooming. The efficiency of the various modes of transmission varies with the agent involved.

Physical examination results will vary with the microbial pathogen involved. Fever may occur, but with peracute disease, animals may be hypothermic. Crying, restlessness, and anorexia may also be evident. Depending on the pathogen, evidence of specific organ involvement may be seen, such as nasal and ocular discharge with respiratory tract disease. Alternatively, multiorgan involvement may occur.

Diagnosis of viral infections of the neonate primarily involves direct detection of the virus, as serology in the neonate will not be useful. This can be done using three basic assays: antigen detection, nucleic acid detection, and viral cultivation. For antigen detection, cellular materials (mucosal swabs, fluid sediment, tissue impressions, and fixed tissues) on glass slides can be probed by fluorescent or immunoperoxidase-labeled specific antibody. Although rapid and inexpensive, these assays have relatively low sensitivity. For some pathogens, specific enzyme-linked immunosorbent assay (ELISA) tests are available. These include feline leukemia virus (FeLV) and parvoviral infections (canine parvovirus type 2 [CPV-2] and feline panleukopenia [FPL]). Sensitivity of these assays is regarded as high. Nucleic acid detection involves polymerase chain reaction (PCR) for amplification of the viral genetic material in biologic samples, including blood, mucosal swabs, feces, and fresh or fixed tissues. These assays are relatively fast and very sensitive. Viral cultivation, done on fresh samples, remains the gold standard but may take several (1 to 4) weeks. Serological analysis of the dam may provide information of previous infection or vaccination status but is often inconclusive.

In any investigation of reproductive disease, the veterinarian should consider the possibility of viral infections that are species specific (canine herpesvirus [CHV]), those that can be transmitted from one species to another (CPV-2), and those that are vector borne (West Nile virus). Such epidemiologic information is valuable both for establishing a diagnosis and for designing control strategies.

Control of neonatal viral infections involves screening for preexisting infections and vaccination (when available) of the dam, minimizing potential exposure during critical periods (Table 16-2) and ensuring adequate colostral intake by the neonates (see Chapter 14). The critical periods are

TABLE 16-1	Effects of population (herd) immunity* on neonatal puppy and kitten survival		
Effects on	**High survivability**	**Low survivability**	
Herd immunity	Increased	Decreased	
Maternal immunity	Increased	Decreased	
Colostral immunity	Increased	Decreased	
Maternal/cohort shedding	Decreased	Increased	
Survival of neonates	Increased	Decreased	

*Defined as 85% or greater of the population that are immune. Immunity is attained by regular vaccination boosters and/or continual boosters from natural infections from subclinical carrier animals.

BOX 16-1   Factors influencing the severity of clinical symptoms in puppies and kittens

- Preexisting maternal infection status (including congenital infections like *Neospora caninum* and CHV)
- Current maternal immune status
- Degree of maternal passive immunity
- Maternal and neonatal nutrition
- Neonatal thermoregulation
- Concurrent neonatal infections and parasitism
- Hereditary defects of the neonate immune system

Modified from Root Kustritz MV: Neonatology. In Root Kustritz MV (ed): *Small animal theriogenology*, St. Louis, 2003, Elsevier, p. 283.

TABLE 16-2	Stages of the naive-susceptible dog/cat and potential outcomes of infection			
Host(s) and outcomes	**Preconception**	**Pregnancy**	**Periparturient**	**Postnatal**
Canine	CDV, CPV-2, CHV, CAV	CPV-2, CHV, CPV-1	CHV	CPV-2, CAV, CCV
Feline	FPL, FHV, FCoV-FIP, FeLV	FHV, FeLV, FPL	FeLV, FIV	FHV, FeLV, FIV, FCV
Outcomes of infection	Immunity, decreased conception	Abortion, congenital infection, immunity	Stillbirth	Neonatal infection, neonatal disease, immunity

preconception, pregnancy, periparturient, and postnatal. The outcome of infection during these periods depends on previous individual animal immunity and viral challenge from the environment.

SPECIFIC VIRAL DISEASES OF PEDIATRIC CANINE PATIENTS

Canine Parvoviruses (CPV-2, CPV-1)

CPV-2

CPV-2 is endemic in most countries of the world. It is carried by a high percentage of dogs as a subclinical infection in the gastrointestinal (GI) tract and is shed intermittently in the feces. The virus can retain infectiousness outside the dog's GI tract for up to 12 months if environmental conditions are optimum (moist, cold). The newer variants of CPV-2 (CPV-2b, CPV-2c) have also acquired the cat as a host, and control efforts must take this into consideration. The virus can be inactivated by disinfectants with oxidizing activity, heat, and diluted bleach (1:30 parts with water).

Infection is spread and acquired by the fecal-oral route. During the first 2 days after ingestion, viral replication occurs in the oropharynx and local lymphoid organs. Viremia from 3 to 4 days postinfection spreads virus throughout the body. Viremia is usually terminated when virus-neutralizing antibodies (IgG) are generated, usually 6 to 9 days postinfection. Clinical symptoms are most severe in puppies and may occur up to age 12 months. Parvoviral enteritis may present acutely or peracutely with anorexia and depression followed by vomiting and profuse, usually hemorrhagic, diarrhea. Newer variants of CPV-2 may cause a mild nonhemorrhagic diarrhea. Pyrexia, depression, anorexia, and dehydration are commonly observed. Intestinal damage in the rapidly developing crypt cells permits bacterial colonization that may result in endotoxic shock characterized by hypothermia, disseminated intravascular coagulation, and jaundice. Mortality rate may be as high as 25% and is a consequence of dehydration, endotoxic shock, electrolyte imbalances, and secondary bacterial infections (see Chapter 15). Mild or subclinical infections are common, especially in dogs aged more than 6 months.

CPV-2 variants can be detected in antemortem samples by in-clinic antigen (Ag) ELISA or by electron microscopy of fecal/diarrheal material. Affected dogs can also be tested by serology, as CPV-specific IgM titers can be detected in serum. Although PCR is available, it may detect dogs that are carriers of CPV-2, and the clinical predictive value may not be as high as the previously mentioned assays. Postmortem detection of CPV-2 uses a combination of histopathology and immunohistochemistry (IHC) for CPV-2–specific antigens. The tissues of choice are the small intestine, mesenteric lymph nodes, and spleen fixed in buffered formalin.

Although there is no specific treatment for CPV-2, viral-bacterial enteritides generally consist of treating dehydration, sepsis, and acidosis/electrolyte imbalances. Intravenous balanced electrolyte solutions, systemic antibiotics (see Chapter 27), and antiemetic therapy may be indicated if vomiting is a significant component of the symptoms. Control measures include disinfection to reduce (dilute) the viral challenge load

TABLE 16-3	Most common viral agents associated with fading puppy and kitten syndromes					
	Puppy			**Kitten**		
	Canine herpesvirus	Canine parvovirus-2	Canine parvovirus-1	Feline herpesvirus	Feline calicivirus	Feline panleukopenia
Nature of the virus	Very labile, temperature sensitive	Very resistant	Very resistant	Very labile	Very resistant	Very resistant
Most common source	Dam	Dam	Dam	Queen	Queen	Queen
Diagnosis	VI, PCR, histopathology (pup), serology (dam)	Histopathology, PCR (pup)	Histopathology (rule out CPV-2)	VI, PCR, histopathology (kitten)	VI, PCR	Histopathology, PCR (kitten)
Control	High levels of hygiene and close adherence to "6-week danger period," no vaccine available	High levels of hygiene, routine vaccination of adult dogs	High levels of hygiene, no vaccine available	High levels of hygiene and routine vaccination of adult cats	High levels of hygiene and routine vaccination of adult cats	High levels of hygiene and routine vaccination of adult cats

VI, Virus isolation.

and immunization with modified live CPV-2 vaccines of adult dogs in the population and the susceptible puppies (Table 16-3). The role of immunization is twofold: the first is protection of individual puppies, and the second is to hyper-immunize adults to minimize viral shedding.

CPV-1

Canine parvovirus type 1 (CPV-1) is also referred to as minute viruses of canines and was initially reported in military dogs with diarrhea. This virus is antigenically distinct from CPV-2 and is more closely related genetically to bovine parvovirus.

CPV-1 is usually a subclinical infection in dogs but may cause enteritis, pneumonitis, myocarditis, and lymphadenitis in puppies aged between 5 and 21 days. Most pups have mild symptoms, but those that worsen may be classified as having fading puppy syndrome. Affected pups may show diarrhea, vomiting, and dyspnea and constantly cry out. Systemic viral infections in naive dams may lead to failure to conceive, fetal death, or abortion.

Because of the similarities of CPV-1 clinical symptoms with CHV and CPV-2, a thorough diagnostic workup is recommended. More specific assays such as PCR or immunoelectron microscopy are required to diagnose CPV-1 presence in fecal matter. Histopathologic changes seen in the thymus, lymph nodes, small intestine, and myocardium are very similar to CPV-2, and without specific IHC or CPV-1–specific PCR, these lesions may be misdiagnosed.

Because there is no vaccine available for CPV-1 control, it is important to maintain a clean whelping environment and keep optimal temperatures for newborn pups.

Canine Distemper Virus

Canine distemper virus (CDV) is a multisystemic viral disease of dogs that affects puppies most commonly aged between 3 and 6 months. The virus can be carried by adult dogs in the respiratory tract and is commonly shed in aerosols. The virus is enveloped and highly susceptible to environmental and chemical inactivation. Although there is only one serotype of CDV, there are numerous strains that vary in their tissue tropism and pathogenicity. Although considered a disease of domestic dogs, many other canids are equally susceptible, as are mustelids (e.g., ferrets). Felines are reported to be infected, but clinical symptoms are rare except in exotic felines (e.g., lions, tigers).

The route of infection with CDV is usually by aerosols, saliva, or grooming. The virus spreads rapidly to the oropharyngeal lymphoid organs, where it then enters the first of two viremic phases. During the first phase, there is generalized immune suppression. There may be fever, anorexia, and mild respiratory symptoms during this phase (7 to 10 days postinfection). During the second viremic phase, the virus is more disseminated to the GI tract, central nervous system, and skin. Hemorrhagic diarrhea may occur 10 to 20 days postinfection. Mortality rate in dogs symptomatic with this form may be as high as 50%. In classic forms of distemper, conjunctivitis is observed first, followed by a dry cough. The cough becomes progressively wet and productive, concurrent with oculonasal discharge. The discharge becomes mucopurulent within several days. Affected dogs are usually pyretic (>104° F, 40° C), depressed, and anorectic. It is estimated that at least 50% of CDV infections are subclinical and that dogs may shed virus for up to 60 days postinfection.

CDV can cause abortion, stillbirth, and birth of weak puppies. Neonatal infection in puppies aged less than 1 week may result in cardiomyopathy and cardiac failure less than 3 weeks postinfection.

CDV presentation is usually classical enough that antemortem diagnostic assays are not conducted. If a definitive diagnosis is of value, then fluorescent antibody-specific CDV staining can be done on either conjunctival smears or whole blood smears. Nucleic acid detection can be done by PCR on whole blood and urine, which offers a good clinical predictive value for a dog with viremia; tissue may be tested postmortem. Serologic detection can identify CDV-specific IgM in serum or CDV-specific IgG in cerebrospinal fluid. Postmortem diagnosis of CDV-induced disease can be verified by histopathology and, if necessary, CDV-specific IHC on fixed tissues from brain, lung, spleen, urinary bladder, and skin.

There are no specific antiviral drugs to treat CDV-induced disease. Treatment is supportive with fluids, expectorants, antiemetics, and antibiotics. Puppies that develop neurologic disease have a poor prognosis. Control measures rely predominately on the use of a modified live virus (MLV) immunization program in dogs. This consists of a thorough vaccination series in puppies, a booster at 6 months, and another booster at age 1 year. Adult dogs in proximity to pregnant dogs and puppies should receive regular boosters to minimize CDV shedding in the environment.

Canine Adenoviruses

The canine adenoviruses (CAV) consist of two predominant serotypes, CAV type 1 and type 2 (CAV-1 and CAV-2). CAV-1 is predominately multisystemic and causes hepatocellular necrosis and vasculitis. The virus is moderately resistant in the environment but susceptible to heat (steam cleaning) and disinfection by quaternary ammonium compounds. Dogs may carry this virus subclinically despite high levels of neutralizing antibodies (immune carriers, see Chapter 14). The antigenically related CAV, CAV-2, is predominately associated with upper respiratory tract disease. It is shed for 8 to 9 days postinfection.

CAV-1 is considered to cause the more serious clinical symptoms in dogs when compared with CAV-2. CAV-1 infects by the oronasal route, where the virus replicates in the oropharyngeal lymph nodes. Viremia occurs wherein hepatocytes and reticuloendothelial cells in other organ systems are the sites of virus replication and subsequent lysis and necrosis. During the acute phase (7 to 9 days) of CAV-1 disease, the virus is excreted in the feces, urine, and oropharyngeal secretions. The occurrence of multisystemic symptoms carries a guarded prognosis. Infection during pregnancy by CAV-1 may result in the birth of dead puppies or weak puppies that die within a few days postwhelping. Carrier dams occur and may act as a source of infection for puppies or other pregnant dogs.

Infections by CAV-2 may result in bronchitis, bronchiolitis, and focal turbinate and tonsillar necrosis. The virus has been reported to be associated with kennel cough syndrome.

The important feature of CAV-2 is its antigenic relatedness to CAV-1 and the use of this strain in vaccines, which provides protective immunity to CAV-1.

The diagnosis of CAV-1 is important to differentiate from the multisystemic CHV (see below). Antemortem diagnosis may be done by virus isolation from fecal samples and oral-pharyngeal swabs in viral transport media. Nucleic acid detection by PCR may be used to detect CAV in the same samples, but the clinical predictive value may be compromised because of the presence of known carrier dogs in the population. Postmortem diagnosis is considered to be the most reliable for CAV-1 disease. Hepatic lesions are pathognomonic and include mottling and fibrinous exudates attached to the liver capsule. The gall bladder may be edematous and hemorrhagic. Histopathology and CAV-specific IHC are confirmatory on the fixed liver tissue.

There is no specific antiviral therapy for CAV-1 disease. Symptomatic supportive therapy for acute liver failure is required for treatment. Immunization with CAV-2 MLV vaccine is an important control measure for CAV-1. This consists of a vaccination series in puppies, a booster at 6 months, and a second booster at age 1 year. Adult dogs in proximity to pregnant dogs and puppies should receive regular boosters to minimize viral shedding.

Canine Herpesvirus

CHV has been recognized as one of the most common and virulent viral infections of neonatal puppies. Recent reports have indicated that this virus may be carried subclinically by up to 70% of some canine populations. As with other herpesviral infections, in particular, feline herpesvirus (see this chapter), CHV can be exacerbated following periods of physiologic, hormonal, and nutritional stress. CHV has several components that are important in control because there is no vaccine available in the United States. The virus is shed predominately in oronasal secretions from carrier dogs to susceptible dogs. This knowledge has been the basis for establishing the 6-week danger period, which includes the 3 weeks before whelping and 3 weeks postwhelping (Figure 16-1).

The effects of CHV can best be described based on what sex is infected and when the dog is exposed. Dogs usually enter adulthood having been infected as puppies and have adequate levels of immunity to control disease. However, if females reach reproductive age and are naive, then they can experience fetal death and mummification early during pregnancy, as well as premature birth and neonatal disease during late pregnancy. Although the female will lose her litter, it is now generally considered that she is immune to subsequent CHV-induced disease.

The puppies whelped by a naive female are susceptible to CHV from other shedding dogs in the vicinity to the female and her litter. The puppies are infected via oronasal secretions from the recently infected female or another dog. The virus infects via the oropharyngeal lymph nodes and rapidly spreads systemically by viremia. Puppies infected at birth or postnatally up to age 3 weeks may develop a systemic disease

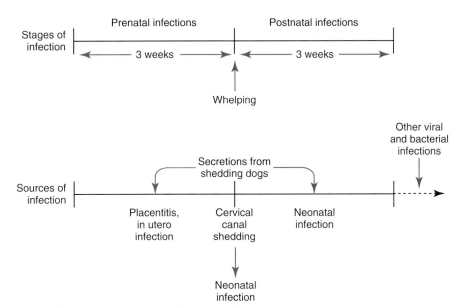

Figure 16-1 The 6-week danger period in relationship to whelping and the various sources of CHV for neonatal infections. (Redrawn from Diagnosis of canine herpetic infections. In *Kirk's current veterinary therapy X*, 1989, Elsevier.)

that is usually fatal. Resistance to systemic disease is age-related and is considered to be directly correlated to the thermoregulatory system of the puppy. The disease has an incubation period of 3 to 7 days. Clinical symptoms include anorexia, abdominal pain, and lethargy.

Male dogs that are infected with CHV can also carry the virus but are usually subclinical. Genital lesions associated with CHV may include hyperemia and lymphoid hyperplasia over the base of the penis. The male may also develop a serous oculonasal discharge, which appears to be one of the major modes of virus spread to susceptible females and her puppies.

CHV has been detected by virus isolation from swabs of vesicular lesions on the genitalia of affected females. These lesions frequently develop during proestrus, indicating that venereal spread may be an important mode of virus spread. Bitches that have fetal death or abort may be tested for CHV-specific neutralizing antibody on a serum sample. Puppies born with clinical symptoms or those developing symptoms during the first 3 weeks can be submitted for necropsy. The puppies will have characteristic petechial hemorrhages on the kidneys.

Swabs in viral transport media from lungs, liver, and kidney can be analyzed by viral isolation. Whole blood can be submitted for CHV-specific PCR. Histopathology can be conducted on the aforementioned tissues, and characteristic intranuclear inclusion bodies can be observed.

Male dogs with genital lesions and serous nasal discharge can be tested for CHV-specific antibodies in serum or by virus isolation using swabs collected in viral transport media.

CHV is regarded as naturally temperature sensitive and does not replicate at elevated body temperatures. Knowing this, as well as the susceptibility of the virus outside the dog's body, allows for a good control measure through sustained superoptimal environmental temperatures for puppies. Once puppies have been infected and demonstrate clinical symptoms, the prognosis is guarded to poor. In some cases, hyperimmune canine serum with CHV antibodies can be administered subcutaneously to assist with management of CHV in a litter if administered early during the course of infection. There is no commercially available vaccine in the United States. A vaccine marketed in Europe has demonstrated good efficacy when administered to the dam. This vaccine would have value in selected canine environments and should be considered for licensure in the United States.

CANINE CORONAVIRUS

Canine coronavirus (CCV) predates CPV-2 by several years as a cause of canine enteritis. The virus is a member of the broader coronavirus family with known pathogens in every mammalian species, including humans. The virus shares common antigens and remarkable similarities in pathogeneses with transmissible gastroenteritis of swine and feline enteric coronavirus (parent virus of feline infectious peritonitis). The virus occurs worldwide, with infection rates ranging from 45% to 100% in some high-density dog populations. CCV is considered to be a primary infection of the GI tract. However, a similar but antigenically distinct coronavirus has been recently reported as the cause of canine respiratory disease. Current studies have indicated that the virulence of enteric CCV has increased, which may be accounted for by the generation of recombinational mutants.

Coronaviral infections of dogs occur very early in the neonatal period and are primarily spread via the fecal-oral route. Maternal antibodies protect the puppy up to about 4 to 5 weeks of age, at which time the puppy becomes susceptible to disease. The virus infects the enterocytes of the small intestine, resulting in epithelial loss and villus atrophy. Colonic epithelium and mesenteric lymph nodes may also become infected, which contributes to the shedding of the virus in the feces. The age range for greatest susceptibility to disease is 5 to 12 weeks of age. The virus is shed in the highest quantity for 16 days postinfection and then intermittently thereafter. The primary clinical symptom is a watery diarrhea that ranges from mild to moderately severe. The severity of the disease can be enhanced by concurrent viral (CPV-2) and bacterial (*Campylobacter* sp.) infections. Recovery usually occurs within 7 to 14 days.

The diagnosis of CCV enteritis has relied on electron microscopy and, to a lesser extent, on virus isolation. Because both techniques are regarded as marginally sensitive, there are a number of false-negative results. Serology has been useful in determining the prevalence of the viral infection in the dog population but has not been widely used to diagnose an acute infection. More recent reports have used CCV-specific IHC on fixed GI tissues from dogs with fatal enteritis. This technique has proven valuable in cases where CPV-2 has not been detected. Molecular detection of CCV by PCR has become an accepted method of viral diagnosis. However, because there is a reasonably high carrier rate with CCV, the clinical predictive value of PCR on fecal preparations or intestinal contents must be interpreted cautiously.

There is no specific treatment for CCV. Puppies with watery, nonhemorrhagic diarrhea can be treated as CPV-2 patients with rehydration and antibiotic therapy. Control of CCV-induced disease depends heavily on vaccination of the dam. This reduces the shedding of the virus and enhances colostral and lactogenic (passive antibodies in dam's milk) immunity. Ultimately, oral vaccines to stimulate mucosal immunity (IgA) will be needed to control the disease associated with this virus. This same type of vaccine will probably be important in controlling the newer CCV variants, which are associated with respiratory disease in 8- to 12-week-old puppies.

SPECIFIC VIRAL DISEASES OF PEDIATRIC FELINE PATIENTS

Feline Herpesvirus

Feline herpesvirus (FHV) is a common respiratory pathogen of cats. The virus is a spherical enveloped virus with a double-stranded (ds) DNA genome and is classified as a member of the Alphaherpesvirinae subfamily of the Herpesviridae family. The virus is highly contagious and is spread via direct and indirect contact. As with other alphaherpesviruses, after acute infection, the virus achieves latency in neural tissue; recrudescence with viral replication and shedding may occur during stressful episodes. The virus targets epithelia of the upper respiratory tract and conjunctiva. Although systemic spread of herpesviruses of other domestic animals occurs, this does not appear to be common with FHV.

Unlike herpesviruses of dogs, horses, swine, goats, and cattle, infection with FHV during gestation does not generally lead to viremia and abortion. Queens infected during gestation have aborted secondary to severe respiratory disease, but no placental lesions were found. Recrudescence of latent infections may occur during queening, leading to exposure of the kittens. Infected kittens may exhibit mild conjunctivitis and serous ocular and nasal discharge; those with insufficient passive immunity may develop severe clinical disease with lower respiratory tract involvement. Secondary bacterial infection may occur following infection, and mortality rates may be high. Affected kittens are inactive, anorectic, and exhibit profuse mucopurulent oculonasal discharge and respiratory distress. In kittens that have not yet opened their eyes, accumulation of purulent material behind the eyelids may occur, leading to noticeable distention.

Viral detection through virus isolation from clinical samples (mucosal swabs antemortem or respiratory tract tissues postmortem) remains the gold standard but may take 2 days to 2 weeks for results. Antigen detection may be done on cells collected from mucosal surfaces or tissue impressions using immunofluorescence. Alternatively, nucleic acid detection on mucosal swabs or tissues using PCR can be done. These latter two assays have a fast turnaround time and are relatively inexpensive. For antigen detection, sensitivity is low to moderate, whereas PCR is high in sensitivity but may detect subclinical or even latent infection.

Antiviral therapy is an option for FHV, although the safety of these regimens in neonatal kittens is not known. In vitro nucleotide analogs such as acyclovir and ganciclovir have shown efficacy. L-lysine is used to minimize recrudescent episodes and functions as an antagonist to arginine uptake, thus inhibiting FHV replication. Administration to infected queens may minimize shedding during the stress of parturition and lactation.

Supportive care is also required and includes fluid replacement, nutritional support, and antibiotics for secondary bacterial infection. Topical antiviral and antibiotic medications may be used for ocular involvement. Most kittens will fully recover unless immunocompromised or secondary bacterial pneumonia occurs. In cases of severe disease with turbinate destruction, chronic rhinosinusitis ("chronic snuffler") may occur.

Vaccination of adults will minimize virus exposure of kittens and enhance maternal immunity for passive transfer. Intranasal vaccines may be used in kittens as young as 3 to 4 weeks of age in populations with endemic infection. During an outbreak, the virus is easily killed with standard detergents. Adults are often subclinical shedders of FHV; thus, contact of adults other than the queen with the kittens should be avoided.

Feline Calicivirus

Feline calicivirus (FCV) is a common pathogen of cats affecting the respiratory tract. It is a small nonenveloped virus with a single-stranded (ss) RNA genome classified in the *Vesivirus* genus of the Caliciviridae family. The virus is very resistant in the environment, and indirect transmission via fomites is a major mode of spread. Replication occurs in the upper respiratory tract epithelia and oral and conjunctival mucosa leading to conjunctivitis, oral ulcers, and typical signs of upper respiratory tract disease. Following recovery from acute infection, a carrier-mucosal infection persists, and viral shedding may continue from the oropharyngeal region for weeks to months. Unlike FHV, latency does not occur.

Less commonly, the virus may exhibit pneumotropism leading to severe interstitial pneumonia. Recently lethal outbreaks associated with systemic spread and multiorgan dysfunction have occurred. Clinical manifestations in these outbreaks have included high fever, depression, anorexia, edema (particularly of the head and limbs), and ulcerative dermatitis of the face, pinnae, and feet. Affected tissues included lungs, pancreas, and liver. Most outbreaks have originated in cats from shelters or rescue facilities, and vaccinated and unvaccinated cats have been affected with significant mortality rates reported.

FCV is rarely associated with abortion in the pregnant queen. It has been isolated from aborted fetuses, indicating transplacental transmission can occur. Viremia occurs in some FCV infections, and the recently characterized isolates from virulent systemic disease could lead to gestational termination, although it has not been described; however, severe signs will be evident in the queen, including edema, ulcerative dermatitis, and hepatic necrosis.

Neonatal kittens may be exposed from subclinically shedding contact animals or via indirect contact with contaminated fomites, including caretakers. Signs may be similar to those described for FHV and require specific diagnostics for differentiation. Primary viral pneumonia can occur with some strains and may have high mortality rates. Affected kittens will exhibit not only the typical signs of upper respiratory tract infection but also severe respiratory distress, and death can be peracute. Although it is likely that infection with strains associated with systemic disease can occur in kittens, specific outbreaks have not been described. In kittens that recover from FCV infection, polyarthritis may be seen associated with mononuclear cell infiltration of joints. Referred to as "limping kitten syndrome," signs are generally self-limiting.

Diagnosis of neonatal FCV infection is similar to that for FHV, involving virus isolation, antigen detection, or genetic detection using PCR on clinical samples.

Treatment for FCV infection is supportive as no specific antiviral therapies currently exist. Control, as for FHV, should emphasize vaccination of adults and, during outbreaks, intranasal vaccination of preweaning-aged kittens. As with FHV, kittens should be isolated from adults other than the queen, as they can be subclinical shedders. During an outbreak, because of the hardy nature of the virus, strict barrier nursing and rigorous disinfection with appropriate reagents (oxidizing agent as active ingredient) are required.

Feline Panleukopenia

Feline panleukopenia (FPL) is an important systemic parvoviral infection of cats associated with replication in and cytopathic effects on rapidly dividing cells, such as bone marrow, lymphoid cells, and intestinal epithelia. In addition, it may target the fetus in utero, and in late gestation and the neonatal period, infection can lead to congenital defects. This agent is one of the smallest animal viruses, barely 18 to 20 nm in diameter. It contains a small ssDNA genome and has a mutation rate similar to RNA viruses. It is extremely hardy in the environment and may persist for as long as 2 years. Following oronasal exposure, the virus spreads systemically via the lymphatic system and blood. Infections are acute, and long-term shedding is uncommon. With the advent of effective vaccines for FPL, reproductive losses resulting from FPL disease have been reduced. However, infections continue to occur among both pedigreed cats and cats from rescue facilities. In one study of 274 kitten deaths in the United Kingdom, 25% were caused by FPL infection.

Infection of the pregnant queen may lead to abortion, stillbirths, fading kittens, or congenital defects depending on the stage of gestation, with the latter resulting from in utero infection in late gestation. These congenital defects may include cerebellar hypoplasia, exhibited by intention tremors and ataxia; hydranencephaly, with abnormal behavior; or cardiomyopathy. Infection in the early neonatal period can lead to similar defects.

Postnatal infection may lead to necrosis of intestinal epithelia and hematopoietic progenitor cells, the classic panleukopenia syndrome, with vomiting, diarrhea, severe depression, and anorexia. Endotoxemia or sepsis may occur secondarily. Peracute deaths may occur in some kittens.

Diagnostics for FPL involve viral detection. Viral antigen can be detected in feces from kittens with diarrhea using commercially available ELISA. Electron microscopy can also be done on fecal samples. For detection in tissues postmortem, virus isolation or nucleic acid detection by PCR is required. Panleukopenia associated with typical signs is also considered diagnostic.

For disease resulting from congenital infections, no specific treatment exists. For cerebellar hypoplasia, the condition is not progressive, and as long as kittens can eat, their overall health will not be affected. More severe neurologic involvement is generally incompatible with a good quality of life. Cardiac damage from FPL infection is also not specifically treatable, and the resultant cardiomyopathy can be life threatening.

Treatment for postnatal infection is supportive, as no specific antiviral therapies exist for parvovirus. Replacement of fluid and electrolyte loss is critical. Transfusion may be required with severe anemia or hypoproteinemia. Treatment of gram-negative sepsis with broad-spectrum parenteral antibiotics will also be necessary. With aggressive treatment, survival is probable.

Control through vaccination of adults is effective. Queens with high levels of neutralizing antibodies will protect kittens in utero, as well as in the neonatal period, through passive transfer. Modified live vaccines should not be used during pregnancy or in kittens aged less than 4 weeks. If an outbreak occurs, adequate disinfection will be critical because of the resistant nature of the virus. Disinfectants must incorporate an oxidizing agent as an active ingredient to be effective. Disinfection of soil is not practical, and objects with porous surfaces, such as carpeting, should be steam cleaned or removed from the environment.

Feline Coronavirus

Feline coronavirus (FCoV) is a common enteric pathogen of cats, and infection in some leads to the fatal disease feline infectious peritonitis (FIP). The virus is an enveloped virus with a helical capsid containing an ssRNA genome of approximately 20 kilobases, one of the largest RNA genomes of animal viruses. As with other RNA viruses, the mutation rate is high and may lead to an FIP-causing phenotype. Most infections target the intestinal epithelia, leading to malabsorption and maldigestion and manifesting as diarrhea. Infection follows oronasal exposure; the virus is shed in feces, and some adults may shed the virus subclinically for extended periods. In populations where infection is endemic, viral infection may be detectable as early as 4 weeks of age.

FCoV is uncommonly associated with reproductive problems in the pregnant queen or with fading kitten syndrome. Postnatal infection of kittens can manifest as enteritis with watery diarrhea. Less commonly, vomiting may be observed. The diarrhea is generally not hemorrhagic, and an associated panleukopenia is not observed, aiding differentiation from FPL infection. Individual kittens in a litter may develop FIP after weaning, but it is uncommon before weaning.

Virus detection via electron microscopy or PCR from diarrheic feces will aid diagnosis of FCoV enteritis. The former, because of its lower sensitivity relative to PCR, is preferable; the high sensitivity of PCR will allow detection of subclinical infections. If FCoV is suspected in cases of abortion or fading kittens, PCR detection on tissues postmortem is optimal for virus identification.

To develop a diagnosis of FIP, a combination of data and tests is required and includes history and clinical signs (multi-cat origin or purebred, fever, weight loss, anorexia), lymphopenia, elevated total protein (TP), decreased albumin: globulin (A:G) ratio, typical effusion (transudate high in TP), and ruling out other etiologies. Coronavirus-specific assays are available but cannot distinguish the enteric virus from that of FIPV. Virus detection assays include antigen detection (effusion sediment, tissue impressions) and genetic detection by PCR. Recently a quantitative PCR to detect viral mRNA in monocytes has been developed. This assay detects efficient viral replication in circulating monocytes, a characteristic of FIPV; however, a recent study has found detectable mRNA in the blood of cats without FIP. Thus, although this assay may provide additional diagnostic information, it is not specific for FIP. Confirmation can only be accomplished through histopathology and IHC.

Treatment of FCoV, both enteric and FIP, is largely supportive and includes fluid and nutritional support. For FIP, treatments using immunomodulation have been tried with minimal success. These include interferon, both feline and human recombinant products, and corticosteroids. The disease is progressive and ultimately fatal.

Infection with FCoV is common and, in the majority of cases, leads to little or no disease. A vaccine is available for FCoV but is not widely recommended. In catteries, early weaning with isolation of the kittens has been recommended as a preventive measure, but this is not feasible for most.

Feline Leukemia Virus

Although uncommon in most breeding catteries, FeLV still occurs in many cat populations. A gammaretrovirus in the Retroviridae family, it is an enveloped virus with a protein core and a diploid ssRNA genome. The capsid is made up of several small proteins, one of which, p27, is detected by commercially available diagnostic ELISAs. Another structural protein, the envelope glycoprotein p15e, has been found to be immunosuppressive through inhibition of a variety of immune functions. As part of its replication cycle, FeLV converts its RNA genome into dsDNA, which integrates into the host cell DNA. Unless virus is cleared early during infection, a persistent infection may occur, leading to neoplasia, bone marrow suppression, and immunosuppression. The majority of cats undergo a latent infection in which the virus remains integrated into host cell DNA.

The virus is transmitted by direct contact between cats, usually via saliva, as shedding in saliva is consistent in persistently infected cats. Therefore, mutual grooming is an important means of transmission. Because of the lability of FeLV, it does not persist in the environment; thus, indirect transmission is not an efficient mode of spread. It can be transmitted in utero to fetuses in pregnant queens and to kittens during parturition by maternal grooming or via milk. After infection, viremia occurs, and if not cleared by the cat's immune response, infection of hematopoietic cells in the bone marrow will occur. Infection that reaches this stage is less likely to be cleared. Resistance increases with age, and kittens are most susceptible to persistent infection.

Infection in utero most commonly leads to pregnancy failure. Pregnant queens that become infected may experience abortion, stillbirths, or fading kittens that die soon after birth. Perinatal infection may also lead to fading kittens, with poor nursing, hypothermia, inactivity, and crying. Rarely kittens infected in utero or during the perinatal period may survive beyond weaning. These kittens may suffer a panleukopenia-like syndrome or may die from septicemia or other infections secondary to FeLV-induced immunosuppression. Long-term survivors may develop any of the typical FeLV clinical syndromes. Infection that occurs in the pre- or perinatal period is likely to affect most or all of the litter; however, it is inappropriate to test only representative littermates.

Diagnosis of FeLV infection involves detection of viral antigen in the queen and her offspring. Initial screening is done most commonly using commercially available ELISA kits. Testing should be done on serum, as saliva and tears may not contain detectable virus for weeks or longer after infection. Positive ELISA results should be confirmed using immunofluorescence on whole blood smears. Animals testing positive by both assays are unlikely to clear the virus. Cats with ELISA-positive results only may clear the virus, but this is unlikely in kittens aged less than 16 weeks as compared with adults. Serial testing in kittens born to infected queens may be necessary to confirm their infection status. Genetic detection by PCR is not routinely done, as antigenemia-negative cats are unlikely to be infected; however, at least one investigation has indicated that a small minority of infected cats may remain latently infected with nonreplicating virus capable of reactivation and detectable only by PCR.

Treatment of FeLV is primarily supportive, including maintenance of hydration and nutrition and broad-spectrum antibiotics. Treatment regimens using various immunomodulators have had little success in improving the health of affected cats. Treatment of affected kittens is unlikely to be successful.

Control involves vaccination and screening of cats to prevent introduction of infected animals into uninfected populations. Screening is done with the ELISA as described above. Vaccines available include a killed whole virus and a recombinant vector vaccine and have reported efficacy rates of 80% to 100%. If infection is identified in a population, disinfection after removal of infected animals is easy and effective using any detergent. The virus is extremely labile and will not persist in the environment or on fomites for longer than minutes to hours.

Feline Immunodeficiency Virus

Feline immunodeficiency virus (FIV) is also a member of the Retroviridae family with a structure similar to FeLV but is a lentivirus related to HIV. It is endemic in domestic cats and causes an immunosuppressive disease. The primary target cell is the T-helper lymphocytes, but the virus also infects cytotoxic T lymphocytes, B lymphocytes, and some epithelial, fibroblast, and neural cell lines. As with FeLV, the replication cycle involves conversion of the RNA genome into dsDNA and integration into host cell DNA. It is shed in saliva and is transmitted efficiently by penetrating bite wounds. Other body fluids are also infectious, and transmission to kittens may occur in utero or via vaginal fluids or milk. The former is not as significant as a mode of transmission as the latter unless the queen is suffering acute infection, has declining CD4+ lymphocyte levels, or is in an advanced disease state. Transmission via milk or grooming by the queen is more likely to result in transmission to the offspring. One study has indicated that the virus is concentrated in milk in early lactation.

Once infection occurs, followed by seroconversion, viral persistence is virtually ensured. The cat may remain asymptomatic for months to years, but viral replication continues at low levels. A progressive immune dysfunction occurs with declining T-helper lymphocyte and cytotoxic T-lymphocyte levels and impairment of cytokine production along with increasing viral levels. Kittens are among the most susceptible to the hematologic changes. Death occurs as a result of multiple disease syndromes, including degenerative, infectious, and neoplastic diseases.

Infection of the pregnant queen may lead to fetal resorption and arrest of fetal development with reduced litter size. Abortion, stillbirths, and fading kittens also may occur. The virus has a predilection for the thymus and leads to thymic atrophy in the kitten. Signs in the neonate are similar to signs in those that fade as a result of FeLV. Those that survive until weaning will ultimately progress to the immunodeficiency state.

Diagnosis of infection with FIV relies on detection of antibody. Screening is done using a commercially available ELISA and is confirmed with Western blot on serum. The diagnosis of infection in kittens can be compromised because of the presence of maternal antibodies. Queens may have antibodies as a result of infection or vaccination. These antibodies interfere with the results often well past the age of weaning, as antibodies from infection cannot be distinguished from maternal antibodies. Virus detection using PCR may be used, but because of the high level of genetic variation of FIV, false-negative results can often occur. Multiple testing may be required to confirm the infection status.

As with FeLV, treatment is largely supportive. Various immunomodulatory therapies have also been tried with FIV with variable success.

Control is also similar to FeLV and involves screening of cats to prevent introduction of infected cats to a household. Most are screened using the ELISA kit; seroconversion may take several weeks to months, thus testing of kittens of unknown history should be repeated during the first 6 months of life. Kittens testing antibody positive should be isolated until their true infection status can be definitively determined by PCR.

A killed vaccine containing two strains of FIV is available, but efficacy rates have been variable. Additionally, because the vaccine antibody response cannot be distinguished from that caused by infection, it is not widely recommended unless the animal is at high risk. If questions arise regarding true infection status versus vaccine-induced antibody, then the kitten can be tested by PCR on whole blood. Kittens born to vaccinated queens will test antibody positive with routine screening because of maternal antibody but should convert to negative status as the antibodies wane.

Disinfection to inactivate FIV is similar to FeLV—the virus is very labile, does not persist in the environment, and is easily inactivated by detergents.

INTERSPECIES VIRAL SPREAD BETWEEN DOGS AND CATS

Virus transmission within a species is considered to be the norm because viral-coded host cell receptors on the virus surface restrict the host range of the virus. Although there are several mechanisms whereby a virus may persist in an animal population, interspecies spread or crossover has become of particular interest. This is because interspecies spread hampers control efforts in a population and may allow for emergence of new strains of multihost viruses. There are three particular types of dogs and cats that are susceptible to interspecies viral and bacterial spread. This susceptibility is directly correlated with the immune status of the host (see Chapter 14). The three types are pregnant animals, neonatal animals, and those animals that have genetic or acquired immunodeficiencies. The viruses that have been reported to cross over include canine distemper to cats, feline calicivirus to dogs, canine coronavirus to cats, and CPV-2 variants to cats. Another source of potential interspecies spread occurs from immunization of high-risk animals with contaminated vaccines. This occurred when a MLV canine vaccine that contained bluetongue virus was used in pregnant dogs. The vaccine was administered to booster maternal antibody but proved to be fatal for the puppies and a high percentage of the pregnant dogs. Nonpregnant dogs that received the contaminated vaccine did not develop clinical symptoms, and there was no evidence that further virus spread occurred.

FADING PUPPY AND KITTEN SYNDROMES

The use of the phrase, "the fading puppy and kitten syndromes" has continued in the pediatric literature. The syndromes are multifactorial in nature and are generally used to describe litters of puppies or kittens that fail to thrive (see Chapter 11). The syndromes can occur from birth up to 9 to 10 weeks of age. The affected neonates decline quickly, and the mortality rate can be high. There are at least three potential causes for these syndromes. They include environmental effects, genetic effects, and infectious microorganisms. The environmental effects include hypothermia or hyperthermia. Neonates that are too cold or too warm are unable to nurse and digest food correctly. Heart rates become erratic, and respiratory systems may collapse. Maternal factors that contribute to these syndromes are dams that are overweight and maternal neglect leading to inadequate colostral antibody intake.

Genetic effects that contribute to the syndromes are congenital deformities or deficiencies of the immune system and low birth weights for puppies and kittens.

Infectious causes of the syndromes have been delineated during the past decade and are summarized in Table 16-3. The most common infections for the puppy are CHV, CPV-2, and CPV-1. The dam is the primary source of infection to her puppies at birth or shortly thereafter. The occurrence of CPV-2–related neonatal deaths has decreased with the use of routine vaccination. Under high challenge environments and in populations of dogs not routinely vaccinated, it is possible to see early CDV and CAV-1 infections occurring with high mortality rates. Newer strains of enteric CCV appear to be more virulent and are

associated with fatal enteritis in puppies as early as 5 weeks of age.

The most common infections for the kitten are FHV, FCV, and FPL. The queen is the primary source of infection to her kittens. The occurrence of these three viruses causing "fading kittens" has decreased with the routine use of vaccines in queens and adult cats in proximity to the kittens. Other feline viruses that may cause neonatal loss are FeLV and FIV. These two viruses can be readily tested for by the Ag ELISA (FeLV) and antibody ELISA (FIV) on all queens as part of their biosecurity screen.

EMERGING VIRUSES TO WATCH

A main theme throughout this chapter has been the awareness of the carrier status of the viruses in the adult population of dogs and cats. These asymptomatic carriers are usually the source of viral infections to puppies and kittens early in life. Other sources of viral infections are the environment where wildlife cohabitate and interspecies infections between animals in the same household or facility. As was mentioned in Chapter 14, the dam and queen are unusually susceptible to infections and to exacerbation of preexisting infections as a result of temporary immune suppression. The immunologically naive neonatal puppy and kitten are equally susceptible to infections. Several viral infections that have emerged during the past few years are more virulent strains of CCV causing enteritis and respiratory disease, more virulent calicivirus strains affecting both dogs and cats, and influenza strains being spread from horses to dogs (canine influenza) and from birds to cats (avian influenza). More virulent strains of CDV have been reported within some dog populations, as well as in large felids. The clinical recognition of unusual outbreaks of viral disease will most likely occur initially in pregnant animals and neonates and then proceed to susceptible animals before involving the general population of dogs and/or cats.

ACKNOWLEDGMENTS

The authors thank Alison McKeirnan for her expertise in companion animal diagnostics and Theresa Pfaff for editorial assistance. The authors also thank Sarah McCord for literature search and library services.

SUGGESTED READINGS

Battersby I, Harvey A: Differential diagnosis and treatment of acute diarrhea in the dog and cat, *Practice* 28:480, 2006.

Birchard SJ, Sherding RG: *Saunders manual of small animal practice,* ed 3, St Louis, 2006, Saunders/Elsevier.

Brownlie J, England GCW: Viral infections with pathological consequences for reproduction in veterinary species. In Jeffries DJ, Hudson CN (eds): *Viral infections in obstetrics and gynecology,* New York, 1999, Arnold-Oxford Univ Press, pp 289-333.

England G: The reproductive tract and neonate. In Ramsey I, Tennant B (eds): *Manual of canine and feline infectious diseases,* Gloucester, UK, 2001, British Small Animal Veterinary Association, pp 185-195.

Evermann JF: Accidental introduction of viruses into companion animals by commercial vaccines, *Vet Clin North Am Small Anim Pract* 38(4):919, 2008.

Evermann JF, Sellon RK, Sykes JE: Laboratory diagnosis of viral and rickettsial infections and epidemiology of infectious diseases. In Greene CE (ed): *Infectious diseases of the dog and cat,* ed 3, St Louis, 2006, Saunders/Elsevier, pp 1-9.

Kennedy M: Methodology in diagnostic virology, *Vet Clin North Am Exotic Anim Pract* 8:7, 2005.

Levy J: Queen and kitten with problems, the fading kitten and neonate. In Rand J (ed): *Problem-based feline medicine,* New York, 2006, Saunders/Elsevier, pp 1126-1144.

Speakman A: Management of infectious disease in the multi-cat environment, *Practice* 27:446, 2005.

Thrusfield M: Companion animal health schemes. In Thrusfield M (ed): *Veterinary epidemiology,* ed 3, Ames, IA, 2005, Blackwell, pp 379-381.

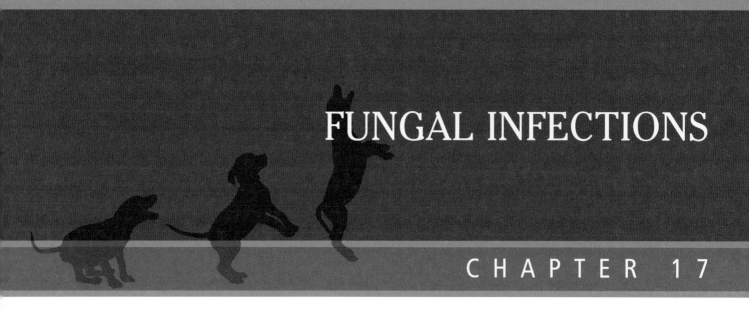

FUNGAL INFECTIONS

CHAPTER 17

Kevin T. Fitzgerald, Kristin L. Newquist

CUTANEOUS FUNGAL INFECTIONS

Dermatophytes

The majority of clinical cases presented are caused by three fungi: *Microsporum canis*, *Microsporum gypseum*, and *Trichophyton mentagrophytes*. Typically *M. canis* is the most common source of dermatophytosis in dogs and cats. Table 17-1 summarizes dermatophytes isolated from hair and skin of dogs and cats.

The dermatophytic fungi are spread through contact with infected hair or scales or contaminated environments or through carriage by fomites. Infective spores enter the environment when contaminated hairs break and are shed. Combs, brushes, clippers, bedding, transport cases, and paraphernalia associated with grooming, moving, or housing of animals can be sources of infection and subsequent reinfection. These spores are small and can be transported by currents of air, on dust, and on other mechanical fomites.

M. canis infections are usually caused by exposure to an infected cat or contact with fomites contaminated by an infected cat. The incubation period is from 1 to 3 weeks. Germination is temperature dependent. Most *Trichophyton* infections are caused through contact with infected rodents, their nests, or contaminated fomites. Dogs and cats are infected by the geophilic fungal organism *M. gypseum* from rooting, sleeping, and digging in contaminated soil. Animals can be exposed by reverse zoonoses from direct contact with infected people.

Dermatophytic infections display spontaneous resolution when infected hairs either enter the telogen phase or an inflammatory reaction is triggered. When hair follicles reach telogen, the production of keratin slows and stops. Dermatophyte infections require actively growing hair to survive. Infective arthrospores remain on the hair shaft, but reinfection of that particular hair follicle does not reoccur until that follicle reenters the anagen phase. Dermatophyte infections are often self-limiting and resolve spontaneously within 3 to 4 months.

Younger animals are predisposed to acquiring and developing symptomatic dermatophyte infections. This is in part because of a delay in development of adequate host immunity and immature immune surveillance machinery. However, there are also differences in puppies and kittens in biochemical properties of the hair and skin (especially sebum), the growth and replacement of hair, in healing properties, and in the physiologic status of the host as related to age that may also play a large role.

Clinical Signs

Dermatophytosis is a diagnosis that must be based on positive culture results or biopsy. In multiple studies of suspected fungal skin cases, only about 15% were positive on culture. Results from all studies of cutaneous diseases of dogs and cats where fungal cultures have been obtained show the prevalence of dermatophytic infections is approximately only 2% of all dermatologic disease cases.

Fungal skin infection is almost always a disease of the follicles in dogs and cats. The most common clinical signs include hair loss, scaling, and crusting. There may be one or many circular patches with variable degrees of scaling. Some animals demonstrate the classic ring lesion with central healing, fine follicular papules, and crusts at the periphery. Pruritus is variable and is usually minimal or absent.

Dermatophytic lesions in puppies typically consist of focal or multifocal areas of hair loss and are clinically indistinguishable from other sources of hair loss. Dermatophytes invade hair shafts and cornified epithelium. As a result, the hair shaft is destroyed and normal keratinization is disrupted. Clinically this results in scaling and hair loss, but fungal skin infections can have a wide array of presentations, particularly if pruritus and secondary bacterial infection are involved. Dogs are more likely than cats to develop the classic ring lesion, a focus of alopecia, follicular papules, scales and crusts, and a central area of hyperpigmentation.

Infections with *Trichophyton* may also cause folliculitis and furunculosis of one paw or leg. Like the facial form, this leg or foot furuncular form can leave significant scars once healed. Generalized infections can present as a seborrhea-like eruption with greasy scales. The dermatophyte version is an exudative, usually fairly well circumscribed, nodular type of lesion that may develop multiple draining tracts. It is most often in dogs associated with *M. gypseum* or *T. mentagrophytes* infections. It can commonly appear as a solitary lesion on the face or on a limb. Although onychomycosis is rare, it is typically produced by *T. mentagrophytes* and presents asymmetrically with only one digit or multiple digits on only one paw involved.

In cats, dermatophytosis can effectively mimic almost any described feline skin disease. More than 90% of the time *M. canis* is the culprit responsible for feline dermatophytosis. *M. canis* is not typically a localized disease in cats.

TABLE 17-1	Dermatophytes isolated from dogs and cats
Most common	
Microsporum	Most common isolate
Microsporum gypseum	Generally from soil contact
Trichophyton mentagrophytes	Soil contact
Less common	
Microsporum persicolor	Sylvatic form
Microsporum fulvum	Rare
Microsporum audouinii	Rare
Trichophyton rubrum	Rare

In kittens, dermatophytes tend to consist of areas of alopecia and scaling. Erythema is variable and hard to detect in both long-haired and dark-haired cats. Lesions usually first appear as areas of hair loss on the face, muzzle, ears, and forelegs. Extent and severity of the lesion are inextricably tied to the health of the kitten. As a result, lesions can be focal, multifocal, or generalized. In some young cats, *M. canis* can produce comedone-like lesions resembling chin acne.

Diagnosis
Wood's lamp

One of the quickest, easiest, and oldest diagnostic tests for fungal identification is the use of the Wood's light or Wood's lamp. This is a light emitting ultraviolet rays (320- to 400-nm wavelength) and is a useful initial test for certain dermatophytes. However, the Wood's lamp is not definitive because only about one-half of all *M. canis* infections will show fluorescence, and other animal-infecting dermatophytes do not fluoresce at all. The characteristic "apple-green" or "Jimi Hendrix–green" fluorescence results from metabolites of the fungal organism that grow only on the hair and never on scale or claw material. In early infections, the whole hair shaft will fluoresce. As the dermatophyte infection clears, only the more distal portion of the hair glows as the proximal portion of the hair shaft is no longer infected. In later stages of infection, only the very tips of hair shafts fluoresce (Figure 17-1).

Direct hair examination (microscopic)

Direct microscopic examination of suspected fungally infected hairs can be time consuming and not very cost effective.

Fungal culture

Fungal culture of affected material (scale and hairs) is the most reliable method to diagnose dermatophytosis and the

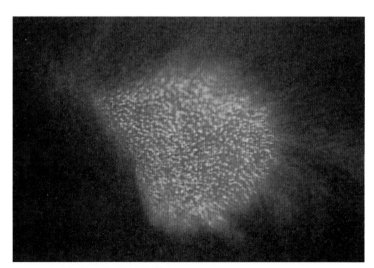

Figure 17-1 Dermatophytosis. Positive Wood's lamp examination of a cat with *M. canis*. Note the apple-green glow. (From Medleau L, Hnilica K: *Small animal dermatology—a color atlas and therapeutic guide*, ed 2, St Louis, 2006, Saunders/Elsevier.)

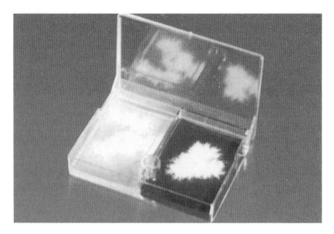

Figure 17-2 Dermatophytosis. *M. canis* growing on several commercially available dermatophyte media. The white colony and red color change of the culture media are suggestive of a dermatophyte. (From Medleau L, Hnilica K: *Small animal dermatology—a color atlas and therapeutic guide,* ed 2, St Louis, 2006, Saunders.)

only way to identify specific fungal pathogens. However, both false-positive and false-negative results are possible. Proper specimen collection techniques are critical for successful diagnosis.

Specimens are best collected by plucking hair near the lesion and active inflammation. Hair can be plucked with a hemostat or forceps or through use of a "brushing" method. This involves a brand-new (mycologically sterile) human toothbrush vigorously combed over suspect areas for 2 to 3 minutes. The bristles of the toothbrush (and their attached hairs) are lightly and repeatedly pressed into the surface of the culture medium.

In kittens, brushing both the face and the hair inside the bell of the ear is extremely important because early lesions often start at these sites. In the case of suspect claw or nail bed infection, special culture techniques may be necessary.

Dermatophyte test medium can be easily obtained for in-house procedures and is best bought as a plate for the toothbrush technique (Figure 17-2). Dermatophyte medium containers are best incubated loosely covered or capped at room temperature protected from ultraviolet light and desiccation, and covered in a container holding a damp paper towel. Colonies of dermatophytes can appear within 5 to 7 days of inoculation. Nevertheless, plates must be maintained for at least 3 weeks before determining a culture negative. Culture plates must be examined daily for medium color change to red. Growth of a white to buff-colored, powdery to cottony mycelium also will be observed. Color change must occur simultaneously as the first colony is visible, never later. All fungi, including nonpathogen fungal growth, will produce a red color change after colonies have growth from several days to a week. Colonies of infectious dermatophytes are never black, brown, gray, or green. Often *M. canis* will fail to grow or sporulate on dermatophyte medium. Recently studies have demonstrated that increased sporulation and

growth can be obtained when plates were incubated at higher temperatures of 70° to 73° F (21° to 23.8° C).

Most colonies will produce spores after 7 to 10 days of growth, which will allow specific identification on microscopy. Spore collection is best accomplished by brushing clear cellophane tape lightly over the colony surface. Place the tape sticky side down onto a drop of lactophenol cotton blue stain on a glass slide. Then add another drop of stain on top of the tape. After a coverslip is placed, the prep can be examined at 100× magnification. Among the hypha strands will be microconidia (spores) that will have characteristic shapes according to their species. If no spores are visible, wait another 4 to 7 days. Certain colonies may not sporulate until they are old and established. The presence of an infectious dermatophyte can only be definitively confirmed by culture results, appearance of the colonies, and microscopic confirmation of fungal elements.

Biopsy—histopathological examination

Demonstration of the organism in a biopsy sample is definitive proof of a true fungal infection.

Treatment

Clinical management and therapeutic regimens for cutaneous fungal infections in puppies and kittens are complicated by the immature immune systems; hepatic, renal, and healing mechanisms of the young; and often the exceedingly small size of these animals.

Healthy dogs and some cats may show spontaneous remission of dermatophyte infections within 3 months. Kittens and cats with seemingly local disease can self-cure, but infections may be prolonged, at least 60 to 100 days. Long-haired cats can have spontaneous remission, but it may take from 1.5 to 4 years. Animals with generalized dermatophytosis typically require systemic therapy. For dogs, sylvatic forms of ringworm (*Microsporum persicolor* and *Trichophyton* species) do not resolve spontaneously and need systemic therapy.

Ideal clinical therapy involves not only treatment of the infected animal but also treatment of all animals exposed and the environment. Topical therapy used in conjunction with systemic treatment results in a faster mycologic cure than systemic therapy alone and reduces contamination on the haircoat and subsequent environmental contamination.

Hair clipping

Clipping of the entire haircoat is optimal in all cases of dermatophytosis because it removes infected, fragile hairs that will spill spores back onto the haircoat and into the animal's environment. Clipping allows for penetration of topical medications and significantly reduces both the amount of medication needed and the duration of the therapy. Short-haired animals with fewer than five focal lesions need not be clipped.

Topical treatment

Localized or spot treatments of dermatophyte infections in companion animals have almost no evidence for their efficacy. More effective than topical "spot" treatment are whole-body shampoos, rinses, or dipping with topical antifungal medications. The most effective topical antifungal whole-body baths, rinses, and dips are lime sulfur, enilconazole, and miconazole. Captan, povidone-iodine, and chlorhexidine are ineffective against dermatophytes when used as whole-body topical treatments.

Lime sulfur has shown superior antifungal activity at 8 oz per gallon of water (a 1:16 dilution). Lime sulfur applied twice weekly at 4 oz per gallon has demonstrated to be effective against dermatophytes if used together with whole-body clipping and aggressive environmental treatment methods. Lime sulfur is virtually nontoxic if applied properly and can even be safely applied to newborn puppies and kittens.

Enilconazole is effective in treating dermatophytosis when used as a sole, whole-body therapy (dipping) following whole-body hair clipping. Enilconazole is generally well tolerated. Side effects can include hypersalivation, anorexia, weight loss, and generalized muscle weakness. There have been anecdotal accounts of severe toxicity in cats after ingestion of enilconazole. It is believed these cases result from cats ingesting the medication by grooming after application of the antifungal agent. It appears that enilconazole is safe for cats if they are fitted with Elizabethan collars for a few hours after treatment and grooming is prevented until the animal is dry. Enilconazole is an effective treatment as a topical medication (10% solution or 100 mg/ml), but it is licensed only for dogs and horses.

Miconazole can be used as a sole therapeutic agent or used together in combination with chlorhexidine. Generally it is used twice weekly as an adjunct topical to systemic therapy rather than as a sole treatment method. As with all medicated shampoos and dips, for optimal therapeutic effects a skin contact time of 10 minutes is recommended for miconazole. Synergism between miconazole and chlorhexidine has been confirmed, and shampoos with this combination have been shown to hasten mycological cure. A list of topical antifungal therapy is included in Box 17-1.

Systemic treatment

Systemic therapy of dermatophytosis is used to hasten resolution of infection. Several drugs have been shown effective in the treatment of dermatophytosis. The appropriate choice for treatment is based on fungal species present, patient species involved, age and size of the patient involved, possible adverse effects and toxicity, and cost. Dogs and cats with multifocal lesions, all long-haired animals, and those in multianimal situations are candidates for systemic antifungal treatment. Animals nonresponsive following 2 to 4 weeks of topical therapy should also be considered for systemic treatment. See Box 17-2 for dermatophyte treatment summary. Itraconazole is currently the systemic treatment of choice for dermatophytosis in dogs and cats. Griseofulvin and ketoconazole both have significant issues of safety and efficacy. Box 17-3 and Table 17-2 list systemic fungal medications and antifungal drug dosages.

Complete resolution of clinical signs is considered a *clinical cure*, and when fungal cultures are sequentially negative 1 week or more apart that is considered a *mycologic cure*.

Vaccines

At present, there is no prophylactic vaccine for feline dermatophyte infection.

Environmental Control

Spores of *M. canis* can remain viable in the environment for several years. The microscopic spores of dermatophytes can be carried by drafts and air currents, contaminate dust, and move in heating vents, and carpets, curtains, and animal bedding can become infective.

Three antifungal disinfectants have proved to be consistently effective in treating dermatophyte-contaminated

---

BOX 17-1   Topical antifungal therapy

- Most consistent topical antifungal agents: lime sulfur, enilconazole, miconazole
- Recommend twice-weekly whole-body rinse or shampoo
- Topical treatment best used together with systemic antifungal
- If topical used alone, do haircoat clip and use lime sulfur
- Animals should not be allowed to lick or groom the solution

---

BOX 17-2   Current dermatophyte treatment summary

Clipping of the haircoat
- Cost effective
- For generalized lesions
- For all long-haired cats

Topical therapy
- As a sole treatment only use lime sulfur or enilconazole
- Topical therapy works best together with systemic therapy
- Topical medications should be used twice weekly
- Do not overlook face, ears, and feet

Systemic treatment
- Itraconazole: daily for 28 days and then 1 week on and 1 week off (pulse therapy)
- Terbinafine: daily or treated like itraconazole, is used in pulse therapy
- Griseofulvin: daily microsize or daily ultramicrosize therapy

- Currently fungal vaccines are not available, effective, or recommended. However, research is promising.
- Lufenuron is not effective.
- Ketoconazole and terbinafine are cost effective. Itraconazole is effective, has fewer side effects, but may be cost prohibitive.

BOX 17-3   Systemic fungal medications

Amphotericin B is the only drug that is fungicidal and has been proven capable of permanently clearing CSF infections. Use of this drug requires hospitalization because it must be given parenterally and can be nephrotoxic in dogs or cats with disseminated infection. Newer forms of amphotericin (lipid complex and liposomal forms) are less nephrotoxic, although much more expensive. Pretreating with heat (at 140° to 158° F, 60° to 70° C for 10 minutes) reduces nephrotoxicity in standard formulations.

Griseofulvin use has decreased largely in part because of its cost, a fairly high potential for toxicity and adverse effects, and the growing availability of safer, more effective drugs. Griseofulvin is poorly water soluble; its absorption is variable; and its uptake is heightened if given with a fatty meal. Dosages shown to be effective against dermatophytes are higher than the recommendations of manufacturers, and significant toxicity has been reported. Animals younger than 6 weeks of age should not receive griseofulvin.

Ketoconazole is moderately effective against *Microsporum canis* and *Trichophyton mentagrophytes* infections. Its action is fungistatic, and it has been used successfully in the treatment of canine and feline dermatophytosis. In long-haired animals it has more variable results. Ketoconazole is best absorbed in an acidic environment. As a result, vitamin C is often recommended to be given concurrently.

Itraconazole is a triazole antifungal. It is fungistatic at lower concentrations and fungicidal at high concentrations. Generally it is well tolerated at recommended dosages, and it is better tolerated than either griseofulvin or ketoconazole by cats and dogs. The most common side effects are anorexia and vomiting. Rarely hepatotoxicity has been documented in cats, and idiosyncratic cutaneous vasculitis has been seen in dogs. This antifungal drug is available for use as a liquid (10 mg/ml), which is helpful in dosing extremely small animals and kittens. Itraconazole has been used in kittens as young as 6 weeks of age. Itraconazole persists in the skin and nails for months after administration. In humans, intermittent or pulse therapy is frequently prescribed for use in onychomycosis. Such intermittent therapy may be useful in animals as well.

Fluconazole may be less effective than itraconazole against fungal infections, and no advantage has been documented for its use against dermatophytes.

Terbinafine is the newest antifungal agent to be given systemically. Terbinafine is a fungicidal drug. Currently it is available as a topical cream and as an oral tablet. It is well tolerated by most animals; vomiting is its most common side effect. In humans, this drug reaches high concentrations in the sebum and the stratum corneum. Fungicidal levels of the drug may persist for several weeks after administration. This would suggest, like itraconazole, that terbinafine intermittent pulse dosing might be effective. At present, no advantage has been documented for this drug over itraconazole for use in animals with fungal infections.

Lufenuron is a benzolphenylurea drug that disrupts the synthesis of chitin. It is used for the control of fleas in companion animals. Currently lufenuron is not recommended in the treatment or prevention of dermatophytes.

environments. These products are lime-sulfur formulation (1:33), 2% enilconazole, and household chlorine bleach (1:10 to 1:100). No fungal strains were shown to be susceptible to chlorhexidine or detergent peroxide disinfectants even when exposed to four times the recommended concentration. Most resistant infections are a result of insufficient decontamination procedures and not variations in fungal strain susceptibility to disinfectant products.

Prevention

The risk of infection for single pet cats living solely indoors is relatively low. The most likely source of infection is introduction of an infected animal or exposure through contact in a contaminated shelter, boarding kennel, grooming facility, or veterinary hospital.

Zoonotic Potential

Dermatophytosis is a zoonotic condition with tremendous potential for transmission. Those most vulnerable are children, elderly people, cancer patients, and those with other immunocompromised diseases (see Chapter 46).

Malasseziasis (*Malassezia* Dermatitis)

Malassezia (*Malassezia pachydermatis*) is normal commensal yeast of the skin. Infection occurs either when hypersensitivity to the yeast develops or when there is overgrowth of the organism. It is a rare condition in cats.

Clinical Signs

Dogs typically demonstrate an unpleasant body odor with the condition. Pruritus may be moderate to intense, and dogs may show local or generalized alopecia, erythema, seborrhea, and excoriations. Chronically affected areas can become hyperpigmented, hyperkeratotic, and lichenified. Generally areas most commonly displaying lesions are the interdigital spaces, ventral neck, axillae, leg folds, and perineal region. Nails may be affected, exhibited as paronychia with a dark brown nail-bed discharge. Simultaneous yeast otitis externa infections are not uncommon.

Although more rarely seen in cats, signs in felines include alopecia, seborrhea, multifocal to generalized erythema, chin acne, and black waxy otitis externa infections with or without pruritus.

Diagnosis

Malasseziasis is best confirmed by cytology and finding more than two round to oval budding yeasts per high-power field. These are best seen on a skin imprint tape preparation. Fungal culture is also possible.

Treatment

Effective topical therapies include ketoconazole baths and dips in lime sulfur. Moderate to severe cases may require ketoconazole or itraconazole. Prognosis is good, particularly when the underlying cause is identified and addressed. Best results are obtained when topical shampoos are combined with systemic medications.

TABLE 17-2	Antifungal drug dosages		
Drug	**Dose**	**Route**	**Frequency**
Amphotericin B	Dog: 0.22-0.5 mg/lb (0.5-1 mg/kg)	IV	q 48 hours
Amphotericin B (lipid complex)	Cat: 0.125-0.25 mg/lb (0.25-0.5 mg/kg)	IV	q 48 hours
	Dog: 0.5-1.5 mg/lb (1-3 mg/kg)		
Flucytosine	Dog: 11.4-22.7 mg/lb (25-50 mg/kg)	PO	q 6 hours
Ketoconazole	Dog: 4.5-13.6 mg/lb (10-30 mg/kg)	PO	q 12 hours
Itraconazole	Dog: 2.2-4.5 mg/lb (5-10 mg/kg)	PO	q 24 hours
	Cat: 4.5 mg/lb (10 mg/kg)		
Fluconazole	Dog: 1-4.5 mg/lb (2.5-10 mg/kg)	PO	q 12 hours
	Cat: 1-4.5 mg/lb (2.5-10 mg/kg)		
Enilconazole	Dog: 4-5 mg/lb (10 mg/kg)	Intranasal	q 12 hours
Clotrimazole	Dog: 1 gm	Intranasal	Once
Sodium iodide	Dog: 20 mg/lb (44 mg/kg)	PO	q 8 hours
Terbinafine	Dog: 4.5-9 mg/lb (10-20 mg/kg)	PO	q 24 hours
	Cat: 4.5-9 mg/lb (10-20 mg/kg)		
Lufenuron	Dog: 2.2-4.5 mg/lb (5-10 mg/kg)	PO	q 24 hours

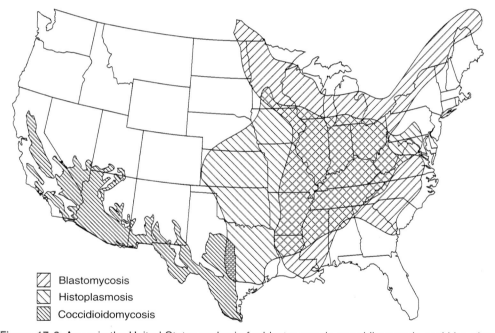

Blastomycosis
Histoplasmosis
Coccidioidomycosis

Figure 17-3 Areas in the United States endemic for blastomycosis, coccidiomycosis, and histoplasmosis. (From Ettinger S, Feldman E (ed): *Textbook of veterinary internal medicine*, ed 7, St Louis, 2010, Saunders/Elsevier.)

Zoonotic Potential

This condition is not contagious either to other animals or to people.

SYSTEMIC FUNGAL INFECTIONS

Histoplasmosis

The causative agent responsible for histoplasmosis is a soil-borne fungus, *Histoplasma capsulatum*. The majority of cases occur most commonly in the Ohio, Missouri, and Mississippi river valleys (Figure 17-3). The organism does best in high nitrogen, and its sporulation happens ideally in soil rich in bird and bat feces or frequently fertilized. However, some totally house-bound, indoor cats have become infected, suggesting that even accumulations of household dust, soil containing houseplants, or greenhouses may serve as possible infectious sources.

The incubation period in susceptible hosts is roughly 12 to 16 days postexposure. Once in mammalian tissues

(98.6° F [37° C]), microconidia convert to a yeast phase in the lung and reproduce by budding. Lymphatic and hematogenous spread of the organism can occur as a result.

If the initial dose of infective spores is large or the animal is in any way immunocompromised, severe clinical disease can occur. An intact, mature cellular immune system will control the infection in most animals.

Clinical Signs

Most dogs affected are young (aged less than 4 years), and no breed or sex predilection has been reported. The main clinical signs described are weight loss, inappetence, and coughing. Dogs may demonstrate a fever unresponsive to antibiotics. For most dogs the disease is limited to the respiratory tree with signs of dyspnea, abnormal lung sounds, and a significant cough. Signs of gastrointestinal involvement may result, including large bowel diarrhea, tenesmus, and fresh blood and mucus in the stool. Splenomegaly, visceral lymphadenopathy, hepatomegaly, icterus, and ascites are not uncommon associated findings. The ocular lesions reported in cats can occur but not as frequently. Neurologic involvement secondary to dissemination of the organism is rare.

Cats may be more susceptible than dogs. There is no breed predilection apparent, and juvenile animals are definitely more vulnerable. Unlike dogs, cats display a wide array of nonspecific signs. In cats, histoplasmosis appears as a slowly progressive disease. Clinical signs include weight loss, inappetence, low-grade fever, and pale mucous membranes. In cats, coughing is uncommon, but dyspnea, abnormal lung sounds, and tachypnea are found in the majority of cats. Ocular lesions including conjunctivitis, granular blepharitis, granulomatous chorioretinitis, retinal detachment, optic neuritis, and blindness are not uncommon in affected cats. Less frequently vomiting, diarrhea, and gastrointestinal signs are reported.

Diagnosis

The most common hematologic sign of histoplasmosis infection for both dogs and cats is a normocytic, normochromic, nonregenerative anemia.

Radiographically dogs and cats with active pulmonary histoplasmosis typically exhibit a diffuse pulmonary intestinal pattern usually associated with granulomatous fungal pneumonia.

There is no consistently reliable antibody detection test for the identification of histoplasmosis in dogs and cats.

Treatment

Currently the cornerstone for treatment of histoplasmosis is itraconazole. Prognosis for localized and pulmonary infections is good; however, long-term therapy may be required. In cats, 6- to 10-month relapses following therapy have been reported. Typically most animals on oral antifungal drugs are treated for at least 4 months. Itraconazole should be given for at least 30 days following resolution of all clinical signs. A list of antifungal drugs used and their dosages is included in Table 17-2.

Ketoconazole, another oral azole antifungal agent, is much less expensive than itraconazole but has increased incidence of toxic side effects and is as effective in cats only about one-third of the time.

Fluconazole has better penetration into the central nervous system (CNS) and eye than itraconazole. It is available in an intravenous form, so it can be used in vomiting or severely ill animals. It is not as effective in people for treating histoplasmosis, but its actual efficacy in treating the disease in animals is unknown.

Zoonotic Potential

Histoplasmosis is not considered a zoonotic disease relative to dogs and cats. It is zoonotic from avian and bat feces.

Blastomycosis

Blastomycosis is a systemic mycotic infection caused by the fungus *Blastomyces dermatitidis*. In the United States the disease has a fairly well-defined endemic area, including the Ohio, Missouri, and Mississippi river valleys; the Mid-Atlantic States; and the Canadian provinces of Ontario, Quebec, and Manitoba (see Figure 17-3). Animal waste, decaying organic and wood products, and low altitudes (less than 500 meters above sea level) appear to create ideal environmental conditions for the growth of this organism. In many studies, proximity to water appears critical; in one report dogs with blastomycosis are 10 times more likely to live within 400 meters of some body of water (pond, lake, creek, stream, river, or marsh).

Infection with *Blastomyces* organisms is caused by the inhalation of spores into the lungs. Incubation period is 5 to 12 weeks. Pulmonary disease develops, and the yeast forms of the organism spread throughout the body to other organs: lymph nodes, testes, skin, subcutaneous tissues, bones, eyes, and brain. Dissemination in the body is generally thought to occur along vascular and lymphatic routes. Lung lesions may have resolved by the time disseminated sites of the infection become apparent.

Dogs are 100 times more likely to become infected than cats. In cats no age, breed, or sex predilection was found with *Blastomyces* infections. Most infections are in dogs aged less than 5 years. Young age and proximity to water are increased risk factors for *Blastomyces* infection in dogs.

Dogs appear to have a shorter prepatent period and develop the disease more quickly than cats exposed at the same time.

Clinical Signs

Canine infections with blastomycosis cause weight loss, anorexia, dyspnea, cough, lameness, and skin lesions. Lymphadenopathy of one or more lymph nodes is not uncommon. Fevers are present in 40% to 60% of infected dogs. The majority of dogs show exercise intolerance; dry, harsh lung sounds; and dyspnea even at rest. The extent of coughing is very variable. Radiographs of the chest are recommended for all dogs suspected of blastomycosis because many will show characteristic lung changes without respiratory signs. Radiographic findings are diffuse, nodular, interstitial, and bronchointerstitial lung changes.

Forty percent of all dogs with blastomycosis have ocular lesions, most commonly uveitis. Chorioretinitis, optic neuritis, retinal detachment, retinal granulomas, vitritis, and vitreal hemorrhage can also be caused by blastomycosis infections. Severe corneal edema can prevent a good eye exam. Glaucoma secondary to angle closure may develop. Lens rupture can occur, requiring enucleation of the affected eye. Keratitis, conjunctivitis, and inflammation of periorbital tissues are commonly observed.

Skin lesions can be found anywhere, but preferred sites seem to involve nail beds, the face, and the planum nasale. The lesions may ulcerate with drainage of purulent or serosanguineous fluid (Figure 17-4). These lesions can become secondarily infected, and well-defined subcutaneous abscesses may develop.

Bone involvement with blastomycosis can occur in up to 30% of infected individuals. Blastomycosis infections of bone typically affect the appendicular skeleton and are osteolytic with periosteal proliferation and soft tissue swelling. The majority of these body lesions are solitary and occur distal to the stifle and elbow. Lameness is the primary clinical sign in these animals and may be the only sign of the disease.

Cats with blastomycosis show similar clinical signs to those displayed by dogs. Weight loss, dyspnea, draining skin lesions, and visual impairment are the findings most commonly described. Eye involvement usually involves a pyogranulomatous uveitis.

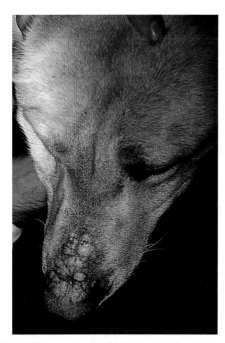

Figure 17-4 Blastomycosis. Multiple draining lesions on the nasal planum of a dog. (From Medleau L, Hnilica K: *Small animal dermatology—a color atlas and therapeutic guide*, ed 2, St Louis, 2006, Saunders.)

Diagnosis

Diagnosis of *Blastomycosis* organisms is best made through identification using cytologic or histologic means. Fine-needle aspirates of enlarged lymph nodes and impression smears of skin lesions or the cytology of draining exudates reveal *Blastomyces* organisms more than half the time.

Treatment

Ease of administration, decreased likelihood of toxicity, and the effectiveness of itraconazole make it the drug of choice for treatment of blastomycosis. Itraconazole should be started at a dosage of 5 mg/kg every 12 hours for the first 5 days. The dose is then reduced to 5 mg/kg/day for the remainder of the treatment. Therapy should continue at least 60 days to be successful and for at least 1 month after all signs of disease have resolved. Dogs showing severe lung involvement need to be treated at least 90 days. About 20% of dogs that respond to therapy show signs of recurrence. Recurrence of disease can be effectively treated with another 60- to 90-day treatment of itraconazole.

Cats with blastomycosis have been safely and successfully treated with itraconazole at 5 mg/kg given every 12 hours. No studies have been performed examining lower dosages. Current recommended dosages for dogs and cats are shown in Table 17-2.

In 85% of eyes enucleated despite the itraconazole treatment, budding, visible *Blastomyces* organisms were found. As a result, blind eyes should be enucleated as soon as they can tolerate the anesthesia in an attempt to eliminate a persistent nidus of infection within the eye.

The best pragmatic indicators of survival are brain involvement and severity of lung disease. Dogs with brain involvement usually die. The severity of lung infiltrates may worsen in the first 2 to 3 days of treatment.

Zoonotic Potential

Blastomycosis is not considered a zoonotic disease.

Cryptococcosis

Cryptococcosis is an important fungal disease of animals. It is the most common systemic mycosis in cats. The infection is usually caused by two encapsulated yeast species of the genus *Cryptococcus* (*Cryptococcus neoformans* and *Cryptococcus gatti*). No cases of transmission have been reported from one affected animal to another.

Avian guano, particularly pigeon, and other avian habitats may provide an infectious environment for *C. neoformans*. *Cryptococcus* organisms have been shown to remain viable for up to 2 years in moist pigeon lofts where droppings are protected both from sunlight and from drying.

Cryptococcus infection most likely occurs through inhalation of airborne organisms. Most infections of feline and canine *Cryptococcus* begin as mycotic rhinitis.

Birman, Siamese, and Ragdoll cats, as well as German Shepherd Dogs and American Cocker Spaniels, are all significantly overrepresented in numbers of reported cases when compared with other breeds. Pulmonary forms of the disease are often followed by hematogenous dissemination and lymphatic transport to other organs. Typically the CNS, eyes, and skin become infected. Cryptococcal organisms have been found to invade almost any body organ and generally cause granulomatous lesions. *Cryptococcus* tends to localize in cooler body areas, the nasal cavity, respiratory passages, and subcutaneous tissues. Cryptococcal organisms do not aerosolize from sites of tissue infection, so the disease cannot spread among people or animals.

Clinical Signs

Canine *Cryptococcus* is predominantly a disease of young adults. Clinical signs in dogs include lethargy and weight loss. In the canine, cryptococcal organisms typically infect the nasal cavity, the CNS, and the eyes. CNS signs associated with *Cryptococcus* are ataxia, head tilt, circling, nystagmus, facial paralysis, and paraplegia. Periorbital swelling and anterior uveitis may be seen. Other ocular signs are optic neuritis, retinal hemorrhage, dilated pupils, and blindness. Usually it is a chronic condition that has caused lethargy, poor appetite, and weight loss.

Cryptococcosis is the most common feline systemic mycosis. Young adult animals seem to be at highest risk of infection. Clinical signs include serous, mucopurulent, or hemorrhagic nasal discharge; snuffling; sneezing; and snorting (Figure 17-5). Firm polyp-like masses may be evident in the nostril. Cats with the nasopharyngeal form may be dyspneic, show open-mouth breathing, and develop secondary otitis media. Signs of lower respiratory involvement are rare. Neurological signs include ataxia, head tilt, and seizures. Ocular signs most commonly seen are peripheral blindness with dilated, unresponsive pupils. Fever is rarely seen in affected cats.

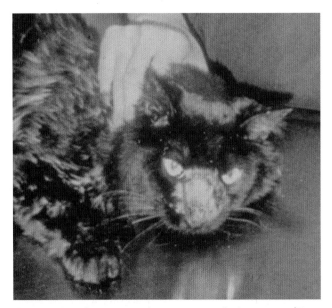

Figure 17-5 Severe nasal cryptococcosis in a cat. (From Nelson R, Couto C (eds): *Small animal internal medicine*, ed 4, St Louis, 2009, Mosby/Elsevier.)

Diagnosis

Appropriate tissue samples for cytology, culture, and histology may be obtained from nasal swabs, nasal flushes, fine-needle aspirates of enlarged lymph nodes or cutaneous masses, bronchoalveolar lavage, pleural fluid, and cerebrospinal fluid (CSF). A definitive diagnosis of cryptococcosis is made by culture and identification of the fungal organisms by a certified laboratory.

Treatment

Immunocompetent animals can be cured. Surgical removal or "debulking" of large aggregations of fungus-infected tissue may help treatment if the affected areas are removed early in the course of the infection. This decreases the area involved and allows antifungal agents to better diffuse into infected tissue. Surgical debridement is not always possible, depending on the size and the location of the lesions.

Serial antigen titer levels are used to gauge the efficacy of therapy. It is recommended that antifungal therapy continue until the antigen titer is zero. This may take extended periods, potentially years. After achieving a zero titer, it is recommended that previously infected animals have titers monitored every 6 months to obtain early diagnosis of recurrence.

Itraconazole is currently the treatment of choice, particularly for cats. This drug is used most frequently because it is more effective than ketoconazole, less expensive than fluconazole, has a high therapeutic index, fewer side effects, and once-daily dosing. It is not as well distributed into the CNS as some other antifungal agents but has been used successfully in both dogs and cats. Cats treated with itraconazole typically require a median of 8 months of therapy.

Amphotericin B is the only drug that is fungicidal and has been proven capable of permanently clearing CSF infections.

Zoonotic Potential

Cryptococcosis is not considered a zoonotic disease, and infected dogs and cats pose no threat to people.

Coccidioidomycosis

Coccidioides is only found in one specific ecological region, the Lower Sonoran life zone (see Figure 17-3). This region possesses sandy, alkaline soil; high environmental temperatures (summer mean, above 79.8° F [26.6° C]; winter mean, 39.2° to 54° F [4° to 12° C]); low annual rainfall (3 to 20 inches); and low elevation (sea level to a few hundred feet). After an outbreak in the San Joaquin Valley of California, the disease in the United States is often known as "Valley Fever." *Coccidioides* outbreaks are also prevalent in Arizona and southwest Texas. The condition is less commonly seen in Nevada, New Mexico, and Utah.

Coccidioidomycosis is highly infectious but typically not contagious. Route of infection is through inhalation. The incubation period is anywhere from 1 to 3 weeks from inhalation to start of respiratory signs. Dogs appear to be the most susceptible of companion animals and have the highest likelihood of development of disseminated disease.

If within 10 days of exposure the disease has progressed beyond hilar lymph nodes, it is said to have "disseminated." Dissemination usually progresses about 4 months after pulmonary signs and can follow a chronic course over months to years. The disseminated form has been documented in a puppy aged 10 weeks.

It is generally held that neonatal transmission occurs from contact of the neonate with the female genital tract or vaginal secretions at birth.

Clinical Signs

In dogs, respiratory clinical signs can be either a dry, harsh cough similar to tracheobronchitis or a productive, wet, moist cough. The dry cough usually represents either hilar lymphadenopathy or diffuse, interstitial, pulmonary disease. The wet, productive cough is usually characteristic of alveolar involvement. Anorexia, fever, and weight loss are seen with both forms. If pulmonary forms of the infection worsen, it can lead to a severe, generalized pneumonia.

In disseminated forms of the disease, clinical signs include fever, anorexia, weight loss, weakness, lameness, localized peripheral lymphadenomegaly, draining skin lesions, seizures, keratitis, uveitis, and acute blindness.

Ataxia, behavioral changes, and seizures have been reported as a result of encroachment on the CNS by granulomatous meningoencephalomyelitis. Paraspinal and/or cranial hyperesthesia are typical in dogs with early CNS localization as a result of meningeal localization and inflammation.

Lameness can occur usually accompanied by painful bone swellings. The bony lesions are usually initially localized to a single site but can progress to multiple locations. Lesions can occur in long bones in the distal diaphysis, metaphysis, and epiphysis. The lesions demonstrate bony lysis and abnormal production. Lesions can be seen in the axial skeleton, but lesions occur 90% more frequently in the appendicular skeleton. Joint infections are not typically seen. However, infected dogs can develop secondary immune-mediated polyarthritis.

In the cat, signs associated with *Coccidioides* organisms closely resemble manifestations found in dogs. However, skin lesions are the most frequent form of the disease in the cat, without bony involvement. Cats show inappetence, fever, and weight loss in addition to the skin lesions. Lung lesions and/or appendicular bony lesions are rarely seen. Chorioretinitis, anterior uveitis, and other ocular lesions appear with the same frequency in cats and dogs.

Diagnosis

A definitive diagnosis of coccidioidomycosis can be made by cytologic or histologic visualization of the organisms. However, lesion location is often limiting, and invasive procedures necessary to obtain such samples may not be possible. Thus diagnosis is often based on history, clinical signs, and serology.

If not demonstrated by biopsy or histology, antibodies to the organism and serology can be used as a presumptive test.

Treatment

The most commonly prescribed drugs used to combat *Coccidioides* infections are the azole drugs ketoconazole, itraconazole, and fluconazole. The use of these drugs for at least 3 months beyond resolution of the clinical signs and normalization of serological titers is recommended.

Ketoconazole has been traditionally the recommended treatment for coccidioidomycosis in dogs. Duration of therapy is variable depending on the site of infection and the extent of its spread. Relapses with ketoconazole therapy are common if the drug is not administered daily for an adequate treatment period. Bone infections and disseminated forms of the disease typically require a minimum of 1 year of treatment. Recommended ketoconazole dosages are included in Table 17-2. Some animals respond poorly to treatment with this drug, and clinical signs can return. Titers should be checked, and if they continue to increase and relapse is evident, an alternative antifungal drug should be selected. In people, ketoconazole appears to be fungistatic, and mycologic cures occur in only 30% of the cases. For these reasons, one of the newer azole drugs (e.g., itraconazole, fluconazole) should be considered. The newer azole molecules (itraconazole, fluconazole) have been shown to be more effective and display fewer side effects than ketoconazole. Cats tolerate itraconazole better than ketoconazole and with much fewer side effects. Recommended dosages for the newer azoles are included in Table 17-2.

Lufenuron, a chitin synthesis inhibitor used and licensed for control of fleas in cats and dogs, has been evaluated for use against fungal infections. It has not been effective for successful treatment of coccidioidomycosis.

Recovery rates vary tremendously with the site and severity of the infection. Complete recovery rates vary in dogs from 90% for infections with pulmonary involvement alone to no recovery for those with multiple bone involvement. Overall a recovery rate of around 60% is sometimes quoted. Untreated dogs with disseminated forms of the infection usually die or are euthanized. Because of poor drug penetration, CNS forms have much worse prognosis. Relapses in cats are common, and some cats show multiple relapses each time the drug is stopped.

Zoonotic Potential

Coccidioidomycosis is typically thought to be noncontagious because the infective arthroconidia are usually not formed in tissues.

Aspergillosis

Aspergillus is a ubiquitous fungi found everywhere in the environment, primarily living and growing in organic debris. Typically it causes either nasal infections or pulmonary and disseminated forms of the disease. Cats can show gastrointestinal mucosal localization. Rarely are solitary lesions found outside the nasal passages. *Aspergillus* is a common contaminant of body and mucosal surfaces and of the respiratory tract. These organisms are generally opportunistic pathogens. Immune competence of the host is the main determinant in whether an animal becomes infected.

Young and middle-aged dogs of mesaticephalic and dolichocephalic breeds are commonly affected by nasal aspergillosis. Dogs with disseminated forms of the infection usually do not display any nasal involvement. Infection is a combination of an animal's underlying immunodeficiency and the fungal organism itself inhibiting an animal's defenses. Bony invasion is typically restricted to the nasal turbinates. Nasal passage infections can involve the cribriform plate, palatine bone, and the bones of the orbit and may result in osteolysis.

Unlike nasal aspergillosis, which has as its primary infectious agent *Aspergillus fumigatus*, the disseminated form most commonly has *Aspergillus terreus* as the source of infection. The causative agent most likely enters the respiratory tract and then spreads hematogenously to other parts of the body. Fungal organisms typically disseminate to the renal glomeruli, intervertebral disks, long bones, and uveal tissues.

In dogs, predisposing factors include particular climate conditions, particular strains of the *Aspergillus* organism, and genetic deficits in mucosal immunity (German Shepherd Dogs). Glucocorticoids should never be given to animals with aspergillosis.

Clinical Signs

Clinical signs of *Aspergillus* infection in dogs include nasal discomfort (pawing at face, dragging nose on ground), mucopurulent nasal discharge, decreased appetite, lethargy, breathing difficulties, and open-mouth breathing. Unilateral infections generally progress to bilateral involvement and destruction of the midline nasal septum. *A. fumigatus* produces an endotoxin responsible for both hemolytic and dermonecrotic activities. The nasal planum can also be sore, depigmented, and ulcerated. Over time, nasal involvement may extend to oculonasal discharge as a result of nasolacrimal duct obstruction, causing epiphora, and facial swelling below the orbits. Pastelike exudates may develop within nasal passages or sinuses as a result of caseous sinusitis in animals with more long-standing infections. Mucosa itself has signs of chronic suppurative inflammation but no actual fungal invasion. Clinical signs of pulmonary aspergillosis include fever, cough, lethargy, inappetence, and mucopurulent nasal discharge.

The most commonly seen clinical signs with canine disseminated forms of aspergillosis is vertebral pain progressing to paraparesis and limb lameness with pronounced swelling and draining sinus tracts. Onset of paraplegia may stem from other infected intervertebral disk rupture or infected intervertebral disk instability. Infected dogs may also show anorexia, weight loss, fever, lethargy, muscle wasting, and vomiting. Dogs may have uveitis and endophthalmitis months before other signs of illness develop.

Nasal *Aspergillus* infections are rarely reported in cats. Systemic immunosuppression does not appear to be critical to the development of *Aspergillus* infections in cats as it does in dogs. Clinical signs of sinonasal *Aspergillus* infections in cats include mucopurulent nasal discharge, epistaxis, and mandibular lymphadenomegaly. Clinical signs usually begin localized to one side, but the disease can become bilateral.

Disseminated feline aspergillosis infections are very uncommon. Affected cats have concurrent immunosuppressive diseases such as feline leukemia virus infection, feline infectious peritonitis, panleukopenia, or underlying neoplasia. Clinical signs of this disease may be nonspecific as in dogs or more typically show signs of gastrointestinal or pulmonary involvement.

Diagnosis

Criteria regarded necessary to make a definitive diagnosis include suspect clinical signs, positive results on cytology and biopsy, a positive serum titer, positive culture results, or a positive titer coupled with radiographic or computer tomography scan changes consistent with fungal rhinitis and turbinate loss. Currently in cats, diagnosis is most often made at necropsy, where findings include pulmonary granulomas, gastrointestinal granulomas and ulcers, and the presence of fungal hyphae in examined tissue samples.

Because *Aspergillus* is often a part of the normal endogenous flora in the nasal cavity of dogs, fungal culture alone can be unreliable and misleading.

Radiographs of bony involvement consistently show osteolysis in long bones and cortical destruction and changes in vertebrae similar to what occurs in diskospondylitis. Infectious organisms can be identified in living tissue through fungal culture, cytology, or biopsy and histopathological evaluation. A single diagnostic test involves examination of aseptically collected urine for the presence of hyphae and branching hyphal elements. Fungal elements may also be detected in lymph node biopsy, synovial fluid, blood, bone, or infected intervertebral disk material. Positive confirmation of fungal culture requires at least 5 to 7 days on Sabouraud dextrose agar medium.

The diagnosis of feline nasal aspergillosis must be based on history and clinical signs accompanied by diagnostic imaging of suspect tissues and histological evidence of pyogranulomatous fungal rhinitis. Currently fungal culture and serology techniques are less than consistent in establishing the concrete presence of *Aspergillus* organisms.

Treatment

Treatment of nasal aspergillosis with newer antifungal medications such as triazoles has been disappointing. No single effective treatment protocol has been identified for *Aspergillus* infections in cats. Systemic therapy is indicated if the fungus has invaded extranasal structures. Results of systemic therapy with antifungal drugs are not as effective as those obtained with topical treatments. Recommended dosages of antifungal treatments for aspergillosis are included in Table 17-2. Amphotericin B is not recommended for treatment of canine nasal aspergillosis infection.

Topical administration of enilconazole and clotrimazole has been shown to be more effective compared with orally administered antifungal drugs. Erosion of the cribriform plate is a contraindication to infusion of large amounts of topical medication under pressure. Administration of topical antifungal medications causes direct damage to fungal membranes and inhibits fungal ergosterol synthesis. Topical administration of clotrimazole is an effective therapy for nasal aspergillosis in dogs. A larger volume of infusate (50 to 60 mg per side) results in a uniform distribution of infusate to all areas of the nasal cavity. Most infusates are 1% formulations of clotrimazole, and 30 ml per side appears adequate for smaller dogs. Surgical intervention of fungal infections has fallen into disfavor. Patients do best when as little damage as possible is done to nasal and turbinate mucosa.

Unfortunately most dogs with disseminated aspergillosis are terminally ill by the time they are first examined. Treatments with supportive fluids, antibiotics, thiabendazole, and ketoconazole have not proven successful. In dogs, itraconazole has proven useful in treatment; however, relapses have been reported once the drug is stopped. Because azole-resistant fungal strains have been recognized, newer triazole compounds like voriconazole and posaconazole are being evaluated.

Indicators for successful therapy include the resolution of pain, ulcerations, epistaxis, and nasal discharge. For some dogs, a mild serous to mucopurulent, crusty discharge can persist in one or both nostrils. Serology is of limited value in assessment of response to therapy. Positive titers may persist in dogs that remain free of disease for 5 years using agar gel immunodiffusion antibody tests. Unlike other fungal infections, relapse is not a common problem in canine aspergillosis once the clinical signs of the infection have been eradicated. Severely ill dogs with disseminated forms of aspergillosis have a poor prognosis. The prognosis for successful resolution of feline sinonasal aspergillosis remains poor.

Zoonotic Potential

No documented instances of infections in people arising from infected dogs or cats have been reported.

Sporotrichosis

Sporothrix schenckii infection is typically caused traumatically, with inoculation of infected soil, plant material, or other organic material infected by the fungus. In dogs, sporotrichosis is usually associated with a puncture wound from an infected thorn or splinter. In cats, the disease is most often identified in intact, adult male cats.

Clinical Signs

Three forms of sporotrichosis have been recognized: cutaneous, cutaneolymphatic, and the disseminated form. Multiple forms may exist in the same infected animal simultaneously. If an animal with recognizable cutaneous lesions also has depression and fever, the clinician should suspect disseminated disease. Often these animals are immunocompromised.

Dogs typically develop cutaneous or cutaneolymphatic forms of the disease; disseminated sporotrichosis is rare. The cutaneous form is multinodular, usually with nodules forming on the head and trunk involving dermal and subcutaneous layers of tissue. The nodules may ulcerate and become secondarily infected with purulent exudate and crust formation. Nasal masses have been reported in the nostrils. Cutaneolymphatic forms are characterized by nodules on the distal aspect of one limb. The infection follows the lymphatic system and ascends proximally. Secondary nodules may form, the so-called "cording" of the lymphatic system, and these may also ulcerate, rupture, and drain purulent exudates. The cutaneolymphatic form is associated with simultaneous regional lymphomegaly.

Cats typically develop lesions in sites commonly injured during cat fights (e.g., head, limbs, tail base), which are inoculated with *Sporothrix* organisms. These draining puncture wounds initially can be mistaken for cat-bite abscesses (Figure 17-6). However, treatment appropriate for cat-bite

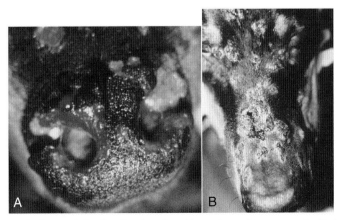

Figure 17-6 A and **B,** Sporotrichosis affecting the skin and nasal mucosa of a Doberman Pinscher. (From Ettinger S, Feldman E (eds): *Textbook of veterinary internal medicine*, ed 7, St Louis, 2010, Saunders/Elsevier.)

wounds (e.g., warm soaks, drainage, antibiotics) is unsuccessful. Affected areas continue to drain, ulcerate, form purulent exudates, and form large crusts. Large necrotic areas may develop. If the disseminated form develops in cats, the lung and liver are predominantly involved.

Diagnosis

A definitive diagnosis is generally made after fungal organisms are visualized in cytology or histopathology samples and subsequently is isolated by fungal culture. A positive result on blood culture of infected cats establishes the presence of the disseminated form of the disease.

The best specimens to be submitted for histopathology are biopsies of intact nodules. Generally, as with cytology, it is easier to determine the presence of *Sporothrix* organisms in cats than in dogs. Dogs may show only a few organisms in infected tissues; therefore histopathology specimens must be carefully examined, and simultaneous fungal culture should also be performed.

Treatment

Treatment of choice for dogs is oral administration of a supersaturated solution of potassium iodide given orally for 30 days past apparent clinical cure. Dogs that exhibit side effects to potassium iodide or signs of iodism (e.g., vomiting, dry haircoat, ocular and nasal discharge) may be treated with alternative drug regimens. Itraconazole has been shown to be safe and effective for treatment of sporotrichosis in people, and dogs have been treated successfully as well. Side effects associated with itraconazole have not been reported in once-daily dosing regimens. If sporotrichosis infections are not treated for an appropriate period, relapses are common.

Recommended dosages for treatment in dogs are included in Table 17-2.

Because cats are more likely to develop toxic side effects from iodides, itraconazole is the treatment of choice. Treatment should be continued for at least 1 month beyond apparent clinical cure. For animals with a poor response to itraconazole treatment, the fungicidal allylamine terbinafine has been used successfully. Terbinafine has few side effects and has been used successfully in cats for infections with *M. canis*. Recommended drug dosages for compounds used to treat sporotrichosis in cats are listed in Table 17-2.

Zoonotic Potential

A feature unique to feline sporotrichosis is the large number of organisms found in the feces, exudates, and tissues of infected cats. As a result, inoculation of the organisms can occur through scratches or punctures caused by the claw or oral cavities of infected cats.

SUGGESTED READINGS

Davidson AP: Coccidioidomycosis and aspergillosis. In Ettinger SJ, Feldman EC (eds): *Textbook of veterinary internal medicine*, ed 6, St Louis, 2006, Saunders/Elsevier, pp. 690-699.

Foil C: Dermatophytosis. In Foster A, Foil C (eds): *BSAVA Manual of small animal dermatology*, ed 2, Gloucester, 2003, British Small Animal Veterinary Association, pp. 169-174.

Greene CE: *Infectious diseases of the dog and cat*, ed 3, St Louis, 2006, Saunders/Elsevier.

Kukanich B: A review of selected systemic antifungal drugs for use in dogs and cats, *Vet Med* 103(1):41, 2008.

Taboada J, Grooters AM: Systemic mycoses. In Ettinger SJ, Feldman EC (eds): *Textbook of veterinary internal medicine*, ed 6, St Louis, 2006, Saunders/Elsevier, pp. 671-690.

DISEASES FORMERLY KNOWN AS RICKETTSIAL
The Rickettsioses, Ehrlichioses, Anaplasmoses, and Neorickettsial and *Coxiella* Infections

CHAPTER 18

Linda B. Kidd, Edward B. Breitschwerdt

CLINICALLY RELEVANT NOMENCLATURE

In the strictest sense, "rickettsial" infection refers to infection with organisms belonging to the genus *Rickettsia*. Historically rickettsial has been used to describe infection with organisms belonging to family Rickettsiaceae. The organisms in this family included obligately intracellular organisms with phenotypic characteristics of both viruses and bacteria. Several genera of bacteria belonged to the family, including (but not limited to) *Rickettsia*, *Ehrlichia*, *Neorickettsia*, and *Coxiella*. Recent genetic analyses of 16S rRNA genes, heat shock and surface protein genes, along with consideration of various phenotypic characteristics, have resulted in dramatic changes in the classification and ultimately the composition of the family Rickettsiaceae. Members of the genera *Ehrlichia* and *Neorickettsia* were entirely removed and placed into the family Anaplasmataceae. Like *Ehrlichia* and *Neorickettsia*, *Coxiella* has also been removed from the family Rickettsiaceae and has been placed in the more distant family Coxiellaceae.

As a result of these taxonomic rearrangements, the family Rickettsiaceae currently includes only the genera *Rickettsia* and *Orientia*, which are intracellular bacteria that live free in the cytoplasm or nucleus of vertebrate host cells. The family Anaplasmataceae includes intracellular organisms that reside within vacuoles of hematopoietic cells (erythrocytes, monocytes, neutrophils, and platelets) and includes (but is not limited to) the genera *Ehrlichia*, *Anaplasma*, and *Neorickettsia*.

Because these organisms no longer share the family name Rickettsiaceae, we propose to limit the term *rickettsioses* or *rickettsial disease* to disease caused by organisms in the genus *Rickettsia*. Accordingly in this manuscript, diseases caused by *Ehrlichia*, *Anaplasma*, *Neorickettsia*, and *Coxiella* are referred to as ehrlichioses, anaplasmoses, and neorickettsial and *Coxiella* infections, respectively.

TICKBORNE RICKETTSIOSES, EHRLICHIOSES, AND ANAPLASMOSES

Several species within the genera *Rickettsia*, *Ehrlichia*, and *Anaplasma* are transmitted to vertebrate hosts through tick vectors. Accordingly the geographic distribution of disease usually follows the distribution of ticks infected with and capable of transmitting a particular organism. It is clinically useful to consider the known geographic distribution of vectors and the disease-causing agents they carry when determining differential diagnoses for infection. For example, for a dog presenting with neutrophilic polyarthritis in Wisconsin, infection with *Anaplasma phagocytophilum* (transmitted by *Ixodes scapularis*) would be a more likely diagnostic consideration, whereas in the southern United States, *Ehrlichia ewingii* (transmitted by *Amblyomma americanum*) would be a more likely differential diagnosis. Therefore practitioners should ensure that tests used to diagnose tickborne diseases (e.g., the "tick panel") are appropriate for organisms prevalent in their area of practice or relevant to a particular patient. The distribution of some tick vectors of clinical significance in the United States can be found at http://www.cdc.gov/Ncidod/dvrd/rmsf/Natural_Hx.htm and http://www.cdc.gov/mmwr/preview/mmwrhtml/rr5504a1.htm.

Despite these considerations, it is important to be aware that these organisms have been very difficult to study in the past because of their complex and highly specialized life cycles. Therefore information regarding their epidemiology and pathophysiology remains incomplete. Recent advancements in molecular biology have led to increased understanding of the spectrum of diseases caused by these agents, the extent of their geographic distribution, and the range of species that are capable of causing disease in people. It is important that veterinarians consider the possibility of infection with a novel vector-borne agent when pets present with atypical clinical signs.

Atypical clinical signs may also be caused by coinfection with multiple organisms. Coinfection with *Ehrlichia*, *Bartonella*, *Rickettsia*, and *Babesia*, or *Anaplasma*, and *Borrelia* has been documented and is likely attributable to coinfection in tick vectors transmitting the agents in a particular geographic location. Atypical clinical signs or failure to respond to appropriate therapy should prompt consideration for testing for additional agents.

Importantly, treatment of infection must begin before clinical confirmation of the causative infectious agent in most cases. Delayed or inappropriate antibiotic therapy results in increased morbidity and mortality. Doxycycline is the treatment of choice for adult animals. Fluoroquinolones are not recommended for treating ehrlichioses or anaplasmoses. Special considerations for the treatment of the pediatric patient are necessary.

Finally, it is important for the veterinarian to be aware that companion animals can serve as sentinels for some of these vector-borne diseases in people. Communication with owners and their physicians regarding a documented infection in a companion animal and the possibility of simultaneous or subsequent human exposure to the same infected vectors can be lifesaving. The role of companion animals as sentinels for disease is particularly important for *Rickettsia rickettsii* and *Coxiella burnetii* because these agents can cause serious morbidity or mortality in people. These organisms are also considered by the U.S. government to be potential weapons for use in bioterrorist attacks.

Rickettsioses: The Spotted Fever Group *Rickettsia*

The genus *Rickettsia* is divided into the spotted fever group (SFG) and the typhus group. The SFG *Rickettsia* includes important causes of emerging and reemerging infectious disease worldwide. These organisms are transmitted by arthropod vectors and primarily infect endothelial cells in vertebrate hosts. Many species of SFG *Rickettsia* have been associated with disease in people, with several being recognized very recently.

R. rickettsii and *Rickettsia conorii* cause Rocky Mountain spotted fever (RMSF) and Mediterranean spotted fever (MSF), respectively, in people. Because of their pathogenicity, these are the best characterized of the SFG *Rickettsia*. *R. rickettsii* also causes RMSF in dogs. Recently we documented infection with *R. conorii* in Italian dogs presenting with signs consistent with a spotted fever–like illness. Therefore *R. conorii* infection should be considered in dogs with a spotted fever–type illness in endemic areas. Evidence suggests that *Rickettsia akari*, *Rickettsia japonica*, and *Rickettsia australis* may also infect dogs. The role of these and other SFG *Rickettsia* as disease-causing agents in dogs is beginning to be elucidated.

As the most pathogenic and well-characterized SFG *Rickettsia* infecting dogs, *R. rickettsii* will be considered in detail here. Although cats can be seroreactive to *R. rickettsii*, clinical disease has not been well characterized. The ability of typhus group *Rickettsia* to cause disease in dogs and cats has also not been well characterized and will not be described here.

Rickettsia rickettsii and RMSF in Dogs

RMSF is a reportable disease in people in the United States. Reporting is also mandatory for dogs in some regions of the country. Natural and experimental infection in dogs has been well documented. As is the case in people, *Dermacentor* ticks are believed to be the primary vector for dogs in the United States. However, *Rhipicephalus sanguineus*, a one-host tick that prefers to feed on dogs, may also play a role in transmitting *R. rickettsii* to dogs. Dogs living outdoors are at increased risk for infection, and most canine cases of RMSF coincide with months of increased tick feeding activity. In dogs, a sex predisposition has not been substantiated across studies. Similarly, studies investigating whether infection is more likely in young dogs (aged less than 2 years) are conflicting. Whether purebred dogs may be at increased risk for infection is also controversial. Springer Spaniels with phosphofructokinase deficiency and German Shepherd Dogs may suffer from more severe disease. The majority of dogs with RMSF do not have a history of a tick bite.

RMSF is an acute illness, with the onset of clinical signs occurring within 2 to 14 days after transmission. In dogs, the most common signs are nonspecific and include fever, anorexia, and lethargy. Although common, it is important to note that fever is not always present. *R. rickettsii* infect endothelial cells and therefore induce vasculitis. The pathologic consequences of vasculitis include disorders of primary hemostasis and edema. Many of the clinical signs of RMSF reflect the presence of vasculitis and systemic inflammation involving several body systems. Ocular signs are common and may include discharge, scleral and conjunctival injection and hemorrhage, conjunctivitis, uveitis, retinal hemorrhage, and retinitis. Respiratory signs can include nasal discharge, epistaxis, tachypnea, dyspnea, and coughing. Gastrointestinal signs may include vomiting, diarrhea, and melena. Cutaneous and mucocutaneous abnormalities can include petechiae, ecchymoses, edema, hyperemia, and necrosis. Orchitis, scrotal edema, hyperemia, hemorrhage, and epididymal pain are often present in intact male dogs. Hematuria may also occur. Myalgia and arthralgia signal muscle and joint involvement. Central nervous system (CNS) signs can be focal or generalized and can include hyperesthesia, ataxia, vestibular signs, stupor, seizures, and coma. Dramatic weight loss, disproportionate to the amount of time the dog has been ill, has also been described. Severe consequences of vasculitis and increased vascular permeability include edema, microvascular hemorrhage or thrombosis, hypotension, and gangrene. As a result, oliguric renal failure, cardiovascular collapse, and brain death can occur terminally.

Typical hematologic findings in dogs include normocytic normochromic anemia and thrombocytopenia. Thrombocytopenia has been identified as one of the most consistent hematologic abnormalities. Thrombocytopenia likely occurs as a result of immune-mediated destruction and sequestration of platelets secondary to vasculitis. Although generally mild, thrombocytopenia can be severe. Leukopenia can occur in the first 48 hours of infection, after which leukocytosis, neutrophilia, monocytosis, lymphopenia, and eosinopenia can occur. Toxic change within neutrophils and metamyelocytes may be observed. Serum chemistry abnormalities can include hypoalbuminemia, azotemia, hyponatremia, hypocalcemia, increased alanine aminotransferase and alkaline phosphatase, mild hyperbilirubinemia, and bilirubinuria. Cerebrospinal fluid analysis may reveal a mild increase in protein and cells with a neutrophilic pleocytosis occurring acutely, followed by a mononuclear pleocytosis later in the course of the disease. Proteinuria may be present secondary to glomerular or tubular damage. Joint fluid analysis is consistent with neutrophilic polyarthritis. Animals rarely develop disseminated intravascular coagulation; however, abnormalities in fibrinogen levels (increases or decreases), elevated fibrin/fibrinogen degradation products, decreased antithrombin, and prolongation of activated partial thromboplastin time or activated clotting time can occur. Thoracic radiographs may show an increased interstitial pattern reflecting pneumonitis.

Because of the nonspecific nature of the clinical abnormalities associated with RMSF, confirmatory testing is necessary for diagnosis and requires serologic testing, direct immunofluorescent testing for *R. rickettsii* antigen in biopsy specimens, and/or polymerase chain reaction (PCR) testing for rickettsial DNA.

Serology is commonly used to diagnose SFG rickettsiosis. Importantly, titers can be negative early in infection, and antibodies can be detected in animals with no history of illness in endemic areas. Therefore seroconversion (a fourfold increase or decrease in antibody titer) must be documented to confirm acute infection. An acute phase sample should be obtained at presentation and a convalescent sample obtained 2 to 3 weeks thereafter. Antibody titers greater than 1:1024 obtained 1 week or more after the onset of clinical signs have also been used to diagnose infection. However, it is important to note that high antibody titers can persist in dogs long after recovery, and therefore high titers in the absence of seroconversion must be interpreted in the context of the individual patient. Notably, serologic cross-reactivity among SFG *Rickettsia* occurs; therefore the species of infecting SFG *Rickettsia* is presumed to be *R. rickettsii*.

Immunohistochemistry and Gimenez staining of tissue samples can also be used to demonstrate SFG *Rickettsia* and therefore can confirm the diagnosis early in the disease course. Importantly, neither determines the species of infecting SFG *Rickettsia*.

Demonstration of rickettsial DNA using PCR also confirms infection. *R. rickettsii* infect endothelial cells and circulate in the bloodstream in very low numbers. Therefore detecting the organism in blood can be challenging. Recently a very sensitive PCR was specifically developed to test dog blood for the presence of SFG *Rickettsia* DNA (Vector Borne Disease Diagnostic Laboratory, North Carolina State University). Importantly, this test can detect *Rickettsia* in

blood before seroconversion and may be useful in confirming infection early. However, it is important to note that rickettsial DNA cannot be demonstrated in the blood of all acutely infected dogs, and a negative test does not indicate a lack of infection. Notably, the species of infecting *Rickettsia* can be confirmed by sequencing the gene product using this test.

Treatment must begin *before* results of confirmatory testing are available and is based on a high index of clinical suspicion by the veterinarian. Response to appropriate antibiotic therapy is rapid and dramatic. The consequences of delayed or missed diagnosis and inappropriate antibiotic therapy can be severe morbidity or death. Doxycycline (5 mg/kg twice a day for 7 to 14 days) is the treatment of choice for RMSF. Chloramphenicol is also effective, but studies in people suggest it may be less effective than doxycycline. The undesirable side effect of bone marrow suppression precludes its use in people and should be considered as a less likely but potential side effect in dogs. Owners should wear gloves and avoid inhaling the drug if it is used to treat RMSF in dogs. Enrofloxacin is also effective in treating RMSF in dogs. Notably, studies suggest chloramphenicol may not be as effective as doxycycline in inhibiting the growth of *A. phagocytophilum*, *Ehrlichia canis*, or *Ehrlichia chaffeensis* in vitro. In addition, fluoroquinolones are less effective in inhibiting the growth of *E. canis* or *E. chaffeensis* in vitro and do not clear infection in dogs infected with *E. canis*. Furthermore, chloramphenicol is inferior to doxycycline for treating human monocytic ehrlichiosis (HME) caused by *E. chaffeensis*. Diseases caused by these organisms in dogs are often differential diagnoses for unconfirmed cases of RMSF presenting acutely. In addition, they may act as coinfecting agents. Therefore doxycycline offers several advantages over other antibiotics that have activity against *R. rickettsii*. Treatment considerations in the pediatric patient are covered later in this chapter.

Other treatment for RMSF consists of supportive care, which may include cautious use of colloids and fluid therapy (exacerbation of edema with fluid therapy is a concern). Treatment of coagulopathies may be necessary, but clinical and hematological improvement following initiation of doxycycline is generally rapid. Short-term immunosuppression with glucocorticoids may be considered in dogs with severe thrombocytopenia with a suspected immune-mediated component. Most clinical signs resolve rapidly after instituting appropriate antibiotic therapy, often within 12 to 48 hours. Residual neurologic signs or gangrenous lesions requiring surgery may occur in severe cases. If rapid response to treatment is not observed, coinfection with *Babesia*, *Ehrlichia*, *Bartonella*, or other organisms or other alternative diagnoses should be considered.

Immunity to natural infection with *R. rickettsii* appears to be permanent. Minimizing tick exposure, routine use of acaricides, and removing ticks from dogs daily are effective means of prevention.

Dogs are sentinels for the disease in people. Therefore veterinarians should notify owners and their physicians when RMSF is diagnosed in a dog (Box 18-1). Owners

BOX 18-1 **Important points regarding Rocky Mountain spotted fever in dogs**

- Most cases of RMSF in the United States occur in geographic association with *Dermacentor* ticks; however, epidemics involving other ticks such as *R. sanguineus* can occur in nonendemic areas. Human cases have been reported from every state except Vermont.
- Most cases of RMSF coincide with peak tick activity, between March and October, but can occur any time of year.
- Most dogs with RMSF do not have a history of a tick bite.
- Misdiagnosis and delayed or inappropriate antibiotic therapy increase morbidity and mortality.
- Appropriate antibiotic therapy must begin before laboratory testing confirms diagnosis.
- Owners and their physicians should be contacted when RMSF is diagnosed in canine patients because illness in dogs can coincide with or precede illness in people.
- Veterinarians should be aware that the agent may be used in bioterrorist attacks, and dogs may be sentinels for such an event.

should be instructed with regard to proper tick removal, and crushing the tick should be avoided to prevent inadvertent exposure to infected hemolymph. Hands should be washed immediately after removal. Contact with infected dog blood by veterinarians and support staff could result in transmission of the organism, although this risk is presumably small. Wearing gloves, washing hands, avoiding aerosolization, and using zoonotic warning labels are recommended for handling samples from suspect cases.

Ehrlichiosis and Anaplasmoses

Members of the genera *Ehrlichia* and *Anaplasma* are obligate intracellular parasites that reside in vacuoles within hematopoietic cells in clusters (morulae). The organisms are transmitted to mammals through the salivary glands of ticks while obtaining a blood meal. Recently there has been a large shift in the taxonomic organization of these organisms that is relevant to the small animal practitioner. Genetic analysis has shown that the agents formerly known as *Ehrlichia equi* and the agent of human granulocytic ehrlichiosis (HGE) are variants of the species *A.* (formerly *Ehrlichia*) *phagocytophilum*; thus they have been renamed accordingly. Furthermore, *Ehrlichia platys* has been reclassified and has been renamed *Anaplasma platys*. Finally, *Ehrlichia risticii* is now classified as *Neorickettsia risticii*.

Although the disease syndrome caused by these organisms is similar, there are apparent differences in their epidemiology, pathophysiology, and response to treatment. For example, the agents that cause granulocytic anaplasmosis and ehrlichiosis (*A. phagocytophilum* and *E. ewingii*) infect neutrophils and appear more likely to cause polyarthritis

than the agents of monocytic ehrlichiosis. Furthermore, infections with *A. phagocytophilum* usually appear to induce more acute disease that responds more rapidly to doxycycline therapy than monocytic ehrlichiosis caused by *E. canis* or *E. chaffeensis*. Notably, *E. ewingii* causes chronic infection in dogs, whereas the extent to which *A. phagocytophilum* induces chronic infection is unknown. It is helpful to keep these differences in mind when determining appropriate diagnostic and therapeutic plans for affected patients.

The following is a brief review of *Ehrlichia* and *Anaplasma* species known to cause disease in dogs and cats.

Canine Monocytic Ehrlichiosis Caused by *Ehrlichia canis* or *Ehrlichia chaffeensis*
Ehrlichia canis

E. canis is a gram-negative obligately intracellular organism that resides in vacuoles within mononuclear cells. It is transmitted by *R. sanguineus*, the brown dog tick. *R. sanguineus* feeds on canid hosts during all three stages of its life cycle. This tick requires dry environments to maintain water balance. Therefore it often infests isolated dry environments of homes and kennels. Although *R. sanguineus* prefers to feed on canids, its proximity to humans results in occasional feeding, and therefore disease transmission to this less-desirable host is possible.

R. sanguineus and *E. canis* have a worldwide distribution. In general, infection appears to be more common in warmer locales. Seroprevalence studies sampling dogs from multiple regions of the United States suggest the disease occurs in most states but is more common in the Southeast. Most cases of HME are caused by infection with *E. chaffeensis*. Because serologic cross-reactivity between *E. chaffeensis* and *E canis* occurs, previous reports of HME attributed to *E. canis* have been disputed. However, recently infection with *E. canis* has been confirmed in people with HME using molecular techniques.

The manifestations of disease caused by *E. canis* in dogs can be characterized as acute, subclinical, and chronic, although distinguishing these phases in the clinical setting may be difficult. It has been hypothesized that variability in the manifestation of clinical disease is likely caused by *E. canis* strain differences, the presence of coinfecting agents, the immune status of the patient, and host genetic factors. Increased susceptibility and disease severity have been reported in German Shepherd Dogs.

After transmission, an incubation period of 8 to 20 days occurs before clinical signs develop. The acute phase of illness lasts 2 to 4 weeks. Clinical signs include anorexia, lethargy, fever, lymphadenomegaly, splenomegaly, hepatomegaly, weight loss, scleral injection, and oculonasal discharge. Neurologic abnormalities may also occur. The most consistent and prominent hematologic abnormality is thrombocytopenia. Evidence suggests the thrombocytopenia associated with *E. canis* infection is caused by vasculitis, immune-mediated destruction, and sequestration. Other hematologic abnormalities that occur during the acute phase include leukopenia and nonregenerative anemia. Transient hypoalbuminemia and proteinuria have been documented during the acute phase in experimentally infected dogs. Glomerular pathology, including minimal change disease and glomerulonephritis, has been associated with proteinuria during this phase. Dogs may recover from the acute phase and clear the infection or progress to the subclinical phase.

The subclinical phase lasts months to years, and dogs appear healthy during this time. Thrombocytopenia can persist in the subclinical phase. Neutropenia and lymphocytosis also occur. Hyperglobulinemia appears to be common during the subclinical phase of infection. Although usually polyclonal in nature, the gammopathy associated with *E. canis* infection can also be monoclonal.

During the chronic phase, nonspecific signs such as weight loss, lethargy, and anorexia can recur. Disorders of primary hemostasis caused by thrombocytopenia and platelet dysfunction are prominent and include epistaxis, petechial or ecchymotic hemorrhages, hematuria, and melena. Fever, lymphadenopathy, and splenomegaly may also be present. Dyspnea resulting from pneumonitis can also occur. Uveitis is common in dogs with *E. canis* infection. Other ocular abnormalities include corneal ulceration, hyphema, retinal hemorrhage, necrotic scleritis, decreased tear production, and orbital cellulitis (Figure 18-1). Importantly, ocular abnormalities can be the only presenting clinical sign. Neurologic signs include ataxia, seizures, head tilt, nystagmus, and conscious proprioceptive deficits. Hematologic findings include nonregenerative or rarely Coombs-positive immune-mediated hemolytic anemia. Like the acute and subacute phases of *E. canis* infection, thrombocytopenia can persist in the chronic phase. White blood cell counts can be normal, increased, or decreased, and pancytopenia may be present. Large granular lymphocytosis, which can be confused with leukemia, is noted on blood smears in some cases. Examination of bone marrow may reveal hypoplasia of the erythroid, myeloid, and/or megakaryocytic cell lines. Hyperplasia, particularly of the megakaryocytic cell line, may occur during the acute phase of the disease. Interestingly, bone marrow

examination can sometimes reveal plasma cell hyperplasia, which can be confused with neoplasia.

Hyperglobulinemia is present in many dogs with chronic ehrlichiosis. This, particularly when monoclonal in nature, along with plasma cell infiltration into the bone marrow can be confused with multiple myeloma. Hypoglobulinemia, presumably resulting from profound lymphopenia, has also been documented in the chronic phase. Hypoalbuminemia, protein-losing nephropathy from glomerulonephritis, and elevations in liver enzymes also occur. Thoracic radiographs may show a diffuse interstitial pattern in dogs with respiratory manifestations of disease.

Clinically it is difficult to determine whether a patient is in the acute or chronic phases of *E. canis* infection. Regardless of the stage of illness, clinical findings in infected dogs may include ocular inflammation, splenomegaly, lymphadenomegaly, petechiae/ecchymosis, and hemorrhages, anemia, thrombocytopenia, leukopenia, proteinuria, and hyperglobulinemia. Anecdotally, the presence of pancytopenia and bone marrow hypoplasia (rather than hyperplasia) suggests a poor prognosis. However, it is important to note that leukopenia, thrombocytopenia, and anemia can occur in any stage of disease, without bone marrow hypoplasia. Therefore pancytopenia should not necessarily be considered a poor prognostic sign. In addition, it is important to note that although recovery can be prolonged, dogs with bone marrow hypoplasia may recover with specific treatment and supportive care.

Morulae in monocytes and lymphocytes may be observed with Giemsa staining, particularly during acute infection. Buffy coat and lymph node smears may be more sensitive than peripheral blood. Serology is often used to document infection with *E. canis*. Serologic cross-reactivity with other ehrlichial agents has been described in detail elsewhere. Of clinical importance, cross-reactivity occurs between *E. canis*, *E. chaffeensis*, and *Neorickettsia helminthoeca*. Healthy dogs that have previously cleared infection with *E. canis* may remain seropositive for prolonged periods. Therefore a positive serologic test may indicate acute, subclinical, or chronic infection or previous exposure to *E. canis*, infection with other ehrlichial agents, or infections that were eliminated immunologically or by previous treatment.

Importantly, *E. canis* antibodies may not be detectable for up to 28 days after infection, after clinical signs are apparent. Therefore a negative test does not exclude the diagnosis, and follow-up testing 2 to 3 weeks later (to document seroconversion) may be necessary. Dogs infected with *N. risticii*, *A. platys*, *A. phagocytophilum*, and *E. ewingii* do not generally develop antibodies that react with *E. canis* antigens. Therefore for seronegative dogs with suspected clinical ehrlichiosis, acute illness (before seroconversion) or infection with another related agent should be suspected.

Recently an in-house enzyme-linked immunosorbent assay that simultaneously tests for *E. canis*, *A. phagocytophilum*, and *Borrelia burgdorferi* antibodies, as well as for *Dirofilaria immitis* infection, has become available. Guidelines with regard to the testing of healthy dogs, sensitivity, and

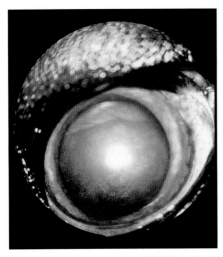

Figure 18-1 Hyphema in a dog with *E. canis* infection.

specificity of this test have been described and are available from the manufacturer or at http://www.cvm.ncsu.edu/docs/PDFS/interpretation_SNAP_4DX_1_07.pdf.

PCR can be used to detect active *E. canis* infection in dogs. Primers that amplify DNA from both *Ehrlichia* and *Anaplasma* species are available (e.g., Vector Borne Disease Diagnostic Laboratory at North Carolina State University). Speciation is performed on genus-specific PCR positive samples. PCR can be a valuable tool in detecting infection before seroconversion, verifying infection in a seropositive dog, and for monitoring response to therapy (see below). It is necessary to use laboratories with excellent quality control to minimize false-positive and false-negative results. PCR can be used to diagnose *Anaplasma* or *Ehrlichia* infection in blood and other tissues such as lymph nodes, bone marrow, and spleen. Notably, splenic aspirates should not be performed in animals at risk for hemorrhage. A negative PCR does not rule out infection.

Currently doxycycline therapy (5 mg/kg orally every 12 hours for 28 days) is the preferred treatment for *E. canis* infection in dogs. Imidocarb dipropionate (5 mg/kg intramuscularly 15 days apart) has also been reported as an effective treatment for *E. canis*. However, a recent study found that imidocarb was not effective in clearing experimental infection. In addition, combination therapy has not been shown to be superior to doxycycline alone. Importantly, enrofloxacin is ineffective against experimentally induced *E. canis* infection. Chloramphenicol has been suggested as an alternative treatment, although no studies regarding its efficacy in naturally or experimentally infected dogs have been performed. In addition, in vitro studies suggest that chloramphenicol is not as effective as doxycycline in inhibiting the growth of *E. canis*. The risk of exposing human companions of infected dogs to chloramphenicol is of concern and is described in the section on RMSF. Additionally, chloramphenicol should be avoided in pancytopenic dogs because of its potential for myelosuppression.

In addition to doxycycline therapy, supportive care may be required, particularly in chronically infected dogs with severe neutropenia, anemia, and thrombocytopenia. In addition to fluid therapy, colloid therapy and nutritional support, transfusions, and treatment for concurrent sepsis may be required. Ocular disease, including uveitis, and neurologic abnormalities require specific therapy. A short course of glucocorticoids may be necessary to treat immune-mediated destruction of platelets, polyarthritis, vasculitis, or meningitis. Specific considerations for the treatment of pediatric patients are discussed later in the chapter.

Generally a rapid response to doxycycline therapy occurs. Resolution of thrombocytopenia can be used to monitor response to therapy. After treatment, platelet counts generally begin to increase within the first 24 to 48 hours. If they do not increase within 1 week of therapy, coinfection with *Babesia*, *Bartonella*, other bacteria, or immune-mediated destruction of platelets should be considered. For responsive patients, platelet counts should be reevaluated 4 to 8 weeks after therapy is complete. Hyperglobulinemia may

take months to resolve. Similarly, antibodies can persist in dogs for prolonged periods. Therefore monitoring response to therapy with serology is not always useful. These patients should be evaluated by PCR to determine whether they are persistently infected or whether antibody production is persisting in the absence of identifiable *E. canis* infection.

Guidelines for the use of PCR for monitoring response to therapy have been determined. It is not clear whether *E. canis* is ever entirely cleared from infected dogs, but more recent studies using long-term administration of doxycycline (3 to 4 weeks) support therapeutic elimination in naturally and experimentally infected dogs. If clinical findings, hyperglobulinemia, and other abnormalities resolve progressively, it has been suggested that the infection may be considered resolved.

With doxycycline therapy and early intervention, the prognosis for *E. canis* is favorable, with resolution of clinical signs occurring in the majority of cases. Ocular abnormalities usually resolve completely with treatment. Anecdotally, animals with chronic ehrlichiosis, severe pancytopenia, and bone marrow hypoplasia or advanced glomerulonephritis may have a worse prognosis, although favorable response to treatment has been documented.

Unlike *R. rickettsii*, infection with *E. canis* does not protect dogs against reinfection (Box 18-2). Minimizing tick exposure and the routine use of approved tick control products on dogs and in infested kennels are necessary to minimize infection in endemic areas. Prophylactic use of doxycycline has been described but is controversial and is discussed elsewhere.

HME is caused by infection with *E. chaffeensis*. However, recent evidence suggests that *E. canis* can also cause HME. Proximity to the vector through exposure to dogs carrying ticks may put people at risk for infection. Direct transmission from a dog to a person has not been described. Proper handling of ticks during removal and using precautions when handling fluids and tissues from infected dogs are recommended as described for *R. rickettsii*. In addition, because the tick vector for *E. canis* is *R. sanguineus*, treatment of infested kennels and buildings may be necessary.

Ehrlichia chaffeensis

E. chaffeensis, a cause of monocytic ehrlichiosis in dogs and people, is a reportable human disease in the United States. Experimental and natural infection has been documented in dogs. The organism is transmitted by *Dermacentor variabilis* and *Amblyomma americanum*. Accordingly the disease is primarily found in the southeast and south-central areas of the United States. In people, disease has been reported in Missouri, Oklahoma, Tennessee, Arkansas, and Maryland. *E. chaffeensis* infection in dogs appears to be more common than *E. canis* infection in endemic areas. Clinical findings in dogs are not well documented. In one study, experimentally induced disease in dogs was subclinical. In naturally infected dogs, clinical findings were similar to those caused by *E. canis*, including lymphadenomegaly, gastrointestinal signs,

Important points regarding *E. canis* infection in dogs

- *E. canis* causes monocytic ehrlichiosis in dogs.
- Acute, subclinical, and chronic phases occur experimentally but are difficult to differentiate clinically.
- Clinical findings include anorexia, weight loss, splenomegaly, lymphadenomegaly, hemorrhagic diatheses, uveitis, and neurologic abnormalities.
- Laboratory abnormalities can include anemia, leukopenia, thrombocytopenia, hyperglobulinemia, and protein-losing nephropathy. Hyperglobulinemia can consist of a polyclonal or monoclonal gammopathy.
- Monoclonal gammopathy, granulocytic lymphocytosis, and infiltration of bone marrow with plasma cells can occur and must be differentiated from neoplasia.
- Dogs may be seronegative during the acute phase of illness, and treatment must be instituted based on a high index of clinical suspicion.
- Titers may persist for long periods after illness and infection is resolved.
- Doxycycline, 5 mg/kg orally every 12 hours for 28 days, is the recommended treatment.
- Resolution of clinical signs occurs in response to therapy. Platelet counts can normalize within 14 days; resolution of hyperglobulinemia may take 6 to 9 months.
- Coinfection with *Babesia* and *Bartonella* spp. should be considered in dogs that fail to respond rapidly.
- Antibody to *E. canis* can be detected after resolution of clinical signs.
- Resolution of clinical and laboratory abnormalities and PCR testing can be used to support therapeutic elimination of infection.
- Reinfection can occur, and preventative measures should be instituted in conjunction with the initiation of doxycycline treatment.

anterior uveitis, epistaxis, thrombocytopenia, anemia, increased total protein, and hypoalbuminemia. However, the presence of coinfection has complicated interpretation of studies of natural disease in *E. chaffeensis*–infected dogs.

The principles of diagnosis are similar to those described for *E. canis*. Whether monocytic inclusions are visible in infected dogs has not been studied. Serology can be used to document exposure to *E. chaffeensis*. Similar to *E. canis*, titers may be negative acutely and may persist following treatment. Serologic cross-reactivity between *E. chaffeensis* and *E. canis* makes distinguishing infection based on serological testing currently impossible. PCR of the blood and other samples from infected dogs can be used to document active infection and may be used to determine the species of infecting *Ehrlichia*.

Doxycycline therapy, as described for *E. canis*, is recommended for *E. chaffeensis* infection in dogs. Few studies regarding treatment of natural infection in dogs exist. However, in one study *E. chaffeensis* DNA could be detected

in the blood for months after treatment with doxycycline. It is not clear whether reexposure or persistent infection was the cause of repeated DNA detection, but failure to interrupt frequent reexposure to infected *A. americanum* ticks was considered likely. The use of chloramphenicol or fluoroquinolones for the treatment of *E. chaffeensis* in dogs has not been investigated, but studies suggest these drugs are not as effective as doxycycline in inhibiting growth in vitro, and enrofloxacin is ineffective in treating experimentally induced *E. canis* infection in dogs. The use of imidocarb has not been investigated. Notably, doxycycline is the treatment of choice for people with HME caused by *E. chaffeensis*.

The zoonotic implications of *E. chaffeensis* infection in dogs await further study, but because infection in humans has been well documented, precautions against human exposure to ticks and infected blood should be followed as described for *R. rickettsii*.

Granulocytic Ehrlichiosis (*E. ewingii* Infection)

E. ewingii infects granulocytes, including neutrophils, eosinophils, and more rarely monocytes. The distribution of the disease is primarily in the central, southern, and southeastern United States and follows the distribution of its vector, *A. americanum*. Similar to *E. canis* and *E. chaffeensis*, *E. ewingii* can induce chronic, nonclinical infection in dogs.

Fever and lameness are the most common clinical signs in dogs naturally infected with *E. ewingii*. Neurologic signs such as ataxia, paresis, proprioceptive deficits, anisocoria, intention tremors, and head tilt may also be seen. Neutrophilic polyarthritis is characteristic of *E. ewingii* infection that may differentiate it from *E. canis* infection. Like infection with *E. canis*, thrombocytopenia is the most common clinicopathologic abnormality. Anemia, leukocytosis or leukopenia, and hyperglobulinemia may also occur.

E. ewingii has not been grown in cell culture, so a specific indirect fluorescent antibody (IFA) that tests for exposure is not available. Cross-reactivity between *E. ewingii* and *E. canis* antigens by IFA may infrequently occur, but coinfection with *E. ewingii* and *E. canis* is more likely in dogs with *E. canis* antibodies. Granulocytic morulae may be identified in neutrophils. PCR is useful to confirm and speciate the infecting organism; however, it should be kept in mind that false-negative results can occur. Therefore clinical signs consistent with granulocytic ehrlichiosis without demonstration of infection cytologically, serologically, or by PCR should not rule out the presence of infection. Of note, therapeutic administration of corticosteroids or immunosuppressive drugs for other diseases has resulted in visualization of morulae or the development of thrombocytopenia in dogs chronically infected with *E. ewingii*.

Treatment with doxycycline as outlined for *E. canis* is recommended. Preventative measures are as outlined for *R. rickettsii*.

In people, disease caused by *E. ewingii* is reportable. Infection has been identified primarily in immunocompromised individuals. Precautions to prevent human infection should be followed as outlined for *R. rickettsii*.

Granulocytic Anaplasmosis (*A. phagocytophilum* Infection)

Anaplasma phagocytophilum

A. phagocytophilum (formerly *E. equi*) causes canine granulocytic anaplasmosis (CGA). Infection also occurs in cats, ruminants, horses, and humans. The tick vector of *A. phagocytophilum* in the United States is *I. scapularis* in the Northeast and upper Midwest and *Ixodes pacificus* on the west coast. The distribution of disease follows the distribution of the tick vector. Similarly, coinfecting agents are those known to infect *Ixodes* ticks, such as *B. burgdorferi. A. phagocytophilum* also occurs in Europe. In the United States, human infection with *A. phagocytophilum* is reportable.

A. phagocytophilum appears to be predominantly an acute disease, although persistent infection has been documented experimentally. The clinical findings are similar to *E. ewingii* and include fever, lameness, joint swelling, and CNS signs, in addition to the less specific findings of anorexia, lethargy, and splenomegaly. Thrombocytopenia, nonregenerative anemia or immune-mediated hemolytic anemia, mild hypoalbuminemia, proteinuria, neutropenia, neutrophilic polyarthritis, and neutrophilic pleocytosis have been documented in association with infection.

The findings of thrombocytopenia and neutrophilic polyarthritis in an *I. scapularis* or *I. pacificus* endemic area should raise clinical suspicion of infection with *A. phagocytophilum*. Granulocytic morulae can be identified in peripheral blood smears, joint fluid, and cerebrospinal fluid in some patients. Seroconversion can be used to document acute infection. Because of frequent exposure to *I. scapularis* or *I. pacificus*, dogs in endemic regions have a high seroprevalence (up to 50%) to *A. phagocytophilum*. Therefore single detection of antibodies can only be used to support exposure, not active infection. Notably, there is little cross-reactivity with *E. canis*; thus appropriate serologic tests must be requested to document infection with *Ehrlichia* spp. versus *Anaplasma* spp. Antibodies to *A. phagocytophilum* are cross-reactive with *A. platys*. PCR is a valuable tool for the diagnosis of *A. phagocytophilum* infection in dogs. PCR may be positive prior to seroconversion and is also useful in verifying active infection in seropositive patients. However, a negative PCR does not rule out infection, and multiple diagnostic modalities may be necessary to diagnose active infection.

Treatment with doxycycline as outlined for *E. canis* is recommended (Box 18-3). Response to doxycycline treatment is rapid in most dogs. A delayed response to doxycycline should suggest the possibility of concurrent infection. There are no reports of the use of chloramphenicol to treat the infection in dogs; however, in vitro studies suggest it may be less effective than doxycycline in inhibiting its growth. Reports on in vitro susceptibility to fluoroquinolones are variable, and studies suggest they are ineffective for the treatment of HGE. Recently rifampin was shown to be an acceptable treatment for human granulocytic anaplasmosis (HGA) in children. Its efficacy and safety for treatment of CGA is not known.

BOX 18-3   **Important points regarding canine granulocytic ehrlichiosis and granulocytic anaplasmosis in dogs**

- *A. phagocytophilum* is transmitted by *I. scapularis* and *I. pacificus* ticks; therefore infection is prevalent in the Northeast, upper Midwest, and in Washington and California.
- *E. ewingii* is transmitted by *A. americanum*; therefore infection is prevalent in the central, southern, and southeastern United States.
- Fever, polyarthritis, and thrombocytopenia are the most common clinical signs.
- Polyarthritis and granulocyte inclusions distinguish *E. ewingii* and *A. phagocytophilum* infection from *E. canis*.
- A rapid, favorable response to doxycycline therapy should be anticipated, but chronic infection may occur.

Measures to prevent reinfection through the use of acaricides are outlined under *R. rickettsii*.

A. phagocytophilum causes HGE in people. Dogs may increase human exposure to tick vectors. The potential for direct transmission from dogs to humans is unknown. Precautions in handling ticks, preventing exposure, and in handling specimens are as outlined for *R. rickettsii*.

Anaplasma platys, Neorickettsial, and *Coxiella* infections

Anaplasma Platys (Formerly *Ehrlichia platys*) in Dogs

The vector for *A. platys* infection has not been proven, but *R. sanguineus* is the suspected tick vector. Infection with *A. platys* in dogs results in primarily subclinical disease, with cyclical thrombocytopenia being the predominant clinical sign. It appears to have a worldwide distribution. More severe disease manifestations including fever, petechia, nasal discharge, lymphadenomegaly, and uveitis may occur with more pathogenic strains outside the United States. Experimentally, coinfection with *A. platys* and *E. canis* causes more severe thrombocytopenia than infection with either agent alone.

Serologic cross-reactivity between *Anaplasma* and *Ehrlichia* spp. does not occur. However, serologic cross-reactivity with *A. phagocytophilum* is likely. Experimentally infected dogs were PCR positive for *A. platys* for 4 to 14 days after infection. Coinfection with many different tick-borne agents has been described, with up to 50% of dogs with *E. canis* infection having antibodies to *A. platys*.

Doxycycline appears to be an effective therapy.

Neorickettsia risticii var. *atypicalis* Infection

There is some evidence that *N. risticii* may cause disease in dogs and possibly in cats. Infection appears to be rare and is described elsewhere.

Neorickettsia helminthoeca in Dogs

N. helminthoeca has a complex life cycle involving the trematode *Nanophyetus salmincola*. This organism infects snails, fish, and birds or mammals during its life cycle. The snail intermediate host is *Oxytrema silicula*. This host and thus the disease were thought to be restricted to the Pacific Northwest of the United States and Canada. However, recently infection has been documented in dogs in Brazil. Dogs develop infection by ingesting raw salmonid and a few types of nonsalmonid fish, including trout. Consumption of salamanders can also transmit infection. *N. helminthoeca* infects histiocytic cells and appears to have a tropism for enterocytes. Therefore acute gastrointestinal signs in the presence of fever in an endemic area should raise clinical suspicion of the disease. Lymphadomegaly, nasal and ocular discharge also occur. Laboratory findings may include thrombocytopenia, lymphopenia and eosinophilia, hypoalbuminemia, and elevated alkaline phosphatase. Organisms are frequently visible on fine-needle aspiration of lymph nodes. Trematode eggs can sometimes be identified in the feces. The disease is rapidly progressive and can be fatal, but response to appropriate treatment is also rapid and favorable. Tetracyclines (oxytetracycline, doxycycline, tetracycline) are considered the treatment of choice. Chloramphenicol, sulfonamides, and penicillin are also reported to be effective, although it has been suggested resistance to these antibiotics may be a concern due to in vitro susceptibility studies of other *Neorickettsia*. There are no reports of use of penicillin in naturally infected dogs. Aggressive supportive therapy is also required. Treating trematode infection with praziquantel is also necessary. Infection has not been reported in pregnant dogs or puppies and so treatment recommendations have not been established. However, penicillin or sulfonamides could be initially considered over more teratogenic antibiotics in these patients. See "Considerations for Treating Rickettsioses, Ehrlichioses and Anaplasmoses in the Pediatric Patient" and "Therapy During Pregnancy" for further discussion.

Coxiella burnetii

C. burnetii is an intracellular organism with two life stages. An intracellular form in mammals lives in macrophages and is resistant to destruction. There is also a small extracellular stage, which is highly stable and can persist in the environment. This form of the organism is highly resistant to temperature, desiccation, light, and many chemicals. *C. burnetii* is found worldwide, except for New Zealand. It can be transmitted to vertebrate hosts through tick bites or through inhalation or ingestion. Importantly, *C. burnetii* is a reportable and zoonotic disease, and is a potential agent of bioterrorism according to the CDC. In animals, the organism concentrates in the placenta, and most transmission to people occurs from exposure during parturition. Urine, milk, and feces also contain the organism. Livestock are the most important sources of infection in people.

C. burnetii has been detected in the vagina and in biopsies of the uterus of healthy cats, and infection in people after exposure to whelping cats and dogs has been described. Despite these reports, a recent study demonstrated that pet ownership was not associated with increased risk of antibody production in people.

Clinical signs in people include fever, malaise, myalgia, gastrointestinal signs, and respiratory signs. Chronic disease develops in 1% to 5% of people and can include chronic fatigue syndromes and severe complications that may develop many years after the initial episode. These include endocarditis, fever, hepatitis, dyspnea, thrombocytopenia, and thromboembolism. Pregnant women infected with *C. burnetii* experience a high rate of complications, including abortion, retarded fetal growth, fetal death, and premature birth.

Disease is usually subclinical in dog and cats. Splenomegaly may be the only clinical sign. Abortion or neonatal death can occur in periparturient animals. In one report, lesions in an affected kitten included granulomatous myocarditis, hepatitis, nephritis, and pneumonia. Thus granulomatous lesions in aborted kittens may indicate infection. Serology, isolation, and PCR have been used to document exposure and infection in dogs and cats.

Treatment of *C. burnetii* infection in people includes tetracyclines, fluoroquinolones, and chloramphenicol. In chronic infection combinations of antibiotics for long periods of time are used. A recent long-term study showed that co-trimoxazole helped reduce the severe complications associated with infection in pregnant women. Studies investigating efficacy of treatment in cats and dogs have not been reported. A mask and gloves should be worn by people exposed to dogs and cats during parturition to help prevent exposure.

Tickborne Rickettsial, Ehrlichial, and Anaplasma Infection in Cats

Very little is known regarding rickettsial, ehrlichial, and *Anaplasma* infections in cats. It has been hypothesized that disease is less frequently identified in cats because they may be resistant to tickborne rickettsial, ehrlichial, and *Anaplasma* infections or remove vectors before transmission as a result of their fastidious nature. Although antibodies to *Rickettsia* have been documented in cats, clinical disease has not. It should be noted that *Ctenocephalides felis* (the cat flea) is a vector for *R. typhi* and *R felis*, two zoonotic pathogens. Conscientious flea control is important to help prevent these rickettsial infections in people.

Serosurveys also suggest that cats are exposed to *Ehrlichia* species. DNA from an *E. canis*–like agent has been amplified from the blood of three cats with disease resembling chronic *E. canis* infection in dogs. Clinical signs of *E. canis*–like infections in cats may include fever, lethargy, and polyarthritis. Interestingly, an epidemiologic association between polyarthritis and antibody to *E. canis* has also been documented in cats. Clinicopathologic abnormalities may include anemia, thrombocytopenia, pancytopenia, hyperglobulinemia, plasma cell infiltration of lymph nodes, bone marrow hypoplasia and dysplasia, and antinuclear antibodies. Serosurveys have documented that cats have been exposed to *A. phagocytophilum*, particularly in endemic areas. In addition, although experimental infection appears subclinical, naturally occurring *A. phagocytophilum* infection has been documented in cats with anorexia, fever, weakness, lethargy, hyperesthesia, muscle and joint pain, lameness, lymphadenomegaly, hyperglobulinemia, and weight loss. For some cats, neutrophilic inclusions are visible during acute infection. Based on these studies, it has been suggested that cats with immune-mediated disease should be tested for ehrlichiosis and anaplasmosis. Interestingly, most cats with ehrlichiosis and anaplasmoses are young adults, and frequently these cats have a history of being feral or rescued. Cats with naturally occurring ehrlichiosis and anaplasmoses appear to respond to doxycycline therapy. The risk of esophageal stricture must be kept in mind with doxycycline therapy in cats. Oral doses should be followed by administration of water.

Considerations for Treating Rickettsioses, Ehrlichioses, and Anaplasmoses in the Pediatric Patient

Few case reports specifically describing tickborne rickettsial, ehrlichial, and *Anaplasma* infections in pediatric canine and feline patients have been published. However, coinfections of *E. canis* with other agents have been described in a 6-week-old and a 5-month-old dog. Disease would be expected in any young animal with clinical signs and potential exposure to vectors. In addition, the risk of perinatal transmission exists and is described below.

Doxycycline is the treatment of choice in adult dogs and people with RMSF, ehrlichioses, and anaplasmoses. Although effective for elimination of infection with *R. rickettsii*, fluoroquinolones should not be used in growing dogs because of the potential for inducing cartilage abnormalities. Although imidocarb has been used to treat canine ehrlichioses, the treatment efficacy has recently been questioned. In addition, the safety of imidocarb in puppies has not been determined. Chloramphenicol has been suggested as an alternative drug for the treatment of tickborne rickettsioses, ehrlichioses, and anaplasmoses in pediatric patients because of the risk of dental discoloration associated with doxycycline. However, in vitro evidence suggests that doxycycline is more effective than chloramphenicol in inhibiting the growth of *E. chaffeensis*, *A. phagocytophilum*, and *E. canis*. In addition, reports of people infected with RMSF and HME suggest superior efficacy of doxycycline compared with chloramphenicol. Importantly, infection with these three agents cannot be differentiated early in the course of disease, when empirical treatment is required. In addition, coinfection is possible. Therefore doxycycline has the advantage of being effective against many tickborne agents that cause similar clinical signs.

The use of doxycycline as first-line therapy in children with RMSF, HGA, HGE, or HME is no longer controversial. It has been established that unlike other tetracycline antibiotics, there is very minimal risk of dental discoloration with short-term doxycycline therapy in pediatric patients. In addition, there is a serious risk of chloramphenicol-induced myelosuppression in people exposed to the drug. Therefore because of its superior efficacy and minimal side effects, doxycycline is considered the treatment of choice in human patients **of any age** with RMSF, HME, HGE, or HGA.

Controlled studies comparing the efficacy of doxycycline with chloramphenicol for the treatment of ehrlichioses and anaplasmoses in naturally infected dogs have not been performed. It is likely doxycycline has superior efficacy in infected dogs, as has been documented in vitro and in people. Importantly, there are no published reports of doxycycline-associated dental discoloration in dogs, and this has not been observed by the authors in a limited number of treated dogs. Although the risk of chloramphenicol-associated myelosuppression is less in dogs than for people, this serious side effect and the risk of exposing human companions to the drug must be considered.

The risk of dental discoloration associated with the use of tetracycline antibiotics in increased with prolonged or repeated use. In people, the optimal duration of doxycycline therapy for infection with *R. rickettsii*, *E. chaffeensis*, *E. ewingii*, and *A. phagocytophilum* has not been established. However, it is important to note that the recommended therapy in people is shorter than for dogs. Current recommendations for human RMSF and for HME are to treat at least 3 days after the fever subsides and until evidence of clinical improvement is noted. This typically results in a minimum total course of 5 to 7 days. Severe or complicated disease may be treated longer. Recommendations for treating human patients with HGA are slightly longer (10 to 14 days) in case coinfection with *B. burgdorferi* disease is present.

The recommended duration of therapy for uncomplicated RMSF in canine patients is short (7 to 14 days). Therefore it is reasonable to consider doxycycline the treatment of choice in pediatric canine patients with RMSF. However, the recommended duration of doxycycline therapy for canine ehrlichiosis and anaplasmoses is currently 28 days. Whether prolonged treatment would increase the risk of dental discoloration in these patients has not been established. In general, canine infection with *A. phagocytophilum* and *E. ewingii* appears to be milder and of shorter duration than that associated with *E. canis* and *E. chaffeensis*. Reports in the literature suggest infection may be cleared in some patients after a 2-week course of therapy. Therefore treating for 14 rather than 28 days with appropriate monitoring for resolution of infection may be considered in pediatric patients when cosmetics are of great concern. Overall the risks and benefits of doxycycline versus chloramphenicol therapy must be determined on an individual patient basis and discussed with owners.

Therapy during Pregnancy

During pregnancy, doxycycline has been associated with the teratogenic effects of bone deformity and dental discoloration. In addition, hepatotoxicity and pancreatitis may occur in the mother. Although also associated with significant teratogenic risk, chloramphenicol is considered the treatment of choice for pregnant women with RMSF and should be considered the treatment of choicc for pregnant dogs with this disease as well. Short-term doxycycline therapy has been used to successfully treat *A. phagocytophilum* and *E. chaffeensis* in pregnant women without complication to the fetus. Given the variable in vitro efficacy of chloramphenicol against these agents, the use of doxycycline could be considered instead of chloramphenicol in severely life-threatening or nonresponsive infections during pregnancy, but that choice must be heavily weighed against the risk of severe bone deformity and other serious complications in the fetus and bitch associated with the use of doxycycline. Interestingly, rifampin has in vitro activity against *A. phagocytophilum* and *E. chaffeensis* and has been used to successfully treat pregnant women with HGA. The efficacy of rifampin for treating ehrlichioses and anaplasmoses in canine patients is unknown.

Perinatal Transmission

There is one report of perinatal transmission of *A. phagocytophilum* in people. Clinical signs resolved rapidly in the neonate with doxycycline therapy. There are no reports of perinatal transmission of rickettsioses, anaplasmoses, or ehrlichioses in dogs. In fact, our laboratory could not find evidence of perinatal transmission of *A. phagocytophilum* using serial evaluation of physical parameters, PCR, blood smears, and serologic testing in puppies born to a bitch acutely infected with *A. phagocytophilum* shortly before whelping. However, the potential for transplacental and transmammary transmission of these agents exists, and close monitoring of puppies born to infected bitches is required. They should be evaluated frequently (twice daily) for fever and other clinical signs of disease. In some cases it may be prudent to monitor for evidence of infection using PCR. Maternal antibodies may theoretically interfere with serologic testing, so caution must be used in interpretation of serologic data. In the case of anaplasmoses and ehrlichioses, blood smears may be monitored for the presence of inclusion bodies.

Supportive Care in the Pediatric Patient

Neonatal animals have unique nutritional and thermoregulatory needs that should be considered. Critical care is considered in Chapter 10.

Prevention in the Pediatric Patient

Prevention of tickborne rickettsial, ehrlichial, and anaplasma infection requires controlling exposure to the tick vector. However, caution should be exercised when applying acaricides and tick repellents to very young animals. Consult manufacturers' recommended guidelines with regard to their use in young animals. Avoiding tick habitat and twice-daily tick removal with appropriate precautions to protect humans from exposure to infected hemolymph and salivary secretions are also recommended.

CONCLUSION

Rickettsioses, ehrlichioses, anaplasmoses, and *Neorickettsia* and *Coxiella* infections are important causes of disease in companion animals and people. Diagnostic testing should be tailored to the geographic locale relevant to the patient's exposure or travel history. Empirical trcatment must begin before confirmation of infection with laboratory testing. Doxycycline is the treatment of choice in most adult and pediatric patients with tickborne rickettsial, ehrlichial, and *Anaplasma* infection. Zoonotic implications of infection must be considered, and veterinarians should implement preventative measures in endemic areas.

SUGGESTED READINGS

Breitschwerdt EB: *Rocky Mountain spotted fever*. In Ettinger SJ, Feldman EC (eds): *Textbook of veterinary internal medicine*, ed 6, St Louis, 2006, Saunders/Elsevier, pp 631-632.

Chapman AS et al: Diagnosis and management of tickborne rickettsial diseases: Rocky Mountain spotted fever, ehrlichioses, and anaplasmosis, *MMWR* 55(RR04):1-27, 2006.

Gorham JR, Forey WJ: Salmon poisoning disease. In Green CE: *Infectious diseases of the dog and cat*, ed 3, St Louis, 2006, Saunders/Elsevier, pp 198-201.

Neer TM et al: Consensus statement on ehrlichial disease of small animals from the Infectious Disease Study Group of the American College of Veterinary Internal Medicine, *J Vet Intern Med* 16:309, 2002.

Neer TM et al: Ehrlichiosis, neorickettsiosis, anaplasmosis, and *Wolbachia* infection. In Greene CE (ed): *Infectious diseases of the dog and cat*, ed 3, St Louis, 2006, Saunders/Elsevier, pp 203-232.

Tissot Dupont H, Raoult D: Q Fever, *Infect Dis Clin North Am* 22:505-514, 2008.

PARASITIC AND PROTOZOAL DISEASES

CHAPTER 19

Craig Datz

Young animals are commonly at risk of a variety of parasitic infections, and morbidity and mortality rates are typically higher than in adults. Resistance to parasitic infection is weak in pediatric patients, as the immune system is not fully developed and the relative parasite burden is high. Successful management depends on a working knowledge of parasites and their life cycles, diagnostic techniques, appropriate therapeutics, and preventative strategies. The information in this chapter is intended as a brief overview of parasitic diseases encountered in puppies and kittens. It is not intended as a comprehensive list of all possible parasites. The list of Suggested Readings at the end of the chapter is a guide to more complete discussions. General guidelines concerning parasite control in dogs and cats are summarized in Box 19-1.

GASTROINTESTINAL PARASITES

Helminths

Roundworms (Ascarids): *Toxocara canis*, *Toxocara cati*, *Toxascaris leonina*

Roundworms are relatively large nematodes (3 to 18 cm long) found in the small intestine. *Toxocara canis* affects virtually all puppies because of prenatal infection. Many kittens are infected with *Toxocara cati* soon after birth by transmammary transmission. *Toxascaris leonina* affects both dogs and cats but is less common.

Pregnant bitches have arrested (dormant) *T. canis* larvae in somatic tissues that become activated after day 42 of gestation. These larvae migrate to the uterus and infect developing fetuses. Postnatal infection may occur as a small amount of larvae are excreted in the milk. Older puppies acquire *T. canis* after ingestion of embryonated eggs, and larvae may undergo hepatotracheal migration before being coughed up and swallowed, leading to maturation in the small intestine. Pregnant queens also have arrested *T. cati*

that migrate during gestation to mammary glands. Neonates commonly acquire larvae by this route, whereas older kittens are infected by ingestion of larvae or paratenic hosts such as rodents. *T. leonina* larvae are acquired by ingestion of embryonated ova or paratenic hosts.

Mild infections may be asymptomatic, whereas moderate numbers of worms cause vomiting, diarrhea, lethargy, and an unthrifty appearance. A rounded, fluid-filled abdomen ("pot belly") is common with heavier worm burdens. Severe complications including intestinal obstruction, intussusception, and death are possible. Larvae migrating through the liver, lungs, and other organs occasionally result in tissue damage.

Roundworm ova are easily identified on routine fecal flotation. Adult worms may be passed in the feces or found in vomitus.

A number of effective anthelmintics are available (Table 19-1). Deworming is ideally started at 2 weeks of age and repeated every 2 weeks for four treatments. Following this, certain heartworm preventatives will control roundworms if continued year-round (see Table 19-1). Prenatal infection with *T. canis* can be prevented in puppies by daily administration of fenbendazole to pregnant bitches starting at day 40 of gestation and continuing through day 14 postpartum. Selamectin also prevents prenatal transmission in puppies if given at days −40, −10, +10, and +40 before and after whelping. Similar studies have not been reported in cats. Roundworm ova persist in the environment for months and possibly years. Removal and proper disposal of feces at least twice a week will decrease the risk of soil contamination.

T. canis and, to a lesser extent, *T. cati* cause visceral larval migrans and ocular larval migrans in humans. Accidental ingestion of soil contaminated with embryonated ova is considered to be the main source of infection, but roundworm ova have also been found in hair samples clipped from the perianal areas of dogs. Households with children or immunosuppressed individuals should be informed of the risk of toxocariasis.

BOX 19-1 **New 2008 CAPC general guidelines for controlling internal and external parasites in U.S. dogs and cats***

Parasite Control Should Be Guided by Veterinarians

- Prescribe control programs to local parasite prevalence and individual pet lifestyle factors.
- Adapt prevention recommendations to address emerging parasite threats.
- Conduct physical examinations at least every 6 to 12 months or as deemed advisable by veterinarian.
- Conduct annual heartworm testing in dogs; test cats before placing on preventatives and thereafter as indicated by history and physical findings.
- Conduct fecal examinations 2 or 4 times during the first year of life and 1 to 2 times per year in adults, depending on patient health and lifestyle factors.

Every Pet, All Year Long

- Administer year-round broad-spectrum parasite control with efficacy against heartworm, intestinal parasites with zoonotic potential, fleas, and ticks.
- Administer anthelmintic treatment to puppies and kittens starting at 2 weeks of age repeating every 2 weeks until regular broad spectrum parasite control begins.

- Maintain pregnant and nursing dams on broad-spectrum control products.

Healthy Lifestyle, Healthy Pets, Healthy People

- Feed pets cooked or prepared food (not raw diets) and provide fresh, potable water.
- Cover sandboxes when not in use and protect garden areas from fecal contamination.
- Pick up feces immediately whenever walking a dog in a public area; remove feces from the backyard environment at least weekly, preferably daily.
- Keep dogs and cats under control; do not allow roaming.
- Practice good personal hygiene when handling animal waste, particularly important for children and other individuals at increased risk.

If Less Than Optimal Control Is Practiced

- Deworm puppies and kittens starting at 2 weeks, repeating every 2 weeks until 2 months of age, and then monthly until the pet is 6 months old.
- Conduct fecal examinations 2 to 4 times a year in adult pets, depending on patient health and lifestyle factors, and treat with appropriate parasiticides.

*From CAPC website: http://capcvet.org/recommendations/guidelines.html. (Accessed 12-8-09.)

TABLE 19-1 **Common drugs used to treat canine and feline parasites**

	Rounds	Hooks	Whips	Tapes	*Giardia*	Heartworms
Pyrantel	X	X				
Fenbendazole	X	X	X	X*	X	
Febantel	X	X	X	X	X	
Emodepside	X†	X†				
Praziquantel				X		
Epsiprantel				X		
Milbemycin	X	X	X			X
Selamectin	X†	X†				X
Moxidectin	X	X	X			X

*Taenia only.
†Cats only.

Hookworms: *Ancylostoma caninum, Ancylostoma tubaeforme, Ancylostoma braziliense, Uncinaria stenocephala*

Hookworms are small bloodsucking nematodes (5 to 15 mm long) that attach to the mucosa of the small intestine. Perinatal infections are common in puppies, whereas kittens generally acquire infections after several weeks of age. *Ancylostoma caninum* is found in dogs, *Ancylostoma tubaeforme* in cats, and both dogs and cats can be infected with *Ancylostoma braziliense* and *Uncinaria stenocephala*.

Both dogs and cats acquire hookworms through larval ingestion and skin penetration. Rodents may contain larvae in tissues and serve as paratenic hosts for cats. As with roundworms, an arrested larval stage in somatic tissues is activated during pregnancy in bitches. *A. caninum* larvae migrate to mammary glands and infect puppies through nursing.

Asymptomatic cases are possible, but diarrhea and weight loss are common with mild to moderate infections. Puppies and kittens with heavy worm burdens become anemic and may die peracutely. Hemorrhagic diarrhea caused by hookworms may resemble other causes of enteritis such as parvovirus. Dermatitis is occasionally reported as a result of larval skin penetration.

Adult hookworms are rarely excreted, so diagnosis depends on identifying ova by fecal flotation.

Many anthelmintics treat both hookworms and roundworms (see Table 19-1). An appropriate schedule for puppies and kittens is every 2 weeks starting at 2 weeks of age for four treatments. Monthly deworming may be continued using heartworm preventatives. Perinatal infection in puppies can be avoided using daily fenbendazole in pregnant bitches from day 40 of gestation through day 14 postpartum.

Humans can acquire larvae through skin penetration, leading to cutaneous larval migrans. *A. braziliense* is the most common hookworm recovered from humans, although *A. caninum* is occasionally reported.

Whipworms: *Trichuris vulpis*

Whipworms are nematodes found in older puppies and adult dogs rather than in neonates. The usual length is 4 to 7 cm, and they are found in the large intestine, where they attach and absorb blood. In the United States, cats are unaffected by *Trichuris vulpis*. Feline whipworms *(Trichuris felis)* have been reported in Australia and Central and South America.

Dogs are infected by ingestion of ova from contaminated environments. Perinatal transmission does not occur. Development of whipworms takes place in the intestines without tissue migration or arrested larval stages. The prepatent period is approximately 3 months, so puppies less than 8 to 12 weeks of age are generally not at risk.

Weight loss and diarrhea of large intestinal origin (i.e., mucus, hematochezia) are the most common signs associated with moderate to heavy worm burdens. Dogs may remain asymptomatic.

Whipworm ova are relatively heavy, and careful fecal flotation techniques with appropriate solutions are necessary for recovery and identification.

Several anthelmintics are effective against whipworms (see Table 19-1). Fenbendazole and febantel are commonly used, although monthly heartworm preventatives containing milbemycin and moxidectin can be used for treatment and control of recurrent infections.

Sporadic cases of human infection with *T. vulpis* have been reported, but in general whipworms are not considered zoonotic.

Tapeworms: *Dipylidium caninum, Taenia pisiformis, Taenia taeniaeformis*

The common tapeworms found in puppies and kittens are large cestodes (15 to 60 cm long) that are anchored to the mucosa of the small intestine. The terminal segments (proglottids) containing eggs or egg packets are able to crawl out of the anus onto the haircoat or are excreted along with feces.

Tapeworms are acquired through ingestion of intermediate (paratenic) hosts rather than by direct fecal-oral exposure. The larval stage of *Dipylidium caninum* (cysticercoid) is found in fleas, and dogs and cats become infected after swallowing infected fleas. A mature worm develops approximately 2 to 4 weeks later. *Taenia* spp. larvae occur in rodents and rabbits. Cats are more likely to acquire *Taenia* as a result of hunting behavior, and adult worm development takes 1 to 3 months.

Other than anal pruritus associated with shedding of proglottids, tapeworms are considered to be harmless parasites. There is one report of acute small intestinal obstruction in an adult cat from a mass of *T. taeniaeformis*.

Direct observation of tapeworm segments is possible. A close examination of the perianal region may reveal proglottids (resembling grains of rice) on the skin or haircoat. Segments are also seen in feces or in the environment. To identify the type of tapeworm, a proglottid is placed in a drop of saline or tap water on a glass slide and squashed or teased apart to release eggs. *D. caninum* occurs in egg packets, whereas *Taenia* ova are spherical and contain six-hooked larvae. Fecal flotation rarely reveals tapeworm ova.

Praziquantel and epsiprantel are effective one-time treatments for tapeworms. Fenbendazole treats *Taenia* but not *Dipylidium* (see Table 19-1). To prevent recurrence, flea control and avoidance of hunting are necessary.

Humans may become infected with *D. caninum* if fleas are accidentally ingested. *Taenia* tapeworms have occasionally been found in humans.

Strongyloides stercoralis, Strongyloides felis, Strongyloides tumefaciens

These worms are uncommon in puppies and kittens but occasionally cause mild to severe clinical signs, including gastroenteritis and pneumonia. Infection occurs through skin penetration or by ingestion of colostrum or milk (transmammary). The worms are small (1 to 5 mm long) and after tissue migration penetrate the mucosa of the small intestine. Eggs often hatch while still in the intestines, so diagnosis relies on identifying larvated ova in fecal flotation or actual larvae in fecal samples (culture or Baermann technique). Treatment options include fenbendazole and ivermectin. There is a slight zoonotic potential, especially in immunosuppressed individuals.

Physaloptera rara, Physaloptera felidis, Physaloptera praeputialis

Several species have been identified in dogs and cats. The worms are 1 to 6 cm long and are attached to the mucosal lining of the stomach. Infected animals may be asymptomatic or have intermittent vomiting. Anemia resulting from blood loss has also been reported. These parasites are acquired by ingestion of paratenic hosts such as beetles and crickets. Ova are rarely found in routine fecal flotation, and definitive diagnosis often involves visualization of the worms during endoscopic examination. Pyrantel, fenbendazole, and ivermectin have been reported to be effective treatments. Humans are rarely infected by ingestion of paratenic hosts but not directly from animals.

Spirocerca lupi

This parasite occasionally affects puppies under 1 year of age but is mainly found in middle-aged dogs. It is very rare in cats. The worms are 3 to 8 cm long and are found in the esophagus, stomach, and arterial walls (including the aorta). Migrating larvae cause hemorrhage and inflammation leading to nodules, which occasionally cause stenosis and neoplastic transformation. Dogs acquire these worms by ingestion of paratenic hosts (e.g., beetles, reptiles, rodents). Clinical features include vomiting, dysphagia, aortic aneurysm, pulmonary osteoarthropathy of the long bones, and esophageal sarcomas. Larvated ova are occasionally found by fecal flotation, but diagnosis may require endoscopy or other imaging techniques. Successful treatment has been reported using either ivermectin or doramectin.

Stomach Worm (Cats): Ollulanus tricuspis

These nematodes are very small (1 mm long) and are located in the stomach wall, leading to gastritis and signs of vomiting, anorexia, and weight loss. Larvae are excreted in vomitus, which can be infective to other cats. Diagnosis is difficult because larvae are rarely identified in feces or vomitus because of digestion and destruction. Tetramisole is reported to be an effective treatment, but this drug is not available in the United States. Humans are not affected.

Protozoa
Coccidia: Isospora canis, Isospora felis

A wide variety of coccidia is found in animals, but *Isospora canis* and *Isospora felis* are considered host specific. Dogs and cats may accidentally ingest other coccidia such as *Eimeria* but do not become infected. The parasites are single-celled organisms with a worldwide distribution.

Puppies and kittens acquire coccidia through ingestion of sporulated oocysts from the environment or paratenic hosts such as rodents. In the intestine, sporozoites excyst and develop through several generations in the intestinal wall. Some migrate to mesenteric lymph nodes or other tissues and form cysts. The prepatent period is approximately 7 to 11 days.

Neonatal and very young animals are at the highest risk of disease associated with coccidial infection. The most common finding is diarrhea, which is usually mild and only rarely hemorrhagic. Vomiting, severe diarrhea, anorexia, depression, dehydration, and death occur in severely affected or stressed animals.

Routine fecal flotation or direct saline fecal smears usually reveal the characteristic oocysts. However, they may be missed in diarrheic samples because of dilution. The size and appearance of the various coccidia can help identify the species.

Medications are not indicated for every animal testing positive for coccidia. In many cases, managing underlying stressful conditions (e.g., crowding, transportation, malnutrition, and other parasites) will decrease or eliminate coccidia infection. The most commonly used drug in puppies and kittens is sulfadimethoxine. Supportive therapy may be nec-essary for those with severe disease. For resistant or recurrent cases, other unapproved drugs have been used, including nitrofurazone, amprolium, quinacrine, and ponazuril. Dietary therapy, such as low-residue, highly digestible diets with or without probiotics, may be successful.

There is no evidence of human infection with *Isospora*.

Giardia: Giardia duodenalis (Giardia intestinalis, Giardia lamblia)

Like coccidia, these single-celled protozoa have a worldwide distribution and generally exhibit host specificity. Two forms are recognizable: trophozoites, which are motile and flagellated, and cysts, which contain dormant trophozoites.

Transmission is by fecal-oral ingestion of cysts. In the stomach and small intestine, trophozoites excyst and attach to the mucosal lining. Eventually more cysts are formed and excreted along with feces. The prepatent period varies from 5 to 16 days.

Many affected puppies and kittens remain asymptomatic or have mild diarrhea. Acute diarrhea, often with mucus or pale soft stools, may be seen along with weight loss in more severe cases. Vomiting is not a common finding but may occur with heavy infections localized in the duodenum.

Giardia organisms are often missed on routine fecal examination. Repeating fecal tests daily for 3 days along with careful lab techniques will increase both sensitivity and accuracy. A direct saline fecal smear with a fresh sample (examined immediately after collection from the animal) may reveal motile trophozoites (tumbling or falling-leaf motion). Fecal flotation can recover cysts, which are small and tend to desiccate (shrink) if samples are not examined within 15 minutes of processing. Enzyme-linked immunosorbent assay (ELISA) tests can be performed both in-clinic and at reference labs, most of which have high sensitivity and specificity. Indirect fluorescent antibody (IFA) and polymerase chain reaction (PCR) testing may be available.

Metronidazole, fenbendazole, and febantel are commonly used, and a combination of medications may be necessary. If resistance is suspected, alternative drugs include quinacrine and furazolidone, but the risk of side effects is increased. A vaccine is available but has not shown consistent results for prevention or treatment. Bathing animals to remove cysts from the haircoat improves treatment efficacy.

Giardia is a common intestinal parasite in people around the world. Limited evidence links canine and feline isolates to human infection, but the usual cause is drinking contaminated water. Cysts may survive for weeks to months in moist environments. Careful cleanup and disposal of feces from dogs and cats will reduce the risk of contamination of households and surrounding areas.

Trichomonas: Tritrichomonas foetus, Pentatrichomonas hominis

These protozoa are pear-shaped, highly motile flagellated organisms. Kittens appear to be more susceptible than puppies to *Tritrichomonas foetus*, whereas *Pentatrichomonas hominis* was recently identified in dogs with diarrhea.

The trophozoite form of *T. foetus* is infective by the fecal-oral route (there is no cyst form, as with *Giardia*). The organism colonizes the large intestine of affected cats. Factors such as stress, crowding, and host susceptibility are involved in the pathogenesis of *T. foetus*.

Diarrhea ranging in severity from mild to liquid is the main sign of infection in cats and kittens. Blood and mucus may be present, and the diarrhea often waxes and wanes over time. Vomiting and weight loss are uncommon. Untreated cats continue to have diarrhea for months to years (median, 9 months).

A fresh saline fecal smear may reveal trophozoites. The motility of the organisms is rolling and jerky. Multiple specimens should be examined over several days to increase sensitivity. A more accurate test is a culture system available for cattle. PCR testing may be available at some labs.

There are currently no approved drugs for treatment of *T. foetus* in cats. Ronidazole, a drug marketed for *Trichomonas* infections in birds, is the most successful treatment to date. Antimicrobial drugs may help improve fecal consistency but rarely cure the infection.

There is no evidence of transmission to humans, but normal precautions should be taken when handling diarrheic feces.

Cryptosporidia: *Cryptosporidium canis, Cryptosporidium felis, Cryptosporidium parvum*

This coccidian parasite is found in many types of animals, and cross-infection is possible. Oocysts and trophozoites are found in affected puppies and kittens.

Transmission is by ingestion of sporulated oocysts. Sporozoites excyst in the intestines and develop into trophozoites in enterocytes. The prepatent period is as short as 3 to 5 days. *Cryptosporidium parvum* may be a primary pathogen but is more commonly a secondary opportunist when animals are in crowded, stressed, or unsanitary conditions.

Diarrhea may be self-limiting in mild cases, and some puppies and kittens remain asymptomatic. In immunosuppressed individuals, anorexia, weight loss, and chronic small-intestinal diarrhea may be observed.

Oocysts may be seen in direct saline fecal smears or fecal flotations, but they are much smaller than other coccidia and are easily missed. Care should be taken in handling suspect specimens because of the zoonotic potential. ELISA, IFA tests, and PCR are available at reference labs. Screening symptomatic puppies and kittens is recommended if more common parasites have been ruled out.

No drugs are approved or reliable for treatment. Paromomycin has been used, but side effects limit its use. Azithromycin has shown promise with fewer adverse reactions. Tylosin is another antibiotic with potential efficacy.

The risk to humans is high, although most infections can be traced to water contaminated with *C. parvum*. Cattle are a significant source. The oocysts are resistant to many disinfectants—concentrated ammonia and formalin solutions have been used. Boiling water may be used to disinfect bowls, toys, and other in-contact objects.

Toxoplasma gondii

Toxoplasmosis occasionally results in gastrointestinal disease in puppies and kittens, although other body systems are more commonly affected. Cats serve as the definitive host, and infection can occur through ingestion of oocysts, paratenic hosts (rodents), and congenital exposure. Mild, self-limiting diarrhea may occur, with shedding of oocysts in the feces. Serologic antibody tests are typically used for diagnosis. No drugs are approved for treatment, but clindamycin and sulfonamides (trimethoprim-sulfa) with or without pyrimethamine are commonly used. Humans are susceptible through ingestion of cysts in raw or undercooked meat or from contact with cats actively shedding oocysts.

Amebiasis: *Entamoeba histolytica*

This protozoal parasite mainly affects humans and primates, but dogs and cats may be susceptible. Transmission is usually from people to pets through cyst shedding in human feces. Clinical signs range from asymptomatic to severe colitis. Direct saline fecal smears may reveal trophozoites, but reference labs can be used for ELISA or special stains. Treatment has not been reported.

RESPIRATORY PARASITES

Helminths

Heartworms: *Dirofilaria immitis*

These large nematodes (15 to 30 cm long) affect dogs, cats, and several other mammals in many parts of the world. The geographic distribution continues to increase with changes in the vector (mosquito) and host populations. Although they are most commonly called "heartworms," the worms are actually located in pulmonary arteries leading to the lungs. When large numbers are present, they may be found in the right ventricle and right atrium of the heart or other blood vessels such as the caudal vena cava.

Mature female worms produce microfilariae, which circulate freely in the bloodstream. Female mosquitoes feeding on infected hosts become infected, and larval stages continue to develop. Mosquitoes then feed on another host and deposit the larvae onto the skin, where they migrate through connective tissues. Eventually the larvae gain access to the venous circulation where they are carried through the right heart to the pulmonary arteries. The migration stops, and the larvae mature into reproducing adults during the next 3 months. The infective period from the time of the mosquito bite to arrival in the lungs is approximately 70 to 90 days, and the prepatent period (time until microfilariae are produced) is typically 6 to 7 months.

Many dogs are asymptomatic, especially if the worm burden is low. Coughing, weight loss, and exercise intolerance may be seen. A more advanced stage of the disease, caval syndrome, includes signs of right heart failure and hemoglobinuria. Cats are more likely to show signs of coughing, vomiting, or respiratory distress, even with one or two adult worms. Fatalities resulting from cardiac or respiratory failure are sometimes observed in dogs, whereas cats may die suddenly as a result of pulmonary thromboembolism. Adult dogs and cats are more likely to be infected with heartworms, but puppies and kittens are susceptible and may show signs starting as early as 6 months of age in endemic areas.

Microfilariae may be directly visualized by microscopic examination of fresh blood (direct smear, filter concentration, modified Knott's test). Antigen testing is more sensitive, and several techniques are available both in-house and at reference labs. Antibody testing is not valid in dogs but can serve as a screening test in cats. False-positive results are seen with all types of serologic tests, so confirmation with a second type of test is essential.

Melarsomine is an adulticidal drug that clears most or all of the worms in dogs. Circulating microfilariae, if present, may be treated with ivermectin. Cats should not receive melarsomine, as fatal thromboembolism may result. In both species, prevention should be started early (6 weeks of age) and continued throughout the animal's life.

D. immitis affects humans through mosquito bites, but there is no direct transmission from animals.

Lungworms (Dogs): *Filaroides (Oslerus) osleri, Filaroides hirthi*

These nematodes are acquired by puppies and dogs through fecal-oral ingestion. The larvae migrate from the intestinal tract to the lungs, where they develop in the parenchyma or cause nodules to form in the airways. Clinical signs range from asymptomatic to a dry hacking cough to pneumonia. Larvae or ova are occasionally detected in fecal flotations, but diagnosis may involve tracheobronchoscopy or transtracheal wash techniques. Fenbendazole is the most common anthelmintic used along with supportive care, and all in-contact dogs should be treated.

Lungworms (Dogs): *Crenosoma vulpis*

This type of lungworm is a parasite of foxes, wolves, and raccoons, but occasionally dogs are infected by ingestion of paratenic hosts (snails and slugs). These small nematodes (5 to 15 mm long) are found in bronchioles and cause a productive cough (elicited on tracheal palpation). Larvae can be found in fecal flotations or with Baermann technique. Fenbendazole or milbemycin may be effective treatments, and there is no zoonotic potential.

Lungworms (Cats): *Aelurostrongylus abstrusus*

Cats around the world may be infected with these small worms (5 to 10 mm long) that are found in the lung parenchyma and bronchioles. The main paratenic hosts are snails, but infected rodents and birds may also transmit the larvae to cats through ingestion. Most cats remain asymptomatic or show signs of coughing. Respiratory distress and pleural effusion are possible complications. Larvae but not ova are

passed in the feces, so diagnosis relies on Baermann technique on fresh stool specimens. Samples obtained by transtracheal wash or bronchoalveolar lavage may contain larvae along with increased eosinophils. Fenbendazole or ivermectin is generally used for treatment. There is no reported zoonotic potential.

Lungworms (Dogs and Cats): *Eucoleus aerophilus* (syn. *Capillaria aerophila*)

These nematodes also have a worldwide distribution. They are medium-sized worms (25 to 30 mm long) and found in the upper airways, where they may lead to signs of coughing and wheezing. The life cycle is direct or possibly through paratenic hosts such as earthworms. Ova are coughed up, swallowed, and excreted in the feces, where they can be detected by routine fecal flotation (must be differentiated from whipworm ova). Fenbendazole or ivermectin may be effective, but treatment in asymptomatic animals is not always necessary. Human cases are sporadically reported.

Lung Fluke: *Paragonimus kellicotti*

Both cats and dogs can be infected with these small trematodes (5 to 15 mm), which are acquired by ingestion of crayfish and possibly other paratenic hosts such as rodents. The larvae migrate to the lungs, where they may cause chronic coughing. Eggs are shed in feces and may be detected by routine fecal flotation. High doses of praziquantel and fenbendazole are effective (Table 19-2). A few human cases resulting from crayfish have been diagnosed.

MISCELLANEOUS PARASITES

Helminths

Urinary Bladder Worm: *Pearsonema plica, Pearsonema feliscati*

Infection with these nematodes is uncommon but has been observed throughout the world. Dogs acquire these worms (15 to 30 mm long) from ingestion of earthworms, whereas cats may be infected from birds or other paratenic hosts. Many cases are asymptomatic, but hematuria, pollakiuria, dysuria, or other signs of lower urinary tract disease may be observed. Ova may be detected by microscopic exam of urinary sediment. Fenbendazole and ivermectin have been reported as effective treatments, although infection is usually self-limiting. Humans are unaffected.

Kidney Worm (Dogs): *Dioctophyma renale*

This is the largest nematode (up to 100 cm long) known to affect dogs. Mink are the definitive hosts, but dogs can become infected by ingestion of paratenic hosts such as earthworms, frogs, and fish. The larvae penetrate the peritoneal cavity and the kidney, where they may cause peritonitis or kidney failure. Ova may be seen in urinary sediment or peritoneal fluid. Effective drugs are not available, so treatment may involve surgical removal of the worms and the

TABLE 19-2	Drug doses			
Drug	**Trade name(s)**	**Dogs (mg/kg)**	**Cats (mg/kg)**	**Interval**
Pyrantel	Nemex, Drontal, Heartgard Plus	5-20	5-20	Once
Fenbendazole	Panacur, Safe-guard	50	50	Daily for 3 days
Febantel	Drontal Plus	25-50	–	Once
Emodepside	Profender	–	3	Once
Praziquantel	Droncit, Drontal, Profender	5	5	Once
Epsiprantel	Cestex	5.5	2.75	Once
Milbemycin	Interceptor, Sentinel	0.5	2	Monthly
Selamectin	Revolution	6	6	Monthly
Moxidectin	Advantage Multi	2.5	1	Monthly

entire kidney if the other kidney is unaffected. There is no zoonotic potential.

Liver Fluke (Cats): *Platynosomum concinnum*

These small trematodes (5 mm long) are acquired by ingestion of paratenic hosts such as lizards and frogs. They are found in the gall bladder and bile ducts and may result in cholangiohepatitis. Ova may be identified with fecal sedimentation techniques, or adult flukes may be detected with ultrasonography of the gall bladder and bile ducts. A high dose of praziquantel along with supportive therapy may be effective. Humans are unaffected.

SUGGESTED READINGS

Barr SC, Bowman DD: *The 5-minute veterinary consult clinical companion canine and feline infectious diseases and parasitology*, Ames, IA, 2006, Blackwell.

Bowman DD et al: *Feline clinical parasitology*, Ames, IA, 2002, Iowa State University Press.

Foreyt WJ: *Veterinary parasitology reference manual*, ed 5, Ames, IA, 2002, Blackwell.

Greene CE: *Infectious diseases of the dog and cat*, ed 3, St Louis, 2007, Saunders/Elsevier.

Zajac AM, Conboy GA: *Veterinary clinical parasitology*, ed 7, Ames, IA, 2006, Blackwell.

APPROACH TO THE FEBRILE PATIENT

CHAPTER 20

James B. Miller

Obtaining a body temperature measurement is important in the evaluation of all patients, especially the critical care patient. A rectal temperature higher than 102.5° F (39° C) is considered elevated in the unstressed dog or cat. The method of measurement must also be taken into account because ear, axillary, or toe web measurements will be lower than rectal temperature.

Too frequently the veterinarian associates any elevation in body temperature with true fever. The assumption often is made that the fever is caused by an infectious agent, even if there is no obvious cause. If the patient's fever resolves after antibiotics are given, the assumption is made that it was caused by a bacterial infection. A normal body temperature often is assumed to mean the absence of disease. This approach to fever, hyperthermia, or normothermia can be misleading and may result in improper diagnoses and therapy (or the lack thereof).

THERMOREGULATION

The thermoregulatory center for the body is located in the central nervous system (CNS) in the region of the anterior hypothalamus (AH). Changes in ambient and core body temperatures are sensed by the peripheral and central thermoreceptors, and the information is conveyed to the AH via the nervous system. Thermoreceptors sensing that the body is below or above its normal temperature (normal "set point") will stimulate the AH to cause the body to increase heat production and reduce heat loss through conservation if the body is too cold or dissipate heat if the body is too warm (Figure 20-1). Through these mechanisms, dogs and cats can maintain a narrow core body temperature range in a wide variety of environmental conditions. With normal ambient temperatures, most body heat is produced by muscular activity, even while at rest. Patients with severe neurologic impairment or cachexia and those under anesthesia may not be able

to maintain a normal set point or generate a normal febrile response.

Thermoregulation in the Neonate

After birth, there is rapid heat loss in the puppy and kitten as a result of decreased environmental temperature and evaporative heat loss. Because the neonate has poorly developed muscles there is little to no ability to generate heat through shivering, and heat production must occur through nonshivering thermogenesis. Heat generation is primarily via the lipolysis of brown adipose tissue. Brown adipose tissue contains numerous mitochondria. Heat is produced when adenosine-5'-triphosphate synthesis is uncoupled from the oxidative process by a protein in the mitochondria. In the neonatal dog or cat, brown adipose tissue is used within the first 2 to 3 weeks of life. This process is only partially able to maintain body temperature, and an environmental temperature of approximately 85° F (30° C) is needed to maintain normal body temperature. Neonatal puppies and kittens cannot generate a true fever in response to pyrogens for the first few weeks of life until shivering thermoregulation can take place and there are increased stores of glycogen in the muscles and liver.

HYPERTHERMIA

Hyperthermia is the term used to describe any elevation in core body temperature above the accepted normal for that species. Hyperthermia is a result of the loss of equilibrium in the heat balance equation such that heat is produced or stored in the body at a rate in excess of heat lost through radiation, convection, or evaporation. The term *fever* is reserved for those hyperthermic animals in which the set point in the AH has been "reset" to a higher temperature. In hyperthermic states other than fever, the hyperthermia is not a result of the body attempting to increase

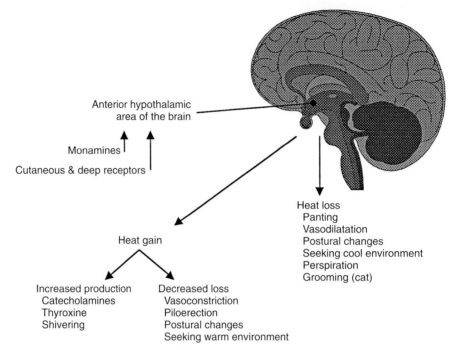

Figure 20-1 Normal thermoregulation. (From Miller JB: Hyperthermia and fever of unknown origin. In Ettinger SJ, Feldman EC (eds): *Textbook of veterinary internal medicine*, ed 6, St Louis, 2005, Saunders/Elsevier.)

| BOX 20-1 | **Classification of hyperthermia** |

True Fever
- Production of endogenous pyrogens

Inadequate Heat Dissipation
- Heat stroke
- Hyperpyrexic syndromes

Exercise Hyperthermia
- Normal exercise
- Hypocalcemic tetany (eclampsia)
- Seizure disorders

Pathologic or Pharmacologic Origin
- Lesions in or around the anterior hypothalamus
- Malignant hyperthermia
- Hypermetabolic disorders
- Monoamine metabolism disturbances

---

its temperature but is caused by the physiologic, pathologic, or pharmacologic intervention in which heat gain exceeds heat loss. Box 20-1 outlines the various forms of hyperthermia.

True Fever

True fever is a normal response of the body to invasion or injury and is part of the "acute phase response." Other parts of the acute phase response include increased neutrophil numbers and phagocytic ability, enhanced T and B lymphocyte activity, increased acute phase protein production by the liver, increased fibroblast activity, and increased sleep. Fever and the other parts of the acute phase response are initiated by exogenous pyrogens that lead to the release of endogenous pyrogens.

Exogenous Pyrogens

True fever may be initiated by a variety of substances, including infectious agents or their products, immune complexes, tissue inflammation or necrosis, and several pharmacologic agents including many antibiotics. Collectively, these substances are called exogenous pyrogens. Their ability to directly affect the thermoregulatory center is probably minimal, and their action is to cause the release of endogenous pyrogens by the host. Box 20-2 lists some of the more important known exogenous pyrogens.

Endogenous Pyrogens

In response to stimuli by an exogenous pyrogen, proteins (cytokines) released from cells of the immune system trigger the febrile response. Macrophages are the primary immune cell involved, although T and B lymphocytes and other leukocytes may play significant roles. The proteins produced are called endogenous pyrogens or fever-producing cytokines. Although interleukin-1 (IL-1) is considered the most important cytokine, at least 11 cytokines capable of initiating febrile responses have been identified (Table 20-1). Some neoplastic cells are also capable of producing cytokines that lead to a febrile response. The cytokines travel via the blood stream to the AH, where they bind to the vascular endothe-

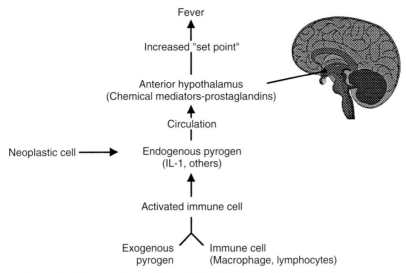

Figure 20-2 Pathophysiology of fever. (From Miller JB: Hyperthermia and fever of unknown origin. In Ettinger SJ, Feldman EC (eds): *Textbook of veterinary internal medicine*, ed 6, St Louis, 2005, Saunders/Elsevier.)

BOX 20-2   Exogenous pyrogens

Infectious Agents
- Bacteria (live and killed)
- Gram positive
- Gram negative
- Bacterial products
- Lipopolysaccharides
- Streptococcal exotoxin
- Staphylococcal enterotoxin
- Staphylococcal proteins
- Fungi (live and killed)
- Fungal products
- Cryptococcal polysaccharide
- Cryptococcal proteins
- Virus
- *Rickettsia*
- Protozoa

Nonmicrobial Agents
- Soluble antigen-antibody complexes
- Bile acids

Pharmacologic Agents
- Bleomycin
- Colchicine
- Tetracycline (cats)
- Levamisole (cats)

Tissue Inflammation/Necrosis

TABLE 20-1   Proteins with pyrogenic activity

Endogenous pyrogen	Principal source
Cachectin/tumor necrosis factor (TNF-α)	Macrophages
Lymphotoxin/tumor necrosis	Lymphocytes (T and B) factor-β (TNF-β; LT)
Interleukin-1α (IL-1α)	Macrophages and many
Interleukin-1β (IL-1β)	other cell types
Interferon-α	Leukocytes (esp. monocyte-macrophages)
Interferon-β	Fibroblasts
Interferon-γ	T lymphocytes
Interleukin-6 (IL-6)	Many cell types
Macrophage inflammatory protein 1α	Macrophages
Macrophage inflammatory protein 1β	
Interleukin-8 (IL-8)	

Adapted from Beutler B, Beutler SM: The pathogenesis of fever. In Bennett JC, Plum F (eds): *Cecil textbook of medicine*, ed 20, Philadelphia, 1996, WB Saunders, p 1535.

lial cells within the AH and stimulate release of prostaglandins (PGs), primarily prostaglandin E_2 (PGE$_2$) and possibly prostaglandin $E_{2\alpha}$(PGE$_{2\alpha}$). The set point is raised, and the core body temperature increases through increased heat production and conservation (Figure 20-2).

Inadequate Heat Dissipation
Heat Stroke

Heat stroke is a common form of inadequate heat dissipation. Exposure to high ambient temperatures may increase heat load at a faster rate than the body can dissipate the heat. This is especially true in larger breeds of dogs and brachycephalic breeds. Heat stroke may occur rapidly in the dog, especially in closed environments with poor ventilation (e.g., inside a car with windows closed), even on moderately hot days. Environmental temperatures inside a closed car exposed to the direct sun may exceed 120° F (48° C) in less than 20 minutes, even when the outside temperature is only 75° F

(24° C). Death may occur in less than 1 hour, especially in the breed types mentioned. Heat stroke will not respond to antipyretics used in true fever. The animal must be treated with total body cooling immediately if a fatal outcome is to be avoided. Water baths and rinses using cool (but not cold) water best accomplish total body cooling. If the water is too cold, a tendency exists for peripheral vasoconstriction, which will inhibit heat loss and slow the cooling process. Cool water, gastric lavage, or enemas have also been suggested. Cooling should be discontinued when body temperature approaches normal to avoid potential hypothermia. In addition to total body cooling, treatment for vascular collapse and shock should be instituted with severe hyperthermia (greater than 107° F [41.6° C]) or when clinical judgment warrants its use. Intravenous crystalloid solutions given at shock doses and glucocorticoids are indicated in an attempt to prevent permanent organ damage and disseminated intravascular coagulopathy.

Hyperpyrexic Syndrome

Hyperpyrexic syndrome is associated with moderate-to-severe exercise in hot and humid climates. This syndrome may be more common in hunting dogs or dogs that "jog" with their owners. In humid environments, a tendency exists toward a zero thermal gradient for dry heat loss, leading to a net heat gain. In addition, severe exercise may cause the cardiovascular system to supply skeletal muscles with adequate blood flow while compromising peripheral heat loss by not allowing proper vasodilation in the skin. Many hunting dogs and dogs that run with their owners will continue to work or run until they become weak, begin to stagger, and then collapse. In suspected cases, owners should obtain a rectal thermometer and monitor their dog's temperature. If increased, in the future the owner should evaluate the dogs' rectal temperature at the first sign of weakness or resistance to further exercise. Owners should be instructed that rectal temperatures greater than 106° F (41° C) require immediate total body cooling, and temperatures more than 107° F (41.6° C) are an immediate threat to permanent organ damage or death.

Exercise Hyperthermia

The body temperature will slowly increase with sustained exercise because of increased heat production associated with muscular activity. Even when extreme heat and humidity are not factors, dogs will occasionally reach temperatures that would require total body cooling. This is especially true in dogs not accustomed to exercise, overweight dogs, or those with respiratory disease. Puppies seen for vaccinations have often been excited and active during the trip. Activity and probable release of catecholamines result in the increased body temperatures obtained on physical examination. These dogs will display features suggestive of attempting to dissipate excess body heat and are neither febrile nor ill.

Seizure disorders as the result of organic, metabolic, or idiopathic causes are encountered frequently. In the young dog and cat, the most common cause of seizures or severe muscle tremors is toxicity (e.g., metaldehyde, organophosphates, and pyrethrins). Hyperthermia associated with severe muscular activity can be life threatening, especially if the seizures are prolonged or occur in clusters. The initial concern of the clinician should be to stop the seizures; however, when significant hyperthermia is present, total body cooling is recommended.

Pathologic and Pharmacologic Hyperthermia

These types of hyperthermia encompass several disorders that lead to impairment of the heat balance equation. Lesions in the hypothalamus may obliterate the thermoregulatory center, leading to impaired response to both hot and cold environments. Malignant hyperthermia has been reported in the dog and cat. It leads to a pharmacologic myopathy that is initiated by pharmacologic agents, including inhalation anesthetics (especially halothane) and muscle relaxants such as succinylcholine. Extreme muscle rigidity results with the production of excess body heat. Removal of the offending causative agent and total body cooling may prevent death.

BENEFITS AND DETRIMENTS OF HYPERTHERMIA

Benefits

Fever is part of the acute phase response and is a normal response of the body. Even poikilotherms such as fish and reptiles will respond to a pyrogen by seeking higher environmental temperatures to increase their body temperatures. It would be logical to think that a true fever is beneficial to the host. Most studies have shown that a fever will reduce the duration of and mortality from many infectious diseases. A fever decreases the ability of many bacteria to use iron, which is necessary for them to live and replicate. Blocking the fever with nonsteroidal antiinflammatory agents in rabbits with *Pasteurella* infections significantly increases mortality rates. Many viruses are heat sensitive and cannot replicate in high temperatures. Increasing the body temperature in neonatal dogs with herpes infections significantly reduces the mortality rate.

Detriments

Hyperthermia leads to an increased metabolic state and oxygen consumption that increase both caloric and water requirements by approximately 7% for each degree Fahrenheit (0.6° C) above accepted normal values. In addition, hyperthermia leads to suppression of the appetite center in the hypothalamus but usually not the thirst center. Animals that have sustained head trauma or a cerebrovascular accident may suffer more severe brain damage if coexisting hyperthermia is present.

Body temperatures greater than 107° F (41.6° C) often lead to increases in cellular oxygen consumption that exceed oxygen delivery, resulting in deterioration of cellular function and integrity. This may lead to disseminated intravascular coagulation with thrombosis and bleeding or serious damage to organ systems, including the brain (cerebral edema and subsequent confusion, delirium, obtundation, seizures, coma), heart (arrhythmias), liver (hypoglycemia, hyperbilirubinemia), gastrointestinal tract (epithelial desquamation, endotoxin absorption, bleeding), and kidneys. Additional abnormalities might include hypoxemia, hyperkalemia, skeletal muscle cytolysis, tachypnea, metabolic acidosis, tachycardia, and hyperventilation.

Exertional heat stroke and malignant hyperthermia may lead to severe rhabdomyolysis, hyperkalemia, hypocalcemia, myoglobinemia and myoglobinuria, and elevated levels of creatine phosphokinase. Fortunately true fevers rarely lead to body temperatures of this magnitude and are usually a result of other causes of hyperthermia that should be managed as medical emergencies.

CLINICAL APPROACH TO THE HYPERTHERMIC PATIENT

When a dog or cat has an increased body temperature, an effort should be made to approach the problem in a logical manner to avoid erroneous conclusions (Figure 20-3). A complete history and physical examination should be performed unless the problem is of extreme nature (temperature greater than 106° F [41° C]) and the animal is obviously attempting to dissipate heat (panting, postural changes) or comatose. In such cases, immediate total body cooling and supportive care should be initiated. In other cases, specific questions concerning vaccination history, previous injuries or infections, exposure to other animals, disease in other household pets, previous geographic environment, and previous or current drug therapy may be beneficial. Through this type of questioning and a complete physical examination, the clinician can frequently decide whether the increased body temperature is true fever. Temperatures less than 106° F (41° C), unless prolonged, are usually not life threatening, and caution should be taken on using antipyretics before a proper clinical evaluation. As stated earlier, the neonate has poorly developed thermoregulation and cannot generate a normal febrile response. In a 1- to 2-week-old "fading" puppy or kitten, infectious diseases such as herpes virus (dog) or bacterial infections that have usually gained entrance via the umbili-

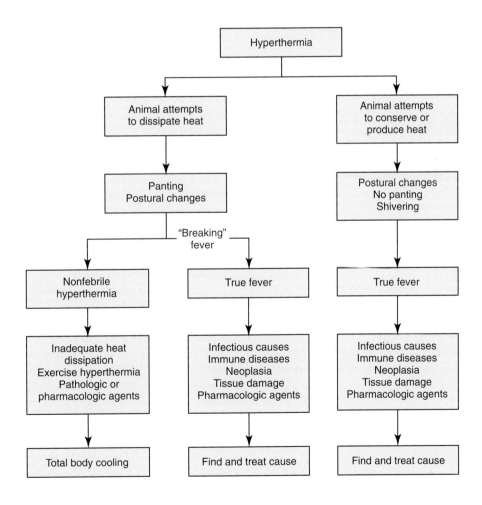

Figure 20-3 Algorithm for treatment of hyperthermia. (From Miller JB: Hyperthermia and fever of unknown origin. In Ettinger SJ, Feldman EC (eds): *Textbook of veterinary internal medicine*, ed 6, St Louis, 2005, Saunders/Elsevier.)

cus (dog and cat) should be considered even though no fever is present.

FEVER OF UNKNOWN ORIGIN

Fever of unknown origin (FUO) is defined in human medicine as a fever that has lasted 3 weeks and has a cause that has not been determined through laboratory evaluation and radiographs. In veterinary medicine, most clinicians consider any animal that does not have any obvious historical or physical finding that would cause a fever to have an FUO. Although research involving a large number of patients with FUO has been completed in humans, little veterinary information suggests the most common causes of FUO in dogs or cats. The information given in this chapter is based primarily on clinical experience. Most young dogs and cats with FUO probably have an infection or suffer from products of those agents. The prevalence of the causative infectious agent varies depending on the area where the clinician practices and the previous travel history of the pet. In the young dog or cat, viral diseases should always be considered even if they are not typical clinical signs. The young cat with an upper respiratory viral infection may show significant fever (105° F to 106° F) (40.5° C to 41° C) before clinical signs. Other viral diseases such as feline leukemia virus, feline infectious peritonitis virus, and feline immunodeficiency virus are common infectious causes of FUO in the young cat. In the young dog, viral diseases including canine distemper and parvovirus infection are common causes of fever. Although bacterial infections are probably the next most common cause of FUO in the dog, in some geographic locations, systemic fungal diseases or rickettsial infections might be more common. Endocarditis, pyelonephritis, pyothorax, and other deep abscesses should be considered in a dog with FUO. Two noninfectious diseases affecting the young dog (especially large breed dogs) that may lead to significant fevers are enostosis (panosteitis) and metaphyseal osteopathy (hypertrophic osteodystrophy). The next most common cause of FUO in the dog and cat is immune-mediated disease. Most immune-mediated diseases occur in young adult dogs. Immune complexes are a potent stimulator for the release of fever-producing cytokines and frequently lead to temperatures of 105° F (40.5° C) or 106° F (41° C). Neoplasia is a rare cause of fever in the young dog or cat with the exception of mediastinal lymphoma in the cat. Another often overlooked cause of fever is tissue trauma. Trauma often causes mild fever (103° F to 104° F [39.6° C to 40° C]) 1 or 2 days postsurgery when there has been significant muscle involvement. This appears more common in the cat. Most of these animals do not have infections and probably should not be treated with antibiotics without additional evidence of infection.

Evaluating for infectious disease, skeletal growth disease, immune-mediated disease, neoplasia (in the cat), and causes of tissue trauma will usually lead to a final diagnosis, even when no obvious cause for the fever exists.

NONSPECIFIC THERAPY FOR FEBRILE PATIENTS

Mild-to-moderate elevations in body temperature are rarely fatal and may be beneficial to the body. As stated before, hyperthermia may inhibit viral replication, increase leukocyte function, and decrease the uptake of iron by microbes (which is often necessary for growth and replication). If a fever exceeds 107° F (41.6° C), a significant risk of permanent organ damage and disseminated intravascular coagulation exists. The benefits of nonspecific therapy versus its potential negative effects should be considered before initiating such management.

Nonspecific therapy for true fever usually involves inhibitors of prostaglandin synthesis. The compounds most commonly used are the nonsteroidal antiinflammatory drugs. These products inhibit the chemical mediators of fever production and allow normal thermoregulation. They do not block the production of endogenous pyrogens. These products are relatively safe, although acetylsalicylic acid is potentially very toxic to the cat, and cyclooxygenase-2 inhibitors are relatively safer. Dipyrone, an injectable nonsteroidal antiinflammatory drug sometimes used in cats, may lead to bone marrow suppression, especially when given over a prolonged period.

Total body cooling with water or fans, or both, in a febrile patient will reduce body temperature; however, the thermoregulatory center in the hypothalamus will still be directing the body to increase the body temperature. This may result in a further increase in metabolic rate, oxygen consumption, and subsequent water and caloric requirements. Unless a fever is life threatening, this type of nonspecific therapy is counterproductive.

Glucocorticoids block the acute phase response, fever, and most other parts of this (adaptive) response. In general, their use should be reserved for those patients in whom the cause of the fever is known to be noninfectious and blocking the rest of the acute phase response will not be detrimental (and may prove beneficial). The most common indications include some immune-mediated diseases in which the fever plays a significant role and glucocorticoid therapy is often part of the chemotherapeutic protocol (i.e., immune-mediated hemolytic anemia, immune-mediated polyarthritis).

Phenothiazines can be effective in alleviating a true fever by depressing normal thermoregulation and causing peripheral vasodilation. The sedative qualities and potential for hypotension caused by the phenothiazines should be considered before administration to the febrile patient.

SUGGESTED READINGS

Asakura H: Fetal and neonatal thermoregulation, *J Nippon Med Sch* 71(6):360, 2004.

Berlin MT, Abeche AM: Evolutionary approach to medicine, *South Med J* 94:26, 2001.

Beutler B, Beutler SM: The pathogenesis of fever. In Bennet JC, Plum F (eds): *Cecil textbook of medicine,* ed 20, Philadelphia, 1996, WB Saunders.

Cunningham JG: *Textbook of veterinary physiology,* ed 2, Philadelphia, 1997, WB Saunders.

Dinarella CA: The acute phase response. In Bennet JC, Plum F (eds): *Cecil textbook of medicine,* ed 20, Philadelphia, 1996, WB Saunders.

Holloway BR: Reactivation of brown adipose tissue, *Proc Nutr Soc* 48:225, 1989.

Johnson KA: Skeletal diseases. In Ettinger SJ, Feldman EC (eds): *Textbook of veterinary internal medicine,* ed 6, St Louis, 2005, Saunders/Elsevier.

Mackowiac PA: Approach to the febrile patient. In Humes HD (ed): *Kelley's textbook of internal medicine,* ed 4, Philadelphia, 2000, Lippincott Williams & Wilkins.

Taylor SM: Exercise-induced collapse in Labrador retrievers: an update, *Proceedings of the 26th ACVIM Forum* 326, 2008.

RADIOGRAPHIC CONSIDERATIONS OF THE YOUNG PATIENT

CHAPTER 21

John S. Mattoon

Radiography of kittens and puppies is technically demanding because of the small patient size. Interpretation of radiographic images can be an even greater challenge, primarily because of unfamiliarity with the immature, developing skeletal system. Use of the basic principles of radiographic interpretation is essential, and doing so at least in part alleviates the uncertainties invariably encountered. This chapter will focus on the important unique radiographic features of puppies and kittens, application of radiographic principles, and interpretation advice; specific diseases are left to the appropriate dedicated chapters.

The basic principles of radiographic interpretation include size, shape, location, number, margination, and opacity of structures imaged. Recall that the five basic radiographic opacities, in increasing order, are air, fat, soft tissue, bone, and metal. The term *summation* refers to the two-dimensional (2D) additive effects of three-dimensional (3D) structures, such as the organs within the abdomen. For example, the caudal pole of the right kidney often overlaps the cranial pole of the left kidney, the area of overlap yielding an increase in soft tissue opacity relative to the nonoverlapping portions. The term *silhouette sign* (or border effacement) is used to describe the effacement of the borders of two touching structures of the same radiographic opacity. For example, if the spleen touches the border of the liver without fat between, the margins of the two organs cannot be distinguished.

Because there are relatively few anatomic and radiographic resources of the neonatal and juvenile dog and cat to use to compare, we must rely on laterality comparison (right vs. left) and on littermates or other age-matched patients for comparison. Further, such resources are of limited value because of the great differences in radiographic appearance that can occur in a relatively short period, not to mention breed differences. Although the neonatal puppy or kitten poses the most difficult interpretation challenge, fortunately these ill or injured patients are often presented by the breeder, who may have access to littermates. Radiographing a littermate for direct comparison can be the most important criterion for the practitioner when deciding normal from abnormal.

RADIOGRAPHIC TECHNIQUES

Radiographic examination of neonatal puppies or kittens is a supreme challenge in patience. Safe manual restraint is nearly impossible when using leaded gloves trying to hold tiny appendages. Because sedation or anesthesia is not routinely performed in such young patients, restraint methods using positioning devices such as foam sponges and tape are needed. Experience has shown us that a well-fed kitten or puppy is the most amenable to radiography. Exercise and play will quickly tire a neonate, which allows the patient to be restrained using positioning foam and tape. Cooing and soothing the patient help but require the radiographer's patience. Your best kitten or puppy "whisperer" may be needed! However, even under the best of circumstances, perfect positioning can be taxing, and it may be necessary to accept less-than-perfect radiographic images, depending on the specific indication for radiography. For example, critical assessment of the cardiac silhouette may be compromised by rotation of a ventrodorsal (VD) or dorsoventral (DV) radiograph; mild patient rotation probably will not hinder a diagnosis of heart failure.

For the youngest puppies and kittens, the lowest radiographic technique that the x-ray equipment is capable of will be necessary, as you might use for a bird or guinea pig. This requires a very low kilovoltage potential (kVp) and corresponding relatively low milliamperage-seconds (mAs). For example, a kVp of 40 or 45 is used for the smallest patients, which is the lowest allowable setting on diagnostic x-ray units. The mAs used depends on the speed of the intensifying screen/film combination. A 400 or 800 speed system may use 1 to 2 mAs, whereas a slower speed higher detail system (e.g., a 100 speed system) may require 4 to 8 mAs to achieve proper film density (blackness).

Given a choice, a slower speed system (e.g., 100 vs. 400 speed) should be used to achieve the best image detail. Use of a higher speed (more efficient) system will noticeably reduce image detail and in some instances may not be capable of yielding a diagnostic image because even the lowest machine setting will be too high and result in over-exposed radiographs. In this circumstance, the focal-film distance (FFD) can be increased, effectively reducing exposure. For example, the conventionally used 40-inch FFD can be increased to 50 inches or more by raising the x-ray tube height. Although a grid is not typically used for imaging of small patients or body parts less than 10 inches in thickness, a grid can be used to effectively reduce x-ray film exposure; this effect can be dramatic. A grid with an 8:1 ratio will reduce x-ray exposure by a factor of 3; a 12:1 grid can do so by as much as a factor of 4.

Once puppies or kittens reach 5 to 10 lb, the radiographic technique will not differ from that of any small patient.

If digital radiography is used, the same basic aforementioned considerations apply. Use the lowest kVp and mAs that allows enough x-ray (photon) density to achieve a mottle-free image. Many digital x-ray units require more radiographic exposure to achieve a diagnostic image than conventional film-screen radiography. Depending on the digital system used, image quality of such small patients may be worse compared with conventional film-screen radiography, exacerbated by magnification (zooming) of images on the viewing monitor.

For neonatal radiography, "whole body" images are routinely made and are acceptable. In larger puppies and kittens, as in adult patients, thorax- or abdomen-targeted radiographs are ideal, based on requirements of patient size, geometric distortion, and conventional film radiography technique differences used to maximize detail of thoracic or abdominal structures (i.e., high kVp technique to maximize image latitude and lung parenchymal detail, with lower kVp and higher mAs technique used to enhance fat and soft tissue contrast for maximum abdominal radiographic detail).

Either VD or DV images are acceptable. In practice, VD images of the thorax/abdomen are usually easiest to obtain. For the lateral image(s), right or left recumbency positions are equally diagnostic. As for radiography of adults, recumbency may be dictated by the type or laterality of the disease process in question. For example, if the VD/DV radiograph indicates left-sided pulmonary consolidation (such as pneumonia), a right lateral recumbent radiograph is indicated to maximize radiographic visualization of the diseased lung. Recall that the nonrecumbent lung is more aerated than the recumbent lung. It is the aerated portions of lung that provide contrast with lung pathology. Left-sided pulmonary consolidation may be completely invisible on a left lateral radiograph as a result of recumbency-induced left lung atelectasis (collapse).

Radiographic assessment of the appendages is perhaps the most challenging aspect of neonatal radiography. In the smallest patients, whole body images may be sufficient to assess the limbs. In the youngest patients, isolating a limb and obtaining two views may be truly challenging. This becomes easier in older, larger patients. The use of tape or loops of gauze to extend and isolate the limb works well. Care must be exercised because the limbs are relatively vulnerable. Although experience has shown that kittens and puppies are often restless and at first intolerant of these procedures, a gentle hand and patience can usually result in acquisition of diagnostic images.

Progressive Puppy Skeletal Ossification and Growth

Figures 21-1 through 21-8 show the radiographic appearance of normal Cardigan Welsh Corgi puppies from a few days after birth to approximately 2 months of age.

3-Day-Old Puppy

In a 3-day-old puppy (Figure 21-1), the heart looks relatively larger than in an adult (increased cardiothoracic ratio), as the lungs are not fully developed and well aerated as they will be later in life. As a result, the normal lung parenchyma shows a mild, diffuse, and unstructured interstitial pattern compared with an adult. Increased cranial thoracic soft tissue opacity is caused by overlying forelimb musculature and the thymus (see Figure 21-1, *A*). The abdomen of this puppy is normal and differs markedly from an adult. There is essentially no abdominal serosal detail, principally because of lack of abdominal fat to provide contrast with the soft tissue abdominal organs. Gastrointestinal gas provides the only contrast visible. The kidneys are not visible because of lack of retroperitoneal fat. The pendulous appearance of the abdomen is also a normal finding in puppies and kittens, caused by relative lack of abdominal wall muscle tone and a relatively large liver. In an adult, this appearance would be diagnostic for abdominal fluid.

Musculoskeletal items of note include open fontanel of the skull, separate centers of ossification of the wings of the first cervical vertebra (atlas), ossification of the hyoid apparatus, and upright and rectangular shape of the vertebrae with apparent widening of the intervertebral disc spaces because of nonossification of the vertebral endplates (epiphyses). The sternum has a similar appearance.

A VD whole body radiograph (see Figure 21-1, *B*) allows adequate visualization of the heart, lungs, and abdomen. There is increased width of the cranial mediastinum because of the presence of the immature thymus. When the puppy is repositioned to remove the overlying paws (see Figure 21-1, *C*), note the shortened, rectangular shape of the vertebral bodies created by nonossified vertebral endplates (epiphyses). The ilial and ischial ossification centers of the pelvis can be seen; the femoral heads are not ossified at this age.

A lateral radiograph of the left forelimb (see Figure 21-1, *D*) shows that the humeral, radial, ulnar, metacarpal, and phalangeal diaphyses are ossified. The humeral head, distal humeral condyle (the lateral portion, the humeral capitulum, and the medial portion, the humeral trochlea, are separate

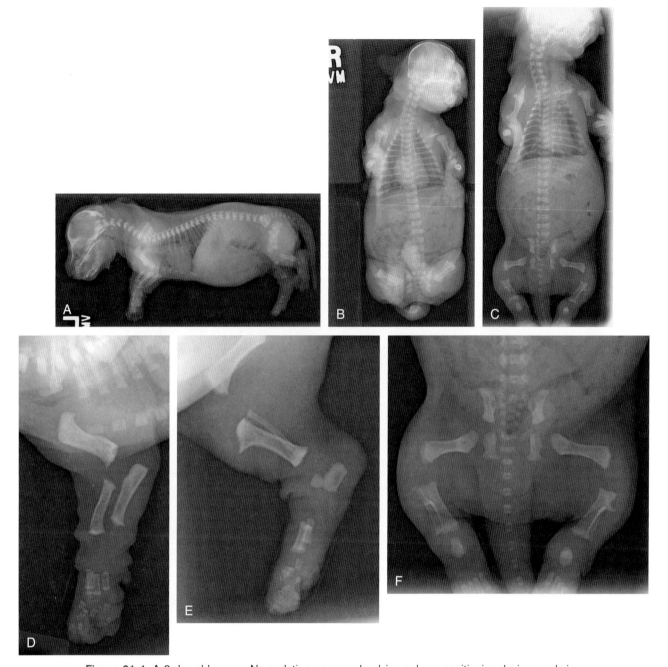

Figure 21-1 A 3-day-old puppy. No sedation was used, relying only on positioning devices, calming and cooing, and patience. **A,** Left lateral whole body radiograph. The puppy was placed in left lateral recumbency, calmed until she was still. **B,** Ventrodorsal whole body radiograph. The puppy was positioned in dorsal recumbency, secured laterally by foam sponges. The thorax is well positioned, except for the overlying forelimbs. Overlying hindlimbs compromise abdominal assessment. If critical assessment of the peripheral lung parenchyma or abdomen were necessary, the overlying paws would need to be repositioned. **C,** Ventrodorsal whole body radiograph. The same puppy as in **B** was repositioned. The abdomen is perfectly positioned, although the thorax is now rotated. **D,** Lateral radiograph of the left forelimb. Tape and a small pad have been used to position the limb for radiography while gently restraining the puppy's body. Note the small ossified clavicular remnant cranial to the shoulder. **E,** Lateral radiograph of the left hindlimb. The limb was passively positioned, extending it while gently restraining the puppy's body. The thin linear radiopaque structures surrounding the pes are tape, used to position the limb for radiography. **F,** Ventrodorsal pelvis.

centers, eventually fusing by approximately 2 months of age to become the humeral condyle), radial and ulnar epiphyses, metacarpal and phalangeal epiphyses, and all the carpal cuboidal bones are not ossified at this early age. Radiographs of the hindlimb (see Figure 21-1, *E*) show that the femoral, tibial, fibular, metatarsal, and first and second phalangeal diaphyses are ossified, as are the calcaneus and talus. The third phalanges are barely perceptible. All the epiphyseal centers are still cartilage models (soft tissue radiographic opacity) and not yet ossified. Note that the patellar, fabellar, and tarsal cuboidal bones are not visible as bony structures. In Figure 21-1, *D* and *E*, the lack of ossification creates a radiographic image of "widened" joints and soft tissue swelling. Therefore assessment for potential trauma or infection is challenging and may require comparison with the contralateral limb.

In a VD pelvic view (see Figure 21-1, *F*), the ilial, ischial, and pubic ossification centers are present, although the acetabular bones and femoral heads are not ossified. The stifle joints appear wide due to lack of epiphyseal ossification; the patellae and fabellae are also not ossified. The tarsi have a similar appearance, due to lack of epiphyseal and cuboidal bone ossification.

12-Day-Old Puppy

In the 12-day-old puppy (Figure 21-2), phalangeal and talus ossification has progressed. The primary difference in the radiographic appearance between the 3-day-old and 12-day-old puppy is identification of early ossification of accessory carpal bones (see Figure 21-2, *C*), the fourth tarsal bones (see Figure 21-2, *D*), and very faint ossification of the central

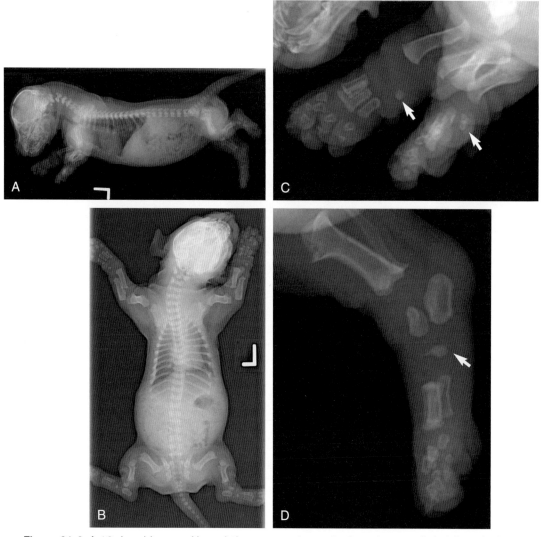

Figure 21-2 A 12-day-old puppy. No sedation was used to make these images. **A,** Left lateral whole body radiograph. **B,** Dorsoventral whole body radiograph. After calming the patient, the dorsoventral radiograph was made by simply positioning the puppy in sternal recumbency. There is now identification of the accessory and fourth tarsal bones and mild progression of ossification of the talus and phalanges. **C,** Close-up lateral view of the carpi showing early ossification of the accessory carpal bone *(white arrows).* **D,** Close-up view of the tarsus showing the earliest ossification of the fourth tarsal bone *(white arrow).*

tarsal bones. The cardiothoracic ratio is considered normal (identical to an adult) with better aeration of the lungs; although poor abdominal detail persists, a very thin stripe of abdominal fat can be seen separating the ventral abdominal body wall from the ventral liver margin, and the abdomen is less pendulous.

26-Day-Old Puppy

A lateral whole body radiograph of a 26-day-old puppy shows further skeletal ossification (Figure 21-3, *A*). The vertebral endplates (epiphyses) are now identified. Abdominal detail is still poor, but the thin layer of fat between the abdominal wall and the ventral margin of the liver is thicker and more evident than at day 12. In Figure 21-3, *B*, note visualization of carpal bones, many long bone epiphyses, vertebral endplates (epiphyses), and maturation of ossification centers noted 2 weeks earlier. The cranial mediastinum is widened by the thymus. Abdominal detail remains poor, but the margins of the spleen can be faintly seen along the

cranial to mid-left abdominal wall. Partial ossification of the humeral head, distal humeral condyle (two parts), distal radial epiphysis, radiocarpal and distal row carpal bones, distal metacarpal epiphyses, and proximal epiphyses of the first phalanges has occurred in the forelimbs (Figure 21-3, *C*). The femoral head, distal femoral epiphysis, and proximal and distal tibial epiphyses are now clearly evident in the hindlimbs (Figure 21-3, *D*). The distal metatarsal and proximal first phalangeal epiphyses are faintly seen as tiny focal areas of ossification. Tarsal bone ossification has progressed.

34-Day-Old Puppy

In a lateral whole body radiograph of a 34-day-old puppy (Figure 21-4, *A*), the lungs are not fully inflated, resulting in a diffuse increased soft tissue interstitial pulmonary pattern, not to be confused with pneumonia. Cranial thoracic soft tissue opacity from the thymus and overlying forelimb musculature can be seen. Abdominal detail remains

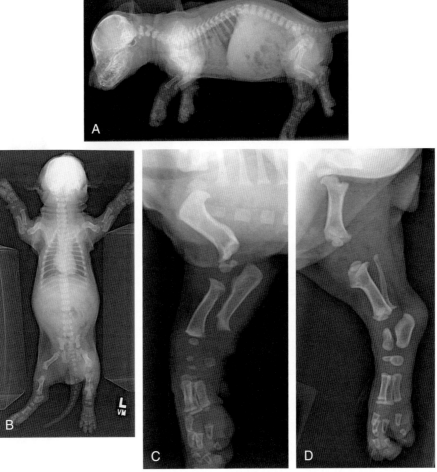

Figure 21-3 A 26-day-old puppy. No sedation was used to make these images. **A,** Left lateral whole body radiograph. Note the concavity of the vertebral endplates (epiphyses). Positioning of the patient is less than ideal for critical evaluation of the cranial thorax, obscured by forelimb musculature. **B,** Ventrodorsal whole body radiograph. The patient was positioned in dorsal recumbency using laterally placed large foam positioning devices. **C,** Lateral radiograph of the left forelimb. **D,** Lateral radiograph of the left hindlimb.

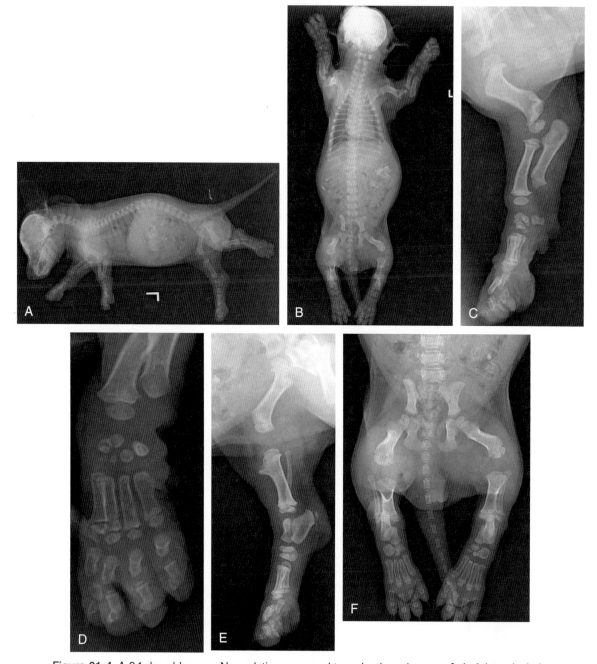

Figure 21-4 A 34-day-old puppy. No sedation was used to make these images. **A,** Left lateral whole body radiograph. **B,** Ventrodorsal whole body radiograph. **C,** Lateral radiograph left forelimb. **D,** Close-up dorsopalmar view right forepaw. The cuboidal bones are distinctly ossified but far from their mature appearance. **E,** Lateral radiograph of the left hindlimb. **F,** Ventrodorsal pelvic radiograph. Skeletal maturation has progressed.

poor, but a small amount of intraabdominal fat is seen along the ventral body wall, separating several loops of small intestine. A VD whole body radiograph shows further skeletal ossification (Figure 21-4, *B*). Cranial mediastinal widening is caused by the presence of the thymus. Abdominal detail remains poor, similar to 1 week earlier. In the forelimbs (Figure 21-4, *C*), the humeral head is similar to what its mature shape will be. The distal medial and lateral portions of the humeral condyle (capitulum and trochlea) are readily

identified as separate centers of ossification that will fuse to each other by approximately 2 months of age. The proximal radial epiphysis is beginning to ossify. Progressive ossification of the distal radial epiphysis, the carpal cuboidal bones, the metacarpus, and phalanges is noted. In the paws (Figure 21-4, *D*), continued maturation of the metacarpal bones and phalanges is evident, but the distal ulnar epiphysis is not yet ossified. Progressive ossification of the diaphyseal and epiphyseal long bones and the cuboidal bones of the tarsus has occurred in the hindlimbs (Figure 21-4, *E*). The apophysis of the calcaneus (calcaneal tuber) is now evident. Still not ossified are the patella, fabellae, and tibial tuberosity. A VD pelvic view (Figure 21-4, *F*) shows that the acetabular bones are not yet ossified, nor are greater trochanters, patella, and fabellae. The coxofemoral joints appear widened, as do all the joints imaged.

42-Day-Old Puppy

A lateral whole body radiograph of a 42-day-old puppy (Figure 21-5, *A*) shows how abdominal serosal detail continues to improve. Note the thin fat stripe between the ventral abdominal body wall and the ventral margin of the liver, as well as increased visualization of the serosal surfaces of the small intestinal loops, separated by mesenteric fat. The liver margin extends well beyond the costal arch, with smooth and sharply defined margins. Whereas in an adult this would indicate liver enlargement, this is a normal finding in puppies and kittens. Note the subcutaneous fat accumulation when compared with the earlier images.

Progressive ossification of skeletal structures has occurred. Note the vertebrae have assumed an adult shape (except the open physes); the intervertebral disc spaces are also near normal in width, without the concavity noted in the earlier studies.

In Figure 21-5, *B*, the thoracic portion of the puppy is mildly rotated with the sternum projected to the left. The thymus can be identified as a roughly triangular soft tissue opacity in the cranial left thorax. Abdominal detail continues to improve. Note the spleen is well visualized along the left lateral body wall by the thin fat opacity along its mesenteric margin.

Joints are becoming more adult-like in appearance as the epiphyseal bone continues to ossify (Figure 21-5, *C*). The distal ulnar epiphysis is now visualized; a tiny focus of ossification of the medial humeral epicondyle is now seen. The

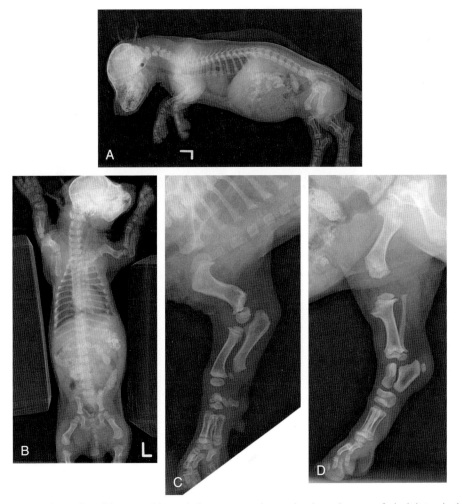

Figure 21-5 A 42-day-old puppy. No sedation was used to make these images. **A,** Left lateral whole body radiograph. Mineral ingesta are noted incidentally in the stomach and colon. Motion artifact is noted with one of the forepaws. **B,** Ventrodorsal whole body radiograph. The nonsedated puppy is securely positioned using laterally placed foam sponges. Bony ingesta are noted in the stomach and colon. **C,** Left lateral forelimb. **D,** Left lateral hindlimb. Note the irregularity of the distal femoral condyle ossification. This irregularity is a normal pattern of ossification; it can be confused with lytic change associated with osteomyelitis.

joints of the pes are becoming more adult-like in appearance (Figure 21-5, *D*). The stifle lags in ossification; the patella, fabellae, and tibial tuberosity have not yet begun to ossify.

49-Day-Old Puppy

In a 49-day-old puppy, progressive skeletal maturation has occurred. The thorax and abdomen (Figure 21-6, *A* to *C*) are otherwise very similar in appearance to the preceding week. In the forelimbs (Figure 21-6, *D*), the medial epicondylar apophysis of the distal humerus and distal ulnar epiphysis have significantly ossified during the past week. The remaining osseous structures are progressively maturing. Progressive ossification of the bony structures of the hindlimb has also occurred (Figure 21-6, *E*); however, the patella, fabellae, and tibial tuberosity are still not apparent radiographically.

55-Day-Old Puppy

At 55 days of age, the thorax is normal (Figure 21-7, *A*). The vertebrae and other osseous structures continue to mature. A VD view (Figure 21-7, *B*) shows persistent widening of the cranial mediastinum caused by the thymus. Abdominal detail is still vastly different from an adult, but progressive fat deposition has resulted in a striking increase in abdominal serosal detail when compared with earlier images, although a typical puppy "pot belly" appearance remains (Figure 21-7, *A* and *C*). In the past 6 days, the olecranon (proximal ulnar apophysis) has been ossifying in the forelimbs. The supraglenoid tubercle ossification center is now visualized within the cranial portion of the scapulohumeral joint, overlying the manubrium (Figure 21-7, *D*). Within the same period, the patella and tibial tuberosity and the head of the fibula also now begin to ossify. Continued

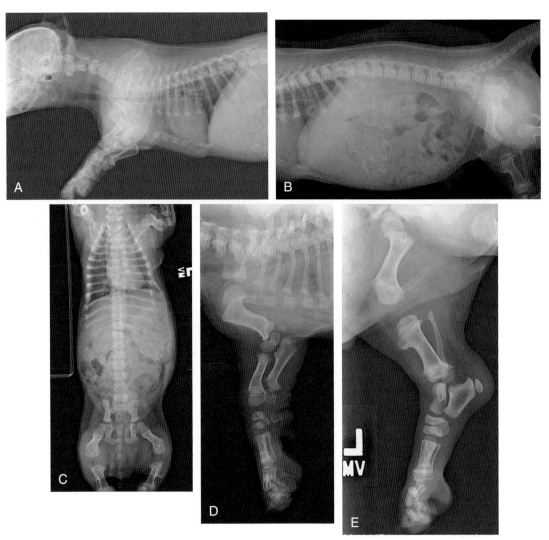

Figure 21-6 A 49-day-old puppy. No sedation was used to make these images. **A,** Lateral thoracic radiograph. This image was made on a small image plate. **B,** Lateral abdominal radiograph. This image was made on a small image plate. **C,** Ventrodorsal whole body radiograph. This image was made on a 14 × 17-in image plate, allowing the entire body to be imaged in one exposure. **D,** Left lateral forelimb. **E,** Left lateral hindlimb.

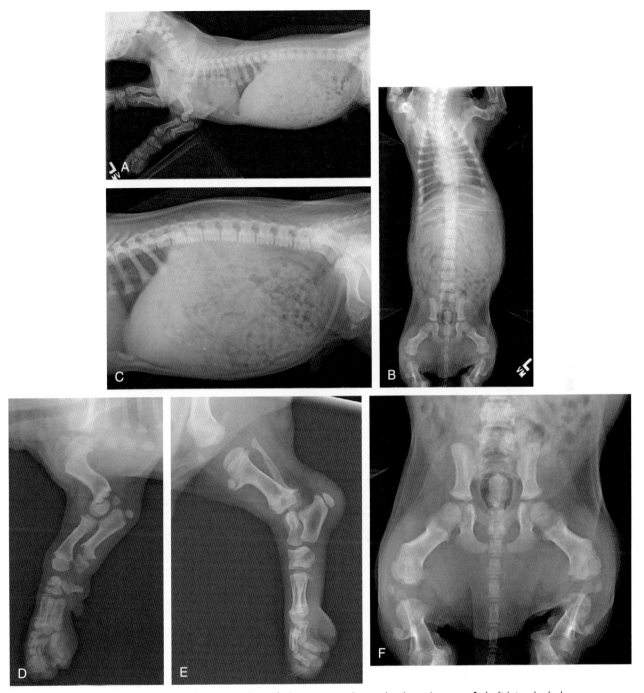

Figure 21-7 A 55-day-old puppy. No sedation was used to make these images. **A,** Left lateral whole body radiograph. Increased opacity noted in the cranial thorax on the lateral view is from the thymus, seen as a soft tissue opacity in the cranial mediastinum on the ventrodorsal view. **B,** Ventrodorsal whole body radiograph. **C,** Left lateral abdominal radiograph. This image is processed to maximize abdominal detail by increasing the radiographic contrast between the abdominal fat and soft tissues of the abdominal organs. **D,** Left lateral forelimb. **E,** Left lateral hindlimb. **F,** Ventrodorsal pelvis. Note the patellae are now evident.

development of the remaining bony structures is evident. A VD pelvic view (Figure 21-7, *F*) will show that the acetabula continue to develop, although considerable ossification will occur during the next 2 months. The femoral heads are nearly completely ossified and have the shape of a mature dog. The patellae are radiographically evident.

62-Day-Old Puppy

Once the puppy reaches 62 days of age, it is now large enough to justify a dedicated thoracic radiograph (Figure 21-8, *A*). The thorax resembles an adult in lateral views, with the exception of the increased opacity of the cranial mediastinum and the immature skeleton. The appearance of the

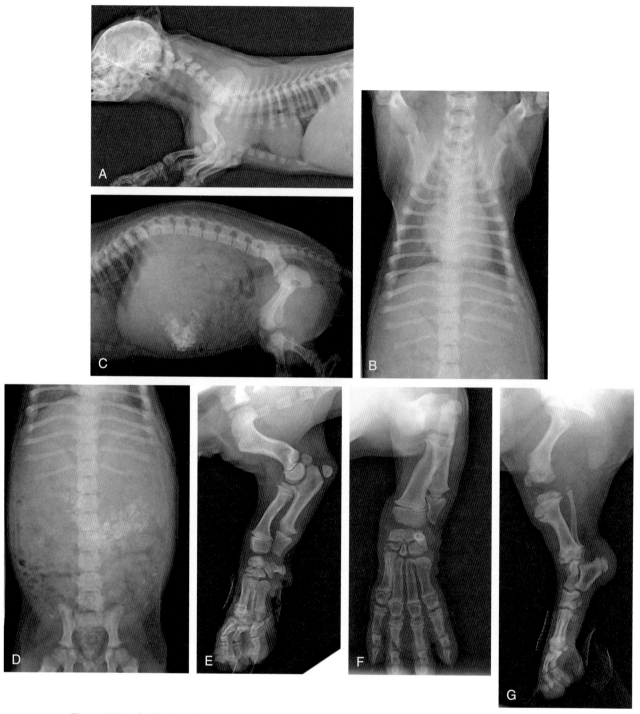

Figure 21-8 A 62-day-old puppy. No sedation was used to make these images. **A,** Left lateral thorax. **B,** Ventrodorsal thorax. **C,** Left lateral abdomen. The stomach is full and contains multiple bone fragments (the puppy had been recently fed). The radiolucent linear structure over the dorsal aspect of the coxofemoral joints represents normal acetabular physes; they can be confused with fractures. **D,** Ventrodorsal abdomen. A markedly distended stomach occupies approximately one half of the abdomen in this recently fed puppy. Note the lucent physis between each ilium and acetabular bone, corresponding to those noted on the lateral radiograph. **E,** Lateral forelimb. The conical conformation of the distal ulnar physis is clearly evident. **F,** Dorsopalmar forelimb (manus). **G,** Lateral hindlimb. Note the patellar ligament and the relatively radiolucent infrapatellar fat pad.

intrathoracic structures closely resembles an adult dog on VD thoracic views (Figure 21-8, *B*) as well. The liver is sharply marginated and extends beyond the costal arch, a normal finding in a puppy or kitten (Figure 21-8, *C*). It is well delineated from the ventral abdominal body wall by an increasing layer of relatively radiolucent fat. Note that the serosal margins of various small intestinal loops are readily seen by surrounding mesenteric fat. There is not yet enough retroperitoneal fat to allow visualization of the kidneys, but there has been a progressive increase in subcutaneous fat layer along the puppy's back. In a VD view, the serosal detail of the abdomen is not as apparent (Figure 21-8, *D*), and the kidneys cannot be seen. The supraglenoid tubercle of the scapula, the medial humeral epicondyle, the olecranon, and the distal ulnar epiphysis have enlarged and continued to ossify (Figure 21-8, *E*). The cuboidal bones appear very well ossified in a dorsopalmar view of the forelimbs (Figure 21-8, *F*). The paired palmar sesamoids of the metacarpophalangeal joints are now visible. The conical conformation of the distal ulnar physis is clearly apparent, as are the normal "flared" appearances of the distal radial and ulnar metaphyseal bone. Rapid maturation of the tibial tuberosity can be noted in the hindlimb (Figure 21-8, *G*), and the patella has developed a mature shape.

ANATOMIC APPEARANCE

Thorax

The neonatal and juvenile thorax does not differ dramatically from the adult. A plethora of congenital and developmental cardiac, pulmonary, and thoracic disorders occur and are discussed in system-specific chapters. Here we will primarily focus on the radiographic appearance of potentially confusing normal anatomy and differences in the juvenile versus the adult thorax.

Although difficult to quantify, the heart of neonatal and, to a lesser extent, older juvenile dogs or cats may appear relatively larger than in the adult (an increase in cardiothoracic ratio). This is probably a result of less fully developed lung (reduced lung volume, less aeration). Semiquantitative and quantitative methods to assess cardiac size can usually be sensibly and reliably applied. In kittens, the width of the heart on the lateral view is usually encompassed by 2 intercostal spaces (ICS), and there should be ample space between the diaphragm and the apex of the heart. In dogs, there is a broader range, with cardiophrenic contact expected, and an increase in the amount of cardiosternal contact compared with cats. Barrel-chested dogs (e.g., Boston Terrier, bulldog) have a wider heart (up to 3.5 ICS) and deep-chested dogs (Borzoi, Afghan) have a narrower heart (as small as 2.5 ICS), whereas normal conformation, such as shepherds and retrievers, are generally about 3 ICS. In the youngest of patients, this may be a difficult assessment as the ribs and costal arches may not be well mineralized. The more quantitative vertebral heart score (VHS) has limitations when used for evaluation of skeletally immature patients because the vertebral ends (epiphyses) are not fully ossified, the vertebral bodies being shorter than in an adult. Thus VHS is larger and will often fall outside the established normal adult range in normal juvenile patients (Figure 21-9). The VHS can probably be used reliably in older juvenile patients, from 6 months of age or older. The VHS for adult cats is 7.5 ± 0.3 vertebral bodies; for adult dogs the VHS is 9.7 ± 0.5.

In addition to evaluation of heart size, it is important to be familiar with the anatomic/radiographic abnormalities that occur with various forms of congenital cardiac disease, as well as the expected pulmonary vascular alterations. As a practitioner, you may be presented with a patient with a congenital heart murmur. Signalment may be important, as certain breeds are predisposed to particular forms of congenital heart disease. It is important to characterize the

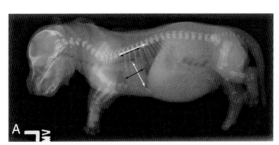
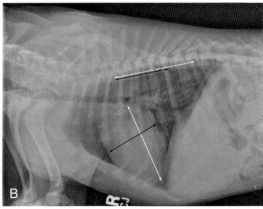

Figure 21-9 Vertebral heart score (VHS) in puppies. The normal values for adult dogs and cats cannot be used for assessment of puppies and kittens because of shortened, immature vertebral bodies that increase VHS. **A,** This normal 3-day-old puppy has a VHS of 11.5, a value significantly larger than the normal adult dog. **B,** This normal 4-month-old dog has a vertebral heart score of 11.2, a value significantly larger than the normal adult dog.

murmur and determine its point of maximum intensity. From here a radiographic examination may ensue. Assessment of heart size, specific chamber and great vessel enlargement, pulmonary vasculature, and lung parenchyma follows. An example case (Figure 21-10) illustrates the importance of knowing the location of specific heart chambers, the great vessels, and evaluation of pulmonary blood vessels.

The congenital cardiac diseases can be simplified and classified into broad groups for the purposes of our radiographic discussion: those that create left-to-right shunts or right-to-left-shunts, pulmonic or aortic stenosis, and atriovalvular disorders.

The combination of radiographic findings described in Figure 21-10 allows confident radiographic diagnosis of a left-to-right patent ductus arteriosus (PDA) with low-grade heart failure. In patients with left-to-right shunts and ventricular septal defects (VSDs; the most common), the heart will be enlarged, and both the pulmonary artery and veins will be larger than normal because of overcirculation through the lungs (see Figure 21-10). Assessment of pulmonary blood vessels can be difficult at times, as published semiquantification parameters using rib width as a guide are often unreliable and misleading. Increased number of vessels visualized and visualization of vessels well into the lung periphery are important clues. Careful review of the artery

and vein pairs to the cranial lung lobes (especially on the lateral view) and caudal lobes (the DV view is best) is essential. In Figure 21-10, *A*, close scrutiny of the cranial lung lobar artery and vein shows that they are symmetrically enlarged, indicative of overcirculation. In addition, pulmonary vascular margins are not as sharply defined as they should be, indicative of an interstitial infiltrate. The pulmonary blood vessels are enlarged, and evaluation of the caudal lobar artery and vein pairs (see Figure 21-10, *B*) shows symmetric enlargement of both, indicating overcirculation. There is increased interstitial pulmonary opacity obscuring pulmonary blood vessel margins and increasing lung opacity in the perihilar region while sparing the lung periphery. This is characteristic of low-grade cardiogenic pulmonary edema.

In right-to-left shunting cardiac anomalies (reverse PDA, tetralogy of Fallot), the right side of the heart enlarges, and the pulmonary blood vessels (artery and vein) will be reduced in size. Severe pulmonic outflow disease (pulmonic stenosis) can also reduce the caliber of both the pulmonary arteries and veins.

Right ventricular hypertrophy will manifest itself as right-sided heart enlargement, although this may not be apparent radiographically in a very young patient. A protruding main pulmonary artery will be present, and in severe

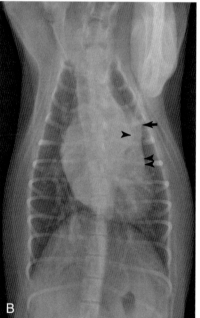

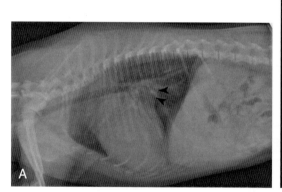

Figure 21-10 Five-month-old German Shepherd puppy with a continuous grade 6/6 heart murmur. **A,** Right lateral thoracic radiograph. The cardiac silhouette is too tall and too wide. The trachea is nearly parallel to the spine. The left atrium is markedly enlarged *(arrowheads)*. The lung has abnormal increased soft tissue opacity, primarily because of increased size of the pulmonary blood vessels. Note the vertebral endplates are fused and normally shaped in the cranial to mid thorax, but open physes can be seen in the caudal and lumbar vertebrae. The right kidney can be seen in the dorsocranial abdomen. **B,** Dorsoventral thoracic radiograph shows the enlargement of the main pulmonary artery *(arrow)* and the left auricle *(two arrowheads)*. A focal enlargement of the proximal descending aorta *(single arrowhead)* indicates enlargement of the ductus arteriosus communication with the aorta. These three "bumps" are characteristic for a left-to-right patent ductus arteriosus.

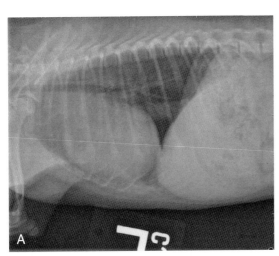

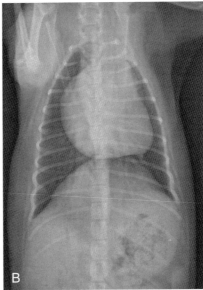

Figure 21-11 Four-month-old Pomeranian puppy with a grade 5/6 ejection murmur loudest at the left cranial base of the heart. In this example, identification of right ventricular enlargement, reduced pulmonary vascular size, and an enlarged main pulmonary artery allows a confident diagnosis of pulmonic stenosis, confirmed with echocardiography. **A,** Left lateral thoracic radiograph. Compare the pulmonary blood vessels for a striking comparison of overcirculation versus undercirculation. Note the liver extends beyond the costal arch, and there is ample intraabdominal fat to allow the liver margins to be seen. **B,** On the dorsoventral view, the heart is greatly enlarged. Note that the head of the spleen can be seen just caudal to the fundus of the stomach, separated from it by intraabdominal fat.

cases of pulmonic stenosis both the pulmonary arteries and veins may be reduced in size, secondary to decreased right-sided cardiac output (Figure 21-11). With aortic stenosis, the left ventricle will enlarge, as will the aortic arch, secondary to a poststenotic dilatation.

Figure 21-11, *A*, shows a heart that is enlarged and round in shape. The trachea is elevated, with increased soft tissue opacity of the cranial thorax. The heart occupies 4 ICS. There is increased cardiosternal and cardiophrenic contact. The pulmonary blood vessels to the cranial lung lobes are reduced in caliber, both the arteries and veins, indicative of undercirculation. Figure 21-11, *B*, also shows the enlarged heart, along with the right ventricle (seen in the 6 to 9 o'clock position), which is primarily responsible for this enlargement. The apex of the heart is easily defined to the left of midline, and the left ventricular border is flattened when compared with the right ventricle. The overall appearance is that of a "reverse D." Pulmonary arteries and veins to the caudal lung lobes are symmetrically reduced in size. The cranial mediastinum is widened, secondary to both the thymus and an enlarged main pulmonary artery (MPA). The characteristic MPA enlargement seen with pulmonic stenosis is mostly hidden from view from silhouetting with the soft tissue opacity of the thymus.

Mitral dysplasia will manifest as a very prominent, enlarged left atrium, with left ventricular enlargement occurring later in the disease process. With time, the pulmonary veins become engorged, larger than the companion arteries,

followed eventually by increased pulmonary opacity, representing cardiogenic edema.

Tricuspid dysplasia will show a greatly enlarged cardiac silhouette secondary to a severely enlarged right atrium. The caudal vena cava will be distended, and eventually ascites will occur. Pleural effusion can also occur, although usually ascites develops before pleural effusion.

It must be stressed that ultrasound plays a primary role in the evaluation of congenital cardiac disease. Although radiography can be very informative and at times essential, its primary purpose is as a screening procedure and in the assessment of heart failure. The radiographic manifestations of specific congenital cardiac diseases are discussed in this text's dedicated cardiology chapter (see Chapter 32).

The normal thymus is radiographically identified in the juvenile dog and cat up to perhaps 4 to 6 months or older, when it slowly involutes. It is a soft tissue opaque structure located within the cranial mediastinum. It is usually best identified on the DV or VD radiographic view as a roughly triangular soft tissue structure within the cranial mediastinum that crosses to the left of midline along the cranial border of the heart (see Figures 21-1 through 21-8). Its appearance has been referred to as a "sail sign," as it resembles the sail of a ship as viewed on the VD or DV radiograph. It causes a normal widening of the cranial mediastinum. Its location is a good reminder of the oblique orientation of the cranial mediastinum, useful in differentiating cranial mediastinal from pulmonary masses in adult patients, particularly large thymomas. On the lateral view, the thymus often can be appreciated as an increase in soft tissue opacity cranial to the heart, with subtle obscuring (silhouetting) of the cranial cardiac margin. This may be mistaken for the presence of pleural effusion. In cats and less frequently in dogs, congenital/developmental branchial cysts can be seen silhouetting as a soft tissue structure with the cranial cardiac border, but these fluid-filled benign structures are usually more focally defined on the lateral view and do not show the typical "sail sign" on the DV/VD view; they may show a more focal cranial mediastinal enlargement just cranial to the heart but are often not large enough to fully appreciate on these views, hidden by normal aortic arch.

Remember, the trachea is an important, always-recognizable radiographic anatomic landmark. When elevated, it can be an indication of increased cardiac size or a cranial mediastinal mass. If ventrally depressed, it is nearly always a sign of esophageal enlargement (Figure 21-12). In some puppies, the trachea is noted to be relatively small in diameter. This may be noticed incidentally when radiographing the thorax for suspected cardiac or pulmonary disease. In patients presented with signs potentially referable to the trachea, this becomes an important consideration. Although congenital hypoplasia of the trachea is a disease entity most commonly seen in brachycephalic breeds (and occasionally in nonbrachycephalic dogs), it has been noted that the trachea can disproportionately grow and become normal over time as the patient matures. Other differential diagnoses must be considered in patients presenting with signs referable to the trachea, such as kennel cough and irritant and parasitic tracheitis, all of which can reduce tracheal luminal size.

An embryologic, congenital malformation of fusion of midline structures, peritoneopericardial diaphragmatic hernia (PPDH), may found incidentally during a radiology examination. Although the clinical importance of PPDH

can be questionable, radiographically it is the appearance of an enlarged heart that can lead to a misdiagnosis. Small intestinal herniation into the pericardial sac may be suspected if borborygmus is auscultated during routine examination of a puppy or kitten. This would prompt a thoracic radiographic examination, in which case the diagnosis of PPDH is usually readily confirmed by the presence of intestinal loops within the pericardial sac. Falciform fat is often contained within the pericardial sac, in which case the cardiac silhouette can be differentiated from herniated fat based on differences in contrast between the soft tissue of the heart and the fat. When liver is present within the hernia, the cardiac silhouette is usually large and globoid in shape and must be differentiated from true heart enlargement (Figure 21-13). Ultrasound or a positive contrast peritoneogram can be used to confirm the diagnosis. Other related radiographic signs may be sternal abnormalities or reduced number of sternebrae.

Abdomen

The abdomen of neonatal and juvenile dogs and cats has reduced serosal detail compared with adults (see Figures 21-1 through 21-8). This is primarily because of a relatively small amount of intraabdominal fat at birth. It is also because of the difference in the type of abdomen fat (brown fat), which has higher water content than adult fat. This is an important concept to remember when viewing the juvenile abdomen because it is mesenteric, omental, falciform, and retroperitoneal fat adjacent to the soft tissue opacity of the abdominal organs that gives us radiographic contrast. In addition, puppies and kittens probably have a bit more abdominal fluid than adults (based on ultrasound observations), and they tend to have "pot bellies" when they are very young. All these features render the puppy and kitten abdomen difficult to reliably interpret and thus emphasize the important role that ultrasound plays in assessment. It is easy to overinterpret the presence of pathologic abdominal fluid in puppies and kittens; likewise, caution must be exercised not to disregard this appearance when the clinical situation dictates. Usually by 6 months of age or so the abdomen has taken on the appearance of an adult, albeit a thin one in most cases (Figures 21-14 and 21-15).

It is also noted that retroperitoneal fat deposition lags behind intraabdominal fat accumulation. This makes radiographic visualization of the kidneys occur later than intraabdominal (peritoneal) organ visualization, as it is the retroperitoneal fat that gives the kidneys radiographic contrast. Visualization of kidneys may occur as early as 3 months or may be considerably longer. This is important to note, as lack of kidney visualization in adults may indicate renal or ureteral pathology (hemorrhage, rupture) in adults (Figure 21-16).

Because of reduced detail of the major abdominal organs, gastrointestinal gas is the only source of contrast within the abdomen and plays a significant role in assessment of abdominal disease in puppies and kittens. Gastrointestinal gas is an important radiographic sign to observe, as it allows

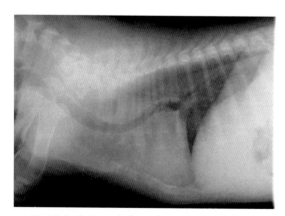

Figure 21-12 Left lateral thoracic radiograph (analog) of a 7-week-old German Shepherd puppy presented for regurgitation. The final diagnosis was a vascular ring anomaly, confirmed with an esophagram. This case illustrates the importance of observing the position of the trachea, as the thoracic trachea is markedly deviated ventrally. A large gas pocket is noted dorsal to the depressed trachea, within the esophagus.

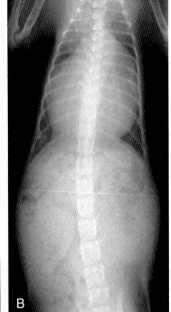

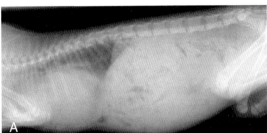

Figure 21-13 Congenital peritoneopericardial diaphragmatic hernia (PPDH) in a kitten. The apparently enlarged cardiac silhouette in these conventional film-screen (analog) radiographs could be mistaken for a congenital heart anomaly. Both images show increased cardiophrenic and cardiosternal contact; the margins of the diaphragm cannot be discerned. Poor serosal abdominal detail is normal for the young age of this patient. **A,** Right lateral whole body radiograph. Note the gas-filled intestinal loops in the most cranioventral abdomen; this is good evidence of herniation, as this is not a normal location for small intestine. **B,** Ventrodorsal whole body radiograph also shows abnormally cranially positioned gas-filled intestinal loops.

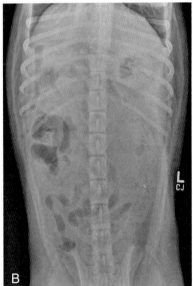

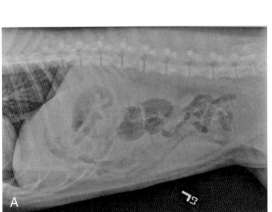

Figure 21-14 A 9-month-old puppy abdomen. By 9 months of age (often as early as 6 months), dog and cat abdomens are considered mature, with overall good serosal detail in normal patients. Although many older juvenile patients remain relatively thin, retroperitoneal fat deposition allows radiographic visualization of the kidneys, as noted in this case. **A,** Left lateral abdominal radiograph shows good detail of the abdomen; the margins of the liver and spleen are easily seen, as is the intestinal tract. The left kidney can be seen ventral to the second through fourth lumbar vertebrae because of the presence of retroperitoneal fat. Note the vertebral physes are closed. **B,** Ventrodorsal abdominal radiograph. The margin of the spleen is seen contained within the left costal arch just caudal to the stomach. The left kidney can be faintly visualized. Various portions of the gastrointestinal tract are seen, including the "C-shaped" cecum in the right midabdomen.

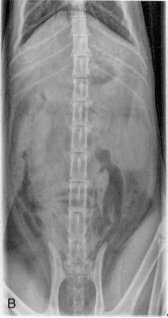

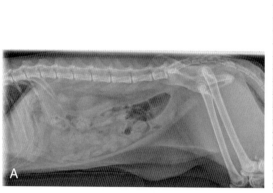

Figure 21-15 A 9-month-old kitten abdomen. There is enough intraabdominal fat to allow radiographic visualization of all the abdominal organs, including the retroperitoneal located kidneys. This cat is thin, but ventral abdominal fat pads are forming. **A,** Left lateral abdominal radiograph. Note visualization of the ventral margin of the liver and small intestine, separated from the ventral body wall by falciform and omental fat. The margin of the urinary bladder is clearly demarcated. Overlapping of the caudal pole of the right kidney with the cranial pole of the left kidney results in a focal area of increased soft tissue opacity, as a result of *summation* of superimposed structures. The triangular area of soft tissue opacity overlying the cranial pole of the right kidney just caudal to the last rib is a result of summation of the head of the spleen with the right kidney. Epaxial musculature can also be seen because of contrast with retroperitoneal fat. Note that the vertebral physes are closed; femoral head, distal femur, and proximal tibial physes remain open at this age. **B,** Ventrodorsal abdominal radiograph. The patient has been positioned using laterally placed foam sponges. There is excellent abdominal detail. The fundus of the stomach is seen separated from the spleen by fat opacity. The spleen is seen along the left lateral body wall.

assessment of the diameter and location of the intestinal tract. As puppies and to a lesser extent kittens have a tendency to ingest foreign objects, familiarity with the appearance of normal bowel is helpful. Fortunately, the juvenile intestinal tract does not differ from the adult in this regard. Key abnormal findings include dilated bowel, be it segmental or diffuse (bowel diameter greater than the height of a vertebral body is suspicious for obstruction or enteritis), and plicated bowel as seen with linear foreign bodies (Figure 21-17).

The liver in neonatal and juvenile puppies and kittens is relatively larger than in adults, extending well beyond the costal arch on lateral radiographs (see Figures 21-1 through 21-8). Liver margins are difficult to identify in neonates, until enough falciform fat accumulates to surround it. By 6 months or so of age, the liver has reached adult proportion, now contained within the rib cage. Hepatomegaly is not a common disease in kittens and puppies, but microhepatia secondary to portosystemic shunts is frequently encountered. In these cases, gas within the stomach helps identify the small liver by being cranially displaced.

Skeletal System

The appendicular skeletal system of the neonatal puppy and kitten presents the greatest radiographic challenge because of incomplete and rapid ongoing ossification. At birth, only primary centers of ossification of long bones (diaphyses) are visualized radiographically. None of the secondary centers of ossification are visible, as they are cartilage models (soft tissue opacity), not yet ossified. These include the epiphyses and apophyses (sites of traction, such as the olecranon or tuber calcaneus) and the cuboidal bones of the carpus and tarsus. It is important to be familiar with the location of secondary centers, as these separate bony islands may be misdiagnosed as fractures (e.g., the supraglenoid tubercle or caudal glenoid ossicle of the scapula, medial epicondyle of the distal humerus, lateral malleolus of the distal fibula, the tibial tuberosity, and the tuber calcaneal apophysis).

The relatively radiolucent cartilage model (soft tissue radiographic opacity) of ossifying secondary centers of ossification yields a radiographic appearance of widened joints and soft tissue swelling. The radiographic absence of these centers at birth, as well as the progressive appearance and

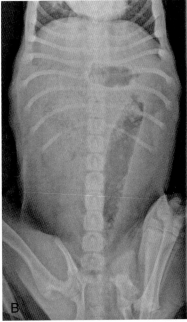

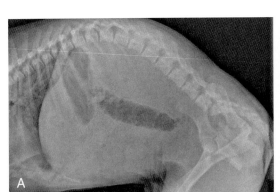

Figure 21-16 Three-month-old puppy presented after being hit by a car. Pelvic trauma was evident clinically, and abdominal radiographs were made. In this case, poor abdominal detail because of the young age of the patient must be considered and differentiated from other causes of reduced detail, namely, traumatically induced hemorrhage or rupture of the urinary system. In this scenario, the clinician must proceed with the assumption that reduced detail is present secondary to intraabdominal hemorrhage or rupture of the urinary system. **A,** Right lateral radiograph of the abdomen. The spine is arched, but fractures are not seen. Leafing of caudoventral lung margins indicates the presence of thoracic fluid, likely hemorrhage. **B,** Ventrodorsal abdominal radiograph. Multiple pelvic fractures are present.

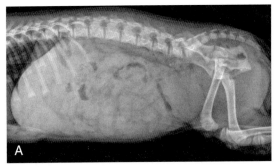

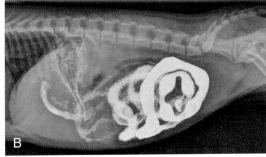

Figure 21-17 Three-month-old Yorkshire puppy presented for vomiting. A representative lateral survey radiograph **(A)** and an upper gastrointestinal examination **(B)** with liquid barium (UGI) administered via orogastric tube are presented to confirm the mildly dilated small intestine both with gas and fluid. Overall detail of the abdomen is poor but is adequate given the 3-month age of the patient. The UGI examination showed irregular intestinal mucosa and gastric mucosal retention of the barium, diagnostic for gastroenteritis. The patient had ingested holiday potpourri. Subsequent radiographs showed normal passage of barium through the intestinal tract; an obstruction was not present.

maturation of them, presents an unfamiliar appearance compared with a skeletally mature patient. Maturation occurs rapidly, with adult-like appearance by 4 months or so of age.

As the secondary centers of ossification mature, they rapidly enlarge and eventually begin to resemble their adult counterparts. The ossification can be irregular, and this appearance can be confused with pathology such as sepsis or osteochondrosis. Figure 21-18 shows an irregular

appearance of the normal humeral head bilaterally in a 4-month-old puppy; the appearance could be mistaken for osteochondrosis, a relatively common disease of juvenile dogs. In this case, the condition is an incidental finding on review of a thoracic radiograph in an asymptomatic patient.

Special attention should be given to the radiographic appearance of the skeletally immature spine. The vertebrae initially appear blocklike with very wide, lucent spaces

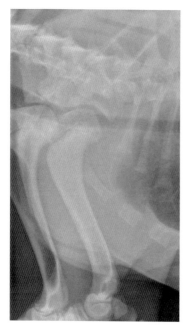

Figure 21-18 Humeral head ossification. The caudal humeral heads are misshapen and flattened in this 9-month-old giant breed dog, an incidental finding noted during a thoracic examination. This is not an uncommon radiographic appearance in larger breed dogs. Ossification will continue as the dog matures until the humeral head is radiographically normal. This normal growth pattern should be differentiated from osteochondrosis (OCD) of the humeral head. With OCD, caudal humeral head flattening is much more focal; clinical signs are usually present, the indication for the radiographic examination.

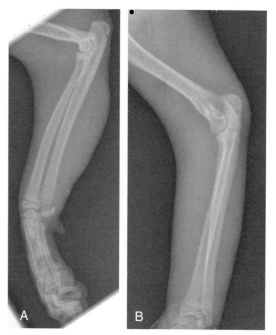

Figure 21-19 Six-month-old cat presented for right forelimb lameness and swelling. The final diagnosis was cellulitis/abscess, without underlying bony involvement. **A,** Lateral radiograph shows a large amount of soft tissue swelling of the caudal antebrachium. Underlying bony changes indicative of osteomyelitis are absent. Note the open physes of the olecranon, the distal radius, and ulna; the proximal radial physes have closed. The secondary centers of ossification are fully formed by this age. **B,** The craniocaudal view of the radius and ulna shows soft tissue swelling without underlying bony involvement. Note the fully formed epiphyses and apophysis and the open physes. The limb was positioned using tape, but the resultant image is obliqued, a result of patient restlessness and lack of sedation.

between them. As the epiphyses appear (vertebral endplates), the size and shape of the vertebrae change, becoming more rectangular. The vertebral epiphyses are initially dished, concave in shape, becoming straight with progressive ossification. The importance of noting this is that certain metabolic diseases manifest by abnormally concave endplates (e.g., hypothyroidism, growth hormone deficiency, nutritional hyperparathyroidism).

Puppy skeletal ossification can be followed in Figures 21-1 through 21-8. Table 21-1 lists the age of appearance of ossification centers and physeal closure in the dog. Table 21-2 lists this information for cats. Note that there are considerable differences between dogs and cats, as well as a considerable range of values. Also note that normal physeal closure dates can be considerably longer in some giant breed dogs and in toy breeds. Finally, breed-specific differences occur.

Once the secondary sites of ossification have matured to the point of being adult-like in appearance, the physes then become a primary focus of radiographic investigation. Diseases affecting the physes include trauma (Salter-Harris classification scheme of physeal fractures), infection, growth arrest abnormalities (e.g., carpal valgus secondary to premature distal ulnar physeal closure), or delayed closure (metabolic disorders).

Interpretation of traumatic musculoskeletal disease is usually straightforward, using comparison with the contra-lateral limb, adjacent vertebrae, and so on to aid confidence of the diagnosis. In nearly all cases of bony trauma or infection, the surrounding soft tissues will be swollen and may be radiographically perceptible even when not apparent on the physical examination. One of the roles of the radiographic examination is to rule in or rule out the presence of bony involvement when limb swelling is present (Figure 21-19). Lysis of epiphyseal or cuboidal bones rapidly occurs with septic arthritis; again, comparison with the contralateral joint is often necessary for a confident diagnosis. Fortunately, blood-borne septic arthritis and osteomyelitis are rare in puppies and kittens; most cases are a result of puncture wounds (bites), unlike the horse and ruminants.

Careful scrutiny of cortical bony margins for subtle misalignment is important in the neonatal patient, as incomplete fractures are a common occurrence because of the relatively soft and compliant bony matrix. This stresses the importance of orthogonal views of the affected limb, as subtle greenstick fractures may be visible in only one image plane.

It is important to keep in mind that trauma can cause unseen damage to the cartilage model of the physes and

Text continued on p. 191

TABLE 21-1	Age of appearance of ossification centers and physeal closure in dogs	
Anatomic sites of ossification	**Age of ossification appearance**	**Age of physeal closure**
Forelimb		
Scapula		
Body	Birth	
Supraglenoid tubercle	7-9 wk	4-7 mo
Humerus		
Diaphysis	Birth	
Proximal epiphysis	1-2 wk	10-13 mo
Distal medial condyle	2-3 wk	6-8 wk to lateral condyle
Distal lateral condyle	2-6 wk	4-6 mo to diaphysis
Medial epicondyle	6-9 wk	6 mo
Radius		
Diaphysis	Birth	
Proximal epiphysis	3-6 wk	6-11 mo
Distal epiphysis	2-4 wk	8-12 mo
Ulna		
Diaphysis	Birth	
Olecranon	7-10 wk	6-10 mo
Distal epiphysis	7-9 wk	8-12 mo
Carpus		
Proximal row*	3-5 wk	3-4 mo*
Distal row†	3-5 wk	
Accessory carpal bone body	2 wk	
Accessory carpal epiphysis	7-10 wk	4-5 mo
Metacarpus		
Diaphyses	Birth	
Distal epiphyses (metacarpi 2-5)	4-5 wk	6-7 mo
Proximal epiphysis (metacarpal 1)	5-8 wk	5-6 mo
Phalanges		
Diaphyses (first, second, third)	Birth	
First phalanx: proximal epiphyses	4-6 wk	6 mo
Second phalanx: proximal epiphyses	4-9 wk	6 mo
Dorsal sesamoid bones MCP/MTP	13-24 wk	
Palmar/plantar sesamoids MCP/MTP	8-13 wk	
Hindlimb		
Pelvis		
Ilium, ischium, pubis	Birth	4-6 mo
Acetabulum	7-12 wk	5-6 mo
Iliac crest	4-5 mo	1-2 y, sometimes never
Tuber ischii	7-12 wk	8-11 mo
Ischial arch	5-6 mo	12 mo
Caudal pubic symphysis	7 mo	5 y
Pubic symphysis		5 y

Continued

TABLE 21-1   Age of appearance of ossification centers and physeal closure in dogs—cont'd

Anatomic sites of ossification	Age of ossification appearance	Age of physeal closure
Femur		
Diaphysis	Birth	
Femoral head	2-4 wk	7-12 mo
Greater trochanter	5-7 wk	6-11 mo
Lesser trochanter	5-11 wk	8-13 mo
Distal epiphysis (medial and lateral condyles) trochlea	2-3 wk	8-11 mo to diaphysis
		3 mo trochlea to condyle
Patella	7-12 wk	
Gastrocnemius sesamoids	13-15 wk	
Popliteal sesamoid bone	18-24 wk	
Tibia	Birth	
Proximal epiphysis (medial and lateral condyles)	2-3 wk	6-12 mo to diaphysis
		6 wk to lateral condyle
Tibial tuberosity	7-11 wk	6-8 mo to condyle
		6-12 mo to diaphysis
Distal epiphysis	2-4 wk	8-11 mo
Medial malleolus	11-13 wk	4-5 mo
Fibula		
Diaphysis	Birth	
Proximal epiphysis	7-10 wk	8-12 mo
Distal epiphysis	2-7 wk	7-11 mo
Tarsus		
Calcaneus	Birth to 1 wk	
Tuber calcaneus	6-9 wk	3-8 mo
Talus	Birth to 1 wk	
Central	2-3 wk	
First	5-7 wk	
Second	4-5 wk	
Third	3-5 wk	
Fourth	2 wk	

Metatarsal and phalangeal ossification similar to forelimb

MCP, Metacarpophalangeal joint; *MTP,* metatarsophalangeal joint.

*Proximal row of carpal bones includes the radiocarpal, central carpal, and intermediate carpal that fuse to form the radiointermediate carpal bone and the ulnar carpal bone.

†Distal row of carpal bones includes the first, second, third, and fourth carpal bones.

Compiled from personal observations and from Ticer JW: *Radiographic technique in small animal practice,* Philadelphia, 1975, WB Saunders; Schebitz H, Wilkens H: *Atlas of radiographic anatomy of the dog and cat,* ed 4, Philadelphia, 1986, WB Saunders.

TABLE 21-2 Age of appearance of ossification centers and physeal closure in cats

Anatomic sites of ossification	Age of ossification appearance	Age of physeal closure
Forelimb		
Scapula		
Body	Birth	
Supraglenoid tubercle	7-14 wk	4-6 mo
Coracoid process	7-14 wk	4-6 mo
Humerus		
Diaphysis	Birth	
Proximal epiphysis	1-2 wk	22-24 mo
Distal medial condyle	4-5 wk	4-5 mo to lateral condyle
Distal lateral condyle	2-3 wk	4-7 mo to diaphysis
Medial epicondyle	7-9 wk	4-6 mo
Lateral epicondyle	7-10 wk	5-7 mo
Radius		
Diaphysis	Birth	
Proximal epiphysis	3-4 wk	5-7 mo
Distal epiphysis	3-4 wk	14-25 mo
Ulna		
Diaphysis	Birth	
Olecranon	5 wk	9-14 mo
Distal epiphysis	3-4 wk	14-23 mo
Carpus		
Proximal row*	3-6 wk	3-5 mo*
Distal row†	3-5 wk	
Accessory carpal bone body	3-4 wk	
Accessory carpal epiphysis	6-9 wk	4-7 mo
Metacarpus		
Diaphyses	Birth	
Distal epiphyses (metacarpi 2-5)	3-4 wk	7-12 mo
Proximal epiphysis (metacarpal 1)	4-6 wk	9-11 mo
Phalanges		
Diaphyses (first, second, third)	Birth	
First phalanx: proximal epiphyses	3-6 wk	4-9 mo
Second phalanx: proximal epiphyses	3-5 wk	4-9 mo
Sesamoid bones of manus	9-26 wk	
Hindlimb		
Pelvis		
Ilium, ischium, pubis	Birth	8-9 mo
Acetabulum	9-10 wk	8-9 mo
Iliac crest	6-8 mo	2 y or greater
Tuber ischium	8-10 wk	2 y or greater
Femur		
Diaphysis	Birth	
Femoral head	2 wk	7-12 mo
Greater trochanter	3 wk	7-14 mo
Lesser trochanter	2 wk	8-15 mo
Distal epiphysis	2 wk	13-20 mo

Continued

TABLE 21-2	Age of appearance of ossification centers and physeal closure in cats—cont'd	
Anatomic sites of ossification	Age of ossification appearance	Age of physeal closure
Tibia		
Diaphysis	Birth	
Proximal epiphysis	2-3 wk	13-21 mo
Tibial tuberosity	7-9 wk	13-22 mo
Distal epiphysis	2-4 wk	9-14 mo
Fibula		
Diaphysis	Birth	
Proximal epiphysis	5-9 wk	13-21 mo
Distal epiphysis	3-4 wk	9-14 mo
Tarsus		
Calcaneus	Birth	
Tuber calcaneus	5-6 wk	7-15 mo
Talus	Birth	
Central	4-6 wk	
First	4-6 wk	
Second	5-6 wk	
Third	4-6 wk	
Fourth	4-6 wk	
Metatarsus		
Diaphyses	Birth	
Distal epiphyses (metatarsi 2-5)	4 wk	7-12 mo
Phalanges		
Diaphyses (first, second, third)	Birth	
First phalanx: proximal epiphyses	3-5 wk	4-9 mo
Second phalanx: proximal epiphyses	4-5 wk	4-8 mo
Sesamoid bones	9-26 wk	
Patella	8-14 wk	
Medial gastrocnemius fabella	22-34 wk	
Lateral gastrocnemius fabella	12-20 wk	
Popliteal fabella	20-26 wk	
Metatarsophalangeal sesamoids	10-16 wk	

*Proximal row of carpal bones includes the radiocarpal, central carpal, and intermediate carpal that fuse to form the radiointermediate carpal bone and the ulnar carpal bone.

†Distal row of carpal bones includes the first, second, third, and fourth carpal bones.

Compiled from personal observations and from Schebitz H, Wilkens H: *Atlas of radiographic anatomy of the dog and cat*, ed 4, Philadelphia, 1986, WB Saunders; Smith RN: Fusion of ossification centres in the cat, *J Small Anim Pract* 10:523, 1969.

result in growth and angular limb deformities, not recognized until long after the inciting event.

Congenital or developmental skeletal disorders can be a most challenging diagnosis because the condition is generally symmetrical and/or generalized. Examples include secondary hyperparathyroidism (nutritional, renal), hypothyroidism, cartilaginous matrix disorders (the Scottish fold), and various forms of skeletal dwarfism. It is in these cases that comparison with littermates or age-matched normal animals is extremely helpful or even essential for a confident diagnosis. Figure 21-20 is an example of nutritional hyperparathyroidism in a cat presented for lameness. Multiple bony abnormalities can be identified radiographically, including generalized reduced bone opacity. Abnormal angulation of the proximal tibias is present as a result of incomplete fractures. One of the femurs is fractured proximally, and the entire femoral cortex is surrounded by bony callus. The limbs are abnormally long, and the humeri, radii, and ulnae are abnormally curved. The lumbar spine is lordotic, and the vertebral epiphyses (endplates) are markedly dished (concave) and sclerotic. The metaphyses of many of the bones are flared.

ACKNOWLEDGMENT

The author thanks Denise Waiting, LVT, for the use of her playful and cooperative Welsh Cardigan Corgi puppies. Their contribution was essential to allow readers to study progressive puppy skeletal ossification and growth.

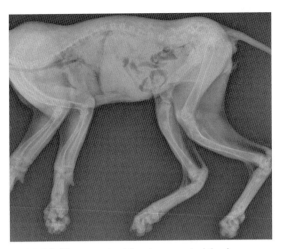

Figure 21-20 Five-month-old cat presented for lameness and unthriftiness. This whole body radiographic examination was made after long bone lesions were identified on dedicated limb radiographs because of the lameness (not shown). This case illustrates a generalized disease process of bony maturation, indicating a metabolic disorder of some type. The final diagnosis was nutritional hyperparathyroidism. This cat also had dorsally located consolidating pneumonia.

SUGGESTED READINGS

Owens JM, Biery DN: *Radiographic interpretation for the small animal clinician*, ed 2, Philadelphia, 1999, Williams & Wilkins.

Schebitz H, Wilkens H: *Atlas of radiographic anatomy of the dog and cat*, ed 4, Philadelphia, 1986, WB Saunders.

ULTRASONOGRAPHY OF THE YOUNG PATIENT

CHAPTER 22

Tomas W. Baker, Autumn P. Davidson

Pediatric dogs and cats often become veterinary patients because of signs referable to the abdominal cavity. Dietary indiscretions, parasitism, and infectious disease (primarily viral, less commonly bacterial) account for most of these presentations. Congenital and developmental disorders should be considered additionally. Abdominal ultrasound provides valuable clinical information about the pediatric peritoneal cavity, great vessels, abdominal viscera, and lymph nodes. This information is obtained in a noninvasive fashion and usually does not necessitate sedation or anesthesia in the pediatric patient. Ultrasound facilitates the initial diagnostic evaluation of the pediatric patient with signs referable to the abdominal cavity. Ultrasound equipment already in place in many small animal veterinary clinics is appropriate for most pediatric cases.

The use of ultrasound during evaluation of the pediatric patient with signs referable to the abdominal cavity provides valuable information obtained in a noninvasive fashion with no confirmed adverse biologic effects. Additionally, minimal or no sedation is generally required to complete an abdominal scan in the pediatric patient. Abdominal ultrasound provides useful data in a short time period. The normal paucity of intraabdominal fat in pediatric patients results in less informative abdominal radiography but actually improves ultrasonographic imaging. (Abdominal fat attenuates the ultrasound beam.) Image quality is improved with small patient size as a higher frequency scanhead can be used. Acquisition of special equipment for pediatric ultrasonography is usually not necessary as scanheads selected for small animal (especially feline) clinical use are appropriate for most pediatric cases.

EQUIPMENT

Pediatric dogs and cats are best evaluated using an ultrasound machine equipped with a curvilinear, phased array, blended frequency scanhead (Figure 22-1, *A*). However, an ultrasound machine with a curvilinear variable frequency scanhead (5.0 to 8.0 MHz) is also satisfactory. Many portable machines now have a high frequency linear scanhead (8.0 to 10.0 MHz) available, which improves image quality and also allows evaluation of smaller, superficial regional anatomy (e.g., thyroid, parathyroid, and cryptorchid testes) (Figure 22-1, *B*).

PREPARATION

The pediatric patient can be placed in dorsal or lateral recumbency for the study. The authors prefer dorsal recumbency within a padded V-trough, which allows less clipping of the haircoat and permits a clockwise scan of the viscera (see below). Optimally, the pediatric dog or cat is gently restrained by assistant(s) holding the forelimbs and hindlimbs (Figure 22-2). Sedation is rarely required for the basic abdominal scan unless marked pain or apprehension is present. By allowing the patient to become accustomed to this positioning before initiating clipping or scanning, struggling and resultant aerophagia are minimized.

Clipping the cranioventral abdominal hair using a No. 40 blade from the arc of the rib cage to the prepuce or pubis is advised unless the patient has scant haircoat along its ventrum. Clipping the hair and wetting the skin with water, tincture of zephiran, or 70% isopropyl alcohol followed by a liberal amount of ultrasound gel permits the best acoustic coupling of the scanhead to the patient, improving the image obtained. The application of 70% alcohol in particular removes cutaneous sebum and dirt and moistens the remaining hair shaft. Care should be taken to avoid excessive chilling of pediatric patients secondary to the application of room temperature liquids followed by evaporation. Electric warming devices (warm water or air blankets) may cause electronic interference with the ultrasound equipment; warm water bottles or their equivalent do not produce such artifact to the image and are superior.

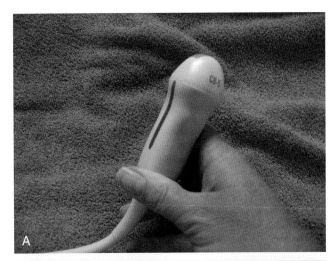

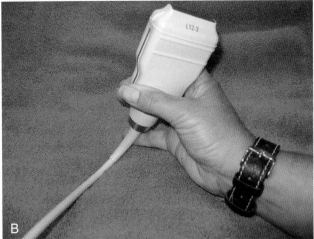

Figure 22-1 A, Curvilinear variable frequency scanhead. **B,** High frequency linear scanhead.

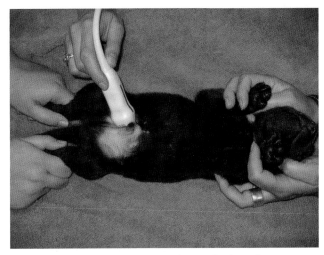

Figure 22-2 Positioning the pediatric patient.

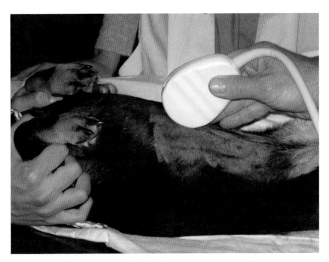

Figure 22-3 Sagittal scanning of the liver.

Fasting the pediatric patient before abdominal ultrasound minimizes gastric ingesta obscuring imaging of the liver and pancreas, as well as gastrointestinal gas accumulation interfering with visualization of other abdominal viscera. Very young dogs and cats should not be fasted for longer than 2 hours. If hypoglycemia is a clinical concern (e.g., toy breeds, sepsis, hepatopathies), an oral balanced electrolyte and glucose solution is superior to food as it will actually displace gas within the gastric lumen. Preventing urination immediately before the examination allows better evaluation of the urinary bladder contents and wall, and provides an acoustic window for the sublumbar region.

Serial evaluations can provide useful information when the clinical status of the pediatric patient has changed or when clinicopathologic deterioration has occurred. Progressive lethargy or obtundation, acute pain, changes in abdominal palpation, and refractory vomiting or diarrhea warrant timely repeat evaluation for ultrasonographic signs that could indicate intussusception, perforation, and/or peritonitis have developed.

THE NORMAL ABDOMEN

Regardless of the clinical history, the abdomen should be evaluated methodically. With the animal in dorsal recumbency, place the scanhead under the xyphoid with the beam in the sagittal plane (Figure 22-3). Visualization of the liver is best achieved by adjusting the depth of the image to include the hyperechoic arc of the diaphragm. Then, in the sagittal plane, pointing the beam toward the patient's right elbow allows visualization of the gall bladder. Fanning the beam from the right to the left elbow maximizes visualization of the liver in the sagittal plane. The gall bladder is seen on the right; the left liver lobes are seen ventral to the stomach. The ultrasonographic appearance of the normal hepatic parenchyma permits differentiation of portal and hepatic vessels. The gall bladder should be thin walled and the fluid within very anechoic. Size can be variable and is usually not correlated with clinical disease in the young animal. The normal-sized liver does not extend caudally beyond the stomach. Turning the beam to transverse allows for visualization of the liver between the gall bladder and stomach. This view is good for evaluation of the hepatic border at its interface with the falciform fat in the near field, echogenicity of hepatic parenchyma, and portal architecture. The portal vessels have very echogenic walls compared with the hepatic veins (Figure 22-4).

After completing evaluation of the liver, resume the sagittal plane; scan clockwise to the upper left quadrant of the patient past the stomach to the spleen. The spleen will be visualized ventrally along the left body wall in the near field. Splenic border, parenchyma, echogenicity, and shape should be evaluated. Splenic parenchyma should be more echogenic and have a more homogeneous echotexture than liver. A transverse image of the spleen can be obtained by scanning to the caudal edge of the left rib cage and pointing cranially in cross-section. This transverse view evaluates the spleen as it follows the left body wall (Figure 22-5).

Following the spleen transversely down the left body wall, you will see the left kidney. Once visualization of the kidney is achieved, turn to the sagittal plane and produce a long axis view of the left kidney. Now evaluate the renal border, cortex echogenicity, corticomedullary interface, and pelvic architecture (Figure 22-6). Dilation of the renal pelvis should be

evaluated and confirmed in both scan planes. The transverse image is best for confirmation of renal pelvic dilation (Figure 22-7). The left adrenal gland is located medial to the left kidney anywhere along its length. Isolation of the left adrenal gland is best achieved by locating the linear aorta and the branching arteries (celiac, cranial mesenteric, and renal). In the sagittal plane, with strong hand pressure, sweep medially from the left kidney to find the aorta. Now find the branching renal artery. The left adrenal gland is located cranial to the left renal artery and caudal to the left cranial mesenteric artery. The left adrenal gland is visualized as a bilobed structure with the phrenicoabdominal vein at its waist (Figure 22-8). This completes evaluation of the upper left abdominal quadrant.

Now with a transverse beam placed perpendicularly in the middle of the abdomen, scan caudally to a large hypoechoic structure, the urinary bladder. Evaluate the ventral bladder wall and urinary bladder lumen contents, and then the dorsal bladder wall. The normal bladder wall is uniform in thickness, and the contents are anechoic. The major vessels (caudal vena cava and aorta) will be located dorsal to the bladder, seen as two large black discs. Sublumbar lymph nodes can be seen at the aortic bifurcation into the iliac arteries, adjacent to the dorsal urinary bladder wall (Figure 22-9, *A*). Sagittal scanning of the urinary bladder

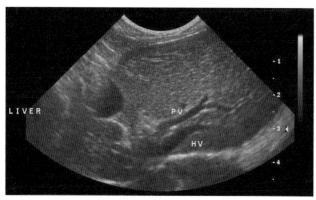

Figure 22-4 Portal veins have hyperechoic wall; hepatic vessels do not. *PV,* Portal vein; *HV,* hepatic vein.

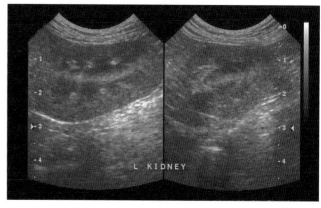

Figure 22-6 Normal kidney, sagittal and transverse.

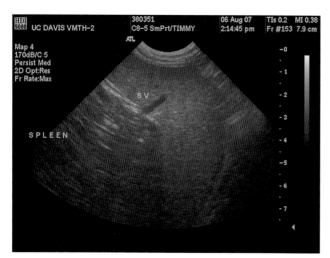

Figure 22-5 Transverse spleen along left body wall.

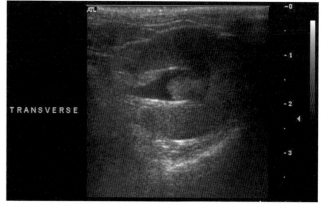

Figure 22-7 Transverse kidney with pelvic dilation.

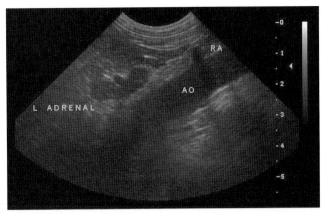

Figure 22-8 Left adrenal gland cranial to renal artery. *AO*, Aorta; *RA*, renal artery.

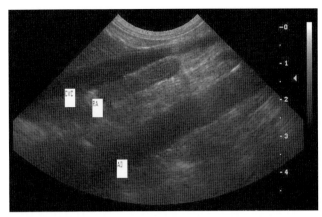

Figure 22-10 Normal right adrenal gland. *CVC*, Caudal vena cava; *RA*, right adrenal gland; *AO*, aorta.

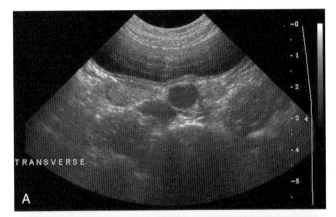

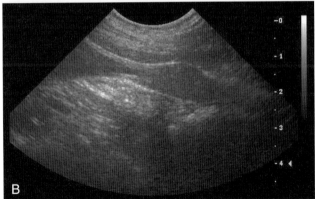

Figure 22-9 A, Transverse urinary bladder with major vessels and sublumbar node. **B,** Normal puppy prostate.

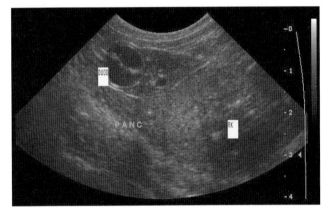

Figure 22-11 Normal right pancreas. *PANC*, Pancreas; *RK*, right kidney; *DUOD*, duodenum.

a fanning technique, as well as the scanhead pointed slightly cranially, the major vessels (vena cava and aorta) will be visualized as two hypoechoic ribbons running across the image from the 8 o'clock position to the 2 o'clock position. The right adrenal gland can be located, visualized, and evaluated for size and shape just lateral to the caudal vena cava (Figure 22-10).

In the transverse plane, return to the right kidney and lateral to the kidney, the duodenum. In the dog, at the cranial pole of the kidney adjacent to the duodenum will be the right limb of the pancreas. The right pancreatic limb border may not be seen but is identified by visualizing the caudal pancreaticoduodenal vein (Figure 22-11). Turning to the sagittal plane, follow the pancreas, scanning medially to the angle of the body and left limb. The pancreatic body is seen caudal to the stomach and cranial to the splenic vein. The left limb of the pancreas is found caudal to the splenic vein and midline to the cranial pole of the left kidney (Figure 22-12). In the cat, in the sagittal plane, the right limb of the pancreas is identified just caudal to the duodenum, which is itself caudal to the gall bladder. Localizing the feline right pancreatic limb varies because the feline duodenum is situated more medially with more cranial flexure than in the canine (Figure 22-13). The normal pancreas is usually not

caudally allows visualization of the urethra (and prostate in the male) (Figure 22-9, *B*).

Evaluation of the upper right abdominal quadrant should include the right kidney, right adrenal, duodenum, and right limb of the pancreas. The right kidney is found at the edge of the right rib cage in the renal fossa of the liver. Obtain images of the right kidney in the sagittal and transverse scan planes. The right kidney should be evaluated as was the left kidney (i.e., renal border, cortical echogenicity, corticomedullary interface, and pelvic architecture). By scanning sagitally between the right kidney and the caudal vena cava with

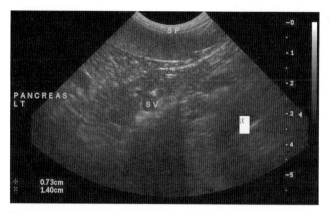

Figure 22-12 Left limb of the pancreas (cursors). *SP*, Spleen; *SV*, splenic vein; *LK*, left kidney.

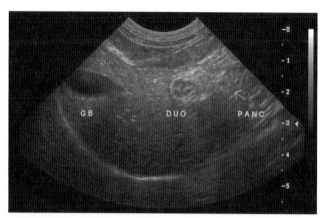

Figure 22-13 Normal feline pancreas *(arrow)*, right limb. *GB*, Gall bladder; *DUO*, duodenum; *PANC*, pancreas.

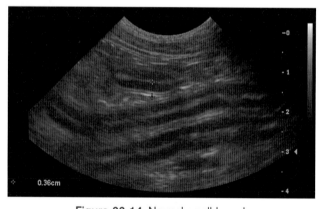

Figure 22-14 Normal small bowel.

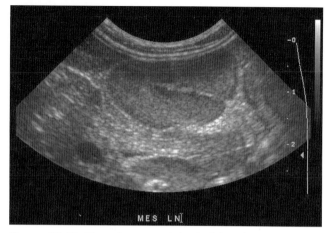

Figure 22-15 Normal puppy abdominal lymph nodes. *MES*, Mesenteric; *LN*, lymph nodes.

the submucosa, which should be 2 times thicker than the muscularis. Outside the muscularis is a bright line, the serosa subserosa. It may take two to three transverse passes with the scanhead perpendicular to the body wall to adequately evaluate the entire midabdomen in a uniform fashion. Having completed the entire abdominal scan, now return to regions of clinical interest using a higher frequency scanhead to improve image quality, and reaffirm changes with documentation (e.g., hardcopy images, videotape).

GASTROINTESTINAL DISEASE

Gastrointestinal signs are a frequent reason for presentation of pediatric patients to a veterinarian. Dietary indiscretion, foreign body ingestion, intestinal parasitism, and infectious (usually bacterial or viral) disease are all common causes for vomiting and diarrhea in the pediatric patient. Physical examination findings, fecal examination for parasites and viral antigens, fecal culture for pathogenic bacteria, and abdominal radiography can all contribute diagnostic information. Abdominal ultrasonography provides additional and complementary information about the presence or absence of fluid in the peritoneal cavity, appearance of gastrointestinal contents, gastrointestinal tract motility, gastrointestinal wall morphology, and mesenteric lymph node appearance and size. Mesenteric lymphadenomegaly is common and not necessarily abnormal in the pediatric patient (Figure 22-15).

Acquired Gastrointestinal Disorders
Gastroenterocolitis

Mild to moderate thickening of the gastrointestinal wall with preservation of wall layering and moderate mesenteric lymphadenomegaly are the most common ultrasonographic findings with nonspecific pediatric gastroenterocolitis, such as that resulting from dietary indiscretion. More severe pathology, such as extensive bowel edema or hemorrhage accompanying infectious gastroenterocolitis, can be associated with changes in fluid volume within the bowel lumen, wall thickening, and loss of normal wall layer ratios. These

well visualized because its acoustic impedance is similar to the surrounding mesentery.

Returning to the transverse plane in the midabdomen, find the major vessels (midline to the kidneys) at the mesenteric root, and scan for the mesenteric lymph nodes around the vessels. Recall that young animals will normally have more visible mesenteric lymph nodes. Evaluate the small bowel for morphology and changes in wall layer ratios (Figure 22-14). The mucosal layer (the thickest black layer outside the lumen) should be 3 times thicker than

changes can be regional or diffuse. Fluid distention of the bowel with generalized decreased motility can be seen with functional ileus accompanying gastroenterocolitis (Figure 22-16).

Intussusception

Intussusception is not uncommon in young dogs and cats, occurring most frequently at the ileocolic junction in dogs and in the jejunum in cats. The classic transverse ultrasonographic appearance of intussusception is a multilayered series of concentric rings representing the invaginated bowel wall layers; the outer layer can be edematous (hypoechoic), and the inner layers may be more normal in appearance (Figure 22-17). Discomfort is typically displayed when scanhead pressure is placed over the affected area of bowel. Doppler evaluation of the bowel and associated mesenteric vessels can provide information about bowel viability. Usually by the time an intussusception is diagnosed in the pediatric veterinary patient, resection rather than reduction is necessary; however, an intussusception can be transient.

Foreign Bodies

Unless radiopaque, gastrointestinal foreign bodies are difficult to confirm radiographically; they are usually suspected clinically based on intraluminal gas and fluid accumulation proximal to the mechanical obstruction caused by

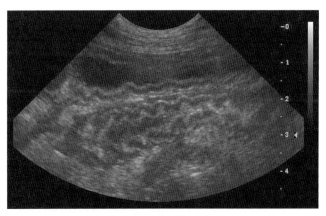

Figure 22-16 Enteritis.

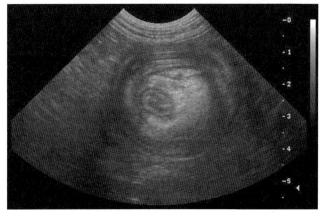

Figure 22-17 Intussusception.

their presence. Ultrasonography can provide supportive information and sometimes confirm the diagnosis if the foreign body has characteristic appearance (such as a ball, a trichobezoar, or a linear foreign body). Typically, a bright interface associated with strong shadowing suggests a foreign body. Fluid dilation proximal to or surrounding the object enhances evidence for a foreign body. Balls have a rounded interface with uniform acoustic shadowing. Trichobezoars have irregular bright interfaces and strong shadowing. Linear foreign bodies produce bowel plication recognized as undulation or corrugation of the bowel wall. Because foreign bodies produce focal bowel abnormalities, effort should be made to localize and follow normal bowel into the area of concern (Figure 22-18).

Congenital Gastrointestinal Disorders

Pyloric stenosis secondary to hypertrophic gastritis has been reported in a pediatric dog. Focal circumferential thickening of the pylorus primarily involving the muscularis is typical.

Enteric duplication or agenesis can be confirmed ultrasonographically in pediatric patients. Duplication is rare and can occur anywhere in the intestinal tract; the clinical signs may be nonspecific. A fluid-filled juxtaintestinal formation with variable peristalsis and contents can be seen. Enteric agenesis usually results in severe clinical signs in the neonatal period. Ultrasonographic findings usually include marked fluid and gas distention of bowel proximal to the defect.

Congenital peritoneopericardial diaphragmatic hernias occur in both the dog and cat; ultrasonography provides an additional modality for their diagnosis. As with other diaphragmatic hernias, careful evaluation for continuity of the echogenic diaphragm differentiates a true hernia from mirror image artifacts. Evaluation of the pericardial contents can be made from the subcostal (across the liver) or intercostal (using the heart as an acoustic window) approach. Abnormal pericardial contents can include falciform fat, liver, gall bladder, and/or small bowel.

Congenital inguinal hernias can similarly be confirmed by ultrasonographic identification of small bowel in the subcutaneous space of the affected groin. This can be a dynamic finding. Mesenteric fat may alternatively be entrapped through the hernia.

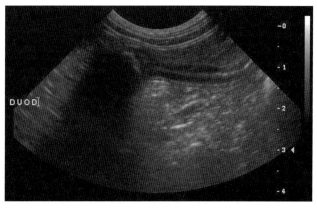

Figure 22-18 Duodenal foreign body. *DUOD*, Duodenum.

Congenital hiatal hernias are more difficult to confirm with ultrasound because of the inherent difficulty imaging the gas-filled stomach and the intermittent nature of the disorder. Stomach wall with characteristic rugal folds can be imaged crossing the diaphragm into the thoracic cavity. Fluoroscopic evaluation can be more informative in these cases.

Congenital Body Wall Evisceration (Celosomy)

A developmental anomaly resulting in extrusion of a portion of the gastrointestinal tract outside of the body wall, occurring within the umbilical canal (omphalocele) or lateral to the umbilical canal (gastroschisis), has been reported in humans and occurs in both dogs and cats. The condition is usually hopeless in small pediatric patients presented to the veterinarian hours after birth; however, a 30% to 70% survival rate is reported in humans with immediate postpartum surgical intervention. Diagnosis is made prepartum with abdominal ultrasound, based on the recognition of fetal gastric wall (rugal) structures or intestinal contents in an abnormal location. Earlier surgical intervention before inevitable septic contamination occurs may improve the prognosis in veterinary patients.

Congenital Portosystemic Shunts

Ultrasonography provides a rapid and noninvasive method for screening patients suspected to have congenital portosystemic shunts. Although scintigraphy is considered the most reliable noninvasive method of documenting a portosystemic shunt, its availability is limited to specialty and university practices, and its use dictates special handling of the radioactive patient for at least 12 hours. The liver may be small and difficult to image in patients with congenital portosystemic shunts. Imaging the liver from the standard ventral approach can be improved in some cases by using the left ventral intercostal and right dorsal intercostal approaches. The presence of ascites can facilitate the study, as can the addition of fluid to the stomach, as well as positioning the patient to shift gas away from the scanhead and shift abdominal organs caudally. Ultrasound evaluation of portosystemic anomalies can be facilitated by positive pressure ventilation under anesthesia for the same reason. Postoperatively, ultrasound can be used to evaluate portal blood flow following surgical banding or coil embolization. Extrahepatic shunts most commonly arise from the portal vein, splenic vein, or left gastric vein in the dog and from the left gastric vein in the cat (Figure 22-19). Identification of a shunting vessel emptying into the caudal vena cava is difficult but confirmatory. Intrahepatic shunts can be difficult to identify because of patient size, bowel gas, and liver size. Clipping the haircoat intercostally on the right can allow for transverse vessel stacking (aorta, vena cava, and portal vein) and visualization of ductal shunts (Figure 22-20). There can be right and left shunting of the ductus.

Traumatic Disorders

Traumatic diaphragmatic herniation can result in the presence of stomach, liver, spleen, small bowel, and falciform fat

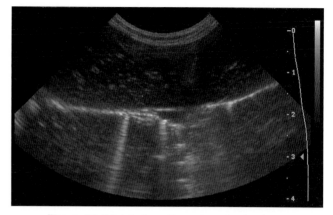

Figure 22-19 Intrahepatic portosystemic shunt.

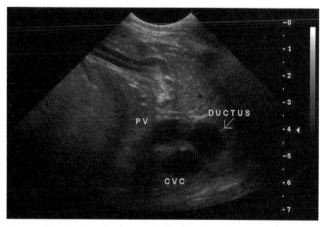

Figure 22-20 Stacked vessels facilitating visualization of portosystemic shunt (ductus). *PV,* Portal vein; *CVC,* caudal vena cava.

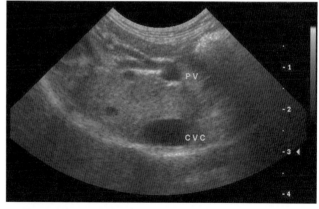

Figure 22-21 "Comet tail" artifact along the diaphragm.

in the thorax, usually accompanied by effusion of fluid, enhancing imaging. Failure to identify a contiguous diaphragmatic image supports the diagnosis. A comet tail artifact cranial to the diaphragm can occur with diaphragmatic disruption accompanied by pleural effusion; thoracic radiography is indicated (Figure 22-21). Positive contrast peritoneography can be used to confirm the diagnosis if ultrasound findings are not conclusive.

Blunt trauma resulting in hemoabdomen is best evaluated with ultrasound. Rupture or crushing trauma to the liver or infarction of the spleen is readily differentiated from normal homogeneous parenchyma. The localization and normal appearance of fluid-filled viscera (urinary bladder, gall bladder) can be reassuring but do not eliminate the possibility of an occult rupture; serial evaluation is advised along with the accumulation of clinical data (e.g., peritoneal fluid evaluation).

GENITOURINARY DISEASE

Young dogs and cats are commonly presented to the veterinarian for perceived genitourinary system disorders. Although gastrointestinal disorders account for most acute presentations, perceived urogenital disorders account for many others. Clinical differentiation between the characteristics of normal pediatric housebreaking with immature renal function and true urogenital disease can be challenging.

Acquired Disorders of the Genitourinary System
Urinary Tract Infection

Puppies are frequently presented to the veterinarian because of owner concerns about difficulty achieving housebreaking and the perception that urination is excessively frequent (pollakiuria). Historical differentiation between a history of true pollakiuria and dysuria associated with cystourethritis and the normal frequency of urination in pediatric dogs with immature renal concentrating abilities can be difficult. A urinalysis/urine culture, with urine obtained by ultrasound-guided cystocentesis can be diagnostic. The bladder can appear normal in those with acute urinary tract infection. Chronic urinary tract infection can induce bladder wall thickening (greater than 1 to 2 mm in a fully distended bladder), especially in the cranioventral portion of the bladder. Similarly, early pyelonephritis can have a normal ultrasonographic appearance; chronic pyelonephritis can produce a dilated renal pelvis, sometimes accompanied by a bright line at the interface, indicating chronicity. Chronic pyelonephritis can also be characterized by irregular renal contour, reduction in renal size, increased cortical echogenicity, and poor corticomedullary definition (Figure 22-22).

Urolithiasis

Cystic calculi (radiopaque or radiolucent), visualized as discrete hyperechoic focal echogenicities in the dependent portion of the bladder, occur most commonly in pediatric patients with urinary tract infection (struvite or triple phosphate uroliths) or portosystemic shunts (ammonium biurate uroliths) (Figure 22-23). Care should be taken not to misinterpret colonic gas as cystic calculi; repositioning the patient should permit differentiation. The presence of a cystic calculus without urinary tract infection in the pediatric patient should prompt evaluation for developmental hepatic

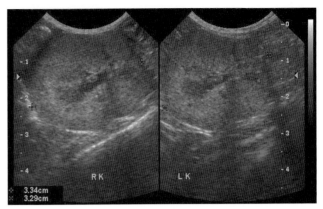

Figure 22-22 Chronic pyelonephritis. *RK*, Right kidney; *LK*, left kidney.

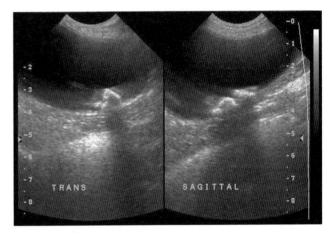

Figure 22-23 Urinary calculi. *TRANS*, Transverse and sagittal views.

vascular anomalies. With the exception of Dalmatians, both urinary tract infection and cystic calculi are more common in female pediatric patients.

Renal Toxicity

Ingestion of nephrotoxic substances (e.g., ethylene glycol, mushrooms, grapes, and raisins) occurs in pediatric canine patients most commonly, less frequently in young felines. Abdominal ultrasound is indicated in uremic patients. Nephrotoxicity from ethylene glycol has characteristic ultrasonographic changes. The renal cortex becomes maximally hyperechoic (the classic expectation for ethylene glycol toxicity) 24 hours postingestion, but a medullary rim sign can be seen as early as 8 hours following ingestion. Ascites and pelvic dilation can be present secondary to aggressive fluid administration and resultant overhydration. Ethylene glycol toxicity does not cause renal morphologic changes; instead it increases the echogenicity of the parenchyma of the cortex. This should help differentiate patients with congenital severe renal dysplasia from those with nephrotoxicities (Figures 22-24 and 22-25).

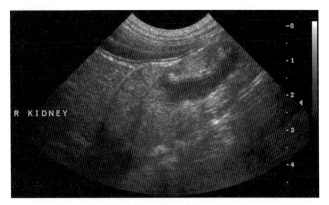

Figure 22-24 Renal dysplasia.

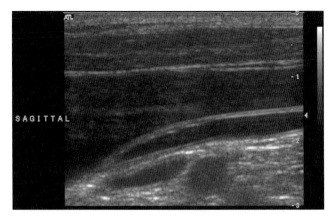

Figure 22-26 Ectopic ureter dorsal to the urinary bladder.

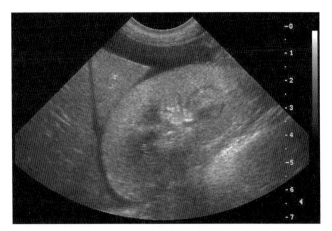

Figure 22-25 Ethylene glycol toxicity.

Ectopic Ureter

Congenital ectopic placement of the distal ureter into the urethra, vestibule, or vagina is usually associated with ureteral dilation and eventually with renal pelvic dilation. Dilation of the ureter improves the sensitivity of the ultrasound study; however, the diagnosis can be elusive. Visualization of a nonvascular, fluid-filled structure with a thin, hyperechoic wall passing dorsal to the urinary bladder or obvious insertion of the structure into the proximal urethra suggests the diagnosis. Monitoring such a structure for a few moments for peristalsis (unique to the ureter) can be rewarding. Visualization of the ureteral jets in the bladder suggests normalcy; however, some ectopic ureters insert initially into the bladder and additionally tunnel distally to terminate in an abnormal site. Visualization of the dilated ureter usually occurs near the urinary bladder (Figure 22-26). Visualization of the bladder neck and proximal urethra may be obscured by pubic bone, making identification of such termination difficult.

Hydronephrosis can eventually result from an uncorrected ectopic ureter caused by flow impedance at the abnormal site of insertion. Urinary tract infection is commonly associated with ectopia, resulting from accompanying urethral sphincter mechanism anomalies, and if not detected and treated, can progress to pyelonephritis and ureteritis. Infection and its associated inflammation in the tract can further alter the ultrasonographic appearance of the kidneys, bladder, ureters, and urethra (see below).

Contrast-enhanced computed tomography is the most sensitive and specific modality for the diagnosis of ectopia but, like double contrast radiography, requires anesthesia, making initial evaluation with ultrasound desirable when ectopia is suspected clinically. The condition is thought to be heritable and is more common in females.

Ureterocele

A ureterocele is an uncommon congenital dilation of the ureter near the bladder, appearing as a cystic structure within the bladder lumen or wall (Figure 22-27). The ureterocele occurs most commonly in association with an ectopic ureter. Diagnosis can be made by scanning the urinary bladder in

Congenital Disorders of the Genitourinary System
Renal Agenesis

Congenital renal agenesis resulting in the absence of a kidney can be confirmed with ultrasound. The contralateral kidney typically has normal internal anatomy but is enlarged as a consequence of obligatory hypertrophy. Renal function of the pediatric patient does not equal that of the adult until 4 to 6 months of age; compensatory renomegaly may not be apparent until that time.

Renal Dysplasia

Until reliable genetic markers are available for all the various breed-specific congenital renal dysplasias, ultrasound provides the best method of screening young dogs and cats for these likely heritable disorders. Screening should take place before puppy or kitten placement. Early ultrasonographic screening is possible in breeds in which morphologic changes are grossly evident (i.e., Persian and other platycephalic cats, Cairn Terriers, German Shepherd Dogs). Dysplastic kidneys tend to be lobular and misshapen with thickened cortices and poor corticomedullary interface. Differentiation between dysplastic kidneys and chronic pyelonephritis can be difficult without clinical input (e.g., age, urinalysis, and urine culture).

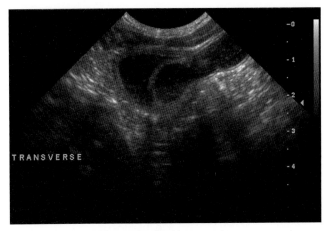

Figure 22-27 Ureterocele.

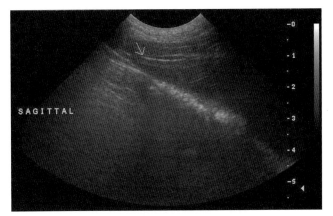

Figure 22-28 Patent urachus *(arrow)*.

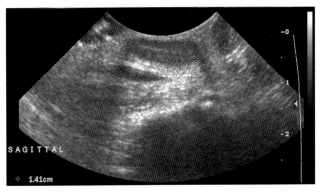

Figure 22-29 Abdominal testicle (cursors) showing hyperechoic slash (median testis).

the transverse plane and watching for strong peristalsis of the adjacent ureter.

Patent Urachus

The urachus permits the flow of urine from the bladder into the allantoic sac of the fetus and normally atrophies at birth. A patent urachus in the neonate is characterized clinically by urine dribbling from the umbilicus. The fluid-filled urachus can be identified ultrasonographically, extending cranially from the cranioventral bladder wall (Figure 22-28). If an incompletely patent urachus is present in the neonate, a urachal diverticulum may result, seen as a divot in the apex of the bladder. Urachal diverticula can predispose the bladder

to recurrent infection because of abnormal bladder flow in the region; surgical excision can be indicated.

Cryptorchidism

Ultrasound localization of cryptorchid testes can confirm the condition in pediatric patients with bilateral involvement whose neutering status is unknown, and assist the surgeon in planning the approach (i.e., inguinal vs. cranial abdominal). Ultrasound can also be helpful in identifying the position of the unilateral cryptorchid testis (whose laterality was identified from palpation and reduction of the scrotal testis to its inguinal ring). A retained testis can be positioned anywhere between the ipsilateral kidney and the scrotum. A common location is between the inguinal canal and the parapreputial subcutis. A systematic evaluation of the region from the caudal renal pole to the inguinal canal can identify an oval, homogeneously echogenic structure with a mildly hyperechoic border representing the parietal and visceral tunics. The epididymis is usually distinctly less echoic than the testicular parenchyma, as in the scrotal testis. The cryptorchid testis will maintain the anatomic structure, the median testes (a hyperechoic slash), and normal testicular echogenicity despite being reduced in size compared with a scrotal testis. Use of a higher frequency linear scanhead can improve image quality to help identify testicular anatomy (Figure 22-29).

SUGGESTED READING

Nyland TG, Mattoon JS: *Small animal diagnostic ultrasound,* ed 2, Philadelphia, 2002, Saunders/Elsevier.

ANESTHESIA IN THE PEDIATRIC PATIENT

CHAPTER 23

Craig A.E. Mosley, Cornelia Mosley

Anesthetizing newborn or very young patients is not uncommon in small animal practice and, when necessary, presents the veterinarian with a unique challenge. Anesthetic procedures may be performed for the correction of life-threatening congenital abnormalities or complications arising during the first weeks of life (e.g., fractures, congenital abnormalities, diaphragmatic hernia), diagnostic procedures, or early spay/neuter surgeries. Cosmetic procedures (e.g., tail docking, ear cropping) may also be performed at this age, but fortunately many of these procedures have become less popular because of ethical and humane concerns.

Several definitions have been given for the neonatal and pediatric phases as they pertain to anesthesia. Small animal patients are considered neonates for the purposes of anesthesia for the first 6 weeks and pediatric patients until 12 weeks old. During the first 12 weeks and beyond, there is a continuum of developmental changes. It is important to consider the impact of these physiologic and anatomic changes on anesthetic management of these patients. In addition, it is important to note that the rate of organ maturity varies among species (dogs, cats), breeds, and individuals; therefore time estimates for organ maturity and development should be viewed only as guidelines and not values with absolute meaning. The organ systems of greatest importance for anesthesia include the cardiovascular, respiratory, hepatic, renal, thermoregulatory, and central nervous systems. Although we normally think of the central nervous system as being relatively immature in neonates, it is now recognized that early nociceptive and painful events can lead to long-term alterations in central pain processing. Therefore it is important that we not only think of the central nervous system in terms of depression and anesthesia but also in terms of pain and nociception.

PHYSIOLOGIC AND PHARMACOLOGIC CONSIDERATIONS FOR PEDIATRIC ANIMALS DURING ANESTHESIA

Cardiovascular System

The cardiovascular system undergoes enormous alterations shortly after birth, from fetal to adult circulation. These changes normally occur without incident in the first days of life, but remnants of fetal circulation may persist (e.g., patent ductus arteriosus, patent foramen ovale), and other congenital heart defects may be detected as heart murmurs during routine auscultation. If a significant murmur is present, additional diagnostics and/or medical intervention may be required before anesthesia.

In general, higher heart rates and lower blood pressure should be expected for the first 4 to 12 weeks compared with adult animals. The cardiovascular system is characterized as a low-pressure system resulting from the lower myocardial contractile mass, decreased ventricular compliance, and a relatively immature autonomic nervous system found in young animals. Normal awake mean blood pressures can be 20 to 40 mm Hg lower than those in adult animals. Consequently lower blood pressures are often tolerated during anesthesia in neonates compared with adults. There are no good guidelines as to what an acceptable blood pressure is in anesthetized neonate and pediatric patients. Current guidelines are based on the lower blood pressure limits for renal autoregulation in adults. The pressure limits for renal autoregulation in neonate and pediatric patients have not been established. However, the authors will often accept mean blood pressures above 40 to 50 mm Hg in neonates and above 50 to 60 mm Hg in pediatrics as being adequate.

The low ventricular compliance may lead to less tolerance for changes (increases and decreases) in preload. Preload is frequently increased by the administration of intravascular fluids and should be maintained without administering excessive fluids to optimize cardiac output and organ perfusion. The immaturity of the autonomic nervous system leads to an impaired ability to change systemic vascular resistance, as well as cardiac contractility in response to cardiovascular challenges (i.e., dehydration and blood loss). Hence the neonate is often incapable of compensating for the vasodilatory effects of commonly used anesthetic drugs (i.e., inhalant anesthetics, acepromazine). In addition, drugs normally used to support the cardiovascular system through their effects on the autonomic nervous system, such as sympathomimetics (dopamine, dobutamine) and parasympatholytics (atropine, glycopyrrolate), are less effective.

Neonates also have higher oxygen consumption, and hence relative cardiac output is greater. Because the neonate and pediatric patient have little means to increase cardiac output through changes in cardiac contractility or alterations in preload, the preservation of cardiac output primarily depends on the maintenance of a relatively elevated heart rate and low system vascular resistance. Drugs that impact these parameters, such as α-2 agonists, are probably best avoided.

Hemoglobin concentrations are usually lower than those of adults because hematopoietic potential does not reach adult levels until around 2 to 3 months. Erythrocyte production is lower with a shorter lifespan. Further, hemodilution is present as a result of an expanding blood volume during that time. However, at birth, hemoglobin levels are actually high with a high percentage of fetal hemoglobin (70% to 80%), and then they decrease as a result of low erythrocyte production.

Respiratory System

The respiratory system changes from neonate to adult are gradual but significant. Pediatric patients have a twofold to threefold higher tissue oxygen demand relative to body weight compared with adults. Pediatric animals commonly have a higher resting respiratory rate because of the elevated oxygen demand. The tidal volume of neonates is similar to adults, but the functional residual capacity (FRC) is lower. The reduced FRC may hasten the development of hypoxia during breath holding in neonates compared with adults.

The work of breathing in neonates is increased as a result of elevated airflow resistance caused by the narrow-diameter airways and the pliable chest wall (increased compliance). Neonates are more susceptible to the muscle-relaxing effects of anesthetics. This contributes to respiratory fatigue and hypoventilation. Assisted ventilation is often necessary in pediatric patients, and capnography can be useful for assessing the ventilatory status of the animal. Finally, ventilatory control in neonates is relatively immature with a decreased responsiveness of the carotid body chemoreceptors to hypoxemia. The neonate and pediatric patient is more prone to developing hypoxia and hypercapnia in the perianesthetic period, and careful attention to respiration, proper respiratory monitoring, and preoxygenation before the induction of anesthesia are all recommended to minimize these risks.

Hepatic and Renal System

The hepatic microsomal and cytochrome P450 enzyme systems are functionally immature for the first 4 to 5 months in pediatric patients. This can lead to slowed elimination of highly metabolized drugs such as nonsteroidal antiinflammatory drugs (NSAIDs) and benzodiazepines. In the case of benzodiazepines, slowed metabolism is likely to be of little clinical significance (for moderately prolonged mild sedation) if only a single dose is used in the perianesthetic period. However, with the repeat administration of drugs with potentially significant side effects (such as NSAIDs), accumulation and toxicities are possible. In general, it is common practice to avoid drugs requiring major hepatic metabolism in neonates or to significantly increase the dosing intervals.

Lower concentrations of plasma albumin are also present for the initial 8 to 12 weeks of life. This can be an important consideration for highly protein-bound drugs, which may exert a greater clinical effect as a result of the higher quantities of unbound or active drug in the plasma. However, this is rarely observed clinically with the commonly used anesthetic-related drugs. This may be in part because most intravenous anesthetic drugs are titrated to effect rather than administered as a single intravenous bolus dose.

Neonates and pediatric patients have little glycogen storage capacity. Therefore excessive fasting before or delays in feeding after anesthesia should be avoided to prevent hypoglycemia. Renal function is also less developed for the first 2 to 8 weeks and is characterized by a decreased glomerular filtration rate, low renal blood flow, and a low concentrating ability. Urine-specific gravity is lower, whereas urine protein and glucose may be higher. In general, this means that during this period of life, animals may not be capable of tolerating large fluid loads and do not have the ability to conserve fluids when faced with decreased intake. Careful attention to hydration status is very important in the perianesthetic period. Because it is sometimes more difficult to assess hydration in neonates based on clinical signs such as skin tenting, serial weight assessments and careful assessment of the volume of fluid administered versus the volume of fluid lost should be made.

Thermoregulation

Pediatric patients have a large surface area–to–body mass ratio and lack significant insulating body fat, predisposing them to hypothermia. In the perianesthetic period, young patients are even more susceptible to hypothermia because of the effects of the anesthetic agents on the thermoregulatory center and loss of peripheral vasomotor tone. During anesthesia, the production of heat is reduced (decreased muscular activity, inability to shiver), and the loss of heat through conduction, convection, evaporation, and radiation is facilitated. All these factors make hypothermia in the perianesthetic period likely. The use of techniques to minimize heat loss (e.g., warm tables, insulation, minimize use of cold fluids, active rewarming—forced warm air, circulating water blankets) should be used preemptively throughout the perianesthetic period. Side effects associated with hypothermia include cardiovascular alterations (bradycardia, hypotension, decreased cardiac output, and arrhythmias), prolonged recovery times and drug metabolism, as well as increased infection rate and decreased wound healing.

Central Nervous System

The central nervous system matures progressively during the first 6 to 8 weeks, with the central nervous system of cats maturing more rapidly than dogs. The peripheral nervous system of dogs may take up to a year to fully develop. Very little is known about the functional level (i.e., consciousness, sensory, and motor coordination) of the central nervous system in dogs and cats. For example, initially it was believed that neonates were incapable of feeling pain. However, it is now known that early pain experiences, such as dewclaw removal, may be associated with an exaggerated pain response later in life in some animals. Pain is generally defined as a sensory and/or an emotional experience associated with tissue damage, and perception of this sensation occurs in the cortex of mammals. Because neonates have questionable cortical activity and sensory coordination, it was believed that neonates do not "feel" pain. However, nociception, the physiological components leading to the sensation and the "feeling" of pain, is active when tissue damage occurs at any stage of life. Nociceptive activity alone can lead to a stress response subsequently leading to alterations in many body systems (i.e., elevated sympathetic tone, increased release of stress hormones, increased metabolic rate). In neonates, acute severe or chronic pain can alter immediate, and perhaps long-term, central and peripheral sensory processing, leading to an exaggerated pain response later in life. Therefore it is important to use analgesics for "painful" procedures (i.e., dewclaw removal, tail cropping), even in the very young patient, to limit the effects of nociceptive activity on the developing central nervous system.

Neonates also appear to have exaggerated responses to many anesthetic drugs. It is unclear whether these exaggerated responses are caused by pharmacokinetic alterations as a result of differences in body water and fat composition or related to an immaturity of the blood-brain barrier.

ANESTHETIC OPTIONS FOR PEDIATRIC PATIENTS

Preoperative Considerations

Preoperative evaluation of pediatric patients should include a thorough physical examination to assess the respiratory (lung auscultations, respiratory pattern and rate), the cardiovascular (heart auscultation especially for murmurs, mucous membranes, pulses), and hydration status of the patient. Normal heart rate and respiratory rate vary depending on size, breed, excitement, and age of the patient. Heart rates

are often greater than 200 beats/min (decreasing with age), and respirations may be 15 to 35 breaths/min. The breathing pattern generally has a greater abdominal component, and this is normal in neonatal animals, but an increased respiratory effort or very fast shallow breathing patterns may require further investigation. Hydration is important to evaluate as these patients are at high risk for dehydration. The patient history (e.g., nursing behavior, diarrhea) plays a particularly important role in addition to the physical examination (heart rate, mucous membranes, capillary refill time, eye position in orbit, skin turgor, and urine color) for the assessment of hydration. Fluid deficits should be corrected before the initiation of anesthesia and can be done with subcutaneous, intravenous (IV), or intraosseous (IO) administration. It is essential to carefully calculate drug doses and fluid requirements based on an accurate weight to avoid complications associated with anesthesia.

Fasting is generally undesirable for neonatal patients as this may exacerbate dehydration and hypoglycemia. Exceptions are patients with delayed gastric emptying, megaesophagus, or cleft palate, for whom a fasting period of 1 to 2 hours may decrease the risk of vomiting, regurgitation, and aspiration. Pediatric patients eating solid food probably require no more than 4 to 6 hours of fasting but should have access to water until 1 to 2 hours before anesthesia.

Common laboratory tests for routine pediatric patients include a packed cell volume (PCV), total protein (TP), blood glucose, and blood urea nitrogen (BUN). However, further testing may be desirable based on the history and clinical examination of the patient. Several biochemical and hematological values in neonatal and pediatric patients differ from those of adults (see Chapters 30 and 9, respectively), and values should be interpreted in light of these differences. Blood glucose should also be monitored periodically in longer anesthetic cases (>45 min) to identify the development of hypoglycemia.

Premedication

Premedication helps improve the quality of induction and recovery, may decrease the amount of drugs used for induction and maintenance, blocks undesirable physiological changes (i.e., bradycardia), and generally provides preemptive analgesia. The selection of premedication drugs and dose depends on the individual case. Factors such as age, temperament, disease status, and the procedure itself may all influence drug and dose selection. In general, selecting agents with minimal side effects and/or drugs that are easily reversed (benzodiazepines, opioids) can minimize the concerns regarding prolonged drug metabolism and elimination.

An opioid is strongly recommended as part of every premedication protocol for which tissue trauma and surgery are expected. For very young (less than 6 to 8 weeks) and/or debilitated patients, opioids alone may provide a suitable level of sedation. The anticipated level of pain and the desired duration of analgesic action should be considered for guiding opioid selection. It may be necessary to administer a follow-up dose of opioid for longer and/or more painful procedures.

All commonly available opioids can be used safely in neonatal and pediatric patients. Opioids may cause a decrease in heart rate, but this can generally be treated by the administration of an anticholinergic drug.

The benzodiazepines are good choices for sedation in neonate and pediatric patients, have very few cardiopulmonary effects, and provide good muscle relaxation. They tend to produce reliable sedative effects in neonatal and pediatric patients, in contrast to their less predictable and sometimes excitatory effects in adults. When used in combination with an opioid, benzodiazepine's sedative effects are frequently even more pronounced. The absorption of diazepam is erratic and inconsistent when administered intramuscularly. The absorption of midazolam is more predictable, and its use is preferred over diazepam for intramuscular administration. All benzodiazepines can be reversed with flumazenil (0.1 mg/kg, IV or IO, titrated to effect).

In healthy slightly older pediatric patients, acepromazine can be used for sedation. However, because of the long duration of action and the potential for an exaggerated hypotensive response, very low doses are recommended. The α-2 agonists are generally not recommended in neonatal patients before anesthesia and should be used cautiously in pediatric patients. The hemodynamic effects may be more pronounced on the immature cardiovascular system, leading to undesirable side effects.

Drug doses are generally reduced in neonatal and pediatric patients, but this is not a universal recommendation. The interaction among body composition (increased volume of distribution, lower fat and muscle mass relative to an adult), immature hepatic and renal function, and apparent increased sensitivity to central nervous system drugs makes it difficult to formulate universal recommendations regarding drug dose alterations. However, in general it is easier to start with lower doses initially and to administer more drugs as needed.

Catheter Placement

Following adequate premedication, intravenous catheter placement is recommended for intravenous fluid and drug support. A catheter placed before induction is ideal and can be critical if complications arise. An intravenous catheter also provides access for the administration of intravenous anesthetic induction agents, and this can be advantageous when a rapid induction and intubation are desired.

Depending on the size of the animal, a 24- to 22-gauge catheter may be used. A local anesthetic cream (EMLA cream, AstraZeneca LP, Wilmington, DE) placed on the skin 30 to 45 minutes before catheterization can greatly facilitate catheter placement in these patients by desensitizing the skin. Sites for catheterization include the cephalic, femoral, and jugular veins. The jugular vein is a relatively easy vein to catheterize, and larger gauge catheters can be used; however, this technique often requires an excellent assistant or some form of chemical restraint. In some very small patients, intravenous cephalic or femoral catheters may be extremely difficult to place. In these situations, fluids can be administered subcutaneously. IO drug and fluid administration is also a very valid option, especially in small and/or dehydrated/debilitated animals, in which IV catheters are hard to place.

Induction

There are two principal techniques used for the induction of anesthesia in neonates and pediatric patients. Historically, most neonates and pediatric patients were induced using inhaled anesthetics. This was performed probably for two reasons: (1) the administration of intravenous drugs is difficult because of the animal's small size; and (2) there are concerns regarding the metabolism of drugs administered systemically, leading to prolonged drug effects. Inhalant anesthetics overcome both concerns because they do not require intravenous access and the drugs are not dependent on metabolism for the cessation of their effects.

However, the cardiovascular side effects (myocardial depression, significant vasodilation) from inhalants are significant at high doses in neonate and pediatric patients. The technique itself can be associated with considerable patient stress. Patient stress can be greatly minimized by using appropriate premedication before initiating mask inductions. Premedications also reduce the subsequent amount of inhaled anesthetic necessary for intubation and maintenance.

Rapid induction with an intravenous agent is recommended when the animal has signs of dyspnea/hypoxemia or is at risk for regurgitation, which is the reason it is often the preferred technique by many anesthetists. Preoxygenation is recommended before induction for all pediatric patients regardless of the specific technique or protocol chosen.

Propofol is an excellent choice for the intravenous induction of anesthesia in neonatal animals. Its metabolism, after a single induction dose, is generally rapid and complete. Hypotension and apnea are common side effects associated with propofol administration, but these can be minimized by carefully titrating the dose to effect.

The combination of ketamine and diazepam (intravenous) or midazolam (intramuscular) is also a good induction method for longer procedures. Ketamine increases sympathetic tone and helps to maintain higher heart rates, which is desirable in pediatric animals. Disadvantages of ketamine include its longer duration of action, extensive hepatic metabolism and renal excretion, increase in salivation seen in some patients, and the potential for "rougher" recoveries after short procedures.

Intubation should be performed very gently to avoid damage to the delicate laryngeal structures. A laryngoscope infant size (00, 0, or 1) can be used to facilitate intubation (Figure 23-1). Endotracheal tube sizes depend on the size of the animal and can range from 2.0 to 6.0 mm (Figure 23-2). Occasionally, intravenous catheters are used as endotracheal tubes if smaller sizes are required. It is important to select the appropriate-sized endotracheal tube because one too large can cause irritation at placement and a tube too

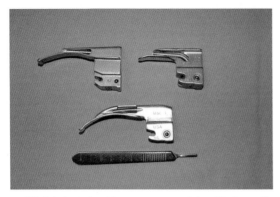

Figure 23-1 Infant-sized laryngoscopes (size 00, 0, or 1) used to facilitate intubation of pediatric dogs and cats.

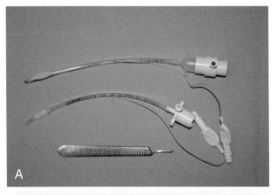

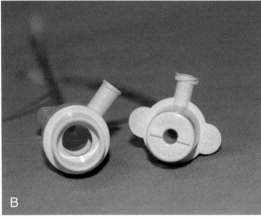

Figure 23-2 Endotracheal tube sizes depend on the size of the animal and vary both in external **(A)** and internal **(B)** diameters (from 2.0 to 6.0 mm).

small can significantly increase the resistance to airflow, increasing the work of breathing and predisposing the patient to obstruction. Endotracheal tube cuffs should be inflated carefully to avoid tracheal irritation. Noncuffed tubes are often used in very small patients, facilitating the use of a larger tube. Occasionally, regardless of the drugs used, endotracheal tube obstructions occur. The smaller tube diameter necessitated by pediatric patients increases the likelihood of obstructions from tracheal secretions, mucus, or kinking of the endotracheal tube. Anticholinergics have

traditionally been used to help limit airway secretions. However, anticholinergics may also thicken tracheal secretions, thereby increasing the risk of endotracheal tube obstructions. Close monitoring for the development of obstructions and methods for suctioning or exchanging tubes should be available.

Anesthesia Maintenance

Anesthesia can be maintained with intravenous or inhalant anesthetic agents. However, maintenance of anesthesia in neonates and pediatric patients is largely done using inhalant anesthetics. Inhalant anesthetics are titratable to effect, require no metabolism for recovery, and produce relatively predictable cardiopulmonary changes. Inhalant anesthesia is best delivered via an endotracheal tube rather than a facemask. Endotracheal intubation protects the airway from accidental aspiration and allows for the use of assisted or controlled ventilation if needed.

Nonrebreathing systems (Bain circuit, Norman elbow, or Ayre's T-piece) are most often used. These systems require high fresh gas flows (200 to 300 ml/kg/min) for proper function, and the absence of an absorber canister and soda lime reduces the resistance of the circuit. The high fresh gas flows required for nonrebreathing systems may contribute to patient hypothermia. Rebreathing systems are generally reserved for patients greater than 5 kg. However, there are several specially designed rebreathing circuits (neonatal and pediatric) with minimal deadspace that can be used safely in patients less than 5 kg.

Close monitoring of the pediatric patient under anesthesia is vital for an optimal outcome. Adverse trends should be promptly identified, diagnosed, and treated because neonate and pediatric patients have less organ reserve compared with adults. Assessment during anesthesia generally includes the following body systems: the central nervous (depth of anesthesia), respiratory, cardiovascular, and thermoregulatory systems. Adequacy of anesthetic depth is based on evaluation of reflexes (e.g., palpebral, withdrawal) and cardiopulmonary responses to surgical stimulation. It should be noted that some reflexes are greatly diminished or absent at birth and only begin to develop during the first few weeks of life.

The two primary functions of the respiratory system are oxygenation (uptake of oxygen) and ventilation (elimination of carbon dioxide). Oxygenation can be assessed using a pulse oximeter. Mucous membrane color is a poor indicator of oxygenation and should not be relied on for the assessment of oxygenation. Ventilation is most easily assessed by simple observation of respiratory rate and tidal volume. However, these parameters can be difficult to assess in pediatric patients with small tidal volumes and rapid respiratory rates.

Capnography can be used as a more reliable method of assessing the adequacy of ventilation but is also prone to erroneous readings in small patients as a result of sampling artifact. Mainstream capnographs are associated with less sampling artifact when compared with sidestream systems. However, mainstream instruments add bulk and deadspace to the endotracheal tube. By using a neonatal airway adapter (available for most capnographs) the deadspace can be minimized. Analysis of arterial blood gas is the most accurate method of assessing the adequacy of oxygenation and ventilation. Arterial blood gas samples are commonly taken from the dorsal pedal, coccygeal, or lingual artery, but it is technically difficult and not readily available in most practices.

The cardiovascular system is monitored by assessing heart rate, rhythm, and blood pressure. Heart rate and rhythm can be determined by using a stethoscope, an electrocardiograph (ECG), a Doppler probe, or an oscillometric blood pressure monitor. Although pulse oximeters and oscillometric blood pressure monitors often report heart rate, they tend to be inaccurate if a rhythm disturbance is present. If pulse oximetry is used in small pediatric patients (<1 kg in body weight), it can be placed across the whole leg to obtain reliable measurements. Blood pressure can be measured using a Doppler probe or an oscillometric method. The Doppler probe in conjunction with a pneumatic cuff and sphygmomanometer can be used to assess blood pressure in most neonate and pediatric patients. Cuff width should be 40% to 60% the circumference of the leg, and cuff sizes 1 or 2 are generally used. Monitoring blood pressure using this method is a relatively easy-to-use and reliable technique, although consistency in use is important for accuracy.

Automated oscillometric blood pressure systems are very simple to use and less prone to operator error. However, some older and human oscillometric monitors are not very reliable for use in neonatal and pediatric veterinary patients. Newer veterinary specific monitors tend to be more reliable. Support with fluids, sympathomimetics (e.g., dopamine, dobutamine), and anticholinergics may be necessary to increase blood pressures and support perfusion. Fluid administration rates should be adjusted to meet the individual patient requirements and range between 5 and 20 ml/kg/hr. A balanced electrolyte solution with or without 2.5% dextrose is frequently used. Dextrose is often added to prevent the development of hypoglycemia. However, this does not mitigate the need to perform periodic glucose assessments in the perianesthetic period.

Small patients are very prone to the development of hypothermia, and every effort should be made to maintain body temperature. Body temperature can be assessed using rectal or esophageal temperature probes. For small pediatric patients (<1 kg in body weight), very thin esophageal probes are available for handheld thermometers. It is important, however, that these are not placed too far down the esophagus. Towels, incubators, radiant heat lamps, warm circulating-water blankets, warm forced-air blankets, warmed fluids and prep solutions, and heated surgical tables and cages can all be used to minimize temperature loss. Microwaved-warming devices should be used cautiously because these can easily be overheated and can produce burns when placed on or near the skin of an anesthetized patient.

Analgesia

All neonatal and pediatric patients should be treated using the same principles of pain management that would be applied to an adult animal. If a painful procedure is performed, appropriate preemptive and balanced analgesia is necessary. The use of analgesics will not only mitigate pain, but analgesics also commonly reduce anesthetic requirements, which will then minimize the cardiopulmonary depression associated with general anesthetics.

Opioids are frequently used for analgesia in neonate and pediatric patients. They tend to be safe and associated with minimal detrimental side effects. The bradycardia associated with opioid administration is not usually pronounced and can easily be treated with an anticholinergic drug. Prolonged duration of action of the opioids, resulting from the immaturity of metabolic pathways, is generally not a significant concern in healthy patients.

Local anesthetics are an excellent option for regional anesthetic/analgesic techniques. Doses should be carefully calculated to avoid overdoses. The volumes available for a regional anesthetic technique are much smaller than what is needed for a larger animal, and this may limit their use in the perioperative period. To increase the available volume, the local anesthetic may be diluted with 0.9% saline to half of its original concentration.

NSAIDs are not generally recommended for use in neonates and pediatric patients. The potential for toxic side effects (renal, gastrointestinal), the role of prostaglandins in early neonatal development, and the potential for accumulation with repeated doses have not been evaluated in this group of patients. Under exceptional circumstances, NSAIDs may be used if the benefits are believed to outweigh the costs. But the owners should be fully informed of the potential for the development of side effects, and the number of doses used should be limited.

Constant-rate infusions (CRIs) of analgesics can be used in neonates but are not recommended for clinical practice because of difficulties involved in properly titrating medications. In adult dogs and cats, the pharmacokinetics of analgesics administered via a CRI varies with the duration of infusion (context-sensitive half-time). It is important to mention that the pharmacokinetics of the analgesics have not been carefully studied in neonatal and pediatric dogs and cats, and CRI should only be used if the clinician has a solid understanding of the pharmacokinetic alterations and associated consequences.

Recovery

Active warming, monitoring, and support of the patient should extend into recovery. Human infant incubators are ideal, providing warmth, humidity, and supplemental oxygen while still providing visual and tactile access to the patient. If the animal is still very sedated and does not actively start nursing/eating following recovery, glucose levels should be determined, and if necessary, intravenous or oral dextrose-containing fluids should be administered.

Postoperative analgesia should be provided. Pain will inhibit the necessary feeding and drinking behavior and prolong healing. Pain assessment in pediatric patients can be very challenging even for very experienced practitioners. There are various grading/scoring scales designed for use in companion animals that can be adapted for use in neonates. One of the simplest to use is the visual analog scale. This scale consists of a 10-cm line with a descriptor: no pain on one end, and the worst pain imaginable on the other. The evaluator then places a mark on the line corresponding to the level of pain he or she believes the animal is experiencing. This score can then be used to assess response to therapy and to provide guidelines for analgesic intervention. It is important to remember that regardless of the scoring system used, there can be significant interindividual differences in pain-scoring assessment that are partly based on the evaluator's own experiences, biases, and beliefs. Despite the challenges associated with pain assessment in neonates, every effort should be made to recognize and eliminate pain and nociception in these patients.

SUGGESTED READINGS

Grubb TL: Anesthesia for the pediatric and geriatric patient. In Slatter D (ed): *Textbook of small animal surgery*, ed 3, Philadelphia, 2003, Saunders.

Grundy SA: Clinically relevant physiology of the neonate, *Vet Clin Small Anim* 36:443, 2006.

Holden D: Paediatric patients. In Seymour C, Duke-Novakovski T (eds): *BSAVA manual of canine and feline anaesthesia and analgesia*, ed 2, Gloucester, UK, 2007, BSAVA.

Pettifer GR, Grubb TL: Neonatal and geriatric patients. In Tranquilli WJ, Thurmon JC, Grimm KA (eds): *Lumb & Jones veterinary anesthesia and analgesia*, ed 4, Ames, IA, 2007, Blackwell.

Rankin DR: Neonatal anesthesia. In Greene SA (ed): *Veterinary anesthesia and pain management secrets*, Philadelphia, 2002, Hanley & Belfus Inc.

SURGICAL CONSIDERATIONS IN THE YOUNG PATIENT

CHAPTER 24

Bernard Séguin

Surgery on immature dogs and cats is routinely performed in clinical practice and is often necessary to correct traumatic injuries or serious congenital problems. As with any other surgical patient, presurgical evaluation of the patient is paramount, and careful consideration needs to be given to differences between immature and mature patients in interpreting the findings. Physiologic differences between immature and mature patients affect many aspects of the management of the surgical patients regarding anesthesia and choice and doses of drugs for example. Specific anesthetic considerations are covered in Chapter 23. This chapter will concentrate on the issues directly related to the surgery of immature dogs and cats. Following sound principles of surgery may be even more important in immature patients because these patients are less forgiving.

PREPARATION OF THE PATIENT FOR SURGERY

Immature dogs and cats have greater insensible water losses and do not have the ability to concentrate urine as much as adult animals. Therefore puppies and kittens have greater fluid requirement relative to body mass than adults. For these reasons, water restriction before surgery should not exceed 1 hour. As well, fasting should be of shorter duration, meaning 4 to 8 hours. The liver store of glycogen is minimal and rapidly declines during fasting. After hepatic glycogen stores are depleted, hepatic gluconeogenesis is responsible to maintain normal glycemia. However, there are decreased feedback mechanisms between hepatic gluconeogenesis and glycemia in puppies and kittens.

Thermoregulation is another challenge that is exacerbated in immature dogs and cats. Puppies and kittens have a larger surface area–to–body weight ratio, with high radiation and evaporative heat losses, an inability to shiver, a small amount of subcutaneous fat, and an immature thermoregulatory system. Appropriate steps can be taken to help limit the loss of heat during anesthesia and surgery. Clipping of the hair should be more conservative (but still adequate), and alcohol or alcohol-containing antiseptics should be avoided if possible. Other means of maintaining the patient's warmth, such as warm water blankets or a Bair Hugger (Arizant Inc., Eden Prairie, MN), should be used.

The skin is very delicate and relatively thin in immature animals. Therefore clipping of the hair should be done very carefully to avoid lacerating the skin.

INTRAOPERATIVE CONSIDERATIONS

Tissues in general are more delicate in puppies and kittens and therefore require very gentle handling. The use of pediatric instruments is, in some instances, necessary to properly handle and manipulate the tissues.

Providing adequate hemostasis should be done more thoroughly because small volumes of blood loss in puppies and kittens can lead to clinically relevant hypovolemia and anemia. Even a small volume of blood loss can be a relatively large amount for a very young dog or cat (the total blood volume of a 1-kg kitten or dog is only 70 to 100 ml). Animals between age 2 and 8 weeks are at greater risk, as hematopoiesis does not begin until age 6 to 12 weeks in response to low levels of hemoglobin. Young animals, irrespective of species, are less able to compensate for hypovolemia. In 1-week-old pigs, a blood loss of only 5 to 10 ml/kg resulted in tachycardia and hypotension. Electrocautery should be used very discriminately because of its deleterious effects on wound healing.

On entering the abdominal cavity, kittens and puppies aged less than 16 to 20 weeks usually have a substantial amount of clear fluid in the peritoneal cavity. The surgeon should not be surprised or alarmed.

When selecting a suture material, the strength of the tissue, the rate of healing of the tissue, and the physical condition of the animal should be considered. In the healthy dog or cat, a rapid gain in wound strength is achieved at 7 to 10 days postoperatively. Most absorbable suture materials provide adequate tensile strength for this period. Soft, non-irritating suture materials, such as polyglactin 910, may be preferred. Polydioxanone, which has a prolonged rate of absorption (180 days), has been reported to cause calcinosis circumscripta in two young dogs. The true significance of this phenomenon is undetermined as it is unknown what incidence of this problem is associated with polydioxanone.

Multifilament or coated nonabsorbable suture materials are best avoided. Suture materials of the smallest possible diameter to achieve successful outcome should be used. In general, sutures of 4-0 to 5-0 are used for most tissues of very young animals, and 3-0 to 4-0 suture material is used for older animals. Obviously the tissue type and the size of the patient will also be critical factors in deciding the suture size.

When suturing skin, fine nonabsorbable suture such as 4-0 or 5-0 nylon should be placed loosely. Skin tension should be alleviated with a subcutaneous or subcuticular closure to avoid sutures pulling through the thin delicate skin.

Specific considerations apply when a fracture of a bone involves a growth plate. Ideally, fixation methods chosen will allow the physis to continue to grow if the potential remains. This topic will be covered in greater depth in Chapter 25. For some surgeries, it is best to delay the onset of the surgery until the animal is older. Specifically, correction of a cleft palate is best attempted when the patient is aged 8 to 12 weeks, and even ideally at least age 16 weeks. Even so, palatoplasty performed in a 16-week-old patient may lead to abnormal maxillofacial growth and development, leading to a narrow maxilla and occlusal problems. Also, the tissues in the older patient will be stronger and less friable, increasing the likelihood of a successful outcome. Until the patient is old enough to undergo the surgery to correct a cleft palate, some patients may need nutritional support by use of a feeding tube.

POSTOPERATIVE CONSIDERATIONS

Protecting the surgical wound from self-trauma or trauma from the licking by the queen or bitch in the nonweaned patient is important. In patients that are weaned, placing an Elizabethan collar is one of the best ways to protect the wound. For nonweaned patients, covering the wound with a bandage may be necessary. It is easy to place a bandage that is too tight around the thorax or abdomen of a puppy or kitten, and care should be taken to avoid this.

Suture removal in a healthy pediatric patient can be done at 7 days postoperatively. In debilitated patients or when electrocautery was used on the edges of the surgical wound, suture removal should be delayed at 10 to 14 days postoperatively.

ELECTIVE GONADECTOMY

Pet overpopulation is an ongoing problem in the United States, where surgical removal of the ovaries and/or uterus or of the testicles of dogs and cats has long been a basis of population control and part of routine veterinary health maintenance programs for animals not intended for breeding. Elective gonadectomy is by far the most common surgical procedure performed in small animals aged less than 12 months in North America.

Optimal age at which to perform ovariohysterectomy (OHE) or castration of dogs and cats is not defined by the veterinary literature. Although most of these elective surgical procedures are delayed until the patient is aged 6 to 7 months (peripubertal), performing gonadectomies as early as age 6 to 14 weeks is gaining more popularity, especially with animal shelters. Although animal shelters have mandatory postadoption spay/neuter policies, reported owner compliance is only 50% to 60%. Preadoption gonadectomy prevents this lack of compliance.

Ovariectomy (surgical removal of the ovaries), OHE (surgical removal of the ovaries and uterus), and tubal ligation (tying off the uterine tubes) are techniques described for surgical sterilization. Tubal ligation is not commonly used in domestic animals anywhere in the world and will not be discussed. OHE is performed more commonly than ovariectomy in the United States and United Kingdom. In the Netherlands and other European countries, ovariectomy has become the procedure of choice for elective neutering.

Ovariectomy appears to offer the same benefits and concerns as OHE. Ovariectomy is reported to be less time consuming and less invasive than OHE but without any differences in reported urogenital problems 8 to 11 years after surgery. Urinary incontinence was a reported finding for both groups without a difference in incidence. In the United States, OHE still is the most common surgical sterilization method.

In pediatric patients, OHE is performed in a routine manner. Figure 24-1 shows a photograph of the ovaries and uterus (top) and testes (bottom) from 7-week-old pups. Note the small size, lack of vasculature, and lack of adipose tissue. For the approach to the OHE, the distance between the umbilicus and pubis is visually divided into thirds. For dogs older than 5 to 6 months, the incision is performed into the cranial third. For younger dogs and in cats, the incision is performed in the middle third.

On entering the peritoneal cavity, it is common to find a substantial amount of serous fluid in the abdomen. Hemoclips can be used to ligate the testicular and ovarian pedicles if the hemoclips are of appropriate size relative to the size of the pedicle. Hemoclips can also be used to ligate the uterus stump if they are of appropriate size. It has been suggested that polydioxanone should be avoided for ligation reasons mentioned earlier. In 6- to 14-week-old male kittens, it has also been suggested not to use castration techniques where the spermatic cord is tied onto itself or the vas deferens and spermatic artery are tied together because the spermatic artery is allegedly too small and fragile.

Fewer surgical complications are reported when gonadectomies are performed before age 12 weeks compared with after age 24 weeks. Additional advantages of pediatric

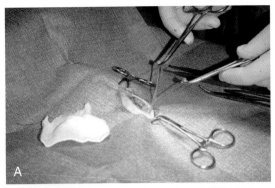

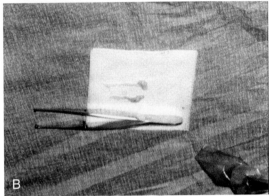

Figure 24-1 Ovaries and uterus **(A)** and testes **(B)** excised from 7-week-old pups. Note the small size, lack of vasculature, and lack of adipose tissue. (Courtesy Margaret Root Kustritz.)

neutering include a quicker recovery and shorter surgery time. However, what are the long-term effects of early-age gonadectomy? Many studies have examined the physical and behavioral effects of early (usually aged <24 weeks) gonadectomies. Although radius and ulna growth plate closure is delayed in both groups, dogs that are neutered at age 7 weeks have a greater delay in closure, resulting in longer bone length compared with dogs neutered at age 7 months. This phenomenon has also been reported in cats where intact cats had earlier growth plate closure.

Whether gonadectomy is performed at age 7 weeks or 7 months, activity levels are increased compared with intact dogs, which leads to a decreased incidence of obesity. In contrast, cats neutered at age 7 weeks or 7 months were more likely to be obese, whereas cats neutered before age 5.5 months were less likely to be hyperactive than cats neutered after age 5.5 months.

The influences of age at gonadectomy on long-term behavior are controversial, with some investigators finding no difference between dogs neutered before age 24 weeks compared with after age 24 weeks; however, other investigators found increased noise phobia and sexual behavior but decreased separation anxiety, escaping behavior, and inappropriate elimination when frightened in dogs neutered earlier than age 5.5 months. With respect to cats, cats neutered at age 7 weeks or 7 months were more affectionate and

less aggressive toward other cats than those left intact. However, cats neutered before age 5.5 months had a higher incidence of shyness but a decreased incidence of sexual behavior and aggression toward veterinarians compared with cats neutered after age 5.5 months.

With respect to effects on the urogenital system, gonadectomy before age 5.5 months results in an increased rate of cystitis and urinary incontinence compared with the same procedure performed in bitches after age 5.5 months. The risk of urinary incontinence is greatest in dogs spayed before age 3 months. Regardless of whether gonadectomy is performed at age 7 weeks or 7 months, vulvar development remains immature compared with intact dogs. However, there is an increased incidence of perivulvar dermatitis and vaginitis in the bitches spayed at 7 weeks compared with those spayed at 7 months.

Pediatric castration in dogs has been shown to cause arrest of the normal development of the balanopreputial fold, resulting in reduced diameter of the pars glandis (penis), prepuce, and os penis. In kittens, complete penile extrusion was not possible even at age 22 months when castration was performed at age 7 weeks. Testosterone is essential for keratinizing the epithelium, allowing the normal separation of the glans penis from the layer of cells lining the prepuce to form the balanopreputial fold. In dogs, the relative risk of developing mammary gland tumors later in life is 0.5% if the spay is performed before the first estrus, 8% if the spay is performed between the first and second estrus, and 26% if the spay is performed between the second estrus and age 2.5 years.

Dogs neutered before age 24 weeks are more likely to contract an infectious disease later in life compared with dogs neutered after age 24 weeks. In contrast, cats were no more or less likely to contract infectious diseases irrespective of age at neutering. However, cats neutered before age 5.5 months had a decreased incidence of asthma, gingivitis, and abscesses.

In conclusion, based on current research, elective gonadectomies in dogs and cats have the most benefits with the fewest risks when performed between age 3 and 5.5 months. For potential canine athletes, postponing gonadectomies until after puberty may be indicated to eliminate tendency toward increased physeal growth.

SUGGESTED READINGS

Aronsohn MG, Faggella AM: Surgical techniques for neutering 6- to 14-week-old kittens, *J Am Vet Med Assoc* 202:53, 1993.

Hosgood G: Surgical and anesthetic management of puppies and kittens, *Compend Contin Educ Pract Vet* 14:345, 1992.

Howe LM: Surgical methods of contraception and sterilization, *Theriogenology* 66:500, 2006.

Root Kustritz MV: Determining the optimal age for gonadectomy of dogs and cats, *J Am Vet Med Assoc* 231:1665, 2007.

Van Goethem B, Schaefers-Okkens A, Kirpensteijn J: Making a rational choice between ovariectomy and ovariohysterectomy in the dog: a discussion of the benefits of either techniques, *Vet Surg* 35:136, 2006.

PEDIATRIC FRACTURE MANAGEMENT

CHAPTER 25

Michael Weh

Fractures encountered in juvenile animals differ from those in adults in several ways. This chapter outlines a systematic method of pediatric fracture assessment, which can guide decision making regarding fracture management. Specifics regarding the treatment of physeal fractures and the use of external coaptation in pediatric patients are discussed. It is not intended to be a comprehensive review of internal fixation or external coaptation. The reader is referred to other textbooks for in-depth discussion of these topics.

The distinct characteristics of pediatric fractures result from the anatomic, biomechanical, and physiologic properties of pediatric bone. Anatomically, perhaps the most obvious difference between adult and pediatric bone is the presence of a growth plate, or physis. Physeal injuries are unique to immature patients. Biomechanically, pediatric bone is able to withstand greater plastic deformation before breaking than adult bone. This results in the classic incomplete "greenstick" fracture, not typically seen in adults. In addition, the presence of a strong periosteum minimizes displacement of fracture ends, even in cases of complete fractures. Physiologically, the robust periosteum and an already activated osteogenic environment result in rapid bone formation and accelerated healing of fractures. These differences in fracture configuration, healing potential, and physical characteristics of bone in pediatric patients dictate a unique approach to fracture management.

FRACTURE ASSESSMENT SCORE

Fracture management has been described as a race between biologic healing of the fracture and mechanical failure of the stabilization used. The more mechanically or biologically favorable the fracture environment, the less robust or long lived need be the stabilization. The fracture assessment score is an objective method of considering all pertinent fracture characteristics to aid in fracture management decision making. It evaluates mechanical factors, biologic factors, and

clinical (patient/client) factors and rates them on a scale of 1 to 10 (Box 25-1). Higher scores are given for factors that predict faster healing, minimal loads on implants, and decreased risk for implant failure. In general, pediatric patients tend to have higher scores for mechanical factors and biologic factors, predisposing them to more rapid healing. However, clinical factors may score lower than in adult patients. An overview of the scoring system is presented in Figure 25-1.

When using the fracture assessment score, it is not critical to come up with an absolute number, as this will probably vary between observers. The important point is that all three factors are considered when making decisions regarding fracture management. Because mechanical factors are the most obvious, and the most easily visualized on the radiograph, the most common error in fracture assessment is to ignore the biologic and clinical factors. This can lead to failure of a fixation that may have appeared appropriate when reviewing radiographs alone.

Mechanical factors that affect bone healing include fracture configuration, patient size, and presence of single limb versus multiple limb injury. This predicts the ability of the fractured limb to share load bearing with the fixation device, as well as the magnitude of load that will be exerted on the limb. Pediatric patients tend to present with a higher proportion of incomplete fractures and simple fractures with contact of fragment ends. These configurations have a higher load-sharing ability than comminuted, nonreconstructable fractures. Thus they have a correspondingly higher assessment score. Larger dogs or dogs with multiple limb injuries can be expected to exert larger forces on the fracture at earlier time points. They will have a lower assessment score than small dogs with single-limb injuries. In general, the mechanical assessment dictates the initial *strength* of implant needed to stabilize a fracture.

Biologic factors that affect the rate of fracture healing include age, health, soft tissue injury, and region of bone

212

Fracture assessment scores

Score 8 to 10

Immediate load sharing and rapid healing are expected with these fractures. These patients tend to have more options for definitive fracture management and overall have a diminished rate of complications. They have a wide range of options for fracture stabilization, including external coaptation, pin and cerclage wire, compression plating, type I external fixation, and interlocking nails.

Score 4 to 7

With these fractures, there is diminished load-sharing ability or a compromised biologic environment, or both. They require stronger implants with a longer fatigue life, and management options are more limited than for higher scores. These fractures can be treated with neutralization plating, type IB or II external fixators, or interlocking nails.

Score 1 to 3

No load sharing exists with these fractures, and there may be significant soft tissue damage as well. The implant must be able to support the entire force transmitted through the limb for an extended period. Options include buttress plating using lengthening plates, plate and rod fixation, type II or III external fixators, external fixator and rod combinations, or interlocking nails.

affected. Because they are "physiologically primed" to produce bone, pediatric patients in good health exhibit significantly accelerated bone healing (higher assessment score) compared with adults or geriatric patients. Fractures resulting from high-velocity injury or open fractures often result in tremendous soft tissue trauma. Soft tissue injury in the fracture region will compromise blood supply to the bone, decreasing healing potential and indicating a lower assessment score. Bones of the distal extremities (radius and tibia) are surrounded by a smaller volume of muscle and soft tissue. Consequently they have diminished extraosseous blood supply and exhibit an increased rate of delayed fracture union, even in pediatric patients. Fractures involving cancellous bone tend to heal more rapidly because of the presence of a large number of osteoblasts and osteoinductive factors compared with cortical bone.

The increased healing potential of growing animals is a great asset in pediatric fracture management. Sometimes this may tempt the surgeon to compromise some mechanical principles of fracture fixation for reasons of expense, available equipment, or time. However, the biologic environment alone cannot compensate for inadequate mechanical fracture stabilization, and the contribution of both factors must be acknowledged when choosing fixation technique. The biologic assessment predicts the required *duration* or *functional lifespan* of the stabilization. Because larger implants have a longer fatigue life, a lower biologic assessment score may indicate use of larger implants. The opposite is true for a high biologic assessment score.

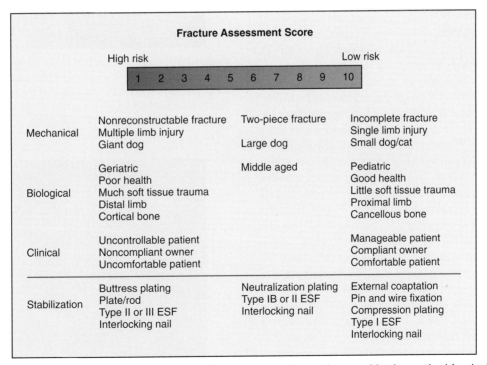

Figure 25-1 The fracture assessment scoring system can be used as an objective method for decision making regarding fracture management.

Clinical factors that affect bone healing include postoperative patient cooperation, patient comfort, and owner compliance. Uncontrollable, active patients tend to be poor candidates for external fixators or external coaptation and will be better served by internal fixation. Owners who are unable or unwilling to perform the postoperative management necessary for casts or external fixators are better off having their pet's fracture managed with internal fixation. Early return to function is important with fracture management. For some dogs, the presence of an external fixator or coaptation will inhibit normal limb use. These dogs may be predisposed to complications such as loss of range of motion or muscle atrophy and may be better managed by internal fixation. Clinical assessment may alter the indicated *strength* or *duration* of fixation (as predicted by mechanical and biologic assessment), or it may dictate alternate management that is *better tolerated* by the patient or client.

The final fracture assessment score can be used to guide fracture management. It is most applicable for diaphyseal fractures, for which many options for stabilization exist. In other applications, such as articular fractures or physeal fractures, the mechanical environment may largely dictate the repair, and there may be little choice in management options.

PHYSEAL FRACTURES

Fractures of the physeal plate are not uncommon in young animals. The zone of hypertrophy in the physis is a focal weak point in the long bone. Ligaments and connective tissue are significantly stronger than the physis in pediatric patients. Thus trauma that would typically result in a sprain or luxation in adults can cause fracture or displacement involving the physis. Physeal fractures are categorized according to the method of Salter and Harris into types I through V, as described in Chapter 42 (see Figure 42-1), primarily in an attempt to prognosticate outcome.

The Salter-Harris system is useful for *describing* most physeal fractures; types I through IV can usually be differentiated radiographically. However, *predicting outcomes* for physeal fractures is more complex, and the Salter-Harris system is limited in this regard. Whereas the articular nature of types III and IV fractures indicates a worse prognosis than type I or II (as a result of the development of degenerative joint disease), the difference in prognosis between types I and II or types III and IV is less clear cut. Type V fractures probably have the worst prognosis because injury to the germinal cell layer of the physis can result in arrested growth and development of angular deformities or length deformities. However, the crushing injury of type V fractures cannot be visualized radiographically, making them very difficult or impossible to diagnose at the time of injury. Moreover, type V fractures often are not a distinct entity; many type I through IV fractures have some degree of type V damage to the growth plate. Any trauma significant enough to cause a fracture (physeal or otherwise) may also cause type V physeal damage to the fractured bone or to a separate bone.

Because of the occult nature of type V physeal fractures, all puppies and kittens with fractures should be reevaluated at least every 2 weeks to assess for the development of angular limb deformities, regardless of the method of treatment. Age at time of injury is a significant factor in prognosis for physeal fractures. Younger animals are at increased risk for growth deformities, and those less than 6 to 7 months old should be monitored more closely. If deformities are diagnosed early, residual growth potential in the limb can be used to aid in treatment. Damage to the physeal plate is of lesser consequence in animals more than 8 to 10 months of age because less growth potential remains.

Principles of Repair
Closed

Physeal fractures should be treated as early as possible after life-threatening injuries have been addressed. If treated early, some type I and II fractures of the tibia or distal radius can be reduced closed and treated with external coaptation (Figures 25-2 and 25-3). Treatment of humeral or femoral physeal fractures with external coaptation is *not*

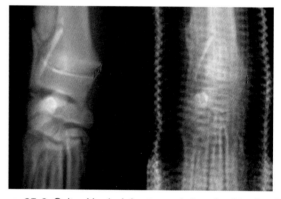

Figure 25-2 Salter-Harris I fracture of the distal radius in a young dog, showing closed reduction and cast stabilization. Displacement is noted by red arrow on the left image. The same two points are marked by the arrow in the right image. Casting material hinders radiographic evaluation.

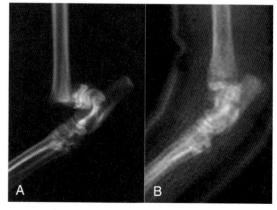

Figure 25-3 Salter-Harris I fracture of the distal tibia in a young cat, showing closed reduction and cast stabilization.

recommended (see following section on External Coapta-tion). If the fracture is significantly displaced or there is greater than 24- to 48-hour delay in treatment, closed reduc-tion will be significantly more difficult or impossible, making open reduction and rigid fixation necessary.

Open

Open reduction is necessary for type III and IV (articular) fractures and for any fracture that cannot be reduced closed. The goal should be anatomic reduction (regarding both articular surface and limb alignment) and stable fixation to allow early return to function (Figure 25-4). This will mini-mize later complications such as degenerative joint disease and developmental abnormalities resulting from altered force distribution or weight bearing.

The germinal layer of cells, critical for continued growth, typically remains on the epiphyseal fragment. Manipulation of fracture fragments should be done as atraumatically as possible to prevent additional injury to this layer. As much as possible, limb manipulation should be used to achieve reduction. If needed, pointed reduction forceps are preferred over blunt bone forceps to avoid crushing damage.

Implants should be placed in a manner that minimizes disruption of physeal growth potential. Smooth implants, such as IM pins and Kirschner wires, should be used when-ever possible. Ideally pins should be directed perpendicular to the physis to avoid inhibiting bone lengthening at the growth plate. Placing implants obliquely or crossing pins over each other in the physis may arrest growth in that loca-tion. For a similar reason, the surgeon should avoid bridging the physis with bone plates, external fixators, screws, or tension bands (Figure 25-5). If it is necessary to place an implant in this manner, it should be removed as soon as possible (i.e., within 2 to 4 weeks, to minimize negative impacts on bone growth).

External Coaptation

External coaptation can be used for emergency fracture management in pediatric patients as it is used in adults. The aim is to reduce instability, to diminish ongoing trauma to the wound and fracture site, and to increase patient comfort. A Robert Jones bandage and a splinted, soft-padded bandage are two treatments among several that can be used in this application. As in adults, soft-padded bandages or slings can also be used postoperatively in pediatrics as a supplement to protect a surgical repair or to minimize perioperative swell-ing or discomfort. These short-term bandaging techniques have been well described by other texts and do not vary significantly in their application to pediatrics.

In certain cases, casts and rigid splints are appropriate for *definitive* fracture treatment. They have a wider range of applications in pediatric patients than adults because of young animals' propensity for robust bone formation and accelerated healing times. Casting can have several advan-tages over open reduction and internal fixation (ORIF) or external fixation. Because there is no surgical approach, soft tissues and blood supply to the fracture site—essential for fracture healing—are not further compromised. This opti-mizes the biologic environment of the fracture. The

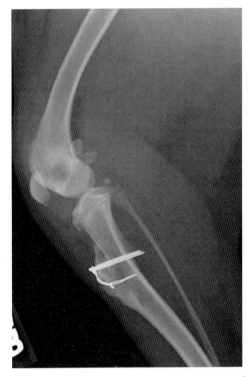

Figure 25-5 Recheck radiograph 8 weeks postoperatively for repair of a tibial tuberosity avulsion in a 7-month-old dog. The tension band has been placed across the tibial tuberosity apophysis, arresting growth at that center. The tibia has con-tinued to grow from the proximal tibial physis, resulting in a patella baja. This illustrates the importance of not bridging the physis with implants in a young dog with significant growth potential.

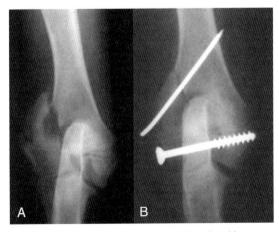

Figure 25-4 Salter-Harris IV fracture of the distal humerus in a young dog. This has been repaired with a lag screw and Kirsch-ner wire. These fractures require anatomic reduction and rigid fixation and are not candidates for closed reduction and external coaptation.

possibility of surgical contamination and infection also is eliminated. Further, casting requires short anesthesia times compared with most open repairs. It may be more cost-effective than ORIF or external fixation, although this is not always the case. The cost of multiple cast changes and anesthesia/sedation must be factored in to obtain a true cost estimate for the entire treatment. Box 25-2 covers recommended casting technique.

Indications/contraindications

Although casting has advantages over ORIF and external fixation, especially in pediatric patients, not all fractures or all patients are amenable to external coaptation. As in adults, successful immobilization of a fracture requires casting of the joint above and below the fracture. Thus casting is used for fractures below the elbow and stifle joints. More proximal fractures cannot be adequately stabilized with this technique.

Attempts at immobilizing the femur and hip joint for femur fractures may have serious consequences. For example, prolonged immobilization of the coxofemoral joint in a puppy using a hindlimb spica splint or Ehmer sling can cause abnormal development of the hip joint similar to congenital hip dysplasia. External coaptation of femur fractures may also result in quadriceps contracture. Also referred to as "fracture disease," quadriceps contracture is one of the most devastating complications of femur fractures in young dogs and cats treated with prolonged immobilization (Figure 25-12). Quadriceps contracture is characterized by complete loss of hock and stifle flexion as a result of muscle contracture, atrophy, and adhesion of the quadriceps muscle to the exuberant callus forming in the femur. Coxofemoral joint function may or may not be compromised. Surgical treatment of quadriceps contracture has uniformly been unsuccessful at returning the leg to function, and arthrodesis and amputation have been recommended as salvage procedures. Because of the high risk of quadriceps contracture alone, splinting and casting are contraindicated for treatment of distal femur fractures. Stifle immobilization for casting of tibial fractures does not typically result in quadriceps contracture.

The suitability of a fracture for casting not only depends on its location but also its configuration and displacement. Fracture biomechanics has been well reviewed in other texts, and similar principles apply to pediatric patients and adults. Casts can counteract bending and rotation at the fracture site. They are relatively ineffective at neutralizing tension/compression and the resultant shear forces across a fracture. Casts do not provide sufficiently rigid immobilization or apposition of fragments for primary bone healing. The fracture heals through secondary bone healing and endochondral ossification. For these reasons, casting must be reserved for cases that would be expected to heal rapidly and to have a lower risk of complications (i.e., a higher fracture assessment score). Fracture fragments should have good angular and rotational alignment, and major fragments should have at least 50% contact at the fracture line (Figure 25-13, *A*).

BOX 25-2   Casting technique

1. Anesthetize animal.
2. Clip affected limb.
3. Apply traction to affected limb for 15 minutes to relax muscle contraction and align major fragments. Tendency is for musculature to deviate distal fragment laterally. If focus is placed on keeping limb in mild varus, this can be countered.
4. Place tape stirrups.
5. Apply stockinette, with enough (5 cm) left at each end to wrap around edges of cast. Excessive stockinette can be removed at narrower portions of the distal limb to prevent folds in the stockinette (Figure 25-6).
6. Apply "doughnuts" made from cast padding or foam to protruding pressure points on the limb. This will help prevent pressure sores from developing.
7. Apply cast padding from ends of toes to above joint proximal to fracture. Under no circumstances should the foot or toes remain uncovered by bandage material. This can compromise venous return and result in swelling of the distal limb. Overlap cast padding 50% (Figure 25-7). Limit number of layers to what is essential to avoid rubbing on casting material. Excess layers will loosen cast, making it ineffective at stabilizing and causing more sores.
8. Apply one layer of Kling gauze, starting distally, overlapping 50%.
9. Using gloves, open fiberglass casting material and soak in cold water. Squeeze out all residual water. Start wrapping distally, proximal to the end of the cast padding. For the first wrap, fold the cast material longitudinally, to create a rounded edge, instead of the sharp edge of the cast material (Figure 25-8). Fold the end of the stockinette with the edge of the cast padding over the rounded edge, and cover the stockinette end with the second layer of casting material. Continue up the limb, overlapping 50% (Figure 25-9). Repeat the longitudinal fold of casting material proximally, and incorporate the stockinette in a similar fashion. For medium-sized dogs, two layers of cast padding overlapped 50% (four layers total) should provide sufficient rigidity. Larger dogs may require three layers overlapped 50% (six layers total). More than this may be too stiff, and cause "stress protection," even in large dogs. Alternatively, the casting material can be applied without soaking in water and then moistened after application by applying a damp layer of Kling gauze to the cast (Figure 25-10). This may make the casting material easier to work with, and it eliminates the time pressure to apply the cast before the casting material hardens.
10. Allow cast to dry (5 to 10 minutes).
11. Bivalve cast with electric saw to facilitate removal for bandage changes (Figure 25-11).
12. Apply three to four pieces of white tape evenly spaced circumferentially around cast to compress the two halves together. Fold stirrups over cast edge. Apply Vetrap to cast, wrapping circumferentially and overlapping.

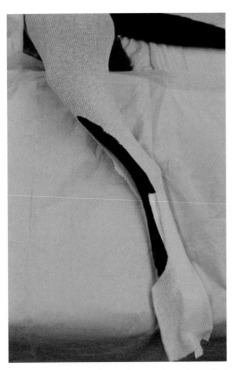

Figure 25-6 Tape stirrups have been placed, and the limb is covered with a stockinette. Excessive stockinette has been removed from the distal limb to avoid excessive folds when compressed with cast padding.

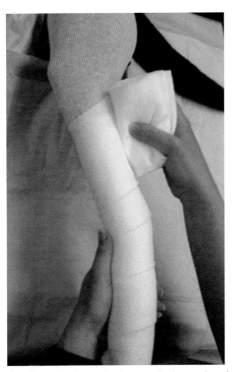

Figure 25-7 Cast padding being applied, overlapping 50% with the underlying layer.

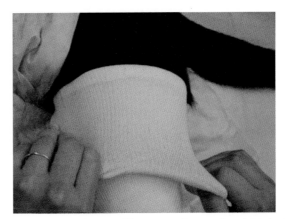

Figure 25-8 The stockinette can be used to fold the layer of cast padding over the edge of the casting material, creating a soft rounded edge.

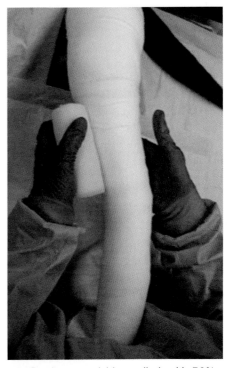

Figure 25-9 Casting material is applied, with 50% overlap of the underlying layer.

Incomplete fractures or radial/tibial fractures with intact ulnae/fibulae are good candidates for casting. Simple closed radius/ulna or tibia/fibula fractures may be casted as well, depending on the configuration and displacement. At the other end of the spectrum, open comminuted fractures with significant displacement are poor candidates for casting. Casting is also contraindicated in articular fractures.

Certain individuals are worse candidates for casting than others. Although most dogs and cats can learn to tolerate casts well, some do not and will continually mutilate the casting material. Species differences exist as well; dogs tend to be amenable to casts, whereas cats generally tolerate them poorly. In addition, some clients are not able to monitor and maintain a healthy cast. Obviously their pets are poor candidates for casting.

Complications and cast management

Complications of casting can be severe, in the worst case resulting in loss of the affected limb. They can be minimized

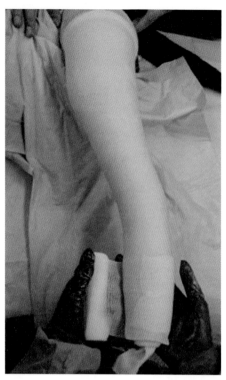

Figure 25-10 The casting material can be soaked in water before application, or it can be moistened after application, by use of a wet roll of Kling gauze wrapped over the cast material.

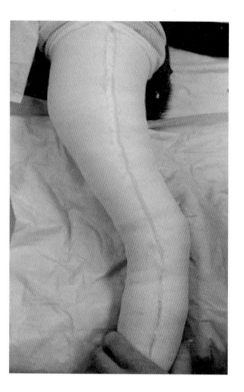

Figure 25-11 The cast has been "bivalved" to facilitate regular removal and inspection. This decreases stiffness somewhat, but wrapping the cast with elastic Vetrap restores cast integrity.

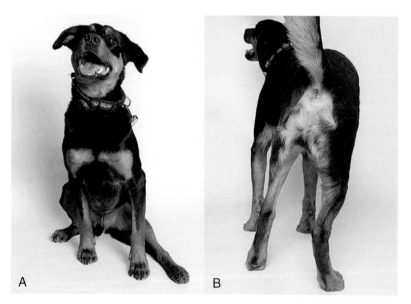

Figure 25-12 A young dog with quadriceps contracture secondary to a distal femur fracture. Note the rigid extension of the left hindlimb. The risk of quadriceps contracture can be minimized by use of internal fixation and early aggressive physical therapy to maintain range of motion during fracture healing.

with proper cast placement, vigilant monitoring, regular cast changes/examination, and removal of the cast as soon as clinical fracture union is observed. As in adult animals, pediatric patients with casts should be monitored regularly to avoid pressure sores, moist dermatitis, or vascular compromise (Figure 25-14). It is wise to observe the animal in the hospital for a day to evaluate for limb swelling after cast placement. This swelling may be caused by trauma from the initial injury or a cast that is too tight. Once the pet is discharged, owners should be advised to monitor for any

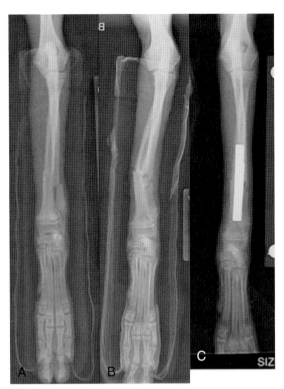

Figure 25-13 Sequential radiographs of a young dog with a radius/ulna fracture showing. **A,** Closed reduction and casting with good apposition and alignment of fracture fragments. **B,** Recheck 9 days after casting, showing loss of alignment and reduction of the radius and ulna. **C,** Compression plating of the radial fracture. Early recheck of the casted fracture diagnosed loss of reduction and facilitated intervention before the fracture progressed to a malunion. Note that the cast does not extend significantly above the elbow in this dog. This may have increased instability of the cast construct and allowed shifting at the fracture line.

moisture on the cast, swelling of toes, or increasing lameness on the limb, all of which indicate need for recheck.

Pediatric patients will also require weekly limb evaluation to monitor cast fit, fracture fragment alignment, and limb alignment (see Figure 25-13, *B* and *C*). In animals younger than 6 months old, the cast may need to be reconstructed every 10 to 14 days. The cast can be cut longitudinally on opposite sides of the cylinder ("bivalved") to facilitate frequent cast changes. This will decrease rigidity of the construct somewhat but should not affect clinical outcome. Even with the best cast maintenance, pediatric patients are at risk for angular or rotational limb deformities as a result of ongoing bone growth. In addition, young animals may develop ligamentous laxity with prolonged immobilization, especially of the carpus joint. This change typically resolves after cast removal.

Joint immobilization has deleterious effects on cartilage health, even after 3 to 4 days. These changes range from

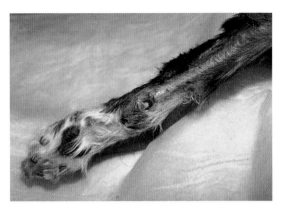

Figure 25-14 Cast sores over the boney prominences such as the ulnar styloid process, accessory carpal bone, calcaneus, and olecranon process are common complications of casts. They can be minimized or avoided by the use of appropriate padding, proper cast fit, and regular recheck examinations.

altered proteoglycan synthesis to cartilage erosion and ankylosis. Fortunately most changes appear to be reversible as long as immobilization is limited to periods of 4 to 6 weeks.

Casted fractures in young animals may heal in as little as 3 to 4 weeks. During this time, owners should be instructed to limit their pet's activity to minimal on-leash walking. Running, jumping, stair climbing, and rough play are not allowed. Ideally the cast should remain in place no longer than absolutely necessary for healing to occur. However, the abrupt transition from cast to unsupported limb may expose the fracture to increased forces too rapidly. Controlled reloading can be facilitated by placing a soft-padded bandage on the affected limb for an additional 1 to 2 weeks. Contrastingly, in some cases the cast can be too rigid, and the fracture becomes "stress protected." Wolff's law says that bone will adapt to the loads placed on it. Lack of force placed on the fracture results in diminished bone production, or even bone resorption at the fracture site, and may proceed to a delayed union or nonunion. If delayed union is diagnosed radiographically, the cast should be weakened to expose the fracture to increased forces. Often these fractures require treatment by ORIF and bone graft.

SUGGESTED READINGS

Akeson WH et al: Effects of immobilization on joints, *Clin Orthop* 219:28, 1987.
Oakley RE: External coaptation, *Vet Clin North Am Small Anim Pract* 29:1083, 1999.
Palmer RH: Decision making in fracture treatment: the Fracture Patient Scoring System. In *Proceedings of ACVS Veterinary Symposium,* Washington, DC, 1994, pp 388-390.
Piermattei DL, Flo GL, DeCamp CE: *Small animal orthopedics and fracture repair,* ed 4, St Louis, 2006, Saunders/Elsevier, pp 737-746.
Simpson AM, Radlinsky M, Beale BS: Bandaging in dogs and cats: external coaptation, *Compend Cont Educ Pract Vet* 23:159, 2001.

PAIN ASSESSMENT AND MANAGEMENT

CHAPTER 26

Turi K. Aarnes, William W. Muir, III

Recognition and treatment of pain in neonates is an emerging science and is controversial. To effectively treat pain in neonates, the maturity and function of many different body systems must be considered (Figure 26-1). Choosing appropriate drug therapy requires consideration of course, cause, and severity of pain and the duration and side effects of the chosen analgesic therapy (Box 26-1). In addition, other medications, concurrent medical problems and medications, and the patient's physical status should be considered when choosing analgesics. Few clinical studies have been conducted investigating pain in neonatal dogs and cats. All too often, pain in neonates and juvenile animals is undertreated.

PHYSIOLOGY AND DEVELOPMENT

Development of Cardiovascular and Respiratory Systems

Parasympathetic innervation of the cardiovascular system is mature at birth. In contrast, sympathetic innervation develops over the first 2 weeks of life and reaches maturity at 14 days in dogs and 11 days in cats. The baroreceptor reflex is active as early as 4 days of age. Normal respiratory rate in dogs and cats occurs at approximately 1 week of age. During the period from birth to 1 week, the respiratory rate is increased. Innervation of the respiratory system is complete and functional by 14 days of age.

Neonates have a much larger metabolic oxygen requirement, and their carotid body chemoreceptors are immature compared with those of adult animals. Because of these factors, neonates are much more susceptible to hypoxemia. The response of a neonate to hypoxemia is a compensatory increase in tidal volume and respiratory rate. However, sleep alters this pattern by disrupting the metabolic and respiratory systems: minute ventilation and metabolic rate

decrease in sleeping puppies and kittens. The result is a relative hypoxemia that is compensated for by a decrease in metabolism.

Tidal breathing in neonates is altered as a result of their increased chest wall compliance. The work of the neonate to move the diaphragm is greater and so is the need to generate increased negative pressure. As a result, respiratory depression that shortens the inspiratory phase negatively affects gas exchange and arterial blood gases (Box 26-2).

Drug Absorption, Metabolism, and Excretion

Absorption of drugs administered orally or transdermally in neonates is altered compared to adults. Gastrointestinal (GI) motility in neonates is irregular and may be related to pressure gradients in the small intestine rather than neuronal activity, until approximately 40 days of age. Generally, GI motility is decreased in the neonate, which results in decreased absorption from the stomach. However, GI permeability is also altered. Immediately after birth, the permeability of intestinal mucosa is increased, but at approximately 10 to 12 hours of age, intestinal mucosal permeability starts to decrease. The skin of neonates contains a greater percentage of water compared to adults and is also thinner, which causes an increase in absorption of drugs delivered transdermally.

Metabolism and excretion of drugs depends on liver and kidney function. Elevations and depressions in different enzyme systems associated with liver function are responsible for most differences in hepatic function in neonates. Alkaline phosphatase and gamma-glutamyltransferase (GGT) are increased in the neonate. However, gluconeogenesis, glycogenolysis, and hepatic elimination are reduced. Cytochrome P-450 activity is approximately 85% of that in an adult at 4 weeks of age and continues to increase until 8 weeks of age. Microsomal enzyme activity matures over a period of months, reaching maturity at approximately 4.5

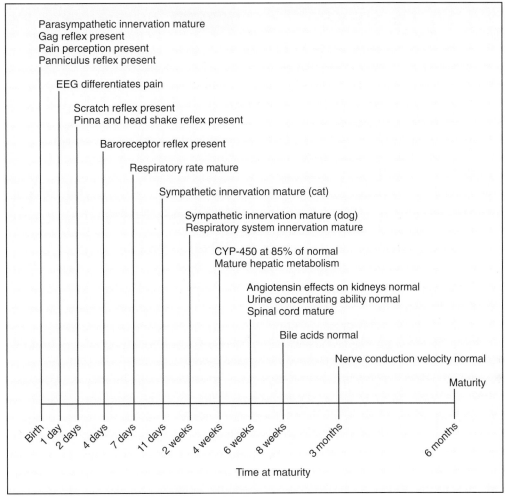

Figure 26-1 Timeline of maturation.

BOX 26-1 Clinical implications of immaturity

- Respiratory depression is more common in neonates, particularly following the administration of opioids.
- Immaturity of the liver and kidneys prolongs drug elimination in neonates.
- Drug-related side effects are more common in immature dogs and cats.
- Skin is thinner and has higher water content, increasing the rate of transdermal absorption of some medications.
- Lower albumin levels, thus potential for more unbound (active) drug.

BOX 26-2 Clinical implications of immature respiratory and cardiovascular systems

- Bradycardia
- Respiratory depression
- Hypoxia

months of age. Regardless, hepatic metabolic activity is adequate by 5 to 8 weeks of age.

Plasma protein levels in neonates are decreased compared with adults. In particular, albumin levels are lower in young animals but reach parity with adult levels by 8 weeks of age. Protein-bound drugs administered to young animals have a higher fraction of unbound and thus active drug in their plasma.

Bile flow in newborn animals is significantly decreased compared with adult animals, and bile acid composition and concentrations gradually increase. By 8 weeks of age, bile flow is comparable with an adult.

The kidneys are functionally and morphologically immature at birth and continue to develop for 2 to 3 weeks after birth. Glomerular filtration rate (GFR) and renal plasma flow (RPF) are lower in the neonate than the adult, and this correlates with a lower arterial blood pressure. As arterial blood pressure normalizes, GFR and RPF increase because GFR and RPF in neonates are directly correlated with arterial blood pressure. The effect of angiotensin on the kidneys does not reach maturity until 6 weeks of age. Urine concentrating ability also matures at approximately 6 weeks of age (Box 26-3).

PHYSIOLOGY AND PATHOPHYSIOLOGY OF PAIN IN NEONATES

Pathophysiology of Pain

The physiology and pathophysiology of pain in neonates is similar to other advanced mammals. Peripheral nociceptors (free nerve endings of primary afferent sensory nerve fibers) transduce mechanical, chemical, and thermal energy (noxious input) into electrical impulses. There are two types of nociceptors (A-mechano-heat receptors and C mechano-heat receptors).

Nociceptive impulses are transmitted to the central nervous system (CNS) by primary afferent sensory nerve fibers. There are two main types of fibers: A-delta and C fibers. The A-delta fibers are comparably large diameter, myelinated axons that conduct impulses rapidly and are associated with "first pain." The C fibers are smaller diameter, unmyelinated axons, with slower conduction velocities, which reinforce the immediate response of A-delta fibers. C fibers mediate second pain.

Primary sensory afferent nerve fibers synapse in the grey matter of the spinal cord dorsal horn, which is organized into layers (laminae). A-delta fibers terminate in lamina I (most important) and lamina V. The C fibers terminate in lamina II. The dorsal horn is the site of modulation of nociceptive input. The primary sensory afferent nerve fibers may form direct or indirect connections with one of three functional populations of dorsal horn neurons (interneurons, propriospinal neurons, and projection neurons). Interneurons are either excitatory or inhibitory and act as relays participating in local processing. Propriospinal neurons extend over multiple spinal segments and involve segmental reflex activity. Projection neurons participate in ascending transmission of nociceptive impulses and extend axons beyond the spinal cord to terminate in supraspinal centers (such as the midbrain or cortex). There are three types of projection neurons: nociceptive specific, wide dynamic range, and complex neurons. Communication in the dorsal horn between primary afferent fibers and dorsal horn neurons occurs by chemical signaling, mediated by excitatory or inhibitory amino acids and peptides produced, stored, and released in the nerve terminals. Glutamate and aspartate are the most important excitatory mediators. Other excitatory neurotransmitters are substance P, neurotensin, vasoactive peptides, calcitonin gene-related peptide, and cholecystokinin.

Development of the Spinal Cord, Pain Receptors, and Pain Recognition

Many tactile and pain-initiated reflexes are present at birth or develop soon thereafter. The neonate's response to noxious stimuli is appreciable from birth to 1 day of age and can be demonstrated by withdrawal from the noxious stimulus. An electroencephalogram (EEG) can differentiate this pain from other stimulation. This withdrawal from noxious stimuli in puppies is slow during the first days of life, suggesting that maturation of nociception occurs after birth. Pain sensitivity (threshold) may be more pronounced in newborns compared with adults because of an increased number of pain receptors and neural reorganization in neonates. A panniculus reflex is present at birth. The scratch reflex and the pinna and head-shake responses to noxious stimuli at the pinna or external ear canal are present at 2 days of age. The gag reflex is present at birth.

Spinal cord maturity occurs at 6 weeks of age in dogs, and the cranial portion develops more quickly than the caudal portion. Complete myelination and maturity of fasciculus gracilis and lateral corticospinal tracts occurs after 6 weeks. Maturation of the feline spinal cord and myelination of nerves occurs earlier than in dogs. Lateral columns in cats are well myelinated at 14 days of age. Dorsal nerve fibers mature rapidly during the first 8 days of life. Nerve conduction velocities in dogs reach maturity between 6 months and 1 year of age, with full maturity in cats reached in 3 months.

The initial noxious stimulus produces transduced electrical signals that are transmitted by afferent sensory neurons to projection neurons in the spinal cord, each of which has receptors that are under developmental control. In addition, these peripheral sensory neurons are overproduced during embryonic development and nearly half of these sensory neurons undergo programmed cell death in the adult. As a result, during postnatal development the perception of pain and its inhibition undergoes waxing and waning based on the neurobiologic development of the animal. This explains large interspecies and interindividual variability in the response to noxious stimuli (Box 26-4).

Projection neurons transmit nociceptive input to supra-spinal centers via tracts that ascend in white matter of the spinal cord: spinothalamic, spinoreticular, spinomesence-phalic, spinocervical, and spinohypothalamic tracts. The spinothalamic tract originates from nociceptive specific and wide dynamic range neurons in laminae I, V, VI, and VII and terminates in lateral and medial nuclei of the thalamus and is believed to be the most important with regard to nociception. The spinothalamic tract is only faintly myelin-ated at birth. Myelination occurs in the external tracts more quickly than in the deeper tracts, with full myelination occurring between 3 and 6 weeks of age. Myelinated fibers in grey matter laminae are present at birth. Diameter increases and myelination of these fibers continues during the neonatal period, with full myelination and density occur-ring at 5 weeks of age.

Nociceptive impulses are subjected to modulation and integration before reaching their ultimate destination, the cerebral cortex. Other supraspinal structures that process and modulate nociceptive input include the reticular formation, periaqueductal grey matter, limbic system, and the thalamus. The thalamus is the major relay station for all sensory input en route to the cerebral cortex. It is especially important for integrating nociceptive impulses and is composed of numer-ous complex nuclei: the lateral thalamic nuclei are involved in sensory discriminative aspects of pain, while the medial thalamic nuclei are involved in motivational affective aspects of pain. The cerebral cortex is the site where the physiologic process of nociception is integrated and ultimately perceived (Figure 26-2). Several discrete cortical regions are preferen-tially activated by noxious stimulation: first and second somatosensory cortices, anterior insular cortex, and anterior cingulate. Neurotransmitters in the thalamocortical region are excitatory (glutamate and aspartate) and inhibitory (gamma-aminobutyric acid [GABA], glycine, monoamines, acetylcholine, and histamine). Differences between the inte-gration of nociceptive impulses in neonates compared with adults are unknown.

Descending inhibitory pathways modulate sensory input and are especially important for nociceptive transmission. The descending inhibitory modulatory system has four tiers, with inhibitory influences located in the following regions: cortical and thalamic structures, periaqueductal grey matter of the midbrain, rostral medulla, and spinal cord dorsal horn. Antinociceptive effects in these regions are mediated by GABA, glycine, serotonin, norepinephrine, and endogenous opioids (enkephalins, endorphins, and dynorphins). This system ensures that the physiologic pain response generated is appropriate for the noxious stimulus initiated.

Physiologic Changes and Responses to Pain

There are two important aspects to the pain experience in animals: the sensory component and the affective (the emo-tional) component. In addition, there is a secondary pain affect, or the consequences associated with chronic pain and homeostatic responses. Pain sensation is more intense in humans than other somatic sensations, which would seem

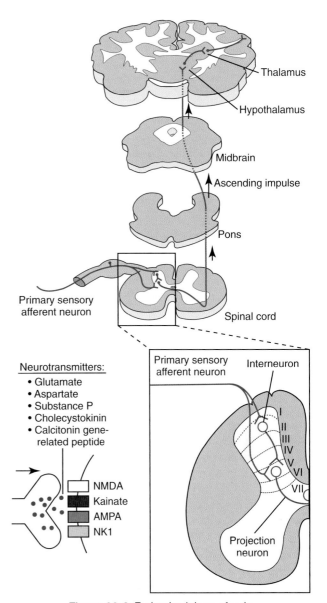

Figure 26-2 Pathophysiology of pain.

to be an evolutionary adaptation. Additional characteristics of pain include quality (e.g., sharp or piercing, dull, throb-bing), persistence, temporal summation, spatial spread of sensation at high pain levels, and unique qualities of the sensation that are intrinsically dependent on the location and degree of tissue injury.

An animal's ability to sense noxious stimuli is present at birth, but the actual sensation of pain in animals is not assessable except by behavioral interpretation. Extrapolation of reports of pain from human studies may result in anthro-pomorphizing and an increase in assignment of pain in animals. Confounding this is the heightened response to what may be considered a nonpainful or mildly painful stimulus in neonates (learning). The nervous system is plastic, and extensive studies of pain in neonatal animals as a model for human neonatal pain show a heightened sensitivity to tissue injury that can result in neural reorganization by for-mation of new primary afferents, increased innervation of wounded tissue, and hyperexcitability of dorsal root ganglia. The long-term result of this neural reorganization is hypersensitivity to sensory input and behavioral modification.

PAIN ASSESSMENT IN NEONATES

Assessment of pain in neonates is difficult because of an incomplete understanding of normal pain behavior in neonates. Neonatal and juvenile dogs appear to be more reactive to noxious stimuli, often demonstrating exaggerated responses compared to adult animals. This may be due to an overproduction of peripheral sensory neurons or evolutionary development of warning systems causing hypersensitivity. While the stimulus itself may be judged to be mild, the experience of the animal may be heightened as a result of innate developmental differences. Neonatal cats are less likely to demonstrate this heightened reaction, possibly the result of an earlier neurologic maturity compared to dogs.

Behavioral and physiologic parameters may be used to assess pain in neonates and are more useful in predicting stressful situations than in adults. Pain behavior in neonates and juveniles includes a change from normal behavior patterns and display of new behaviors such as positioning the painful area in such a way as to limit pressure or stimulation. In neonates, this may include a change in sleeping and eating patterns. Because this constitutes the majority of a neonate's time, a decrease or increase in these behaviors may be indicative of pain perception. Increased vocalization (whining, whimpering, and crying) may also be an indicator of pain. Physiologic indicators of pain in neonates include changes in heart rate, respiratory rate, blood pressure, and oxygen saturation (Box 26-5).

PAIN CONTROL

Sedatives

Acepromazine

Acepromazine is a phenothiazine tranquilizer that blocks dopamine receptors in the CNS and depresses the reticular-activating system, resulting in sedation. Acepromazine also blocks alpha-adrenergic receptors. Acepromazine is not an analgesic but potentiates the effects of analgesic drugs, most

notably, opioids. Acepromazine is metabolized by the liver and eliminated by the kidneys and as a result has a longer half-life in young animals. The duration of effect in adult animals is typically 4 to 8 hours and would reasonably have a longer duration of action in neonates and juveniles.

Acepromazine causes sedation without significant respiratory depression. Although systemic blood pressure can be reduced as a result of vasodilation, acepromazine administration can also result in vagally-induced bradycardia. In addition, acepromazine has antiemetic, antihistaminic, antisympathetic, antiarrhythmic, and antishock properties because of its dopamine inhibition in the chemoreceptor trigger zone.

Caution should be used when administering acepromazine to animals that are predisposed to seizures or with a seizure history because it can lower the seizure threshold. The consequences of this effect remain speculative. The dose of acepromazine should be decreased in neonates or those animals with hepatic insufficiency caused by its slower metabolism and potentially long duration. Acepromazine is a safe and effective tranquilizer in juvenile animals (Table 26-1).

Benzodiazepines

Diazepam and midazolam are the most common benzodiazepines used in veterinary medicine. They are used for their anxiolytic, muscle relaxant, antiseizure, and appetite stimulant properties. Diazepam is administered intravenously in a solution of ethyl alcohol, propylene glycol, and a preservative. Midazolam is water-soluble and can therefore be administered intramuscularly. Diazepam and midazolam are metabolized by the liver and eliminated in the urine. The duration of effect for diazepam and midazolam is approximately 1 to 4 hours.

Benzodiazepines potentiate the effects of GABA, the most abundant inhibitory neurotransmitter in the brain. The binding of GABA to the $GABA_A$-receptor results in an influx of chloride into the cell, hyperpolarization, and inhibition of excitability. Benzodiazepines bind to an accessory site on $GABA_A$-receptors and facilitate the binding of GABA, which causes an increase in the frequency of chloride channel opening and an increased state of hyperpolarization, and inhibition. Thus benzodiazepines produce agonist effects by enhancing GABA's affinity for the receptor, thereby improving inhibitory effects. Benzodiazepines demonstrate a high margin of safety but have limited potency in animals. Although most GABA receptors occur in the brain, benzodiazepine-specific receptors are also located in the kidney, liver, lungs, and heart.

Benzodiazepines have minimal effects on the cardiovascular and respiratory systems. Bradycardia and hypotension have been reported after intravenous (IV) administration as a result of sympathetic suppression. Benzodiazepines can cause significant CNS depression in very young animals. The dose of benzodiazepines should be decreased in neonates or those animals with hepatic insufficiency caused by their potentially long duration of effect (see Table 26-1).

| BOX 26-5 | **Pain assessment in neonates** |

- Change in normal behavior
  - Not eating
  - Change in sleeping patterns
- Display of new behaviors
  - Positioning away from painful area
- Increased vocalization
- Changes in heart rate, respiratory rate, blood pressure, and oxygen saturation
- Owner assessment: quality-of-life questionnaire

TABLE 26-1 Drugs useful for treating pain in neonates

Drug	Dose
Phenothiazine Tranquilizers	
Acepromazine	0.01-0.05 mg/kg IM, SC
Benzodiazepines	
Diazepam	0.1-0.4 mg/kg IV
Midazolam	0.1-0.4 mg/kg IV, IM
Alpha-2 Agonists	
Medetomidine	0.02-0.04 mg/kg IM (dogs)
	0.01-0.02 mg/kg IM (cats)
Xylazine	1-2 mg/kg IM
Opiates	
Morphine	0.2-1 mg/kg IM
Oxymorphone	0.02-0.2 mg/kg IV, IM, SC
Hydromorphone	0.02-0.2 mg/kg IV, IM, SC
Fentanyl	0.002-0.004 mg/kg IV, IM
Fentanyl patches	12.5 µg/hr for dogs and cats 2.5-5 kg body weight
	25 µg/hr for dogs and cats 5-10 kg body weight
	50 µg/hr for dogs 10-20 kg body weight
	75 µg/hr for dogs 20-30 kg body weight
	100 µg/hr for dogs greater than 30 kg body weight
Meperidine	0.2-0.5 mg/kg IV
	1-2 mg/kg IM
Methadone	0.1-0.5 mg/kg IV
Buprenorphine	0.005-0.02 mg/kg IV, IM
	0.01-0.02 mg/kg SL or buccal (cats)
Butorphanol	0.02-0.05 mg/kg IV
	0.2-0.4 mg/kg IM
Nalorphine	0.05-0.1 mg/kg IV
Pentazocine	0.5-1 mg/kg IV
Other Drugs Useful for Treating Pain in Neonates	
Ketamine	1-2 mg/kg IV
	4-20 mg/kg IM
Gabapentin	1-4 mg/kg PO
Tramadol	1-4 mg/kg PO BID to QID
Nonsteroidal Antiinflammatory Drugs	
Carprofen	2.2 mg/kg PO or SC BID
Deracoxib	1-2 mg/kg PO SID (dogs only)
Etodolac	5-10 mg/kg PO SID (dogs only)
Firocoxib	5 mg/kg PO SID (dogs only)
Flunixin meglumine	0.25-1 mg/kg IV or IM once (dogs only)
Ketoprofen	0.5-2.2 mg/kg IM, SC, PO SID
Meloxicam	0.2 mg/kg on the first day, then 0.1 mg/kg SC or PO SID
Tepoxalin	10 mg/kg PO SID (dogs only)
Glucocorticoid Steroids	
Prednisone/ prednisolone	0.1-0.2 mg/kg PO SID-BID

IM, Intramuscular; *SC,* subcutaneous; *IV,* intravenous; *SL,* sublingual; *PO,* by mouth; *BID,* twice a day; *QID,* four times a day; *SID,* once a day.

TABLE 26-2 Reversal drugs

Drug	Dose
Benzodiazepines	
Flumazenil	0.01-0.1 mg/kg IV
Alpha-2 Antagonists	
Yohimbine	0.1-0.3 mg/kg IV
	0.3-0.5 mg/kg IM
Atipamezole	0.05 mg/kg IV (dogs only)
	0.025-0.05 mg/kg IM
Tolazoline	0.5-5 mg/kg IV SLOW
Opioids	
Naloxone	0.005-0.015 mg/kg IV
Naltrexone	0.05-0.1 mg/kg SC
Nalorphine	0.05-0.1 mg/kg IV

IV, Intravenous; *IM,* intramuscular; *SC,* subcutaneous.

Conversely, benzodiazepine administration in healthy, juvenile animals may result in a release of inhibition (suppressed behavior), resulting in excitation and mania, anxiety, and potentially aggression.

Flumazenil is a concentration-dependent competitive antagonist of benzodiazepines. Flumazenil is metabolized in the liver and excreted in the urine. Reversal of the effects of benzodiazepines occurs approximately 1 to 2 minutes after injection. Flumazenil has a short half life, lasting from 1 to 3 hours, so another dose may be necessary (Table 26-2).

Alpha-2 Agonists

Xylazine and medetomidine are the most commonly used alpha-2 agonists in dogs and cats. Alpha-2 agonists cause pronounced sedation and analgesia by stimulating alpha-2 receptors in the CNS and by decreasing norepinephrine release. Alpha-2 agonists depress internuncial neuron transmission without affecting the neuromuscular junction, resulting in central muscle relaxation. Selectivity of medetomidine for the alpha-2 receptor is more than 10 times that of xylazine. Xylazine and medetomidine are metabolized in the liver and excreted by the kidneys.

Alpha-2 agonists have significant effects on the cardiovascular and respiratory systems, particularly in neonates. Decreased activity of the sympathetic nervous system and increased parasympathetic tone result in bradycardia, which can be profound and can also result in atrioventricular (AV) block. First- and second-degree AV block are common, and third-degree AV block may occur. Vasoconstriction occurs as a result of both alpha-1 and alpha-2 stimulation, but blood pressure eventually decreases below normal because of a decrease in central sympathetic output. Additional side effects include respiratory depression (particularly in neonates), hypothermia, and urination. Vomiting is a common side effect of xylazine administration to cats (see Table 26-1).

Yohimbine is a relatively specific competitive antagonist for xylazine and works by blocking alpha-2 receptors and enhancing the release of norepinephrine. Tolazoline blocks both alpha-1 and alpha-2 receptors, thereby antagonizing the sedative effects of alpha-2 agonists but relaxing vascular smooth muscle and potentially aggravating hypotension. Atipamezole is a specific competitive alpha-2 antagonist. Yohimbine, tolazoline, and atipamezole are metabolized by the liver and excreted in the urine. Reversal of sedation, muscle relaxation, and analgesia caused by alpha-2 agonists typically occurs approximately 3 to 10 minutes after injection (see Table 26-2).

Opiates

Opioids include a variety of natural and synthetic products that produce analgesic effects based on their combination with distinct opioid receptors. The most potent opioid analgesics activate mu receptors and include morphine, hydromorphone, oxymorphone, fentanyl, methadone, and meperidine. Buprenorphine is classified as a partial mu agonist. Butorphanol is a kappa receptor agonist and mu receptor antagonist.

Opioid-induced analgesia in human newborns and neonates is under extensive investigation. Significant differences in the sensitivity to opioid-induced analgesia are observed in neonates during maturation compared to adults. The source of these differences is unknown. Maturity of the CNS and the blood-brain barrier, end-organ sensitivity to opioids, and solubility of different opioids have been postulated as the cause of the differences between age-related effects of mu opioid agonists. Studies have also indicated differences in side effects from adult patients, although these differences are seemingly related to differences in drug metabolism and physiology between neonates and adults. The most notable example of these differences is the development of respiratory depression. Respiratory depression, although a concern in adults, is a much more important issue in neonates, since even a small change in tidal volume or respiratory rate in a neonate can result in life-threatening hypoxia. Most opioids have low bioavailability so are not suitable for oral use in cats and dogs.

Mu Receptor Agonists

Mu receptor agonists are considered the most potent of the opioid analgesics. Mu receptor agonists produce analgesia by binding to mu receptor sites primarily in the brain and dorsal horn of the spinal cord, although evidence suggests that peripheral sites may be important (e.g., joints). Mu receptor agonists have potent effects on the CNS and their administration can result in sedation, especially in young animals. The cardiovascular and respiratory side effects of mu receptor agonists include bradycardia (from medullary vagal nuclei stimulation), hypotension (more likely with morphine and meperidine administration from histamine release), and respiratory depression (particularly in young animals). These cardiovascular and respiratory side effects are dose-dependent and decrease with maturation; cardiovascular and

respiratory depression is more likely to occur in dogs or cats younger than 1 week of age. Other effects include nausea, salivation, vomiting, decreased GI motility, and occasionally excitement. The decreased GI motility associated with opioid administration is of particular concern in neonates because of the resultant decreased absorption of concurrently administered oral drugs, as well as nutrients. Hypothermia may occur in dogs, whereas hyperthermia is more common in cats. Mu receptor agonists are metabolized by the liver and excreted in the urine. Metabolism is primarily by glucuronidation. Cats are unable to metabolize (glucuronidate) morphine through this pathway. The duration of action and side effects of morphine may be accentuated in cats.

Morphine

The efficacy and potency of other opioids are usually compared to morphine. Morphine is a mu receptor agonist, although not the most potent mu receptor agonist. Morphine has fewer effects on the cardiovascular system than other mu receptor agonists and is likely to cause severe vomiting, especially when administered rapidly via IV. Morphine can cause respiratory depression in very young animals. In addition, morphine can cause a release of histamine, which may be responsible for induced hypotension and agitation in dogs. Morphine requirements in dogs and cats less than 1 week of age are typically lower than those of older animals (see Table 26-1).

Oxymorphone

Oxymorphone is a semisynthetic mu opioid agonist that has similar effects and side effects to morphine without causing histamine release. It is 5 to 10 times more potent than morphine (see Table 26-1). Oxymorphone is also less likely to cause hypersalivation, nausea, and vomiting than morphine.

Hydromorphone

Hydromorphone is a semisynthetic opioid similar to oxymorphone and approximately seven times more potent than morphine (see Table 26-1). Histamine release is also possible with hydromorphone, although the effect is typically mild and not likely to result in hypotension. Hydromorphone, like oxymorphone, is less likely to elicit vomiting but has been reported to cause hyperthermia in cats.

Fentanyl

Fentanyl is an ultrashort-acting synthetic opioid that is 100 times more potent than morphine. Fentanyl is available in an injectable form and a transdermal patch. Significant respiratory depression may occur in very young dogs and cats (younger than 1 week of age) when high doses of fentanyl are administered. The comparatively short duration of action when administered parenterally makes this drug ideal for use as a constant rate infusion. There are minimal cardiovascular effects associated with fentanyl, although bradycardia may occur. Respiratory depression is less likely to occur compared to morphine. Excessive doses of fentanyl may cause increased anxiety (similar to other mu opioid agonists) in cats. Fentanyl patches provide a means for continued drug effects. Fentanyl is gradually absorbed from a transdermal patch placed on the skin and produces analgesic effects lasting from 48 to 72 hours. The onset of analgesia occurs in 8 to 12 hours. Fentanyl patches are available in 12.5, 25, 50, 75, and 100 µg/hr patches (see Table 26-1).

Meperidine

Meperidine is a synthetic opioid that is approximately one-fifth to one-tenth as potent as morphine. It has a shorter duration of action than morphine, especially in dogs (see Table 26-1). Similar to morphine, meperidine can cause histamine release and result in vasodilation. Meperidine has vagolytic and negative inotropic effects. Repeated meperidine administration is discouraged in human neonates because of an accumulation of toxic metabolites that cause seizures. The relevance of this observation to veterinary medicine is undetermined.

Methadone

Methadone is a synthetic opioid that has potency and duration of effect similar to morphine (see Table 26-1). Evidence suggests that methadone may possess clinically relevant *N*-methyl-D-aspartate (NMDA) antagonist activity and act as a serotonin reuptake inhibitor, which could enhance its analgesic properties. Methadone causes less sedation and less vomiting than morphine.

Partial Mu Receptor Agonists: Buprenorphine

Buprenorphine is a synthetic partial mu receptor agonist. Buprenorphine binds tightly to opioid receptors (high affinity) and as such is not easily displaced from mu receptors by antagonists. Buprenorphine is at least 10 times more potent than morphine in cats and has a long duration of action. However, its onset of analgesic effect is significantly delayed, especially when administered intramuscularly. Analgesic efficacy in dogs is controversial. Buprenorphine is less likely to cause sedation, GI, cardiovascular, and respiratory side effects. It is useful for mild-to-moderate pain, but its partial mu agonist effects make its use for moderate to severe pain in dogs questionable. Buprenorphine can be administered buccally or sublingually in cats with excellent absorption (see Table 26-1).

Agonist-Antagonists
Butorphanol

Butorphanol is a synthetic opioid that is classified as a kappa receptor agonist and mu receptor competitive antagonist. Butorphanol has high affinity for opioid receptors and is not easily displaced. Butorphanol is ½ to 3 times more potent than morphine and has a shorter duration of action (0.5 to 3 hours), with minimal sedation (see Table 26-1). Cardiovascular and respiratory side effects are minimal compared with mu receptor agonists, and butorphanol produces antitussive and antiemetic effects. Butorphanol produces minimal esophageal sphincter constriction and is less likely to depress

GI motility compared to mu opioid receptor agonists. Butorphanol is used for mild-to-moderate pain and seems to be more effective for visceral pain than musculoskeletal pain.

Low doses of butorphanol may be used to reverse the side effects of the mu receptor agonists because of its competitive mu receptor antagonist effects.

Nalbuphine

Nalbuphine is a synthetic opioid that is classified as a kappa receptor agonist and mu receptor antagonist. Nalbuphine is similar to butorphanol in its effects and side effects. It is useful for mild pain, has a short duration of action, provides minimal sedation, and has few effects on the cardiovascular or respiratory systems (see Table 26-1). Unlike the other opioid analgesics, it is not a controlled drug because of its low abuse potential.

Nalorphine

Nalorphine is a synthetic opioid that produces kappa receptor agonist and mu receptor antagonist effects. Nalorphine is used most commonly to reverse the effects of the mu receptor agonists (see Table 26-1).

Pentazocine

Pentazocine, like butorphanol, is a synthetic opioid that is a kappa receptor agonist and mu receptor antagonist. Its duration of effect and efficacy is undetermined. It is especially effective as an analgesic and mild sedative in cats (see Table 26-1).

Mu Receptor Antagonists

The effects of mu receptor agonists can be antagonized by the administration of naloxone or naltrexone. Naloxone and naltrexone are mu receptor antagonists that cause competitive inhibition of all mu receptor agonists. Naltrexone may be more effective in antagonizing the excitatory effects of the mu opioid agonists compared with naloxone. The duration of action of naloxone is approximately 1.5 to 3 hours, and the duration of action of naltrexone is approximately 4 hours. Naloxone and naltrexone are metabolized by the liver and excreted by the kidneys (see Table 26-2).

Ketamine

Ketamine is an NMDA antagonist and dissociative anesthetic. Ketamine inhibits GABA and also blocks serotonin, norepinephrine, and dopamine in the CNS. Ketamine is used in higher doses to induce anesthesia and in lower doses (less than 50 µg/kg/min) as an adjunct to opioid administration for the treatment of severe pain or long-term pain management and to reduce the cardiovascular and respiratory side effects of high doses of opioids (see Table 26-1). Ketamine is metabolized in the liver and excreted by the kidneys.

Ketamine may cause an increase in salivation, especially when administered to cats. Ketamine can cause tachycardia and an increase in cardiac output and in higher doses can cause respiratory depression or an apneustic breathing pattern. The respiratory side effects and apneustic breathing may be pronounced and result in life-threatening hypoxia when administered to neonates. Ketamine also can cause a significant increase in cerebral blood flow and can lower the seizure threshold. Ketamine produces poor muscle relaxation, and administration of a muscle relaxant should be considered when administering ketamine for analgesia.

Gabapentin

Gabapentin is structurally related to GABA but does not appear to have affinity for or bind to GABA sites. Gabapentin's effects seem to be associated with NMDA receptors, although the mechanism for its action is unknown. Gabapentin has been used to decrease seizure activity, as an analgesic for the prevention of allodynia, and in the treatment of neuropathic pain (see Table 26-1). Gabapentin is not metabolized and is excreted in the urine unchanged. No data are published on the safety of gabapentin administration in young animals, although it is reported to be teratogenic and fetotoxic at high doses. Sedation is the most common side effect of gabapentin administration. Other effects are lethargy, somnolence, and diarrhea. Gabapentin has not been evaluated as an analgesic in neonatal dogs or cats.

Tramadol

Tramadol is a synthetic mu opioid agonist that also inhibits serotonin and norepinephrine reuptake (similar to alpha-2 agonists), which contribute to its analgesic properties. Tramadol is not a controlled drug in the United States and is available in an oral formulation (see Table 26-1). Tramadol is metabolized in the liver and excreted in the urine. No data exist on its efficacy or safety in neonates and juvenile dogs and cats, although tramadol is reportedly fetotoxic.

Tramadol has been associated with cardiac and respiratory depression, although these effects are minimal. The CNS effects of tramadol include agitation, anxiety, and tremors. Seizures, vomiting, and diarrhea have been reported. Caution should be used when administering tramadol to animals with a history of seizure or head trauma or in animals being treated with other drugs that may lower the seizure threshold. Naloxone may be administered to partially antagonize tramadol.

Steroids and Nonsteroidal Antiinflammatory Drugs
Nonsteroidal Antiinflammatory Drugs

Nonsteroidal antiinflammatory drugs (NSAIDs) inhibit inflammation and produce analgesia by decreasing prostaglandin synthesis by inhibition of cyclooxygenase (COX) and in some cases 5-lipoxygenase (LOX). Prostaglandins cause vasodilation, increase vascular permeability, and sensitize pain receptors to noxious stimuli. In addition, prostaglandins are responsible for regulation of renal blood flow, protect GI mucosa, and aid in platelet aggregation. COX has two clinically relevant isoforms: COX-1 and COX-2. Both

---

BOX 26-6 Issues with nonsteroidal antiinflammatory drugs in young animals

- Reduced hepatic clearance leads to longer half-lives and longer duration of effects and side effects.
- Developing kidneys at risk for renal papillary necrosis.
- Diarrhea and vomiting.
- Gastrointestinal ulcer formation.
- Lower albumin levels, thus more unbound (active) drug.

---

are constitutively expressed in select tissues, although COX-2 is upregulated in the inflammatory cascade. Differences between NSAID effects, efficacy, and toxicity are related to COX enzymes and the inhibitory effects on preexisting COX activities in the patient. LOX products (leukotriene B [LTB], leukotriene D [LTD], and leukotriene C [LTC]) are responsible for recruitment of immune mediators and alteration of vascular permeability.

NSAIDs have minimal effects on normal cardiovascular and respiratory systems. Side effects are typically the result of COX-1 inhibition, are dose-related, and typically include GI ulceration, renal papillary necrosis, and inhibition of platelet aggregation.

NSAIDs should be used with caution in young animals (younger than 4 months of age) because of their reduced clearance and metabolizing organ immaturity (Table 26-3). Administration of NSAIDs to immature dogs or cats could result in significantly prolonged clearance and longer effects and side effects. NSAIDs could impact the development of organ maturation or cause significant damage to young organs (renal papillary necrosis) (Box 26-6).

Carprofen

Carprofen is a reversible inhibitor of COX and is considered COX-2 selective but does exhibit some COX-1 inhibitory activity. Carprofen is labeled for use in dogs older than 6 weeks of age. Oral and injectable formulations are available and can be administered once daily, or by dividing the dose in half, twice daily (see Table 26-1). Carprofen is metabolized by the liver and excreted in the feces, with some urine excretion.

Carprofen has been associated with reversible liver toxicity in Labrador Retrievers when given chronically or in high doses.

Deracoxib

Deracoxib is a COX-2 selective NSAID for use in dogs. It is only available in an oral formulation and is typically administered once daily for the treatment of pain and inflammation associated with arthritis or acute postoperative pain (see Table 26-1). Deracoxib should be administered with food. Deracoxib is metabolized in the liver and excreted

TABLE 26-3	Manufacturer recommendations for NSAIDs in neonates
Drug	**Recommendations**
Carprofen	Safe use in dogs younger than 6 weeks of age has not been evaluated. Not recommended or approved for use in cats.
Deracoxib	Safe use in dogs younger than 4 months of age has not been evaluated. Not recommended or approved for use in cats.
Etodolac	Safe use in dogs younger than 12 months of age has not been evaluated. Not recommended or approved for use in cats.
Firocoxib	Not recommended for use in dogs weighing less than 12.5 lb. Not recommended or approved for use in cats.
Flunixin meglumine	Not recommended or approved for use in dogs and cats.
Ketoprofen	Not recommended or approved for use in dogs and cats.
Meloxicam	Safe use of oral and injectable formulations in dogs younger than 6 months of age has not been evaluated. Safe use of injectable formulation in cats younger 4 months of age has not been evaluated. Oral formulation is not recommended or approved for use in cats.
Tepoxalin	Not recommended for use in dogs younger than 6.6 lb. Safe use in dogs younger than 6 months of age has not been evaluated. Not recommended or approved for use in cats.

in the feces and should not be used in young pups that are still nursing or younger than 6 weeks of age.

Etodolac

Etodolac is a nonselective COX inhibitor labeled for use in dogs. Etodolac is available as an oral preparation and is not recommended for dogs younger than 12 months of age (see Table 26-1). Etodolac is metabolized in the liver and excreted in feces. In addition to the GI side effects, keratoconjunctivitis sicca can occur.

Firocoxib

Firocoxib is a COX-2 selective NSAID for use in dogs. It is only available in an oral formulation and is typically administered once daily for the treatment of pain and inflammation associated with arthritis or acute postoperative pain (see Table 26-1). Firocoxib is metabolized in the liver and excreted in the feces. Firocoxib is not recommended for use in animals younger than 7 months because of hepatic and thalamic changes in growing juveniles. In addition, the manufacturer does not recommend the use of firocoxib in dogs weighing less than 12.5 lb because of the possibility of inaccuracy of dosing.

Flunixin meglumine

Flunixin meglumine is a nonselective COX inhibitor for use in dogs. Available as an injectable formulation and oral paste (used mainly in horses), administration of flunixin meglumine in small animal practice has decreased as the result of the wide availability of COX-2 selective NSAIDs, which have fewer GI side effects (see Table 26-1). Administration of flunixin meglumine to young dogs and cats is not recommended. Flunixin meglumine is still widely used to reduce ocular inflammation and is an effective antiinflammatory and antipyretic. Flunixin meglumine is metabolized by the liver and excreted in the feces.

Ketoprofen

Ketoprofen is a nonselective COX inhibitor in dogs and cats, although it is labeled for use only in horses. Available in both injectable and oral formulations, administration of ketoprofen in small animal practice has decreased as the result of the wide availability of COX-2 selective NSAIDs, which have fewer GI side effects. Ketoprofen is not recommended for use in young dogs and cats. When administered orally, ketoprofen should not be given with food because of decreased absorption (see Table 26-1). Ketoprofen is excreted by the kidneys unchanged and as a conjugated metabolite. Use of ketoprofen in the perioperative period has been associated with increased hemorrhage, in addition to the GI side effects associated with many NSAIDs.

Meloxicam

Meloxicam is a COX-2 selective inhibitor approved for use in dogs and cats. Meloxicam is available as an injectable and oral (liquid) formulation and is typically administered once daily for the treatment of postoperative pain and pain associated with osteoarthritis (see Table 26-1). Meloxicam is not recommended for use in dogs and cats younger than 6 weeks of age. It is metabolized by the liver and excreted in the feces. GI side effects are the most common adverse effects associated with meloxicam administration, although renal toxicity should always be considered.

Tepoxalin

Tepoxalin is a nonselective COX inhibitor and LOX inhibitor. The LOX inhibitory effects reduce the production of leukotrienes, most notably LTB_4. LTB_4 is thought to contribute to GI inflammation, and LOX inhibition is purported to decrease the GI side effects of the other NSAIDs. However, as a nonselective COX inhibitor, the GI side effects may still be substantial. The long-term effects of LOX inhibition in neonates are unknown at this time, and like the other NSAIDs, caution should be used when administering tepoxalin to young, developing dogs and cats (see Table 26-1).

Glucocorticoid Steroids

Glucocorticoid steroids are used for the treatment of pain associated with inflammation. Glucocorticoids produce anti-inflammatory effects by inhibiting phospholipase A_2, which is the precursor of arachidonic acid in the inflammatory pathway. Its inhibition results in decreased prostaglandin and leukotriene production. The result is an increase in the pain threshold and a decreased sensitivity to pain-causing substances such as histamine and bradykinin. In addition to their effects on prostaglandins, glucocorticoids also reduce COX levels.

COX inhibition is not selective, so glucocorticoid steroids can result in the same side effects as NSAIDs, including GI ulceration. In addition, endogenous glucocorticoids play a role in electrolyte and fluid homeostasis, which can be disrupted with long-term administration or sudden withdrawal of exogenous glucocorticoids. Hepatopathy and liver failure may occur with prolonged use. Glucocorticoids can disrupt wound healing and cause immunosuppression and should be used with caution in perioperative patients (see Table 26-1).

Local Anesthetic Techniques

Epidural

The spinal cord extends the entire length of the spinal column at birth in the dog, although the vertebral column and the spinal cord grow and develop at different rates, and becomes the same as an adult between 4 and 6 months of age. The vertebral column outgrows the spinal cord in length, although the degree to which this occurs is highly variable. In the fully grown dog, the spinal cord extends to approximately L6-L7, although the length of the spinal cord in small dogs may be one vertebral space longer, ending at L7-S1. The end of the spinal cord in cats is more variable and may be located anywhere between L7 to S3.

The typical site for epidural administration of drugs is between L7 and S1. The landmarks for performing an epidural at this area are the craniodorsal iliac crests, the spinal process of L7, and the median sacral crest.

A 22-g Tuohy needle may be used for small dogs and for cats. In larger dogs, a 20-g spinal needle is recommended. The landmarks are palpated, and the needle is inserted after clipping and sterile preparation of the needle placement site. Resistance is felt through the skin and as the needle passes through the supraspinous and interspinous ligaments. The needle is advanced farther, resistance is again felt, and a

distinctive "pop" will be felt as the needle passes through the ligamentum flavum. No fluid should flow out of the needle if the needle is in the epidural space (Figure 26-3).

Local anesthetics or opioids may be used to infiltrate into the epidural space (Box 26-7). Administration of local anesthetics will result in hindlimb paralysis, dilation of the anus, and an inability to urinate. Administration of opioids produces hindlimb analgesia but does not affect motor activity and the ability to ambulate, urinate, or defecate.

Lidocaine is recommended for caudal epidural anesthesia in neonates. The recommended dose of lidocaine 2% is 0.2 ml/kg/body weight. Preservative-free morphine is recommended for caudal epidural analgesia. The dose is 0.2 ml/kg/body weight.

BOX 26-7   Epidural drugs, doses, and equipment

Opioids
Morphine (preservative-free): 0.1 mg/kg
Morphine: 0.1 mg/kg diluted in 0.1 ml/kg saline
Fentanyl: 1-10 mg/kg diluted in 0.2 ml/kg saline

Local Anesthetics
Lidocaine 2%(without epinephrine): 0.2 ml/kg

Alpha-2 Agonists
Xylazine: 0.1-0.4 mg/kg
Medetomidine: 0.015 mg/kg diluted in 0.1 ml/kg saline

Ketamine
Ketamine: 0.5-1 mg/kg

Epidural Equipment
For small patients (dogs ≤ 5 kg and all cats): 22-g needle or 22-g Tuohy needle
For larger patients (>5 kg): 20- or 22-g spinal needle

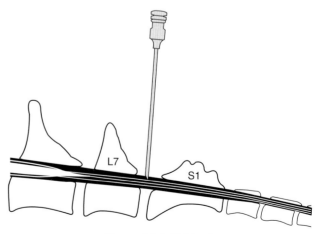

Figure 26-3 Epidural.

Infiltration of Local Anesthetics

Use of a "pain buster" or "soaker catheter" has been advocated for infusion of local anesthetics. A local anesthetic infuses into the area from a pump or reservoir (bulb), which is attached to tubing and a multifenestrated catheter. Rates of administration range from 0.5 to 5 ml/hr.

Caution should be used with these systems because the reservoir is likely to be too big for the size of a neonate, systemic absorption is unpredictable, and neurotoxic effects of long-term local anesthetic can occur.

Topical Local Anesthesia

Creams

Liposomal encapsulated lidocaine creams can be used for topical application of local anesthetics. Liposomal encapsulation extends the release of lidocaine. Liposomal lidocaine cream has an effect in 20 to 30 minutes. Topical anesthesia may also be accomplished by application of a eutectic mixture of local anesthetics (EMLA), consisting of lidocaine and prilocaine. The anesthetic effect of EMLA is demonstrable for as long as 60 minutes after application in dogs and cats. Adverse effects of EMLA include local irritation (swelling, redness, and pruritus) and systemic effects caused by absorption of lidocaine and prilocaine (neurologic and cardiovascular side effects, methemoglobinemia). The use of EMLA in cats has been a concern because of the presence of prilocaine and their increased susceptibility to methemoglobinemia. However, a recent study demonstrated that healthy cats do not have an increased risk of methemoglobinemia with the use of EMLA cream. Liposomal encapsulated lidocaine creams, in contrast to EMLA, do not contain prilocaine and as such are less of a concern when used in cats.

Lidocaine Patches

Transdermal lidocaine patches may be applied over incisions to provide extended pain relief and a protective covering. In addition, the application of lidocaine may be helpful for the treatment of neuropathic pain. Systemic absorption of lidocaine from the transdermal system is variable but tends to be low. The lidocaine patch is effective for 24 hours. These patches can be replaced when no longer effective. Side effects of lidocaine patches have not been reported.

Alternative Approaches to Pain Therapy

Cryotherapy

Cryotherapy is a form of thermotherapy in which cold temperature is applied to an area to limit the inflammatory phase of tissue injury and reduce pain. The objective of cryotherapy is to reduce the inflammatory response and provide analgesia by mitigating the inflammatory cascade, and decreasing pain transmission and muscle spasm.

The results of this inflammatory phase are increased vascular permeability, vasodilation and increased blood flow to the area, and tissue edema. Cryotherapy reduces the tissue metabolic rate, limiting tissue injury, tissue heat, and cellular hypoxia. Reduction of temperature in joints also reduces the rate of cartilage degradation by impairment of collagenase, hyaluronidase, protease, and elastase.

Cryotherapy results in analgesia by decreasing nerve conduction velocity in the affected area and overstimulation of the cold receptors that result in prevention of pain transmission to the spinal centers. Cryotherapy decreases muscle spasm by decreasing muscle guarding as the result of a decrease in the firing rate of the motor neuron.

Cryotherapy should only be used in the acute phase of inflammation to minimize the inflammatory response. Use of cryotherapy is discouraged during the proliferative phase of inflammation because it may impair wound healing.

Cryotherapy may be performed in several different ways, depending on the location of the injury, depth of penetration desired, stage of tissue repair, and physiologic goals. It is important to observe the skin for response to cold. Application times of 20 to 30 minutes may be appropriate for some areas and injuries but may need to be longer to ensure sufficient cooling of the injured tissue.

Ice packs are an easy, inexpensive method of providing cryotherapy. Crushed ice can be placed in a plastic freezer bag, wrapped in a thin towel or cloth, and applied to the desired location. Commercially available ice packs also can be used. Cold immersion using an ice bath is also cost effective, although it is most appropriate for cryotherapy of an extremity, since the animal can stand with only the affected limb in the bath. Ice massage is another method of cryotherapy. The affected area should be stretched gently and a large piece of ice is applied to the area parallel to the muscle fibers. The ice is used to massage the affected muscle or tissue in a slow motion, applying even pressure. Ice massage is typically performed for 5 to 10 minutes, at which point the skin should be red and numb. A cold compression unit is another method, in which cold water circulates within a fabric sleeve to ensure maximal contact with the area, and still allow movement. Cold compression units are also commercially available.

Acupuncture

Acupuncture is a procedure in which fine-gauge needles are inserted to provide stimulation or analgesia at specific anatomic points. The theory of acupuncture is that stimulation of specific anatomic points results in a change in the energy and blood flow to that area, which alters the sensation of pain. Low frequency electrical stimulation can be applied to the needles, and this electrical simulation is transferred through the patient. These electrical impulses result in the release of neurotransmitters and endogenous opioids that reduce pain transmission and alter the sensation of pain. Electrical stimuli are provided for 10 to 20 minutes, the analgesic effects may last from hours to days, and the procedure does not seem to have any long-term side effects.

| BOX 26-8 | Acupuncture points and equipment |

Equipment

Acupuncture needles 26-30 g
Acupuncture electrostimulator

Acupuncture Points

Forelimbs

Shoulder: LI15, SI3, SI9, SI9, BL10, BL11, BL60, TH4, TH14, GB21
Humerus: LU5, SI3
Elbow: LU5, SI3, PC3
Radius/ulna: SI3
Carpus, digits: HT3, SI3, TH4, TH5, Baxie

Hindlimbs

Hip: BL25, BL32, BL40, GB29, GB30, GB31, GB39, Bai Hui, Xiyan, Heding

Femur: SP10, GB29, GB30, GB31, Xiyan, Heding
Stifle: ST35, ST36, SP9, BL23, GB34, GV4, Xiyan, Heding
Tibia/fibula: ST40, GB34, Xiyan, Heding
Tarsus, digits: ST41, ST44, BL60, BL62, GB34, GB41, LV3, Bafeng, Xiyan, Heding

Neck and Back

Cervical and thoracic spine: LU5, LU7, LI4, SI3, SI9, BL10, BL11, BL60, TH5, GB20, GB21, GB39, GV14, Huatuojiaji
Lumbar and caudal spine: BL23, BL25, BL28, BL32, BL40, BL54, BL62, KI3, GB29, GB30, GB31, GV4, GV14, Huatuojiaji

---

Acupuncture points and needle placement are determined by the area being treated (Box 26-8).

CONCLUSION

Neonatal pain has important consequences on behavioral and social development in dogs and cats. Pain in neonates should be treated after consideration of developmental physiology and species-specific differences in drug pharmacodynamics. Future clinical studies need to focus on the diagnosis and efficacy of pain management in neonates.

SUGGESTED READINGS

Gaynor J, Muir W: *Handbook of veterinary pain management*, ed 2, St. Louis, 2008, Mosby.

McMahon S, Koltzenburg M: *Wall and Melzack's textbook of pain*, ed 5, 2005, Churchill Livingstone.

Muir W, Hubbell J, Bednarski R, Skarda R: *Handbook of veterinary anesthesia*, ed 4, St. Louis, 2006, Mosby.

Flecknell P, Waterman-Pearson A: *Pain management in animals*, St. Louis, 2000, Saunders.

PHARMACOLOGIC CONSIDERATIONS IN THE YOUNG PATIENT

CHAPTER 27

John Mata, Mark G. Papich

Treatment of neonates in small animal medicine presents challenges for clinicians because of the marked anatomic and physiologic differences between puppies and kittens and adult animals. Current guidelines for the treatment of puppies and kittens have been extrapolated from other species, including human neonates, and from a small number of studies. Therefore many of the recommendations in this chapter are provided to make practitioners aware of pharmacological considerations that may require dosage adjustments in young animals.

DRUG ABSORPTION

Puppies and kittens can be exposed to drugs in utero through placental transfer. Neonates can also be exposed by ingesting compounds in their mother's milk during nursing or through direct administration. Each source of exposure can be problematic for a developing fetus or a young animal because of differences in proportions and physiology compared with more mature animals. Although current veterinary drug reference handbooks provide little guidance for administration of medications to young animals, there are some basic considerations that are helpful for clinicians when administering drugs to pregnant or nursing mothers and young puppies or kittens.

Transplacental Transfer

The transfer of drugs from mother to fetus has been demonstrated for a number of drugs, which is a greater concern for drugs with high lipid solubility or that reach high systemic concentrations. The main forces that favor drug transfer from mother to fetus are the lipid solubility of the drug and a steep maternal-fetal drug concentration. However, other properties of the drug may also affect the extent of drug transfer; a list of properties and effects are presented in Table 27-1.

Transfer from Milk

Like transplacental transfer of drugs to the fetus, the transfer of drugs from mother's milk to the neonate can also be a concern. The transfer of the drug to milk is similar to placental transfer of drugs. Weakly acidic drugs that are non-ionized and nonprotein bound rapidly transfer from the maternal circulation to milk. Animal milk tends to be more acidic than the plasma pH, therefore drugs that make their way into milk may accumulate because they become ionized and "trapped" in the milk. The neonate may receive a significant dose of drug while nursing, although the amount of drug is generally less than 2% of the maternal dose. It is important to note, however, that the drug present in milk is not necessarily bioavailable and depends again on possible interactions in the neonate's gastrointestinal tract that might limit drug absorption. Examples of drugs that cross the placenta include anesthetics, such as lidocaine; salicylates and nonsteroidal antiinflammatory drugs (NSAIDs); beta-lactam antibiotics; many narcotics; and anticonvulsants, including phenytoin and diazepam (Table 27-2).

Oral Absorption

Within the absorptive region of the neonatal small intestine, the surface area is sufficiently large relative to the size of the animal to allow a highly bioavailable drug to be rapidly absorbed. This absorption may lead to higher-than-anticipated peak plasma drug concentrations after oral administration of a medication. The increase in the rate of absorption combined with increased intestinal permeability in young animals can produce plasma concentrations that may reach toxic levels with some drugs. Drugs that normally have limited oral bioavailability can reach systemic circulation in the neonatal animal. These drugs include aminoglycosides, carbenicillin (and other acid-sensitive beta-lactams), and enteric sulfonamides. However, the practitioner should also consider other factors that may limit absorption of drugs in

TABLE 27-1　Drug effects on fetus

Drug property	Effect on drug exposure to the fetus
Molecular weight (MW)	<500 MW is likely to pass through the placenta. >1000 MW is unable to pass in significant concentrations.
Lipid solubility	Only lipid-soluble drugs cross the placental barrier.
Ionization	Only nonionized drugs are able to cross the placenta. Weak acid drugs are more likely to transfer.*
Protein binding	Only unbound substances are likely to cross the placenta. Decreased maternal albumin increases the amount of free drug and may increase fetal exposure for highly bound drugs.

Data from Syme MR, Paxton JW, Keelan JA: Drug transfer and metabolism by the human placenta, *Clin Pharmacokinet* 43(8):487-514, 2004.
*Because fetal circulation is generally more acidic than maternal circulation, weak acid drugs can ionize in the fetus and be trapped. This results in fetal accumulation of weak acid drugs.

TABLE 27-2　Drugs to avoid in the preterm and lactating animal

Preterm	Lactating
Glucocorticoids	Aminoglycosides
Aminoglycosides	Anticancer drugs
Anticancer drugs	Chloramphenicol
Organophosphates	Tetracyclines
Chlorinated hydrocarbons	
Tetracyclines	

puppies and kittens. For example, intestinal permeability will be substantially reduced after the ingestion of colostrum or exogenous supplementation of either hydrocortisone or adrenocorticotropic hormone (ACTH) in the mother before giving birth.

Very young animals also have decreased gastric emptying time and irregular peristalsis that can partially protect against the increase in maximum systemic drug concentrations. Decreased gastric emptying in young dogs has been observed in multiple breeds, independent of size. Reduced gastric emptying may decrease the likelihood of reaching toxic drug concentrations by slowing the rate of absorption and thus reducing peak plasma concentrations. However, gastric emptying time has been shown to be shorter in puppies 12 weeks of age compared to older animals, so it may not be prudent

to assume that decreased gastric emptying time will provide protection from high peak plasma concentrations. As a puppy develops, the rate increases to become higher than would be expected in an adult animal. This means that the practitioner should be aware that oral drugs with a narrow therapeutic index may present a problem for neonates, particularly when toxicity occurs because of peak plasma concentrations. Further, the practitioner must consider that if the peak concentration is reduced because of gastric emptying time, the net effect may result in increased steady-state plasma concentration and a reduced dose or dosing interval may be warranted.

Gastric pH is also a consideration for oral administration of drugs to newborns. Although pH in adult animals is quite acidic, the pH of newborns is closer to neutral. Mean gastric pH has been found to be stable at 5.85 until the seventh day of life. After day 7, gastric pH was shown to decrease to 3.45 and then increase to a mean of 4.95 through the eighteenth day. These types of changes will likely affect absorption of mildly acidic or basic drugs and either limit or increase bioavailability depending on pKa. For example, when pH is less acidic, drugs, such as beta-lactam antibiotics (weak acids), will be ionized and thus less bioavailable. Also, high gastric pH may decrease the bioavailability of drugs, such as ketoconazole and itraconazole, that require an acid environment for absorption. In contrast, weak bases, including the aminoglycoside antibiotics and fluconazole, have greater bioavailability. It is ultimately up to the practitioner to weigh the margin of safety versus the likelihood that the drug absorption might be significantly different from that expected in the adult.

A consideration for giving medications to nursing puppies and kittens includes the reduced absorption of concomitant administration of drug when milk may be present in the stomach. Milk can both decrease gastric emptying time and may also interact with drugs directly. Drugs likely to have reduced bioavailability include enrofloxacin and doxycycline. These interactions may lead to reduced absorption and result in lower peak plasma concentrations.

Newborn puppies and kittens can also be expected to have reduced hepatobiliary function, reduced capacity for drug metabolism through the cytochrome P-450 system, and reduced glucuronidation up to 4 to 6 weeks of age. These differences in phase I and II metabolism tend to lower absorption of fat-soluble drugs and vitamins. Also, reduced metabolism reduces the clearance of some drugs, including lidocaine and theophylline, that rely on P-450 metabolism. Other drugs, including morphine and many NSAIDs, may have reduced clearance as a result of reduced glucuronidation. Neonatal puppies and kittens also require time for their intestinal flora to be fully colonized; therefore an altered response to drugs that require activation in the intestine can be expected.

Absorption from Extravascular Sites

A common route of administration of drugs in puppies and kittens is by subcutaneous (SC) injection. This is often a preferred route because of the reduced muscle mass in young animals, which can make intramuscular (IM) injections more problematic. As muscle mass develops, the accompanying increase in blood flow also contributes to a more rapid absorption after IM injection. There are a number of physiologic differences between puppies and kittens relative to adult animals that contribute to changes in the absorption of drugs. Reduced fat and increased total body water may enhance SC drug absorption. Absorption likely decreases after either SC or IM administration if the animal is hypothermic.

Topical formulations are becoming more common in small animal medicine. These formulations are often designed to provide the drug at a rate that depends on the hydration state of the skin. Because skin hydration is greatest in the neonate, the rate of absorption will be higher and these patients may reach higher than expected peak plasma concentrations. This increase in peak plasma concentrations in neonatal and young animals could result in adverse effects with drugs that have a low therapeutic index.

DRUG DISTRIBUTION

One obvious difference between neonates and adult animals is the difference in proportion of head-to-body sizes. Body weight is also distributed differently in puppies and kittens, and these differences lead to changes that can present challenges to drug therapy. For example, the proportion of extracellular fluid as a percentage of total body weight changes significantly during the life of a maturing puppy. As seen in Figure 27-1, the changes occurring in the growing puppy (and similarly in the kitten) are a result of the total water alterations as a proportion of body weight. This water is found primarily in the extracellular fluid compared to percent intracellular fluid and will have significant effects on the

absorption and distribution of drugs within the animal, including decreased plasma concentrations and longer half-lives. Plasma concentrations of water-soluble compounds are lower in pediatric patients compared with adults because the volume into which the compound is distributed is greater in the young. Unbound lipid-soluble compounds have the same type of distribution because they are distributed into the total body of water.

A second factor important to the distribution of lipid-soluble drugs is the relative lack of fat in neonates and puppies compared to adult animals. Because fat acts as a reservoir for many lipid-soluble drugs, the absence of significant fat stores results in higher plasma concentrations of these types of drugs.

A number of biologic functions are reduced in young animals and will contribute to differences in drug distribution compared to adult animals. Hepatic gluconeogenesis, glycogenolysis, protein synthesis, and bile acid metabolism are reduced in neonates, with adult values occurring after 8 weeks of age. These decreases can contribute to the changes observed in drug metabolism and will alter the distribution of drugs that are protein bound in the circulation.

ELIMINATION

Kidney function and therefore drug clearance may be attenuated in puppies and kittens. The glomerular filtration rate (GFR) and renal tubular function increase as the puppy or kitten matures, increasing from about 20% of adult values at birth to full adult values over a period of 2 to 3 months. Reduced kidney function results in reduced drug clearance of drugs that undergo renal elimination. Under these conditions, with multiple-dose therapies, reduced clearance will produce a higher steady-state drug concentration for drugs

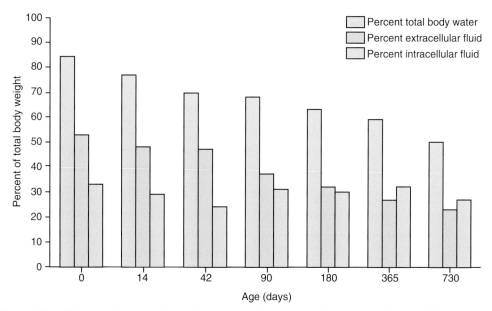

Figure 27-1 Changes in proportion of body weight in extracellular vs. intracellular fluid in maturing puppy. (Adapted from Boothe DM, Hoskins JD: Drug and blood component therapy. In Hoskins JD: *Veterinary pediatrics: dogs and cats from birth to six months*, ed 3, Philadelphia, 2001, Saunders, Table 3-2.)

with a sufficiently long half-life. The impact of reduced renal clearance can require the practitioner to adjust the neonate's recommended drug regimen.

For example, consider the effect that reduced clearance might have on beta-lactam antibiotics such as amoxicillin. The beta-lactam antimicrobials are often the drug of choice for puppies and kittens because of their high therapeutic index. The peak plasma concentrations will be lower than expected because of the greater volume of distribution in puppies compared to adults, and the practitioner may need to select a higher dose for a puppy or kitten. Lower rate of renal clearance and reduced hepatic function will affect the amount of circulating drug and will have its greatest impact on steady-state concentrations. Therefore, to compensate for the reduced clearance, the clinician may have to consider giving an adult dose of the drug and extending the dosing intervals.

DRUG RESPONSES

Adverse responses to drugs and drug formulations are more likely in puppies and kittens than in their adult counterparts. For example, administration of a drug formulation likely to cause a large shift in osmolality can result in a number of clinically significant adverse effects. Intravenous (IV) administration of hypertonic solutions containing sodium bicarbonate and radiocontrast materials in young animals can result in intraventricular hemorrhage and necrotizing enterocolitis.

Although pharmacokinetic differences contribute significantly to therapeutic failure in puppies and kittens, pharmacodynamic differences are also important to drug response in this population. A lack of response from drugs, such as atropine, isoproterenol, dopamine, and dobutamine, as well as anticholinergic drugs, has been demonstrated. The lack of drug response may be due in part to the immaturity of innervation in the developing animal.

There is relatively little information on the risks to the fetus associated with giving medications during pregnancy; much of the information available is limited to human medicine. However, there are some general guidelines that have been developed that may be helpful in assessing the impact of drug therapy in this population. Table 27-3 shows drug categories and a description of the effects of the different categories. Table 27-4 lists the general safety of a variety of drugs for use in neonates.

ANALGESIA

Management of pain is important in the small animal practice, and this holds true for pregnant, neonatal, and young dogs and cats. Without effective pain management, there is a risk of permanent hyperalgesic response. In nursing bitches or queens, there is also a risk that ineffective treatment may lead to aggressive behavior toward the young. In addition, inappropriate selection of analgesics in pregnant or nursing bitches or queens may result in congenital defects of the fetus or young animal.

TABLE 27-3	Drug category and description of effects
Drug category	**Description**
A	Adequate, well-controlled studies in pregnant women have not shown an increased risk of fetal abnormalities.
B	Animal studies have revealed no evidence of harm to the fetus; however, there are no adequate and well-controlled studies in pregnant women.
	or
	Animal studies have shown an adverse effect, but adequate and well-controlled studies in pregnant women have failed to demonstrate a risk to the fetus.
C	Animal studies have shown an adverse effect, and there are no adequate and well-controlled studies in pregnant women.
	or
	No animal studies have been conducted, and there are no adequate and well-controlled studies in pregnant women.
D	Adequate well-controlled or observational studies in pregnant women have demonstrated a risk to the fetus; however, the benefits of therapy may outweigh the potential risk.
X	Adequate well-controlled or observational studies in animals or pregnant women have demonstrated positive evidence of fetal abnormalities. The use of the product is contraindicated in women who are or may become pregnant.

From US Food and Drug Administration: *FDA Consumer magazine* 35(3), May-June 2001.

ANTIBIOTICS

The unique differences between neonates and adult animals require dosage adjustments for many antibiotics. A general recommendation is to decrease the drug dose by 30% to 50% or to increase the dosing interval by 2 to 4 hours. Table 27-5 provides the recommended modifications of antimicrobial drug therapy in puppies and kittens.

FORMULARY

Table 27-6 is a general formulary with estimated drug dosages for pediatric dog and cat patients. These dosages have been adjusted using the best knowledge to date on pediatric physiologic differences from adult dogs and cats. It

Text continued on p. 243

TABLE 27-4	Safety of drugs in neonates*	
Drug	**Recommendation†**	**Comments**
Antimicrobial Drugs		
Amikacin	C	Aminoglycosides are relatively more toxic than other classes of antimicrobials (nephrotoxicity, ototoxicity).
Amoxicillin	A	Not shown to be harmful to neonates.
Ampicillin	A	Not shown to be harmful to neonates.
Carbenicillin	A	Not shown to be harmful to neonates.
Cephalosporins	A	Not shown to be harmful to neonates.
Chloramphenicol	C	Anemia: dose-related, anorexia and diarrhea in cats at high or prolonged dose, use at lower dose/increased interval.
Ciprofloxacin	D	Toxicity is dose-related. Quinolones have been associated with articular cartilage defects.
Clavulanic acid	A	Not shown to be harmful to neonates.
Clindamycin	B	Lincosamides can cause severe, often fatal diarrhea caused by altered GI flora.
Cloxacillin	A	Not shown to be harmful to neonates.
Dicloxacillin	A	Not shown to be harmful to neonates.
Doxycycline	B	Tetracyclines accumulate in growing teeth and bones.
Enrofloxacin	D	See Ciprofloxacin.
Erythromycin	A	Not shown to be harmful to neonates. Can cause GI disturbances.
Gentamicin	C	See Amikacin.
Hetacillin	A	Not shown to be harmful to neonates.
Kanamycin	C	See Amikacin.
Lincomycin	B	Not shown to be harmful to neonates. Lincosamides cause severe, often fatal diarrhea caused by altered GI flora.
Metronidazole	C	High dose or prolonged use may produce neurotoxicity.
Neomycin	C	An aminoglycoside used in topical solutions and ointments. Allergic/hypersensitivity reactions common.
Oxacillin	A	Not shown to be harmful to neonates.
Oxytetracycline	D	May disrupt GI flora; potentially nephrotoxic; photosensitivity and hepatotoxicity rarely.
Penicillin G	A	Not shown to be harmful to neonates.
Streptomycin	D	See Amikacin.
Sulfonamides	B	Use may result in renal crystalluria, keratoconjunctivitis, hypoprothrombinemia, thrombocytopenia, and anemia.
Tetracycline	D	May disrupt GI flora; potentially nephrotoxic; photosensitivity and hepatotoxicity rarely; accumulates in growing teeth and bone.
Trimethoprim	B	Use may result in renal crystalluria, keratoconjunctivitis, hypoprothrombinemia, thrombocytopenia, and anemia.
Ticarcillin	A	Not shown to be harmful to neonates.
Tobramycin	C	See Amikacin.
Tylosin	B	Not shown to be harmful to neonates.
Antifungals		
Amphotericin-B	C	Use may result in conjunctival hyperemia, chemosis, and iritis. Toxic to retina if injected into vitreous.
Griseofulvin	C	Use may result in bone marrow suppression and neurologic signs. Can be used safely in puppies and kittens once they are eating on their own but the dose should be calculated carefully according to body weight (not to exceed 25 mg/kg PO BID).
Ketoconazole	B	Dose-related hepatoxicity.
Miconazole	B	Not shown to be harmful to neonates. May develop irritation or hypersensitivity to the agent or other ingredients: redness, pruritus after topical application.

*The recommendations in this table are based on the best available information regarding the use of these drugs in puppies and kittens. Practitioners should use their best judgment when administering any drug to young animals and should follow established protocols when available.

Continued

TABLE 27-4	Safety of drugs in neonates—cont'd	
Drug	**Recommendation†**	**Comments**
Antiparasitic Drugs		
Amitraz	C	A rinse for treatment of canine demodicosis. Side effects include sedation, bradycardia, hypotension, pruritus, and hyperglycemia. Most of the side effects are due to alpha-2 adrenergic receptors and are reversible with yohimbine.
Fenbendazole	B	May be toxic to liver and bone marrow in dogs, particularly at high doses.
Dichlorvos	D	Should not be administered to puppies or kittens.
Ivermectin	A	Generally safe; some collie dogs show high sensitivity to ivermectin.
Levamisole	C	A nicotinic agonist; no information available.
Mebendazole	A	Not shown to be harmful to neonates.
Piperazine	A	Piperazine is safe but not in large doses. Ataxia caused by GABA-mimetic effect seen in young animals given high doses.
Praziquantel	A	Not shown to be harmful to neonates.
Pyrantel	A	Not shown to be harmful to neonates. At recommended doses, adverse effects are not common.
Thiacetarsamide	D	Nephrotoxic.
Anticancer Drugs		
Azathioprine	C	Adverse effects include neutropenia, thrombocytopenia, and anemia.
Doxorubicin	C	Extravasation produces severe tissue necrosis. May produce hydrochloride malformations.
Chlorambucil	C	Myelosuppression is most common adverse reaction.
Cisplatin	C	Renal toxicity and myelosuppression are more common side effects; not to be used in cats.
Cyclophosphamide	C	Myelosuppression is most common side effect; less common: mild alopecia, hemorrhagic cystitis.
Methotrexate	C	Most common side effects include nausea, vomiting, and diarrhea; less frequently: myelosuppression.
Vincristine	C	Use may produce peripheral neuromuscular weakness and constipation secondary to autonomic neuropathy. Myelosuppression may occur. Extravasation results in severe tissue necrosis.
Analgesic Drugs		
Acetaminophen	D	Unsafe in small animals.
Aspirin	C	May cause bleeding problems.
Carprofen	B	Safety has been tested in puppies >6 weeks of age.
Meloxicam	B	Safety in puppies and kittens not established.
Ketoprofen	B	Safety in puppies and kittens not established.
Ibuprofen	C	Safety in puppies and kittens not established.
Indomethacin	C	Safety in puppies and kittens not established.
Salicylates	C	Safety in puppies and kittens not established.
Anesthetic and Preanesthetic Drugs		
Acepromazine	B	Use may cause hypotension, bradycardia, or CNS depression in neonates.
Atropine	B	Anticholinergic; use may cause tachycardia.
Butorphanol	B	Use may cause sedation, ataxia, anorexia, or diarrhea.
Codeine	B	Use may cause respiratory depression.
Diazepam	C	Known to cause fatal hepatic necrosis in cats after receiving oral diazepam.
Fentanyl	B	Generally safe at recommended doses; adverse effects can be treated with naloxone.
Glycopyrrolate	B	See Atropine.
Isoflurane	B	Depression seen in neonates after a cesarean section. Hepatic and renal effects reversibly depressed.
Ketamine	B	Profuse salivation may occur in cats; seizures are common in dogs with use of ketamine alone.
Lidocaine	B	Use may result in prolongation of PR and QRS intervals, hypotension, and decreased myocardial strength; methemoglobinuria in cats.
Meperidine	B	May cause tachycardia. Large doses will induce excitement and seizures in cats.

TABLE 27-4	Safety of drugs in neonates—cont'd	
Drug	**Recommendation†**	**Comments**
Anesthetic and Preanesthetic Drugs		
Morphine	B	Use may cause neonatal sedation and respiratory depression, hyperexcitability, hypotension, cerebral hemorrhage, and edema. Adverse effects can be treated with naloxone.
Naloxone	A	Used to reverse opioid effects in neonates after cesarean delivery. Not shown to be harmful to neonates.
Nitrous oxide	B	Use may cause hypoxemia, distention of gas-filled spaces, pernicious anemia, and neurologic dysfunction.
Oxymorphone	B	See Morphine.
Pentobarbital	D	Safety in puppies and kittens not established.
Thiopental	D	Safety in puppies and kittens not established.
GI Drugs		
Antacids	A	Not shown to be harmful to neonates. May affect absorption of other drugs.
Cimetidine	B	Adverse effects uncommon with recommended doses.
Dimenhydrinate	B	Safe, if used short term at recommended doses.
Diphenhydramine	B	Safe, if used short term at recommended doses.
Diphenoxylate	C	Studies have reported adverse effects in laboratory animals.
Loperamide	C	Constipation, bloating, and sedation are common side effects. Paralytic ileus, toxic megacolon, and pancreatitis are rare. Opioids and cats = excitement.
Methscopolamine	C	Safety not established in puppies and kittens.
Metoclopramide	B	Not shown to be harmful to puppies and kittens.
Misoprostol	C	Use may cause serious diarrhea.
Prochlorperazine	B	Not shown to be harmful to puppies and kittens.
Ranitidine	B	Safety not established in puppies and kittens.
Sucralfate	A	Not shown to be harmful to neonates. May impair absorption of other oral medications.
Sulfasalazine	B	Side effects are rare. Toxicity may develop with long-term use.
Cardiovascular Drugs		
Atropine	B	Anticholinergic; may cause tachycardia.
Captopril	C	Age-related sensitivity has been reported.
Digitalis	B	Safety is comparable to that of adult animals.
Furosemide	B	Can be used safely in young animals. Dehydration is the major concern.
Dopamine	B	Not shown to be harmful to puppies and kittens.
Heparin	B	Use may predispose to intraoperative or postoperative hemorrhage.
Hydralazine	B	Hypotension most common side effect; tachycardia, GI upset in cats.
Isoproterenol	C	Tachycardia and arrhythmias possible.
Lidocaine	B	Probably safe; tachycardia.
Procainamide	B	Probably safe; bradycardia possible.
Propranolol	C	Use may cause neonatal hypoglycemia.
Quinidine	B	Probably safe; may cause bradycardia.
Theophylline	B	Probably safe; not shown to be harmful to puppies and kittens.
Thiazide diuretics	B	Probably safe; not shown to be harmful to puppies and kittens.
Warfarin	D	Safety not established in puppies and kittens.
Anticonvulsant Drugs		
Diazepam	B	Can be used safely in puppies and kittens.
Midazolam	B	Can be used safely in puppies and kittens.
Phenobarbital	B	Probably safe at recommended doses.
Phenytoin	D	Adverse effects have been reported a low doses.
Primidone	C	Extreme care is warranted in cats; risk of hepatic disease with long-term use.
Valproic acid	C	Generally safe but not the preferred therapy; the clinical dose has not been established in cats.

Continued

TABLE 27-4	Safety of drugs in neonates—cont'd	
Drug	**Recommendation†**	**Comments**
Muscle Relaxants		
Methocarbamol	C	Safety in puppies and kittens not established.
Pancuronium	B	Not shown to be harmful to puppies and kittens.
Succinylcholine	B	Not shown to be harmful to puppies and kittens.
Endocrine Drugs		
Betamethasone	B	Corticosteroid use is associated with suppressed immune function.
Cortisone	B	See Betamethasone.
Dexamethasone	B	See Betamethasone.
Diethylstilbestrol	D	Diethylstilbestrol has been involved in cases of immune-mediated thrombocytopenia in dogs. Safety in puppies and kittens not established.
Estradiol cypionate	D	Use can lead to bone marrow depression.
Flumethasone	C	See Betamethasone.
Mitotane	D	Use may induce hypoadrenocorticism.
Prednisolone	B	See Betamethasone.
Stanozolol	D	Masculinization of physical appearance and behavior possible with prolonged use.
Testosterone	D	See Stanozolol.
Thyroxine	B	Generally safe; overdose will produce signs of hyperthyroidism.

GI, Gastrointestinal; *GABA*, gamma-aminobutyric acid; *CNS*, central nervous system.

†*A*, Demonstrated safe use in puppies and kittens; *B*, Use in puppies and kittens would not likely pose additional risks compared to adult use; *C*, Caution should be exercised when using this drug in puppies and kittens; *D*, Adverse effects likely based on known toxicities; use not recommended.

TABLE 27-5	Recommended modifications of antimicrobial drug therapy in puppies and kittens	
Drug group	**Dosage adjustment for neonate**	**Comments**
Penicillins	Minimal Amoxicillin 6-20 mg/kg PO q12h Amoxicillin + clavulanic acid 12.5-25 mg/kg PO q12h Ampicillin 22 mg/kg IV q8h Ampicillin/Sulbactam 22 mg/kg IV q8h	Increase initial dose.
Cephalosporins	Minimal Cephalexin/Cefazolin 10-30 mg/kg PO q8-12h	Avoid use in first weeks of life. Try to avoid use.
Fluoroquinolones	Increase dose in kittens	
Aminoglycosides	Lengthen dose interval	Avoid use in puppies. Do not use in kittens.
Tetracyclines	Minimal	Avoid use.
Chloramphenicol	Reduce dose	Avoid use.
Sulfonamides	Reduce dose	
Trimethoprim	Reduce dose and lengthen dose interval	
Macrolides	No change	
Lincosamides	No change	
Metronidazole	No change	

PO, By mouth; *q* (as in q12h), every; *IV*, intravenous.

TABLE 27-6	General formulary for estimated drug dosages for pediatric dogs and cats		
Generic name	**Trade name**	**Indications**	**Dosage**
Anthelmintics			
Fenbendazole	Panacur (Hoechst-Roussel)	Ascarids, hookworms, whipworms, *Giardia*, *Taenia*	50 mg/kg/day PO for 3 consecutive days
Ivermectin	Ivomec, Heartgard (Merck AgVet)	Ascarids, hookworms, whipworms, heartworm preventive	200 µg/kg PO as anthelmintic but not approved, 6 µg/kg PO monthly for heartworm preventive
Metronidazole	Flagyl (Searle, Geneva Pharmaceuticals)	*Giardia, Trichomonas*	15 mg/kg PO twice daily
Milbemycin oxime	Interceptor (Novartis)	Heartworm preventive, ascarids, hookworms, whipworms	0.5 mg/kg PO monthly
Praziquantel	Droncit (Miles)	Tapeworms	Dogs: 5 mg/kg PO, SC, IM Cats: 1-3 lb: 11 mg, 3-11 lb: 22 mg, >11 lb: 33 mg
Praziquantel + pyrantel pamoate	Drontal (Bayer)	Ascarids, hookworms, tapeworms	See package insert (cats)
Praziquantel + pyrantel pamoate + febantel	Drontal Plus (Bayer)	Ascarids, hookworms, whipworms, tapeworms	See package insert (dogs)
Pyrantel pamoate	Nemex (Pfizer)	Ascarids, hookworms	15 mg/kg PO
Sulfadimethoxine	Albon (Hoffman-La Roche), Bactrim (Pitman-Moore)	Coccidia	55 mg/kg PO first day, then 12.5 mg/kg PO twice daily for 14-21 days
Thiabendazole	Mintezol (Merck)	*Strongyloides*	50-100 mg/kg PO once daily for 3-5 days
Antiemetics			
Chlorpromazine	Thorazine (SmithKline Beecham Pharmaceuticals)	Effective phenothiazine	0.5 mg/kg IM q8h 0.05 mg/kg IV (dogs)
Diphenhydramine	Benadryl (Parke-Davis)	Effective antihistamine, give before travel	2-4 mg/kg PO q8h 2 mg/kg IM q8h
Metoclopramide	Reglan (AH Robins)	Gastric motility disorders, esophageal reflux, give 30 minutes before meals and at bedtime	0.2-0.4 mg/kg PO, SC q8h 1-2 mg/kg q24h CRI Do not exceed single doses of 1 mg/kg
Ondansetron	Zofran (Glaxo Wellcome)	Selectively inhibits serotonin 5HT3 receptors; does not stimulate gastric or intestinal peristalsis, and has little effect on blood pressure, heart rate, or rhythm	0.1-1.0 mg/kg PO or 0.1-0.2 mg/kg IV q12-24h
Prochlorperazine	Compazine (SmithKline Beecham Pharmaceuticals)	Effective phenothiazine	0.1 mg/kg IM q6h

Continued

TABLE 27-6	General formulary for estimated drug dosages for pediatric dogs and cats—cont'd		
Generic name	**Trade name**	**Indications**	**Dosage**
Antimicrobials			
Amikacin	Many	Systemic infections	10-20 mg/kg IV, IM, SC q24h
Amoxicillin	Many	Combine with aminoglycoside for systemic infections	22 mg/kg PO q12h
Ampicillin	Many	Combine with aminoglycoside for systemic infections	10-20 mg/kg PO q6-8h 5-10 mg/kg IV, IM, SC q6-8h
Cefadroxil	Cefa-Tabs (Fort Dodge Laboratories)	Combine with aminoglycoside for systemic infections	22 mg/kg PO q12h
Cefoxitin sodium	Mefoxin (Merck)	Combine with aminoglycoside for systemic infections	22 mg/kg IV, IM
Cephalexin	Keflex (Dista Products)	Combine with aminoglycoside for systemic infections	20 mg/kg PO, SC, IV q8h
Cephradine	Velosef (Bristol-Myers Squibb)	Combine with aminoglycoside for systemic infections	10-20 mg/kg PO q8h
Chloramphenicol	Many	*Salmonella, Campylobacter, Yersinia*	50 mg/kg IV, IM, SC, PO q8h in dogs, q12h in cats
Clindamycin	Antirobe (Pharmacia & Upjohn)	*Campylobacter, Toxoplasma, Cryptosporidium*	3-5 mg/kg PO, IV, IM q12h
Erythromycin	Many	Can cause vomiting, anorexia	10 mg/kg PO q8h
Gentamicin	Many	Systemic infections, *Shigella, Yersinia, Salmonella*	2 mg/kg IM, SC q8-12h
Metronidazole	Flagyl (Searle, Geneva Pharmaceuticals)	Anaerobic infections	7.5 mg/kg PO, IV q8-12h
Trimethoprim-sulfadiazine	Septra (Glaxo Wellcome)	*Salmonella, Yersinia*	15 mg/kg PO, IM, SC q12h
Tylosin	Tylan (Elanco)	Intestinal bacterial overgrowth	20-40 mg/kg PO q12h in dogs 5-10 mg/kg PO q12h in cats
GI Protectants			
Bismuth subsalicylate	Pepto Bismol (Procter & Gamble)	Nonspecific diarrhea	10-20 mg/kg q8-12h
Sucralfate	Carafate (Marion Merrell Dow)	GI ulceration, give 60 minutes before acid blockers	100-1000 mg PO q6-8h in dogs 100-200 mg PO q6-8h in cats
Cimetidine	Tagamet (SmithKline Beecham Pharmaceuticals)	GI ulceration, inhibits hepatic microsomal enzymes, avoid in animals <3 months of age	5 mg/kg PO, IV, IM q8-12h
Ranitidine	Zantac (Glaxo Pharmaceuticals)	GI ulceration, does not inhibit microsomal enzymes, avoid in animals <3 months of age	2-4 mg/kg PO, IV, SC q12h can be used as CRI
Famotidine	Pepcid (Merck)	GI ulceration, does not inhibit microsomal enzymes, avoid in animals <3 months of age	0.5-1.0 mg/kg PO q12-24h
Omeprazole	Prilosec (Procter & Gamble)	GI ulceration	0.5-1.0 mg/kg PO q24h

TABLE 27-6	General formulary for estimated drug dosages for pediatric dogs and cats—cont'd		
Generic name	**Trade name**	**Indications**	**Dosage**
Miscellaneous			
Diphenoxylate	Lomotil (Searle)	Antidiarrheal	0.06-0.1 mg/kg PO q6-8h in dogs
Loperamide	Imodium (McNeil Consumer)	Antidiarrheal, narcotic	0.08 mg/kg PO q6-8h in dogs
Lactulose	Cephulac, Chronulac (Marion Merrell Dow)	Laxative, hepatoencephalopathy	1 ml/4.5 kg PO q8h in dogs 0.25-1.0 ml PO q12-24h in cats, adjust dose to 2-3 bowel movements per day, can be used as retention enema in hepatoencephalopathy
Dioctyl sodium sulfosuccinate	Colace (Bristol-Myers Squibb)	Laxative, 50- and 100-mg capsules	50-200 mg q PO q24h in dogs 50 mg PO q24h in cats
Bran		Fiber source, laxative, colitis	1-2 tbsp in 400 gm of food q12-24h
Psyllium	Metamucil (Procter & Gamble)	Fiber source, laxative, colitis	1-3 tsp in food q12-24h

CRI, Constant-rate infusion; *IM,* intramuscular; *IV,* intravenous; *PO,* by mouth; *q* (as in q6h), every; *SC,* subcutaneous; *tbsp,* tablespoon; *tsp,* teaspoon.
From Magne ML: Selected topics in pediatric gastroenterology, *Vet Clin Small Anim* 36:533, 2006, p 536.

should be kept in mind these dosages are reasonable estimates and complete pharmacologic studies have not been performed in pediatric patients.

SUGGESTED READINGS

Gillette DD, Filkins M: Factors affecting antibody transfer in the newborn puppy, *Am J Physiol* 210:419, 1966.

Malloy MH, Morriss FH, Denson SE, et al: Neonatal gastric motility in dogs: maturation and response to pentagastrin, *Am J Physiol* 236:E562, 1979.

Root Kustritz MV: Neonatology. In Root Kustritz MV: *Small animal theriogenology,* St Louis, 2003, Butterworth-Heinemann.

Weber MP, Stambouli F, Martin LJ et al: Influence of age and body size on gastrointestinal transit time of radiopaque markers in healthy dogs, *Am J Vet Res* 63:677, 2002.

TOXICOLOGIC CONSIDERATIONS IN THE YOUNG PATIENT*

CHAPTER 28

Michael E. Peterson

RELEVANT PHYSIOLOGIC DIFFERENCES IN PEDIATRIC PATIENTS RELATIVE TO ADULTS

Pups and kittens may be exposed to toxins through various routes: ingestion (including the ingestion of mother's milk), topical exposure, inhalation, and ocular exposure. In dogs and cats, the first 12 weeks of life is a time of significant developmental changes. Physiologic alterations associated with these maturation stages can predispose the pediatric patient to be more susceptible to adverse reactions. All aspects of drug disposition—absorption, distribution, metabolism, and excretion—are affected by these dramatic developmental changes as the neonate matures (Table 28-1).

After oral exposure, toxin absorption occurs primarily in the small intestine. The pediatric patient has a decreased gastric emptying time and irregular intestinal peristalsis and therefore tends to have a slower rate of absorption. These factors may result in the development of lower peak plasma toxin concentrations. The decreased rate of absorption may actually protect against toxic drug concentrations. However, these protective mechanisms may not be present in neonates before colostrum is absorbed. Before colostrum absorption, the permeability of the intestinal mucosa is increased, which also increases the rate of toxin uptake, including the uptake of compounds that normally would not reach the systemic circulation. Intestinal permeability rapidly decreases after colostrum ingestion. This closure may be induced by endogenous release of hydrocortisone or adrenocorticotropic hormone (ACTH). Exogenous supplementation of these hormones to the mother within 24 hours prepartum prevents the increase in permeability and uptake of colostrum.

Several other factors may affect small intestinal drug absorption in pediatric patients. Newborns have a neutral gastric pH, and the rate of progression to adult levels depends on the species involved. Achlorhydria (increased gastric pH) may cause decreased absorption of many compounds that require disintegration and dissolution or that need to be ionized in a more acidic environment (e.g., weak acids). Milk diets can interfere with absorption of toxic compounds by reducing gastric motility or interacting directly with the toxins. The "unstirred water layer" adjacent to the surface area of the mucosal cells is thicker in the neonate compared to the older pediatric patient, and this may limit the rate of absorption of some compounds. Absorption of fat-soluble compounds increases as biliary function develops. Both extrahepatic metabolism and enterohepatic circulation may be altered as microbial colonization of the gastrointestinal (GI) tract occurs. Absorption from the rectal mucosa is rapid in neonates.

Absorption of xenobiotics administered parenterally to pediatric animals varies from that in adults. As muscle mass develops, with its accompanying increase in blood flow and maturation of the vasomotor response, the rate of absorption after intramuscular administration of xenobiotics is altered. Subcutaneous administration of potentially toxic drugs may exhibit variable absorption rates relative to the patient's age. Smaller amounts of body fat but greater water volume may result in quicker absorption of xenobiotics compared to that in adults.

It is suspected that environmental temperature influences subcutaneous absorption. This is especially true in neonates whose thermoregulatory mechanisms are poorly functional. If the neonate is in a cold environment, subcutaneous xenobiotic absorption tends to be reduced. The same thing would be expected for a patient that presents in a hypothermic state. Intraperitoneal exposure to xenobiotics may exhibit rapid absorption in the pediatric patient.

Percutaneous absorption of xenobiotics may be greater in pediatric patients. Percutaneous absorption is directly related to skin hydration, which is highest in neonates. Topical

*Some sections of this chapter are modified from Peterson ME, Talcott PA: *Small animal toxicology*, ed 2, St Louis, 2006, Saunders/Elsevier.

TABLE 28-1	Altered xenobiotic disposition in pediatric patients
Alteration	**Impact**
Increased intestinal permeability	Increased oral uptake, toxic plasma concentrations
Increased gastric pH	Increased oral uptake of weak bases and acid-labile compounds, prolonged and elevated plasma levels, toxic plasma concentrations
Altered peristalsis (decreased gastric emptying time)	Decreased absorption, lower plasma levels of toxin
Decreased plasma proteins	Toxin may accumulate, leading to more unbound compound and thus a potentially longer half-life
Decreased body fat	Increased plasma levels; decreased accumulation of lipid-soluble toxins
Increased total body water (more extracellular fluid)	Decreased plasma concentrations, longer half-life
Increased uptake of volatile gases	High plasma concentrations, increased response and toxicity
Increased dermal absorption	Higher or prolonged plasma exposure levels, toxicity increased
Immature P-glycoprotein system	Poor ability to clear toxins with this system

exposure to potentially toxic lipid-soluble compounds (e.g., hexachlorophene and organophosphates) places the pediatric patient at higher risk of significant absorption.

Volatile gases are absorbed rapidly from the pediatric respiratory tract because of greater minute ventilation. Young animals are more sensitive to the effects of inhaled gases.

The two major differences between adult and pediatric patients relative to xenobiotic distribution are in body fluid compartments and toxin or drug binding to serum proteins. Body fluid compartments undergo tremendous alterations as the neonate grows. As the neonate matures, significant changes occur in both the percentage of total body water and the ratio of compartmental volumes. Although both the percentage of total body water and the volume of the extracellular vs. the intracellular compartment decrease as the animal ages, the change in the ratio of extracellular to intracellular volume is significantly greater. Daily fluid requirements are greater in neonatal and pediatric patients because a larger proportion of their body weight is represented by body water. The net effect on xenobiotic distribution depends on these differences in body compartments. Most

water-soluble compounds are distributed into extracellular fluids. Plasma concentrations of these compounds are lower in pediatric patients compared to adults because the volume into which the compound is distributed is greater in the young. Unbound lipid-soluble compounds have the same type of distribution because they are distributed into total body water. Changes in xenobiotic distribution directly alter the half-life of the xenobiotic. Increases in distribution directly decrease the plasma concentration, a fact that may potentially protect the pediatric patient from toxic xenobiotic concentrations.

Distribution of lipid-soluble compounds that accumulate in the fat (e.g., some organophosphates and chlorinated hydrocarbons) may be decreased as the result of a smaller proportion of body fat in the pediatric patient. Xenobiotic plasma concentrations may be higher, but the half-life is shorter. The movement of many fat-soluble compounds may be facilitated by their high tendency to bind to plasma proteins. This binding decreases their ability to be distributed to target tissues.

Predicting the distribution of highly protein bound compounds is complicated in the pediatric patient. Most compounds are bound to serum albumin, and basic toxins have a high affinity for alpha-1-glycoproteins. Both of these proteins are available in lower concentrations in pediatric patients. Additionally, differences in albumin structure and competition with endogenous substrates (e.g., bilirubin) for binding sites may decrease protein binding. If bound toxins are displaced, the risk of toxicity increases as the concentration of free pharmacologically active compound rises. When a compound has a narrow therapeutic index and is highly protein bound, these age-related changes are significant. Xenobiotic half-life may rise because of increased amounts of compound that are unbound, allowing free distribution to the tissues and decreasing the plasma concentration. Despite the increased volume of distribution, the half-life of a compound may be "normalized" by the increased clearance of free toxin.

Pediatric patients also have differences in regional organ blood flow that may alter toxin disposition. Significant differences in renal blood flow can result in alterations in toxin excretion. Proportionally greater blood flow to the heart and brain in pediatric patients increases the risk of adverse effects that may result from lower exposures to cardiac and central nervous system (CNS) toxins. Neonatal patients have an increased permeability of the blood-brain barrier. This protects the brain from deficiencies in nutritional fuels in stressful states because oxidizable substrates, such as lactate, can pass from the blood into the CNS. However, this mechanism also increases the potential for CNS exposure to toxins. Brain cells that are normally protected in adults are at higher risk of exposure to toxins in the neonate.

Pediatric metabolism is significantly different than the adult. Hepatic and renal excretion is limited in neonatal and pediatric animals, thus decreasing toxin elimination. Absorption of xenobiotics by young animals may be manifested by decreased clearance. Near-term and neonatal puppies have incomplete hepatic metabolism. Both phase I (e.g., oxidative) and II (e.g., glucuronidation) reactions are reduced. Maturation of various metabolic pathways occurs at different rates. Neonatal puppies may not manifest phase I activity until the ninth day of life; this activity steadily increases after day 25 until it reaches adult levels at day 135. Because hepatic xenobiotic metabolism is decreased, plasma clearance of toxins is decreased, plasma half-life is increased, and toxic plasma compound concentrations may result. Until biliary function matures, the absorption of fat-soluble compounds may be impaired.

The oral bioavailability of compounds with a significant first-pass metabolism is probably greater in pediatric patients. Xenobiotics whose toxicity is generated from toxic metabolites may be less hazardous because there is decreased formation of active components. For example, children younger than 9 to 12 years of age have a lower incidence of hepatotoxicity after overdose of acetaminophen than adults. Pediatric hepatic metabolizing enzymes (e.g., cytochrome P-450) do appear to be inducible by phenobarbital and other drugs.

Alterations in toxin excretion manifest in several ways. Pups have reduced renal excretion, which decreases the clearance of renally excreted parent compounds and the products of hepatic phase II metabolism. As pups age, glomerular filtration rate (GFR) and renal tubular function steadily increase. The total number of glomeruli remains constant. Adult levels of GFR and tubular function are attained by 2½ months of age. If normal levels of body fluids and electrolytes are maintained, pediatric renal tubular resorption is equivalent to that in adults. In this pediatric renal environment, water-soluble toxins have decreased clearance and extended half-lives. An example of this phenomenon is the recommendation that pediatric patients require higher doses (as a result of the increased volume of distribution) and longer dosing intervals (as a result of increased distribution and decreased clearance) of gentamicin. One can anticipate alterations in excretion in sick or dehydrated pediatric patients.

MATERNAL TRANSFER OF TOXIN

Almost all xenobiotics cross the placenta and reach pharmacologic concentrations in the fetus after exposure of the mother. Drugs administered to the mother may cross the placenta by passive diffusion, facilitated transport, and active transport. Protein-bound xenobiotics do not cross the placenta. Factors affecting the pharmacokinetic and xenobiotic effects on mother and fetus are (1) altered maternal absorption, (2) increased maternal unbound xenobiotic fraction, (3) increased maternal plasma volume, (4) altered hepatic clearance, (5) increased maternal renal blood flow and GFR, (6) placental transfer, (7) placental metabolism, (8) placental blood flow, (9) maternal-fetal blood pH, (10) preferential fetal circulation to the heart and brain, (11) undeveloped fetal blood-brain barrier, (12) immature fetal liver enzyme activity, and (13) increased fetal unbound xenobiotic fraction.

Passive diffusion is the most common route in which xenobiotics enter milk. Xenobiotics pass through the mammary epithelium by passive diffusion down a concentration gradient on each side of the membrane. The higher the dose received by the mother, the more xenobiotic will pass into the milk. Generally, milk proteins do not bind xenobiotics well. Since milk (pH 7.2) is slightly more acidic than plasma (pH 7.4), compounds that are weak bases are more likely to pass into milk than weak acids. The more lipid soluble the xenobiotic, the greater the quantity and the faster the transfer into milk.

MANAGEMENT OF TOXICOSIS

Toxicologic History

There is an art to acquiring a good toxicologic history. If the history is to provide any type of working diagnosis, the veterinarian's interview must be meticulous, caring, and thorough in scope. The veterinarian must be a calming influence if a reliable account of events is to be obtained. Specific criteria characteristic of a toxicologic history include *what* poison or poisons are involved, *when* the exposure occurred, *how much* poison the animal was exposed to, and the *route* of the exposure It is particularly relevant to inquire about the entire litter, particularly if they are still together. Additionally, what is the mother's condition and is there a possibility that she has been exposed to a compound that could be a problem for her offspring (regardless of whether she is exhibiting clinical signs of toxicosis)? Obtaining packaging containers for known exposures is significant in identifying the compounds involved and quality available to be ingested. Some aids in obtaining an organized history are outlined in Boxes 28-1 and 28-2.

Some toxic exposures manifest specific clinical syndromes called *toxidromes*. A list of common toxidromes can be found in Table 28-2.

Decontamination Procedures

The goal of decontamination is to prevent the continued absorption of the toxicant. Owners and staff should be advised to protect themselves from toxic exposure when decontaminating a patient; this principle is particularly true with dermal toxins and toxins that are easily volatilized.

Exposure assessment should always be attempted to estimate the dose compared to the known toxicity of the compound. If the dose approaches the toxic range, then vigorous decontamination procedures are justified. Various chemical or physical properties of individual toxins may indicate or preclude particular decontamination techniques. Examples of such restrictions would be the high risk of aspiration pneumonia following emesis after ingestion of volatile hydrocarbons.

This is a critical factor. There is a significant decrease in recovery of toxins with a variety of decontamination techniques as the time from exposure increases. Therefore most

TABLE 28-2   **Common toxidromes**

Toxin	Symptoms	Treatment
Narcotics	Respiratory depression, miosis, altered mental status or coma	Naloxone
Organophosphates, cholinergics	*SLUDGE* mnemonic: *s*alivation, *l*acrimation, *u*rination, *d*iarrhea, *g*astrointestinal cramping, *e*mesis. Also bronchorrhea, bronchospasm	Atropine, pralidoxime
Tricyclic antidepressants	Seizures, prolonged QRS, altered level of consciousness, dysrhythmia	Sodium bicarbonate
Anticholinergic	Flushing ("red as a beet"), dry skin and mucous membranes ("dry as a bone"), hyperthermia ("hot as a hare"), delirium ("mad as a hatter"), mydriasis, tachycardia, urinary retention	Supportive care
Sympathomimetic	Mydriasis, anxiety, tachycardia, hypertension, hyperthermia, diaphoresis	Quiet environment and benzodiazepines

BOX 28-1   **Sample items for a prepared toxicology history form**

- Animal's name
- Sex
- Age
- Weight
- Other medications presently given
- Other pertinent medical history
- Suspected poison involved
- Maximum amount of toxin suspected (worst-case scenario)
- Was the original container found?
- Potential route of exposure suspected
- When did possible exposure occur?
- When were clinical signs first noted?
- Describe initial clinical signs.
- Could other poisons be involved?
- Could other animals have been exposed?
- Describe the animal's environment (where animal is kept, how long left alone, hobbies of owner, anything that might lead to poisoning).

BOX 28-2   **Key items in the toxicologic history**

- *Listen* to the client. Avoid any bias or preconceptions.
- At the same time, *observe the animal*. Although you cannot always believe the client, you can believe clinical signs of the animal.
- Identify and *treat immediate life-threatening problems* (e.g., arrhythmias, seizures). Do not wait for confirmation of poisons involved to initiate supportive therapy!
- *Identify* the animal's entire home environment. Could other poisons or other animals or children be involved?
- *Identify* any current medications, underlying conditions, or pertinent previous medical history for the animal (e.g., heart disease, kidney problems, pregnancy).
- *History of the exposure event.* How long ago, what toxin, what concentration, how much? Does the occupation or hobby of the owner predispose to the presence of any particular poisons in the home?
- If possible, *identify the poison* (or poisons). Estimate the mg/kg dose for the exposure and establish a worst-case scenario. Estimate the risk for the animal and the possibility of a toxic or lethal exposure.
- Establish an exposure/onset of clinical signs *time-line*. Is the animal getting better, deteriorating, or showing no signs?
- Establish a *minimum database*.
- Treat the patient, *not* the poison.

decontamination procedures for GI exposures are of little value in exposure occurring over 1 hour before treatment.

Ocular and dermal exposure decontamination techniques are the same as in an adult, with the caveat that extremely young animals are at higher risk of hypothermia.

GI decontamination techniques have recently been reviewed by the American Academy of Clinical Toxicology (AACT); both animal and human data were examined with the following recommendations (Table 28-3). These recommendations in the next section come from position papers prepared using methodology agreed on by the AACT and the European Association of Poisons Centres and Clinical Toxicologists (EAPCCT). All relevant scientific literature was identified and reviewed critically by acknowledged experts using set criteria. Well-conducted clinical and experimental studies were given precedence over anecdotal case reports and abstracts were not considered. The position papers were subjected to detailed peer review by an international group of clinical toxicologists chosen by the AACT and EAPCCT, and final drafts were approved by the boards of the two societies.

Induction of Emesis

Induction of emesis (in this review using syrup of ipecac) "should not be administered routinely in the management

TABLE 28-3	Decontamination recommendations
Method	**Recommendation**
Emesis	Only recommended in first hour of ingestion
Cathartic	Not recommended
Gastric lavage	Generally not recommended, usually when toxin in chunks
Single-dose activated charcoal	Not recommended
Multiple-dose activated charcoal	Recommended for specific toxins
Whole bowel irrigation	Recommended for sustained-release toxins

of poisoned patients. In experimental studies the amount of marker removed by ipecac was highly variable and diminished with time. There is no evidence from clinical studies that ipecac improves the outcome of poisoned patients and its routine administration in the emergency department should be abandoned. There are insufficient data to support or exclude ipecac administration soon after poison ingestion …"

Gastric Lavage

"Gastric lavage should not be employed routinely, if ever, in the management of poisoned patients. In experimental studies, the amount of marker removed by gastric lavage was highly variable and diminished with time. The results of clinical outcome studies in overdose patients are weighed heavily on the side of showing a lack of beneficial effect."

Single-Dose Activated Charcoal

"Single-dose activated charcoal should not be administered routinely in the management of poisoned patients. Based upon volunteer studies, the administration of activated charcoal may be considered if a patient has ingested a potentially toxic amount of a poison (which is known to be absorbed to charcoal) up to one hour previously. Although volunteer studies demonstrate that the reduction of drug absorption decreases to values of questionable clinical importance when charcoal is administered at times greater than one hour, the potential for benefit after one hour cannot be excluded. There is no evidence that the administration of activated charcoal improves clinical outcome. Unless a patient has an intact or protected airway, the administration of charcoal is contraindicated."

Multiple-Dose Activated Charcoal

"Although many studies in animals and volunteers have demonstrated that multiple-dose activated charcoal increases drug elimination significantly, this therapy has not yet been shown in a controlled study in poisoned patients to reduce morbidity and mortality. Further studies are required to

establish its role and the optimal dosage regimen of charcoal to be administered. Based on experimental and clinical studies, multiple-dose activated charcoal should be considered only if a patient has ingested a life-threatening amount of carbamazepine, dapsone, Phenobarbital, quinine, or theophylline. With all of these drugs there are data to confirm enhanced elimination, though no controlled studies have demonstrated clinical benefit. Although volunteer studies have demonstrated that multiple-dose activated charcoal increases the elimination of amitriptyline, dextropropoxyphene, digitoxin, digoxin, disopyramide, nadolol, phenylbutazone, phenytoin, piroxicam, and sotalol, there are insufficient clinical data to support or exclude the use of this therapy. The use of multiple-dose activated charcoal in salicylate poisoning is controversial. Data in poisoned patients are insufficient presently to recommend the use of multiple-dose charcoal therapy for salicylate poisoning. Unless a patient has an intact or protected airway, the administration of multiple-dose activated charcoal is contraindicated. It should not be used in the presence of an intestinal obstruction." (Author note: These recommendations are generally based on adult data. However, the younger the patient the more likely that multiple-dose activated charcoal will be of some benefit. Young patients have decreased gastric emptying time, irregular intestinal peristalsis, good enterohepatic recirculation, and poor p-glycoprotein capabilities, therefore leaving the toxin more susceptible to charcoal binding.)

Cathartic

"The administration of a cathartic alone has no role in the management of the poisoned patient and is not recommended as a method of gut decontamination. Experimental data are conflicting regarding the use of cathartics in combination with activated charcoal. No clinical studies have been published to investigate the ability of a cathartic, with or without activated charcoal, to reduce the bioavailability of drugs or to improve the outcome of poisoned patients. Based upon available data, the routine use of a cathartic in combination with activated charcoal is not endorsed. If a cathartic is used, it should be limited to a single dose in order to minimize adverse effects of the cathartic." In patients with a small body mass, sodium abnormalities can occur with multiple doses of a cathartic (usually with activated charcoal).

Whole Bowel Irrigation

"Whole bowel irrigation (WBI) should not be used routinely in the management of the poisoned patient. Although some volunteer studies have shown substantial decreases in the bioavailability of ingested drugs, no controlled clinical studies have been performed and there is no conclusive evidence that WBI improves the outcome of the poisoned patient. Based upon volunteer studies, WBI should be considered for potentially toxic ingestions of sustained-release or enteric-coated drugs particularly for those patients presenting greater than two hours after drug ingestion. WBI should be considered for patients who have ingested substantial amounts of iron as the morbidity is high and there is a lack of other options for gastrointestinal decontamination."

Manual Removal

Manual removal techniques would include endoscopy or surgery. Treatment approaches for enhancing elimination would be peritoneal dialysis or hemodialysis (charcoal hemoperfusion).

Many toxins have specific antidotes, and a list of common antidotes can be found in Table 28-4.

MOST COMMON INQUIRIES TO POISON CENTERS FOR PEDIATRIC PATIENTS

Common exposures in pediatric canine and feline patients are listed in Box 28-3.

Rodenticides

Rodenticides (bromethalin, anticoagulants, and unknown) are commonly available, and dogs are intoxicated more frequently than any other domestic animals. The veterinarian should read the product label to identify the exact compound involved. The majority of anticoagulant rodenticides inhibit the recycling of vitamin K_1, blocking the victim's ability to clot. More than half of the victims exhibit anorexia, weakness, coughing, epistaxis, and dyspnea. Laboratory tests show prolonged clotting times and possibly thrombocytopenia.

Administration of vitamin K_1 is therapeutic but may take a few hours to work.

Nonsteroidal Antiinflammatory Drugs

Nonsteroidal antiinflammatory drugs (NSAIDs; human and animal products) are a common cause of toxicity in puppies and kittens. These animals have extensive enterohepatic recirculation of NSAIDs, which increases their toxicity. NSAIDs are particularly a problem for cats because cats are deficient in glutathione hepatic pathways, thereby prolonging the half-life of these compounds. The most common clinical manifestations are GI. Clinical signs include vomiting, depression, diarrhea, anorexia, ataxia, bloody stool, polyuria, polydipsia, and tachypnea. There is no specific antidote, and treatment is largely supportive.

Antidepressants

Antidepressants generally are tricyclic antidepressants (TCAs) or serotonin reuptake inhibitors or monoamine oxidase inhibitors (MAOIs). Once ingested, clinical signs usually develop within 60 minutes, but their anticholinergic activity can inhibit GI motility, slowing further uptake. These drugs are highly protein bound. Several compounds have toxic metabolites. Life-threatening clinical signs are related to the compound's effects on the CNS and cardiovascular aberrations. Clinical signs include ataxia, lethargy, hypotension, disorientation, vomiting, dyspnea, mydriasis, hyperactivity, urine retention, ileus, seizures, and cardiac arrhythmias.

TABLE 28-4	Common antidotes
Toxin	**Antidote**
Acetaminophen	*N*-Acetyl cysteine
Anticoagulants (warfarin-like)	Vitamin K
Anticholinergics	Physostigmine
Benzodiazepines	Flumazenil
β-blockers	Glucagon
Calcium channel blockers	Calcium, glucagon
Carbamate pesticides	Atropine
Carbon monoxide	Oxygen
Cyanide	Cyanide antidote kit
Digoxin	Digibind
Ethylene glycol	Ethanol
Iron	Deferoxamine
Isoniazid	Pyridoxine
Lead	Dimercaprol, EDTA, DMSA
Mercury	Dimercaprol, DMSA
Methanol	Ethanol, fomepizole
Methemoglobin	Methylene blue
Narcotics	Naloxone
Organophosphate pesticides	Atropine, pralidoxime
Tricyclic antidepressants	Sodium bicarbonate

DMSA, Dimercaptosuccinic acid; *EDTA,* ethylenediaminetetraacetic acid.

BOX 28-3	The most common groups of toxicants (both serious and not-so-serious) for animals under 1 year of age

Dogs
Rodenticides (bromethalin, anticoagulants, and unknown) were the top category
NSAIDs (human and animal products)
Antidepressants
Herbicides
Mushrooms
Silica gel
Cleaning products
Chocolate
Amphetamines (prescription and illicit)
Birth control pills

Cats
Flea products (sprays, spot-ons, collars, dips) far and away the #1 category
NSAIDs
Silica gel
Insoluble calcium oxalate plants
Liquid potpourri

Courtesy Tina Wismer, DVM, DABVT, DABT; ASPCA Animal Poison Control Center.
NSAIDs, Nonsteroidal antiinflammatory drugs.

Herbicides

Herbicide exposure from pesticide-treated plants is unlikely to result in intoxication in puppies and kittens. Exposure to concentrates can induce clinical signs, and treatment is supportive. Acute exposures rarely induce altered biochemical profile data, unlike long-term feeding trials. Vomiting is a common nonspecific clinical sign.

Mushrooms

Mushroom ingestion can occur year round. Common clinical signs are those of GI distress, including abdominal pain, vomiting, and diarrhea. A wide variety of toxins are available with mushroom ingestion. These compounds can affect the GI tract, nervous system (excitation, hallucinogenic, and muscarinic), kidneys, red blood cells, and liver. A confirmed diagnosis is difficult to obtain, and clinicians should become familiar with the mushroom species (and the expected clinical signs) available in their geographic region.

Silica Gel

Silica gel is used as a desiccant and often comes in paper packets or plastic cylinders. They are used to absorb moisture in a variety of packaging. Silica is considered "chemically and biologically inert" when ingested. Clinical signs, although rare, would consist of GI upset manifested as nausea, vomiting, and inappetence.

Home Cleaning Products

The list of home cleaning products is extensive, highlighting the need for the owner to bring in the toxin container if possible.

Methylxanthines (Chocolate)

The active (toxic) agents in chocolate are methylxanthines, specifically theobromine and caffeine. Methylxanthines stimulate the CNS, act on the kidney to stimulate diuresis, and increase the contractility of cardiac and skeletal muscle. The relative amounts of theobromine and caffeine vary with the form of the chocolate (Table 28-5).

The LD50s of theobromine and caffeine are 100 to 300 mg/kg, but severe and life-threatening clinical signs may be seen at levels far below these doses. Based on National Animal Poison Control Center experience, mild signs have been seen with theobromine levels of 20 mg/kg, severe signs have been seen at 40 to 50 mg/kg, and seizures have occurred at 60 mg/kg. Accordingly, less than 2 oz of milk chocolate per kg of body weight is potentially lethal to dogs. Clinical signs occur within 6 to 12 hours of ingestion. Initial signs include polydipsia, bloating, vomiting, diarrhea, and restlessness. Signs progress to hyperactivity, polyuria, ataxia, tremors, seizures, tachycardia, premature ventricular contractions (PVCs), tachypnea, cyanosis, hypertension, hyperthermia, and coma. Death is generally due to cardiac arrhythmias or respiratory failure. Hypokalemia may occur later in the course of the toxicosis. Because of the high fat content of many chocolate products, pancreatitis is a potential sequela.

TABLE 28-5	Selected sources of theobromine and caffeine	
Product	Theobromine (mg/oz)	Caffeine (mg/oz)
Cacao beans	300-1500	–
Unsweetened baking chocolate	390-450	47
Cacao powder	400-737	70
Dark semisweet chocolate	135	22
Milk chocolate	44-60	6
White chocolate	0.25	0.85
Cacao bean hulls	150-255	–
Cacao bean mulch	56-900	–

Amphetamines

Amphetamines (prescription and illicit) have a minimum oral lethal dose of 20 to 27 mg/kg for amphetamine sulfate and 9 to 11 mg/kg of methamphetamine hydrochloride in dogs. Victims generally manifest hyperactivity, restlessness, mydriasis, hypersalivation, vocalization, tachypnea, tremors, hyperthermia, ataxia, seizures, and tachycardia.

Birth Control Pills

Birth control pills generally are packaged with 21 tablets of estrogen and/or progesterone and possibly 7 placebo pills. Estrogen could cause bone marrow suppression at levels greater than 1 mg/kg. Some oral contraceptives also contain iron. Decontamination is not necessary unless the level of estrogen is greater than 1 mg/kg or the level of iron is greater than 20 mg/kg.

Flea Products

Flea products (sprays, spot-ons, collars, or dips) are still a major problem for inducing toxicity, although much less now that organophosphates are no longer the mainstay of treatment for flea control. These compounds reversibly alter the activity of sodium ion channels in nervous tissue. Clinical signs result from allergic, idiosyncratic, and neurotoxic reactions. The majority of toxicities are due to pyrethrin and pyrethroid flea products applied to cats. Cats are much more sensitive than dogs, and dog products have several times higher concentration of the active ingredient (cat products often are 2%, whereas dog products often are 45% to 65%). The most common problem is misapplication of a dog product onto a cat, or splitting a large dog product onto several cats.

Calcium Oxalate Plants

Insoluble calcium oxalate plants are generally overrated as a toxic exposure; the calcium oxalate contained in the plant is an irritant to the mucous membranes, which generally inhibits ingestion of large volumes.

Liquid Potpourri

Liquid potpourri may contain essential oils and cationic detergents. Since product labels may not list ingredients, it is wise to assume that a given liquid potpourri contains both ingredients. Essential oils can cause mucous membrane and GI irritation, CNS depression, and dermal hypersensitivity and irritation. Severe clinical signs can be seen with potpourri products that contain cationic detergents. Dermal exposure to cationic detergents can result in erythema, edema, intense pain, and ulceration. Ingestion of cationic detergents may lead to tissue necrosis and inflammation of the mouth, esophagus, and stomach. Treatment is symptomatic and supportive.

SUGGESTED READING

American Academy of Clinical Toxicology: Position papers on gastrointestinal decontamination, www.clintox.org/Pos_Statements/Intro.html.

EFFECTIVE USE OF A VETERINARY MEDICAL DIAGNOSTIC LABORATORY

CHAPTER 29

Patricia A. Talcott

Veterinary medical diagnostic laboratories commonly offer a variety of tests in areas such as pathology and histology, serology and immunology, virology, bacteriology, mycology, parasitology, endocrinology, toxicology, molecular diagnostics, nutrition, and immunohistochemistry. These subunits within the diagnostic laboratory have the capabilities of testing for a variety of infectious organisms and substances by using highly specific and sensitive analytical instruments and techniques. Diagnostic personnel within the diagnostic laboratory work together to fine-tune the diagnostic approach to a case to maximize the use of the submitted samples with the goal to achieve a successful outcome—a diagnosis. Additionally, many veterinary medical diagnostic laboratories have close established contacts and working relationships with clinical experts present in associated veterinary teaching hospitals. This close working relationship helps the diagnosticians narrow down or sometimes expand the list of potential problems that might exist in the case at hand.

GETTING STARTED

A veterinarian's first contact with a veterinary medical diagnostic laboratory should be via the telephone (Box 29-1). In most veterinary medical diagnostic laboratories, there is a section head who oversees each unit within the laboratory. Section heads are generally veterinarians with advanced degrees (e.g., MS, PhD, board certification) in their specialty area. Most diagnostic laboratories have a daily consulting pathologist who triages the incoming telephone calls and cases. The pathologist can decide to consult directly with the caller or can transfer the call to the appropriate section within the diagnostic laboratory.

Veterinarians who call diagnostic laboratories are often seeking advice on cases, and questions can range from discussion regarding differentials, appropriate sample collection and submission, interpretation of results, to treatment options for the affected patient(s). Good communication in the early stage of a case between the veterinary practitioner and the laboratory personnel is one of the most useful tools in a case workup and will almost always guarantee proper sample collection and accurate selection of initial tests. The often-mentioned statement, "Laboratories run tests, veterinarians make diagnoses," says it all. Consulting with laboratory personnel to determine the laboratory's capabilities, costs of analyses, turnaround times, method of sensitivity (e.g., some laboratories may be able to test for a substance by a particular method, but the method may not be sensitive enough to provide reliable and accurate clinical interpretation), and interpretation abilities is critical so that everyone involved in the case is well informed. The consultant can help expand or narrow the focus of the investigation, so that the sample submitter does not ask "to test for everything" but rather focuses on some select differentials to target for testing.

During the telephone consult a veterinarian can pass along critical pieces of history regarding the case that may be too cumbersome to write on the accession forms. The telephone consult can also provide necessary information regarding packaging, preserving, and shipping the samples. Some laboratories are open for Saturday deliveries, but many are not. The veterinarian should know this in case samples arrive later than expected and are potentially perishable. Many laboratories have much of this information on Internet websites, but the veterinarian should contact the laboratory directly to make sure that all information on the website is current and correct. A list of the American Association of Veterinary Laboratory Diagnosticians (AAVLD)–accredited veterinary medical diagnostic laboratories located in the United States and Canada can be found at http://www.aavld.org/mc/page.do?sitePageId=33930&orgId=aavld (Table 29-1).

Completing paperwork to accompany the samples is sometimes time consuming but essential to the case. It allows

252

BOX 29-1   Maximizing diagnostic laboratory results

- Discuss with diagnostician exactly what testing you are requesting.
- Contact laboratory for recommendations on sample requirements before collection.
- Provide detailed history, including affected and unaffected animals.
- Complete description of the clinical problem in all affected animals
- Suspected differential diagnosis
- Guidelines for submission of a complete carcass to the laboratory

---

the consultant to refresh his or her memory of any previous telephone contacts and may provide additional pieces of information that were not apparent at the time of initial contact. The accession sheet also provides the laboratory with critical pieces of information that are necessary for internal tracking and appropriate billing. A typical laboratory accession sheet requests the following pieces of information: owner and submitting veterinarian's name, address, and contact information (including telephone and facsimile numbers and e-mail address); number of animals affected and/or dead (age, breed, sex, and weight); animals at risk; number and type of animals on the premise; duration of problem; location of lesion(s); clinical history; disease conditions suspected; date the samples were collected; amount and type of specimens collected; and tests desired. The information provided on the paperwork should be complete and legible, and the accession sheet should be placed in a zip-lock baggie in case accompanying tissue specimens leak in transit.

Samples submitted to each unit within the laboratory should be individually packaged and labeled to avoid any confusion about specimen identification and type. Some analyses require unique specimen handling; this is why initial contact with the laboratory is essential to make sure that all samples are submitted appropriately. For example, some samples should be wrapped in foil to protect light-sensitive compounds from degrading; some samples should be frozen to prevent volatile compounds from escaping; and some samples should be wrapped in foil instead of traditional plastic bags to prevent potential contamination by organic chemicals. All specimens should be double bagged and submitted in appropriate shipping containers to prevent leaking and that comply with the shipping standards of the shipping carrier.

ARRIVAL AT THE DIAGNOSTIC LABORATORY

At most veterinary medical diagnostic laboratories, mail is opened in a central processing unit. There, the accession sheet with the appropriate information is reviewed by the consultant, and samples are routed to appropriate section

units for the testing requested. If there is insufficient information on the accession sheet or if there is confusion regarding the samples submitted and tests requested, the consultant will contact the submitting veterinarian and request additional information to clarify what should be done with the specimens.

Test methods within the laboratory range from simple visualization (e.g., identification of plant parts) and easy bench-top wet lab procedures, to the use of highly sensitive modern analytical chemistry instrumentation and techniques. In many cases, several analyses have to be performed on the same set of submitted specimens. Therefore it is sometimes necessary to send multiple specimens of the same type of sample.

Many techniques used in the laboratory, particularly within the toxicology section, are very specific and potentially very time consuming and expensive. Thus it is crucial to obtain appropriate samples along with a detailed case history to make sure that what the laboratory tests for is reasonable and fits with the clinical presentation. Most veterinary medical laboratories provide routine testing for the most commonly encountered and important diseases in a variety of animal species. Some laboratories can provide very specialized testing for unusual agents. Because of intensive networking between the veterinary medical diagnostic laboratories in the United States and worldwide, a veterinary diagnostician can identify a suitable laboratory in a very short time to test for a substance and provide the best advice regarding diagnostic workup of a particular case.

PITFALLS

There may be many reasons that a diagnostic laboratory cannot confirm a clinician's suspicions. However, there are some common problems that diagnostic laboratories routinely encounter. Many times the wrong sample is collected for the test requested. This can be minimized by making sure the veterinarian has collected a complete set of specimens or by calling the laboratory in advance. Another common problem that hampers a diagnostic service, particularly within the toxicology unit, is insufficient sample volume is submitted for the test(s) requested. Most toxicology tests are designed to be run on a minimum sample volume; below this volume there is decreased sensitivity and accuracy. It is always better to submit too much than to submit too little. Insufficient history and information regarding test selection is also often a limiting factor in securing a successful outcome.

When performing a necropsy, the veterinarian should collect as complete a selection of tissues as possible. Both fixed and fresh tissues should be collected. It is critical that a veterinarian not limit tissue selection to those systems only abnormal by clinical examination or gross postmortem inspection; the laboratory may pick up interesting and perhaps important changes or lesions in tissues or systems that were thought to be unaffected. A complete set of tissues collected from postmortem examination should include, but is not limited to, the brain, eyeball, thymus, thyroid, heart,

| TABLE 29-1 | AAVLD-Accredited veterinary medical diagnostic laboratories |

Arizona	Arizona Veterinary Diagnostic Lab 2831 N. Freeway Tucson, AZ 85705	Phone: 520-621-2356 Fax: 520-626-8696 http://microvet.arizona.edu
Arkansas	Veterinary Diagnostic Laboratory Arkansas Livestock and Poultry Commission Shipping Address: One Natural Resources Drive Little Rock, AR 72205 Mailing Address: PO Box 8505 Little Rock, AR 72215	Phone: 501-907-2430 Fax: 501-907-2410 http://www.arlpc.org
California	CA Animal Health & Food Safety Lab System University of California, Davis Shipping Address: West Health Science Drive Davis, CA 95616 Mailing Address: PO Box 1770 Davis, CA 95617-1770	Phone: 530-752-8709 Fax: 530-752-5680 http://cahfs.ucdavis.edu
Colorado	Colorado State University Veterinary Diagnostic Lab Shipping Address: Fort Collins, CO 80523 Mailing Address: CSU DLab Fort Collins, CO 80523	Phone: 970-297-1281 Fax: 970 207-0320 http://www.dlab.colostate.edu
Connecticut	Connecticut Veterinary Medical Diagnostic Laboratory Department of Pathobiology & Veterinary Science University of Connecticut Shipping Address: 61 N. Eagleville Road, Unit-3089 Storrs, CT 06269-3089 Mailing Address: 61 N. Eagleville Road, Unit-3089 Storrs, CT 06269-3089	Phone: 860-486-4000 Fax: 860-486-2794 http://www.patho.uconn.edu
Florida	Animal Disease Laboratory Florida Dept. of Agriculture Shipping Address: 2700 N. John Young Parkway Kissimmee, FL 34741 Mailing Address: PO Box 458006 Kissimmee, FL 34745	Phone: 321-697-1400 Fax: 321-697-1467 http://doacs.state.fl.us
Georgia	Athens Veterinary Diagnostic Laboratory College of Veterinary Medicine University of Georgia Athens, GA 30602-7383	Phone: 706-542-5568 Fax: 706-542-5977 http://www.vet.uga.edu
	Veterinary Diagnostic and Investigational Laboratory University of Georgia Shipping Address: 43 Brighton Road Tifton, GA 31793 Mailing Address: PO Box 1389 Tifton, GA 31793	Phone: 229-386-3340 Fax: 229-386-7128 http://www.vet.uga.edu
Illinois	Illinois Dept. of Ag. Animal Disease Lab 9732 Shattuc Road Centralia, IL 62801	Phone: 618-532-6701 Fax: 618-532-1195 http://www.agr.state.il.us
	Animal Disease Lab Illinois Dept. of Ag. Shipping Address: 2100 South Lake Storey Rd. Galesburg, IL 61401 Mailing Address: 2100 South Lake Storey Rd. PO Box 2100X Galesburg, IL 61401	Phone: 309-344-2451 Fax: 309-344-7358 http://www.agr.state.il.us/AnimalHW/ labs/index.html

TABLE 29-1	AAVLD-Accredited veterinary medical diagnostic laboratories—cont'd

	College of Veterinary Medicine Veterinary Diagnostic Laboratory Shipping Address: PO Box U Urbana, IL 61802 Mailing Address: 2001 South Lincoln Ave. Rm. 1224 Urbana, IL 61802	Phone: 217-333-1620 Fax: 217-244-2439 http://www.cvm.uiuc.edu/vdl/
Indiana	Animal Disease Diagnostic Lab Purdue University 406 South University St. West Lafayette, IN 47907	Phone: 765-494-7440 Fax: 765-494-9181 http://www.addl.purdue.edu
Iowa	ISU-College of Vet Med Vet Diagnostic Lab 1600 S. 16th Street Ames, IA 50011	Phone: 515-294-1950 Fax: 515-294-3564 http://www.vdpam.iastate.edu
Kansas	Kansas State Veterinary Diagnostic Laboratory Kansas State University 1800 Denison Ave., Moiser Hall Manhattan, KS 66506	Phone: 785-532-5650 Fax: 785-532-4481 http://www.vet.ksu.edu/depts/dmp/
Kentucky	Murray State University Breathitt Veterinary Center Shipping Address: 715 North Drive Hopkinsville, KY 42240 Mailing Address: PO Box 2000 Hopkinsville, KY 42241-2000	Phone: 270-886-3959 Fax: 270-886-4295 http://breathitt.murraystate.edu/bvc
	Livestock Disease Diagnostic Center Shipping Address: 1490 Bull Lea Rd. Lexington, KY 40511 Mailing Address: PO Box 14125 Lexington, KY 40512	Phone: 859-253-0571 Fax: 859-255-1624 http://ces.ca.uky.edu/lddc/
Louisiana	LA Animal Disease Diagnostic Laboratory Shipping Address: 1909 Skip Bertman Dr. Rm. 1519 Baton Rouge, LA 70803 Mailing Address: PO Box 25070 Baton Rouge, LA 70894	Phone: 225-578-9777 Fax: 225-578-9784 http://laddl.lsu.edu
Michigan	Diagnostic Center for Population and Animal Health Michigan State University Shipping Address: 4125 Beaumont Road Rm. 122 Lansing, MI 48910-8104 Mailing Address: PO Box 30076 Lansing, MI 48909-7576	Phone: 517-353-0635 Fax: 517-353-5096 http://www.animalhealth.msu.edu
Minnesota	Veterinary Diagnostic Laboratory University of Minnesota 1333 Gortner Avenue St. Paul, MN 55108-1098	Phone: 612-625-8787 Fax: 612-624-8707 http://www.vdl.umn.edu
Mississippi	Mississippi Veterinary Research and Diagnostic Laboratory System Mississippi State University Shipping Address: 3137 Highway 468 West Pearl, MS 39208 Mailing Address: PO Box 97813 Pearl, MS 39288	Phone: 601-420-4700 Fax: 601-420-4719 http://www.cvm.msstate.edu
Missouri	Veterinary Medical Diagnostic Lab University of Missouri Shipping Address: 1600 East Rollins Road Columbia, MO 65211 Mailing Address: PO Box 6023 Columbia, MO 65205	Phone: 573-882-6811 Fax: 573-882-1411 http://www.cvm.missouri.edu/vmdl

Continued

TABLE 29-1   **AAVLD-Accredited veterinary medical diagnostic laboratories—cont'd**

Montana	Montana Department of Livestock Montana Veterinary Diagnostic Laboratory Shipping Address: South 19th and Lincoln Bozeman, MT 59718 Mailing Address: PO Box 997 Bozeman, MT 59771	Phone: 406-994-4885 Fax: 406-994-6344 http://www.discoveringmontana. com/liv/lab/index.asp
Nebraska	Veterinary Diagnostic Center Fair Street, E. Campus Loop Shipping Address: PO Box 82646 Lincoln, NE 68501-2646 Mailing Address: PO Box 830907 Lincoln, NE 68583-0907	Phone: 402-472-1434 Fax: 402-472-3094 http://vbms.unl.edu/nvdls.shtml
New Mexico	New Mexico Department of Agriculture Veterinary Diagnostic Services Shipping Address: 700 Camino De Salud NE Albuquerque, NM 87106 Mailing Address: PO Box 4700 Albuquerque, NM 87196-4700	Phone: 505-841-2576 Fax: 505-841-2518
New York	Animal Health Diagnostic Center College of Veterinary Medicine Cornell University Shipping Address: Upper Tower Road Ithaca, NY 14853 Mailing Address: PO Box 5786 Ithaca, NY 14852	Phone: 607-253-3900 Fax: 607-253-3943 http://diaglab.vet.cornell.edu/
North Carolina	North Carolina Department of Agriculture & Consumer Services Rollins Laboratory Shipping Address: 2101 Blue Ridge Road Raleigh, NC 27607 Mailing Address: 1031 Mail Service Center Raleigh, NC 27699-1031	Phone: 919-733-3986 Fax: 919-733-0454 http://www.ncvdl.com/
North Dakota	Department of Veterinary Diagnostic Services North Dakota State University Shipping Address: 1523 Centennial Blvd., Van Es Hall Fargo, ND 58105 Mailing Address: PO Box 5406 Fargo, ND 58105	Phone: 701-231-8307 Fax: 701-231-7514 http://www.vdl.ndsu.edu/
Ohio	Animal Disease Diagnostic Lab 8995 E. Main Street, Building 6 Reynoldsburg, OH 43068	Phone: 614-728-6220 Fax: 614-728-6310 http://www.ohioagriculture.gov/addl
Oklahoma	Oklahoma Animal Disease Diagnostic Laboratory Oklahoma State University Shipping Address: Center for Veterinary Health Sciences Farm and Ridge Road Stillwater, OK 74078 Mailing Address: PO Box 7001 Stillwater, OK 74076-7001	Phone: 405-744-6623 Fax: 405-744-8612 http://www.cvm.okstate.edu
Oregon	Veterinary Diagnostic Laboratory Oregon State University Magruder Hall, Room 134 Shipping Address: 30th and Washington Way Corvallis, OR 97331 Mailing Address: PO Box 429 Corvallis, OR 97339-0429	Phone: 541-737-3261 Fax: 541-737-6817 http://www.vet.orst.edu/
Pennsylvania	Department of Agriculture Pennsylvania Veterinary Laboratory 2305 N. Cameron Street Harrisburg, PA 17110-9408	Phone: 717-787-8808 Fax: 717-772-3895 http://www.padls.org

TABLE 29-1	AAVLD-Accredited veterinary medical diagnostic laboratories—cont'd	
	Pennsylvania State University PADLS - Penn State Animal Diagnostic Laboratory Orchard Road University Park, PA 16802-1110	Phone: 814-863-0837 Fax: 814-865-3907 http://www.padls.org
	University of Pennsylvania PADLS - New Bolton Center 382 West Street Road Kennett Square, PA 19348	Phone: 610-444-5800 Fax: 610-925-8106 http://www.padls.org
South Carolina	Clemson Veterinary Diagnostic Center Shipping Address: 500 Clemson Road Columbia, SC 29229 Mailing Address: PO Box 102406 Columbia, SC 29224-2406	Phone: 803-788-2260 Fax: 803-788-8058 http://www.clemson.edu/lph
South Dakota	Animal Disease Research and Diagnostic Laboratory South Dakota State University Shipping Address: Animal Disease Research Building, North Campus Drive Brookings, SD 57007-1396 Mailing Address: Box 2175, North Campus Drive Brookings, SD 57007-1396	Phone: 605-688-5171 Fax: 605-688-6003 http://vetsci.sdstate.edu
Tennessee	CE Kord Animal Disease Diagnostic Laboratory Ellington Agricultural Center Shipping Address: 440 Hogan Rd., Porter Building Nashville, TN 37220 Mailing Address: PO Box 40627 Nashville, TN 37204	Phone: 615-837-5125 Fax: 615-837-5250 http://www.state.tn.us/agriculture/ regulate/labs/kordlab.html
Texas	Texas Veterinary Medical Diagnostic Laboratory (TVMDL) TVMDL-College Station Shipping Address: 1 Sippel Road College Station, TX 77843 Mailing Address: PO Box 3040 College Station, TX 77841-3040	Phone: 979-845-3414 Fax: 979-845-1794 www.tvmdlweb.tamu.edu
	TVMDL – Amarillo Shipping Address: 6610 Amarillo Blvd., West Amarillo, TX 79106 Mailing Address: PO Box 3200 Amarillo, TX 79106-3200	Robert Sprowls Phone: 806-353-7478 Fax: 806-359-0636 http:tvmdlweb.tamu.edu
	TVMDL – Gonzales Shipping Address: 1812 Water Street Gonzales, TX 78629 Mailing Address: PO Box 84 Gonzales, TX 78629	Phone: 830-672-2834 Fax: 830-672-2835 http://tvmdlweb.tamu.edu
	TVMDL – Center Shipping/Mailing Address: 635 Malone Drive Center, TX 79535	Phone: 936-598-4451 Fax: 936-598-2741 http://tvmdlweb.tamu.edu
Washington	Washington Animal Disease Diagnostic Laboratory Washington State University Shipping Address: 155 N Bustad Hall Pullman, WA 99164-7034 Mailing Address: PO Box 647034 Pullman, WA 99164-7034	Phone: 509-335-9696 Fax: 509-335-7424 http://www.vetmed.wsu.edu/ depts_waddl
Wisconsin	Wisconsin Veterinary Diagnostic Laboratory University of Wisconsin 445 Easterday Lane Madison, WI 53706	Phone: 608-262-5432 Fax: 847-574-8085 http://www.wvdl.wisc.edu
Wyoming	Wyoming State Veterinary Laboratory 1174 Snowy Range Road Laramie, WY 82070	Phone: 307-742-6638 Fax: 307-721-2051 http://wyovet.uwyo.edu/

Continued

TABLE 29-1	AAVLD-Accredited veterinary medical diagnostic laboratories—cont'd	
Canada	Animal Health Laboratory University of Guelph Shipping Address: Door P2, Building 49, McIntosh Lane Guelph, Ontario N1G 2W1 Mailing Address: PO Box 3612 Guelph, Ontario N1H 6R8 CANADA	Phone: 519-824-4120 ext. 54502 Fax: 519-821-8072 http://ahl.uoguelph.ca/
	Animal Health Branch 1767 Angus Campbell Road Abbotsford, BC V3G 2M3 CANADA	Phone: 604-556-3003 Fax: 604-556-3010 http://www.agf

From The American Association of Veterinary Laboratory Diagnosticians website, http://www.aavld.org/mc/page.do?sitePageId=33930&orgId=aavld. (Last accessed December 10, 2009.)

lung, spleen, kidney, liver, urinary bladder, pancreas, lymph nodes, skin, adrenal glands, various sections of the gastrointestinal tract, ovaries, placenta, testes, and skeletal muscle. In a multiple-animal outbreak, samples from more than one animal should be collected and submitted. The submitting veterinarian can ask that tests be run in a particular order, so tissues can be saved fresh or frozen until a particular test is requested.

REPORTING

The diagnosticians within the laboratory typically interpret any results in light of the historical, clinical, and pathological findings. For example, a variety of types of information are necessary to prove chronic chlorpyrifos (organophosphate) toxicosis in a cat. Clinical signs may include vomiting, anorexia, and depression, all of which are fairly nonspecific abnormalities. Identification of the compound in vomitus or blood confirms exposure. Depressed cholinesterase activity in blood or brain (if the test is performed postmortem) indicates that the exposure to chlorpyrifos was significant.

Most diagnostic laboratories can report results to veterinarians by facsimile and will also provide a hard copy of the report. Some laboratories allow access to online results. In cases involving malicious poisonings, multiple-animal outbreaks, and potential risks to the public, it might be judicious to report findings to an appropriate regulatory agency (e.g., state or federal department of agriculture or local law enforcement agency). The diagnosticians should be able to assist and direct the veterinarian to the appropriate agency or individual in these cases.

CONCLUSION

A veterinarian's approach to using a diagnostic facility should be thoughtful, logical, and insightful. Do not think that the diagnostic laboratory can test for everything—regardless of what one sees on the television shows; there is no such test as the "poison screen." A veterinarian should refine his or her approach to the use of a diagnostic laboratory so that it is systematic and reasonable and uses all aspects of the diagnostic laboratory to maximize efforts at an affordable price to achieve a successful resolution to the case. Using full-service veterinary medical diagnostic laboratories provides a veterinarian with the opportunity to use multiple specialties' expertise and potentially expedite the finding of a definitive diagnosis.

SUGGESTED READINGS

Galey FD, Talcott PA: Effective use of a diagnostic laboratory. In Peterson ME, Talcott PA (eds): *Small animal toxicology*, ed 2, St. Louis, 2006, Elsevier, pp 154-164.

Galey FD: Diagnostic toxicology. In Plumlee KH (ed): *Clinical veterinary toxicology*, St. Louis, 2004, Mosby, pp 22-27.

Diagnostic toxicology. In: *Veterinary toxicology: basic and clinical principles*, St. Louis, 2007, Elsevier, pp 1063-1138.

CLINICAL CHEMISTRY OF THE PUPPY AND KITTEN

CHAPTER 30

M. Elena Gorman

Neonates have decreased functional capacity of many organ systems because of incomplete development of these organs at birth. As they age, organ function increases and variations in enzyme levels and the products related to normal metabolism, filtration, and function of these organs will change in accordance to appropriate growth of the animal. Serum chemistry can be useful to detect often subtle abnormalities of these organ systems, and although reference ranges have been established for the normal parameters of most of these analytes, these values have often been obtained from adult animals. Because of variations in enzymology and functional capacity of neonatal organ systems, care must be taken when interpreting any changes in chemistry values when using standard adult reference ranges.

This chapter focuses on the typical development and acquisition of normal biochemical constituents in puppies and kittens and illustrates the many differences between adult and neonatal biochemical parameters. Although published reference ranges are provided (Tables 30-1 to 30-5) based on the available research in current literature, it is recommended that reference intervals be established for each laboratory because of the lack of standardization among reference laboratories. Practitioners, however, may use these ranges as guidelines for interpretation of serum biochemical results in puppies and kittens aged less than 1 year. Hereditary conditions affecting biochemical parameters of young dogs and cats are shown in Table 30-6.

GLUCOSE

Glucose in the blood is closely regulated and normally maintained by three major mechanisms: intestinal absorption, hepatic production, and, to a lesser degree, renal production. In young animals with reduced development of normal organ, mainly hepatic, function, there is reduced potential for gluconeogenesis and glycogenolysis. Therefore, much of the plasma glucose concentration in young animals is obtained via ingestion, which makes neonates particularly sensitive to hypoglycemia during incidents of stress, illness, and reduced intake.

In puppies, glucose levels are lowest immediately after birth and then significantly increase after approximately 3 days with normal suckling. No significant variations are noted in glucose from day 8 until post-nursing. Glucose concentration then gradually decreases over time and levels off to normal adult levels at approximately age 9 months. The lower glucose values identified in young puppies, immediately after birth, are likely caused by insufficient blood sugar regulation feedback mechanisms and decreased hepatic functional capability.

In contrast to puppies, glucose levels have been shown to be higher immediately after birth in kittens with a gradual decline throughout the growth period to reach normal adult concentrations soon after weaning.

Hypoglycemia

Decreased glucose absorption secondary to starvation, maldigestion, and poor nursing or agalactia of the queen or bitch are the most common causes of hypoglycemia in neonates. Disease states such as diarrhea, dehydration, or hypothermia may exacerbate hypoglycemia in these patients. A syndrome known as transient juvenile hypoglycemia is well recognized and of particular concern in miniature and toy breeds of dogs; therefore, special consideration must be taken to inhibit decreased intake in these breeds postweaning. Inadequate glycogen and protein stores, decreased gluconeogenesis resulting from decreased hepatic function, and suboptimal epinephrine-mediated response to hypothermia and hypoglycemia are implicated in this syndrome.

Sepsis is another significant cause of hypoglycemia in animals. Neonates may be more susceptible to sepsis as a result of inadequate developing immune function and the inability to rely on normal mobilization of glycogen and protein stores as previously mentioned.

Liver dysfunction should always be considered in cases of persistent hypoglycemia in puppies and kittens. This may include primary causes such as portosystemic shunts (PSSs) in either species or acquired dysfunction secondary to infectious disease, for example, hepatitis in puppies or feline infectious peritonitis (FIP) in kittens.

Common causes of hypoglycemia in neonates are listed in Box 30-1.

Hyperglycemia

Hyperglycemia secondary to excitation, stress, or fear resulting from transient catecholamine release is common in cats and dogs regardless of age but may be particularly pronounced in cats. Likewise, chronic stress resulting in cortisol-induced gluconeogenesis is also relatively common in small animals and may accompany a variety of disease states. Postprandial hyperglycemia may occur in puppies and kittens within 1 to 4 hours after digestion of a meal.

Certain drugs may cause transient hyperglycemia in animals, including neonates, after administration. These compounds include anesthetizing agents such as medetomidine, xylazine, and ketamine, as well as analgesics such as

---

TABLE 30-1 Serum IgG and IgM concentrations in normal, colostrum-fed puppies and kittens

	Puppies		Kittens	
	IgG (mg/dl)	IgM (mg/dl)	IgG (mg/dl)	IgM (mg/dl)
Day 0	34.1-221.4	≤20.3	0	28-112
Day 1	≤2331.4	≤35.3	111-4273	31-88
Day 2	≤4031.3	2.5-38.9	350-1500	–
Day 7	41.3-625.1	4.4-54.3	161-648	–
Day 14	83.6-358.3	10.2-74.7	581-1881	–

Adapted from Levy JK, Crawford PC, Werner LL: Effect of age on reference intervals of serum biochemical values in kittens, *J Am Vet Med Assoc* 228(7):1033-1037, 2006; Casal ML, Jezyk PF, Giger U: Transfer of colostral antibodies from queens to their kittens, *Am J Vet Res* 57(11):1653-1658, 1996; Poffenbarger EM et al: Use of adult dog serum as a substitute for colostrum in the neonatal dog, *Am J Vet Res* 52:1221-1224, 1991.

BOX 30-1 Common causes of hypoglycemia and hyperglycemia in puppies and kittens

Hypoglycemia
Decreased intake
- Starvation
- Poor nursing or agalactia
- Maldigestion

Decreased production
- Infectious disease
- Portosystemic shunt

Sepsis
Insulin administration

Hyperglycemia
Catecholamine induced
- Fear
- Pain

Glucocorticoid induced
Postprandial
Diabetes mellitus
Drugs
- α_2-Agonists
- Opioids
- Ketamine

TABLE 30-2 Puppy biochemical parameters from birth to approximately 8 weeks of age

	Days 1-3	Days 8-10	Weeks 4-5 Days 28-33	Weeks 7-8 Days 50-58
Albumin (g/dl)	1.76-2.75	1.71-2.5	2.17-2.97	2.38-3.22
ALP (U/L)	452-6358	195-768	153-490	153-527
ALT (U/L)	9.1-42.2	4.1-21.4	4.3-17.4	10.3-24.3
Bilirubin (mg/dl)	0.04-0.38	0.01-0.18	0.02-0.15	0.01-0.11
BUN (mg/dl)	29.5-118	29.1-66.7	13.1-46.2	16.8-61.4
Calcium (mg/dl)	10.4-13.6	11.2-13.2	10.4-13.2	10.8-12.8
Cholesterol (mg/dl)	90-234	158-340	177-392	149-347
Creatinine (mg/dl)	0.37-1.06	0.28-0.42	0.25-0.83	0.26-0.66
GGT (U/L)	163-3558	–	–	–
GLDH (U/L)	1.8-17.0	0.2-17.7	1.2-9.0	1.6-7.3
Glucose (mg/dl)	76-155	101-161	121-158	122-159
TP (g/dl)	3.7-5.77	3.26-4.37	3.71-4.81	4.04-5.33
Triglycerides (mg/dl)	45-248	52-220	36-149	39-120
Phosphorus (mg/dl)	5.26-10.83	8.35-11.14	8.66-11.45	8.35-11.14

Adapted from Center SA et al: Effect of colostrum ingestion on gamma-glutamyltransferase and alkaline phosphatase activities in neonatal pups, *Am J Vet Res* 52(3):499-504, 1991; Kuhl S et al: Reference values of chemical blood parameters for puppies during the first 8 weeks of life, *Dtsch Tierärztl Wschr* 107:438-443, 2000; Harper EJ et al: Age-related variations in hematologic and plasma biochemical test results in Beagles and Labrador retrievers, *J Am Vet Med Assoc* 223(10):1436-1442, 2003.

TABLE 30-3   Puppy biochemical parameters up to 12 months of age

	2-3 Months	4-6 Months	7-12 Months
Albumin (g/dl)*	2.6-3.7	2.6-3.7	2.6-3.7
ALP (U/L)	88-532	126-438	4-252
ALT (U/L)	≤29	≤32	5-45
Amylase (U/L)*	≤1683	≤1683	≤1683
AST (U/L)	7-19	3-23	2-26
Bilirubin (mg/dl)	0.01-0.13	0.01-0.13	≤0.3
BUN (mg/dl)*	9.8-37.3	9.8-37.3	9.8-37.3
Calcium (mg/dl)	10.4-13.6	10-13.2	10.4-12
Chloride (mEq/L)*	99-120	99-120	99-120
Cholesterol (mg/dl)	99.6-499.6	99.6-499.6	135-278
CK (U/L)	31-255	40-192	≤134
Creatinine (mg/dl)	0.39-0.49	0.27-0.88	0.21-0.89
GGT (U/L)	≤6.2	≤4.3	≤3.2
Globulins (g/dl)	1.9-2.5	2.2-3.5	2.2-4.5
Glucose (mg/dl)	97.1-166.2	97.1-166.2	76-119
GLDH (U/L)	1.6-9.6	1.9-8.7	1.2-8.0
LDH (U/L)	68-290	≤442	9-269
Lipase (U/L)	≤241	≤139	≤154
Magnesium (mEq/L)*	1.4-5.2	1.4-5.2	1.4-5.2
Phosphorus (mg/dl)	6.4-11.3	5.6-9.6	3.5-7.8
Potassium (mEq/L)	4.5-6.3	3.9-6.1	4.2-5.6
Sodium (mEq/L)	140-156	139-159	138-158
Total protein (g/dl)	4.3-5.8	4.5-7.3	4.9-6.7
Triglycerides (mg/dl)	19.1-205.5	19.1-205.5	40-169
TLI (μg/L)	5-35		

Adapted from the following sources:

Harper EJ et al: Age-related variations in hematologic and plasma biochemical test results in Beagles and Labrador retrievers, *J Am Vet Med Assoc* 223(10):1436-1442, 2003.

Kley S et al: Establishing canine clinical chemistry reference values for the Hitachi 912 using the international federation of clinical chemistry (IFCC) recommendations, *Comp Clin Path* 12:106-112, 2003.

Kraft W, Hartmann K, Dereser R: Dependency on age of laboratory values in dogs and cats. Part 1: Activities in serum enzymes, *Tierärztl Prax* 23:502-508, 1995.

Kraft W, Hartmann K, Dereser R: Age dependency of laboratory values in dogs and cats. Part II: serum electrolytes, *Tierärztl Prax* 24:169-173, 1996.

Laroute V et al: Quantitative evaluation of renal function in healthy Beagle puppies and mature dogs, *Res Vet Sci* 79(2):161-167, 2005.

Vajdovich P et al: Changes in some red blood cell and clinical laboratory parameters in young and old beagle dogs, *Vet Res Commun* 21(7):463-470, 1997.

* Parameters for which significant age variation was not found in puppies.

morphine, fentanyl, and butorphanol, commonly used for elective procedures such as spays and neuters of puppies and kittens.

Juvenile or type 1 diabetes mellitus is more common in young dogs, and it has not been well documented in feline medicine. Juvenile diabetes is discussed in more detail elsewhere in this text but should be suspected in puppies with persistent hyperglycemia, glucosuria, and clinical signs of disease (see Chapter 45).

Common causes of hyperglycemia in neonates are listed in Box 30-1.

PROTEIN

Serum proteins can be divided into two major categories: albumin and globulins. Albumin and the majority of globulins are synthesized by the liver in response to cytokine stimulation. Nutritional intake of proteins may also affect serum concentrations. Plasma also contains coagulation proteins that are also, primarily, produced by the liver. The majority of these coagulation proteins are not present in serum samples as they have been "consumed" by clot formation.

Age-associated increase of total protein and albumin is well described in animals. These increases are attributed to normal immune stimulation resulting in an elevated globulin fraction and increased albumin production resulting from improved liver function and intestinal absorption. As a result, in mammals, total protein concentrations are low at birth, increase dramatically after absorption of colostrum, and then decrease over 1 to 5 weeks as colostrum is metabolized. Total protein concentration then gradually increases to achieve adult levels within 6 months to 1 year.

Albumin

Albumin has a half-life of approximately 8 days in dogs and cats. It accounts for approximately 75% to 80% of the colloidal osmotic activity of plasma and is also a negative acute phase protein. It is important in the transport of many endogenous and exogenous molecules, including hormones, unconjugated bilirubin, and several drugs.

Globulins

Globulins are further classified into alpha (α)-, beta (β)-, and gamma (γ)-fractions. Most acute phase proteins are either α- or β-globulins, and, depending on the inflammatory process and type of globulin, variable increase and decrease of certain globulins may aid diagnosis of disease, response to therapy, and prognosis. The γ-globulin fraction contains the immunoglobulins of which IgG, IgM, IgE, and IgA are measurable in serum.

Puppies are born hypogammaglobulinemic with only a small amount of IgG and IgM and no detectable IgA in serum at birth. Therefore, total protein concentration in puppies is initially low, particularly precolostral intake. Protein concentration then steadily increases during the first year of life and is stable from age 1 year onward. Decreased

TABLE 30-4 **Kitten biochemical parameters from birth to 8 weeks of age**

	Day 0	Day 1	Day 7	Week 4 Day 28	Week 8 Day 56
Albumin (g/dl)	2.5-3.0	1.9-2.7	2.0-2.5	2.4-4.9	2.4-3.0
ALP (U/L)	184-538	1348-3715	126-363	97-274	60-161
ALT (U/L)	7-42	29-77	11-76	14-55	12-56
Amylase (U/L)	310-837	310-659	187-438	275-677	407-856
AST (U/L)	21-126	75-263	15-45	15-31	14-40
Bilirubin (mg/dl)	0.1-1.1	0.1-1.6	0.0-0.6	0.0-0.3	0.0-0.1
BUN (mg/dl)	26-45	34-94	16-36	10-22	16-33
Calcium (mg/dl)	9.4-13.9	9.6-12.2	10.0-13.7	10.0-12.2	9.8-11.7
Cholesterol (mg/dl)	65-141	48-212	119-213	173-253	124-221
CK (U/L)	91-2300	519-2654	107-445	125-592	102-1512
Creatinine (mg/dl)	1.2-3.1	0.6-1.2	0.3-0.7	0.4-0.7	0.6-1.2
GGT (U/L)	0-2	0-9	0-5	0-1	0-2
Glucose (mg/dl)	55-290	65-149	105-145	117-152	94-143
LDH (U/L)	176-1525	302-1309	117-513	98-410	62-862
Lipase (U/L)	12-43	21-131	8-46	4-86	6-70
Phosphorus (mg/dl)	5.9-11.2	4.9-8.9	6.7-11.0	6.7-9.0	7.6-11.7
TP (g/dl)	3.8-5.2	3.9-5.8	3.5-4.8	4.5-5.6	4.8-6.5
TS (g/dl)	3.1-4.4	3.2-5.2	3.0-4.6	4.0-6.0	4.1-6.2
Triglycerides (mg/dl)	23-132	30-644	129-963	43-721	16-170

Adapted from Levy JK, Crawford PC, Werner LL: Effect of age on reference intervals of serum biochemical values in kittens, *J Am Vet Med Assoc* 228(7):1033-1037, 2006.

TABLE 30-5 **Kitten biochemical parameters up to 12 months of age**

	<3 Months	4-6 Months	7-12 Months
ALT (U/L)	10-50	≤77	≤85
ALP (U/L)	≤564	37-333	21-197
Amylase (U/L)*	≤1800	1800	≤1800 (≤2200 Oriental breeds)
AST (U/L)	≤20	≤30	≤30 (≤40 Oriental breeds)
Bilirubin (mg/dl)[†]	≤4	≤4	≤4
BUN (mg/dl)[‡]	17-35	17-35	17-35
Calcium (mg/dl)*	9.2-12.0	9.2-12.0	9.2-12.0
Chloride (mEq/L)	97-125	102-122	104-124
Creatinine (mg/dl)	0.16-1.26	0.33-1.21	—[§]
CK (U/L)	≤188	≤160	≤128
GGT (U/L)*	≤4	≤4	≤4
GLDH (U/L)*	≤7	≤7	≤7 (≤16 Oriental breeds)
Glucose (mg/dl)[‡]	70-150	70-150	70-150
LDH (U/L)	68-280	≤442	9-269
Lipase (U/L)	≤280	≤280	≤280
Magnesium (mEq/L)*	1.2-5.2	1.2-5.2	1.2-5.2
Potassium (mEq/L)	3.7-6.1	4.2-5.8	3.7-5.3
Phosphorus (mg/dl)	6.5-10.1	6-10.4	4.5-8.5
Sodium (mEq/L)*	143-160	143-160	143-160
Total protein (g/dL)[‖]	–	3.3-7.5	3.3-7.5
TLI (µg/L)	17-49[¶]		

Adapted from Kraft W, Hartmann K, Dereser R: Dependency on age of laboratory values in dogs and cats. Part 1: Activities in serum enzymes, *Tierärztl Prax* 23:502-508, 1995; Kraft W, Hartmann K, Dereser R: Age dependency of laboratory values in dogs and cats. Part II: serum electrolytes, *Tierärztl Prax* 24:169-173, 1996; Kraft W, Hartmann K, Dereser R: Age dependency of laboratory values in dogs and cats. Part III: bilirubin creatinine & proteins in serum, *Tierärztl Prax* 24:610-615, 1996.
* Parameters for which significant age variation has not been found in kittens.
[†]Adult values reached after 1 week of age.
[‡]Adult values reached after 8 weeks of age.
[§]Reference ranges have not been reported for kittens over 6 months of age; 0.8-2.3 mg/dl (adult).
[‖]Adult levels are reached between 6 months and 1 year of age.
[¶]Data from Steiner JM: Diagnosis of pancreatitis, *Vet Clin North Am Small Anim Pract* 33:1181-1195, 2003.

TABLE 30-6 Hereditary conditions affecting biochemical parameters of young dogs and cats

Condition	Mode of Inheritance
Benign familial hyperphosphatasemia in Siberian Huskies	Likely autosomal (exact mode of inheritance not known)
Musculodystrophy	X-linked
Hyperchylomicronemia in cats	Believed to be autosomal recessive
Pancreatic acinar atrophy and exocrine pancreatic insufficiency in German Shepherd Dogs	Autosomal recessive
Severe combined immunodeficiency	
Basset Hounds	X-linked
Jack Russell Terriers and Cardigan Welsh Corgis	Autosomal recessive
IgA deficiency	Unknown
Hypercholesterolemia in Rottweilers and Dobermans	Unknown
Hereditary renal dysplasia in Lhasa Apsos	Autosomal recessive
Congenital dwarfism	Autosomal recessive
Hyperkalemia in posthemolysis in Akitas, Japanese Shibas, and Jindos	Believed to be autosomal recessive

total protein in puppies aged 8 weeks or less is likely caused by inefficient ability of the liver to synthesize it. Therefore, there is no compensation for increased blood volume that occurs during nursing and inadequate reabsorption ability from metabolites in the gastrointestinal tract. Puppies may also have higher intravascular water content than adults, resulting in a dilutional effect of their serum analytes.

In puppies, 5% to 10% of maternally derived IgG, and possibly IgM, may be transferred transplacentally. The remainder of IgG is transferred in the colostrum, resulting in an initial spike in globulins immediately after colostral ingestion. Because IgM circulates as a pentamer, it is unlikely that IgM is absorbed through the colostrum because of the large size of the molecule. This is supported by studies showing that puppies given adult canine serum subcutaneously at birth have higher IgM concentrations than puppies given the same serum orally. Additional information pertaining to passive transfer of maternal antibodies can be found in Chapter 2. The half-life of IgG and IgA in puppies is 10 days and 4 to 5 days, respectively. Therefore, a decrease in globulins and an increase in albumin within the first 6 weeks of life are identified as a result of degradation of maternally derived antibodies and increased synthesis of albumin as normal liver function develops. This leads to a peak in the albumin to globulin (A/G) ratio at 6 to 8 weeks, after which the A/G ratio decreases, consistent with a slight

increase in globulin fraction likely related to maturation of the immune system.

Breed differences in protein concentration have been reported in some studies. For example, Greyhounds have also been shown to have lower total protein concentrations as a result of decreased α- and β-globulin production than other breeds of dogs. Thus potential breed differences must be taken into account when interpreting biochemical results.

In kittens, approximately 25% of serum immunoglobulin concentration in newborns is attributable to transplacental absorption. However, unlike in puppies, IgG and IgA are not present in kitten serum at birth. Colostral absorption of maternal antibodies occurs within a very short timeframe in kittens. It is detected at 12 hours after birth but does not occur at 16 hours after birth. After colostral absorption, IgG and IgA concentrations peak within the first day of life and then decrease steadily as maternal antibodies decrease. The half-life of maternally derived IgG and IgA in kittens is 4 days and 1 to 2 days, respectively. Postweaning, IgG increases gradually as the kitten's production capacity by the developing immune system increases. IgA increases at a slower rate than IgG but then increases markedly at age 6 weeks. Unlike IgG and IgA, IgM may be detected in small amounts at birth (28 to 112 mg/dl), and, similar to other immunoglobulins, it increases steadily after the first few days of life.

Hypoproteinemia

Panhypoproteinemia may occur with gastrointestinal disorders, blood loss, liver dysfunction, or renal disease. However, it is important to note that many of these diseases may result from infectious or inflammatory causes resulting in increased globulins secondary to inflammation, thus masking an underlying loss of protein.

Disorders involving the intake and assimilation of protein are common causes for hypoproteinemia in animals. Intestinal malabsorption may result in a protein-losing enteropathy as both albumin and globulins leak through the intestinal wall into the lumen and are then digested and excreted. This may result from a variety of inflammatory conditions and is commonly associated with intestinal parasites in young animals, particularly those causing blood loss (e.g., whipworms). Exocrine pancreatic insufficiency results in the maldigestion of nutrients, including proteins, because of decreased production of digestive enzymes by the pancreas, in this case, trypsin. Because the liver uses amino acids obtained from protein digestion for the production of albumin, malnutrition or maldigestion of proteins results in decreased production of albumin despite normal liver function.

Severe liver dysfunction may result in decreased production of all proteins; however, hypoalbuminemia is typically detected primarily.

Protein-losing nephropathy may result in a net loss of both albumin and low molecular weight globulins because of defective protein tubular resorption of these molecules. Likewise, glomerular disease may result in a generalized loss of protein fractions.

Blood loss or hemorrhage secondary to trauma, coagulation disorders, including warfarin and brodifacoum intoxication, viral disease (e.g. parvovirus), and intestinal parasitism (mentioned previously) results in proportional loss of all blood constituents, including protein. In response to blood loss, interstitial fluid moves into the vascular space to increase blood volume. This results in dilution of the remaining blood constituents and further decreases total protein concentrations in both serum and plasma.

Hypoglobulinemia is most commonly associated with a failure of passive transfer in young animals, including puppies and kittens. As previously mentioned, there is a narrow window for absorption of immunoglobulins by the gut in animals (less than 24 hours). Failure of passive transfer is typically diagnosed by measuring IgG in serum via radial immunodiffusion (RID) method. An enzyme-linked immunosorbent assay is also available but is not as commonly used for measuring IgG in puppies and kittens because of difficulties in interpretation of results.

An inherited deficiency of B lymphocytes has been reported as an X-linked trait in Basset Hounds and also as an autosomal recessive trait in Cardigan Welsh Corgis and Jack Russell Terriers (see Table 30-6). This syndrome, known as severe combined immunodeficiency syndrome (SCID), results in a marked decrease in immunoglobulin production and occurs with profound lymphopenia in affected puppies. Selective immunoglobulin deficiencies have also been identified in other breeds of puppies, including IgA deficiency in German Shepherd Dogs, Beagles, and Shar-Peis (see Table 30-6).

Causes of hypoproteinemia are listed in Box 30-2.

BOX 30-2 Common causes for abnormalities of serum protein values in puppies and kittens

Hypoproteinemia
Maldigestion or malabsorption
- Inflammatory bowel disease
- Exocrine pancreatic insufficiency

Starvation, anorexia, or agalactia
Blood loss
Liver dysfunction
Renal disease
Failure of passive transfer
Congenital immunoglobulin deficiency
- Combined immunodeficiency syndrome
- IgA or IgG deficiency

Hyperproteinemia
Dehydration
Inflammation
Infectious disease
- Viral
- Bacterial
- Protozoal

Hyperproteinemia

Increased hepatic synthesis of albumin does not occur; therefore, hyperalbuminemia, often accompanied by hyperglobulinemia, is usually caused by hemoconcentration secondary to dehydration. Hyperglobulinemia is commonly seen with inflammation and is caused by both increased production of immunoglobulins and increased production of acute phase proteins. In dogs, C-reactive protein has been found to be the most common acute phase protein and is a sensitive, although nonspecific, indicator of inflammation in this species, often preceding changes in the leukocyte profile.

Kittens with FIP commonly exhibit hyperproteinemia secondary to hyperglobulinemia. In kittens with the wet form of FIP, an A/G ratio greater than 0.8 in effusions has been shown to be predictive for ruling out FIP. Similar to C-reactive protein in dogs, the acute phase protein α1-acid glycoprotein (AGP) is a very sensitive indicator of inflammation in cats. AGP levels greater than 1 to 5 g/L (RR < 0.48 g/L) in serum, plasma, or effusion samples are also found to aid in distinguishing cats with FIP from cats with other diseases with similar clinical signs.

Causes of hyperproteinemia are listed in Box 30-2.

LIPIDS

Lipids in plasma are divided into five categories: cholesterol, cholesterol esters, triglycerides, phospholipids, and long-chain fatty acids (LCFAs). LCFAs are obtained through the diet where they are absorbed from the digestive tract and then are incorporated into triglycerides by the intestinal epithelial cells. They may also be synthesized by the liver, adipose tissue, and mammary glandular tissue from glucose. Lipids are transported throughout the body attached to proteins. LCFAs combine with albumin for transport to tissues, whereas triglycerides and cholesterol attach to proteins, forming lipoproteins. These lipoproteins are broken down into very-low-density lipoproteins (VLDL), low-density lipoproteins (LDL), intermediate-density lipoproteins (IDL), and high-density lipoproteins (HDL), which can be differentiated by density and electrophoretically. The function of these lipoproteins is to transport aqueous insoluble lipids (e.g., cholesterol and triglycerides) through blood to tissues for metabolism, storage, or secretion. Cholesterol may be synthesized by the liver, or it may be absorbed from the intestine by animals eating animal protein. Cholesterol is predominantly transported by LDLs and HDLs in the bloodstream and is cleared from the serum by uptake by the liver. In the liver, cholesterol may be converted into bile acids or excreted directly into the bile.

Neonates are predominantly reliant on dietary absorption of lipids because of their decreased liver capacity to synthesize triglycerides and cholesterol. Nursing is an important source of lipids in neonates as milk contains a high content of fat, thus providing a high-calorie form of energy. In fact, plasma triglycerides have been shown to increase by twofold within 4 hours of a fat-rich meal. As a result, cholesterol is higher in nursing animals versus adults because of the high fatty acid content in milk. On ingestion of dietary fat, fatty acids are converted to triglycerides and transported through the blood in chylomicrons. Similarly, triglycerides formed by the liver are transported by VLDLs. Cellular uptake by myocytes and adipocytes for storage and transfer of lipids by lipoproteins is facilitated by interaction with several key enzymes and cell surface receptors that regulate the flux of lipids and the concentration of lipoproteins within plasma.

In puppies, cholesterol and triglyceride concentrations are highest at less than 8 weeks of age because of ingestion of milk fat during nursing. Postweaning, cholesterol and triglyceride concentrations gradually decrease but may peak again at age 5 to 6 months. After 6 months, values typically decrease until adult levels are reached.

For kittens, triglyceride and cholesterol concentrations are highest in nursing kittens, and upper reference limits in these kittens have been suggested to include triglyceride values up to 963 mg/dl and cholesterol values up to 521 mg/dl. These concentrations begin to decrease postweaning, because of withdrawal of milk consumption, to reach adult values by approximately age 9 to 12 months. Cats have been shown to have 5 to 6 times the levels of HDL versus LDL for lipid transport. Certain lipoproteins, particularly LDL, have been shown to decrease in preadolescent kittens (approximately 20 weeks of age) and are significantly lower than in adolescents (age 9 to 12 months). This is likely because of increased uptake of cholesterol to meet the needs of rapid tissue growth, sexual development, and steroidogenesis.

Hypolipidemia

Starvation or malnutrition, including poor nursing ability, in neonates is a serious cause of hypolipidemia, particularly hypotriglyceridemia. As the majority of lipids are obtained via ingestion of milk fats in these animals, lipid stores are rapidly depleted, and severe energy imbalances may ensue. Maldigestion and malabsorption of fats secondary to gastrointestinal disease may result in hypotriglyceridemia and, possibly, hypocholesterolemia in animals. Syndromes such as pancreatic insufficiency and inflammatory bowel disease with lymphangiectasia or the presence of gastrointestinal parasites may be responsible for marked decreases in serum and plasma lipid concentrations.

Hypocholesterolemia is commonly associated with liver dysfunction, as the liver is the major site of cholesterol synthesis. Disease may be acquired, secondary to infectious causes, toxic insult, or hypoxia, or it may be associated with a congenital defect such as PSS.

Causes for hypolipidemia are summarized in Box 30-3.

Hyperlipidemia

Hyperlipidemia occurs most commonly in young and adult animals postprandially as a result of increasing triglyceride concentrations after gastrointestinal absorption. To avoid this syndrome, a 12-hour fast before sampling is recommended in adults to minimize the amount of circulating chylomicrons, which may turn the serum milky white and

---

BOX 30-3 **Common causes of lipid imbalances in puppies and kittens**

Hypolipidemia
Malnutrition
- Starvation
- Poor nursing
- Agalactia
Maldigestion and malabsorption
- Inflammatory bowel disease
- Exocrine pancreatic insufficiency
- Lymphangiectasia
Liver dysfunction
- Infectious disease
- Portosystemic shunt

Hyperlipidemia
Postprandial
Liver disease
Cholestasis
Primary hypercholesterolemia in Dobermans and Rottweilers
Congenital hypothyroidism
Primary hypertriglyceridemia in kittens
Nephrotic syndrome

---

lyse red blood cells, thus adversely affecting laboratory evaluation of both biochemical parameters and blood counts. However, this practice may be risky in young animals, particularly in miniature and toy breeds of puppies because of their propensity for developing hypoglycemia as mentioned previously.

Although liver failure is associated with decreased production of cholesterol in animals, other forms of liver disease may be accompanied by hyperlipidemia, particularly in disorders associated with cholestasis. Because the liver is the major route of cholesterol secretion, hypercholesterolemia and hypertriglyceridemia may result from decreased hepatic uptake and excretion of cholesterol into the bile and decreased lipoprotein production.

In animals with nephrotic syndrome, renal loss of albumin stimulates production of cholesterol and, occasionally, triglycerides in an attempt to increase plasma oncotic pressure.

Primary/congenital hyperlipidemia is described in dogs and cats (see Table 30-6). For example, primary hyperlipidemia secondary to hypercholesterolemia with normotriglyceridemia has been reported in some dog breeds such as Doberman Pinschers and Rottweilers. Fasting hypertriglyceridemia (>5 mmol/L or >454.54 mg/dl) with severe hemolytic anemia may be associated with idiopathic hyperlipidemia in kittens, a congenital condition in cats caused by a defect in lipoprotein lipase, the enzyme necessary for cellular uptake of triglycerides by myocytes and adipose. Elevated chylomicrons and VLDLs with or without low LDL and HDL are also identified in affected kittens. Clinical signs of this syndrome include weakness, inappetence, peripheral neuropathy (hindlimb paralysis), retinal disease (lipemia retinalis), tachycardia, and tachypnea resulting from anemia.

Congenital hypothyroidism with hypercholesterolemia has been reported in puppies and kittens. The mechanism is not completely understood; however, it may be associated with decreased hepatic metabolism of lipids and decreased fecal excretion of cholesterol. This disorder is discussed in more depth in Chapter 45. Some common causes for hyperlipidemia are summarized in Box 30-3.

LIVER

Several enzymes are commonly used for the detection of liver abnormalities in animals. These abnormalities may include direct injury to or necrosis of the liver parenchyma or alterations in the functional capacity of the liver, including synthesis and excretion of manufactured compounds. Alteration in serum hepatic enzyme activity may provide nonspecific indications of the types of liver injury or dysfunction present. However, it is important to note that alterations in many of these enzymes are nonspecific and not sensitive.

Hepatic enzymes may be divided into two major categories: hepatocellular leakage enzymes and inducible enzymes. Inducible enzymes are attached to cell membranes; therefore, their serum activities usually do not increase as a direct result of cell injury or cell death. Increases of these enzymes in serum involve the increased production of an enzyme by cells that normally produce the enzyme and are stimulated to increase enzyme activity and release from the cell. Changes in normal activity of inducible enzymes occur more slowly because of the time required to manufacture these compounds in response to increased stimulation. Leakage enzymes are present in cytosol and/or organelles. They escape from the cells as a result of direct injury to the cell membrane or organelles, and, in contrast to inducible enzymes, serum changes in these enzymes may happen relatively quickly.

Because of the decreased functional capacity of the liver, nonspecific nature of many of these enzymes, and growth of other tissues, many enzymes are noted to be significantly different between young animals and adults. For example, alkaline phosphatase (ALP), alanine aminotransferase (ALT), aspartate aminotransferase (AST), lactate dehydrogenase (LDH), γ-glutamyltransferase (GGT), amylase, and lipase are found in feline colostrum, which is reflected in higher activities in colostrum-fed kittens.

Breed differences have also been seen in both dogs and cats for many of these enzymes. For example, Oriental breeds of cats have higher enzyme activity than other cat breeds of ALT, AST, glutamate dehydrogenase (GLDH), and α-amylase. In dogs, growth patterns are strikingly different between breeds, and differences in many enzymes may occur based on when adulthood is reached.

Common analytes related to detection of hepatocellular damage and liver damage are outlined below with differences between young animals according to species listed as appropriate.

Alanine Aminotransferase

ALT is a cytosolic/leakage enzyme and is considered relatively liver specific in both puppies and kittens. Abnormalities in this and most other enzymes are typically caused by increased concentrations in the serum relative to normal serum values. Neonates typically have values that are lower than adult parameters; therefore adult values should not be used to interpret ALT in young animals.

In puppies, ALT has been shown to increase with age and is likely a reflection of cell growth, adaptation, and differentiation of organs and metabolism. ALT activities are lowest in puppies aged less than 8 weeks and remain lower than adult levels until approximately age 6 months when adult values are obtained.

ALT activity is mildly increased in kittens, increasing with age until adult values are reached by approximately age 6 months. As previously mentioned, ALT is also found in feline colostrum and is reflected in higher activities in colostrum-fed kittens versus kittens deprived of colostrum after birth.

A significant breed-associated difference in ALT has been noted in Oriental breeds. In these patients, normal ALT activity may be nearly twice the activity of other breeds (≤140 U/L vs. ≤85 U/L, respectively).

Elevations in serum ALT often result from hepatocellular injury by damage to the cell membranes and subsequent release of the enzyme into the extracellular space. However, the degree of enzyme elevation does not correlate with the degree of tissue disease, nor does it equate to the functional capability of the liver. Therefore any abnormality in this, or any liver parameter, should be more fully investigated.

Glutamate Dehydrogenase

GLDH is a cytosolic enzyme. It occurs in high concentration in the liver and in very low concentrations in other tissues, such as muscle and kidneys. Therefore it is considered relatively liver specific in dogs and cats, and leakage of this enzyme occurs with damage to hepatocellular membranes.

GLDH is moderately higher in puppies aged 8 weeks or less than in adults.

In kittens, GLDH has not been shown to exhibit age dependence. However, Oriental breeds may normally have activities up to twice that of other breeds (≤16 U/L vs. ≤7 U/L, respectively).

Alkaline Phosphatase

ALP is an inducible enzyme that is synthesized by the liver, osteoblasts, intestinal epithelium, renal epithelium, and placenta. Because of the very short half-life (approximately 6 minutes) of intestinal, renal, and placental ALP in dogs and of intestinal ALP in cats, serum ALP is considered a reflection of liver or bone activity in these species and may also be associated with endogenous or exogenous corticosteroid induction in dogs.

Elevation of ALP, relative to adult values, in healthy young animals may be explained by the osseous isoenzyme bALP, which is increased in serum during bone growth.

ALP is also elevated in healthy young animals because of ingestion of colostrum in milk, which is a rich source of ALP in nursing puppies and kittens, as colostral enzymes are not blocked by gastrointestinal barriers. Bone growth in young animals may result in ALP values up to 4 times normal adult values; thus ALP must be interpreted carefully in light of the timeframe (according to age) and breed (large vs. small breed) of the patient.

In 1- to 3-day-old puppies, ALP activities are 30 times higher (respectively) than adult values, and then ALP decreases at 8 to 10 days. As mentioned previously, this dramatic increase immediately after suckling is caused by high levels of ALP in colostrum. The method most commonly used to measure colostral transfer in animals is RID. Because IgG evaluation by RID may take 2 or more days for test results, measurement of ALP in serum or plasma may provide some information on passive transfer status as a surrogate marker of colostrum ingestion in puppies.

ALP activities are highest in the first 16 weeks of life, peaking at 3 months, during which bone growth is progressing, and then become stable at 1 year. However, adult values of ALP in giant breeds may not be reached until age 2 years or later.

ALP in kittens is highest after ingestion of colostrum and, like in puppies, has been shown to be a predictor of passive transfer of colostral antibodies in kittens. For this interpretation, ALP concentrations higher than 1500 U/L on day 1 after birth and higher than 500 U/L on day 2 after birth are relatively sensitive and specific for predicting adequate colostral antibody ingestion in kittens. ALP remains above the adult reference range in cats and decreases to adult values between age 1 and 2 years.

Pathological elevations of ALP may occur with hepatocellular injury, cholestasis, and, in dogs, by induction of this enzyme by various drugs such as phenobarbital and corticosteroids. ALP is a very sensitive indicator of cholestasis, particularly in cats, and may actually precede the development of hyperbilirubinemia and icterus in affected animals. In dogs, the corticosteroid-inducible fraction of ALP (cALP) may also be increased during times of stress, secondary to endogenous corticosteroid release. The bone isoenzyme of ALP may be elevated beyond the normal reference range for growing animals secondary to bone trauma or developmental disorders, such as panosteitis, which result in increased osteoblast activity.

A rare but reported incidence of hyperphosphatasemia has been identified as a familial defect in Siberian Huskies (see Table 30-6). The ALP levels in serum of affected puppies are reported to be greater than 5 times those of age-matched controls, mainly as a result of induction of the bone isoenzyme. However, clinical or radiographic signs of disease are absent. The exact mode of inheritance for this syndrome is unknown.

γ-Glutamyltransferase

GGT is located primarily in cells that have absorptive or secretory functions. It is an inducible enzyme and is associated with numerous tissues, including renal epithelium, mammary tissue, liver, intestine, and pancreas. Greater GGT activity occurs in renal and hepatic tissues as transport processes are not fully developed in neonates.

GGT is highest in canine kidneys, pancreas, and small intestine and is eliminated in urine, pancreatic secretions, and the luminal intestine, respectively. Therefore in puppies postweaning, serum GGT activity is believed to reflect the enzyme derived from other tissues, mainly liver. Similar to ALP, GGT activities are markedly increased in day-old puppies after suckling and colostrum ingestion, with values being approximately 100 times higher than adult values. The enzyme then decreases to below presuckling values by day 10 after birth. Therefore GGT may also be used as a surrogate marker of colostrum ingestion in puppies. Postweaning GGT values decrease slightly to below adult values and then increase to reach adult values by approximately 6 months of age.

No clinically significant age dependence has been shown for GGT throughout aging in kittens. Unlike in puppies, GGT has not been shown to be useful as a predictor of passive transfer in this species.

Pathologic elevations in GGT are most commonly associated with cholestasis and enzyme induction of the hepatocytes or biliary epithelium in animals. In dogs, including puppies, GGT activity may also increase secondary to induction by exogenous glucocorticoid administration.

Aspartate Aminotransferase

AST is a leakage enzyme and is not liver specific, being found in most tissues and in erythrocytes. However, it is present at highest concentrations in myocytes (both skeletal and cardiac) and hepatocytes. Both cytosolic and mitochondrial isoenzymes of AST exist, but more severe cellular injury is required for release of the mitochondrial isoenzyme to occur. Therefore the magnitude of AST release is usually less than that of ALT release after hepatocellular damage.

In puppies, reports of AST activity are variable with no age dependence to a slight increase with age in puppies up to 6 months.

Age differences in kittens are more consistent than those reported in puppies with slight increases exhibited up to age 4 to 6 months. Oriental breeds have also been shown to have greater enzyme activity (≤40 U/L vs. ≤30 U/L for other breeds).

Moderate elevations of AST may occur with nonspecific hepatocellular damage, muscle trauma, including trauma after birth, and hemolysis.

Lactate Dehydrogenase

LDH activity is found in many cell types and is therefore not liver specific. As other parameters are much more specific for detection of damage to a particular tissue, LDH is not commonly evaluated in small animal chemistry profiles. However, as age-related differences are noted in puppies and kittens, these results will be briefly discussed.

In puppies, LDH is highest during suckling, likely because of the enhanced use of lactose as a glucose precursor during the neonatal period. Adult values are obtained soon postweaning.

In kittens, LDH activity is highest in those aged less than 1 year.

Elevations in LDH activity may result from hemolysis, muscle damage, or hepatocellular injury. Early increases in LDH after birth may be associated with the trauma of birth itself.

Bilirubin

Bilirubin is formed by the breakdown of hemoglobin by the mononuclear phagocyte system in the body. Two forms of bilirubin are identified: unconjugated bilirubin is present in red blood cells and, when free in serum, is transported to the liver for conjugation by albumin, whereas conjugated bilirubin is formed within hepatocytes, which renders the molecule water soluble. Hepatic conjugation of bilirubin is discussed more thoroughly in Chapter 37.

Young animals, within the first few days of life, typically have bilirubin concentrations that are significantly higher than adult levels. This neonatal hyperbilirubinemia is not completely understood. The process may involve increased bilirubin load secondary to relative polycythemia, decreased lifespan of fetal erythrocytes, increased enterohepatic circulation, and transition from maternal bilirubin metabolism to dependence on immature neonatal hepatic uptake and conjugation.

Bilirubin concentration is elevated in puppies aged 1 to 3 days and then decreases to adult levels rapidly thereafter. Serum may be grossly icteric during the first few days of life, and then icterus resolves rapidly.

As in puppies, bilirubin in kittens is also slightly higher than adult levels during the first week of life, and serum may be grossly icteric for 1 to 2 days after birth. Icterus should resolve shortly thereafter, and bilirubin levels are similar to adults at age 1 week.

Neonatal hyperbilirubinemia is common in young animals less than 1 week of age. Therefore elevations in this parameter in the first few days after birth must be interpreted accordingly. Causes for pathologic hyperbilirubinemia are similar to those identified in adult animals. Hemolysis caused by infectious organisms, acquired or congenital erythrocyte membrane abnormalities, and immune-mediated disease results in increased levels of total bilirubin. In the initial stages of hemolysis, hyperbilirubinemia is caused by increased unconjugated bilirubin released from lysed red blood cells. As hemolysis progresses, increased bilirubin overwhelms hepatic uptake, conjugation, and secretion capacities. Thus both conjugated and unconjugated bilirubin levels are often elevated in serum.

Decreased hepatic uptake of bilirubin, as a result of loss of functional hepatic mass, ultimately results in decreased conjugation and secretion of bilirubin. Therefore hepatocellular disease may result in increased concentrations of both unconjugated and conjugated bilirubin. Cholestasis secondary to obstruction of bile flow through the liver typically results in increased levels of conjugated bilirubin in serum and plasma. Often other parameters such as ALP and GGT are also elevated in animals with cholestasis.

MUSCLE

Numerous enzymes are found within myocytes of animals including ALT, AST, LDH, and creatine kinase (CK). CK, along with AST and LDH, is most commonly associated with muscle injury. Therefore it is possible that early increases in these enzymes in neonates may be associated with the trauma of birth.

Creatine Kinase

CK is a cytosolic enzyme found in numerous tissues, although its activity is highest in skeletal muscle, cardiac muscle, and the brain. The enzyme is critical to energy production in myocytes, and its activity varies with age and breed in healthy animals. CK has been shown to be higher in young animals relative to adult values, likely a result of normal development of the musculature.

In puppies, CK activity is highest in those less than 3 months of age and decreases as puppies reach adulthood. Day-old puppies may have 5 times more CK activity in serum than adult dogs. CK then decreases with age, and puppies at age 6 months have values approximately twice those of adults. Adult values are typically reached by approximately age 7 months. Serum CK is increased in young kittens and decreases to adult levels at between 6 and 12 months of age.

As mentioned above, abnormal elevations in CK are the result of direct injury to the musculature and leakage of the enzyme from the cytoplasm of damaged myocytes. Traumatic injury and congenital muscular growth abnormalities may result in dramatic increases in serum and plasma enzyme levels. For example, in puppies with canine X-linked muscular dystrophy, CK levels are markedly elevated and may be approximately 100 times normal values (see Table 30-6).

EXOCRINE PANCREAS

Pancreatic function in mammals is divided into two broad categories: the endocrine pancreas, which is primarily responsible for glucose homeostasis, and the exocrine pancreas, which is responsible for secretion of enzymes used for digestion of carbohydrates, proteins, and lipids. Evaluation of the exocrine function in young animals is often geared toward ruling out disorders related to exocrine pancreatic insufficiency and less commonly to inflammatory conditions affecting the pancreas. Both aspects of exocrine and endocrine pancreatic function are discussed in more detail in Chapters 37 and 46, respectively. However, as some age-dependent variations of commonly measured biochemical parameters evaluating normal pancreatic function have been reported, these enzymes will also be briefly mentioned here.

Pancreatic enzymes and their zymogens (the inactive form of the enzyme) are stored in acinar cells. Therefore, injury to cell membranes may result in transient increases in the normal levels of these enzymes. Amylase and lipase are the most commonly measured parameters to assess pancreatic function and secretion as they are readily evaluated in either serum or plasma. Unfortunately, these enzymes are not specific to pancreatic tissue nor are they sensitive indicators of disease in animals.

Amylase

Amylase is responsible for the digestion of carbohydrates in animals. The enzyme is found in greatest quantities in the pancreas, liver, and small intestine. It is filtered by the glomerulus and resorbed by the renal tubular epithelium.

No age dependence has been reported for amylase activities in puppies; therefore adult values may safely be used to interpret normal pancreatic function for this species.

In kittens, serum amylase activity has been shown to be lower relative to adult values. Breed-associated differences have also been identified, with Oriental breeds having statistically higher levels of amylase than other breeds of cats.

Lipase

The pancreas, the gastric and duodenal mucosa, and adipose are known sources for lipase in mammals. Lipase is responsible for the digestion of ingested fats, and similar to amylase, lipase is also cleared from plasma by the kidneys.

Lipase has been shown to be highest in neonatal puppies and then decreases in those aged 3 to 6 months, followed by a progressive increase to adult values.

Lipase has been shown to increase with age in young kittens. Lipase has also been shown to be higher in colostrum-fed kittens compared with those deprived of colostrum. However, this difference is transient, resolving within a few days postpartum.

Trypsinogen

The proteolytic enzyme trypsin is formulated by the zymogen trypsinogen in the small intestine. The zymogen is secreted exclusively by the pancreas; therefore testing for trypsinogen is specific for pancreatic disease. Detection of trypsinogen is performed by assaying trypsin-like immunoreactivity (TLI). As the TLI concentration in serum depends on pancreatic mass, it is used, most commonly, for the detection of pancreatic insufficiency in dogs and cats. Injury to pancreatic parenchyma results in leakage of trypsinogen into the extracellular space. Therefore serum TLI may be used to detect pancreatic injury; however, this assay has been shown to be poorly associated with pancreatitis in cats or the severity of this disease in dogs. Age-related variations in TLI have not been reported in dogs or cats.

Decreased Pancreatic Enzyme Activity

Exocrine pancreatic insufficiency (EPI) has been shown to occasionally result in decreased values of amylase and lipase. However, because these enzymes are not tissue specific, their production by other tissues may actually result in values within normal reference ranges. Thus EPI cannot be definitively ruled out by the presence of normal amylase and lipase activities in serum. However, TLI has shown to be highly sensitive and specific for the detection of EPI in animals. Therefore subnormal values for TLI along with appropriate clinical signs of disease may be interpreted as consistent with a diagnosis for EPI.

Early-onset EPI is associated with certain breeds of dogs. In German Shepherd Dogs, an autosomal recessive trait resulting in development of pancreatic acinar atrophy with subsequent development of EPI has been elucidated (see Table 30-6). Chows Chows and Rough-coated Collies also exhibit a tendency for developing EPI at a young age, indicating that a congenital predisposition may also occur in these breeds. EPI is diagnosed in dogs with TLI concentrations of 2.5 μg/dl or lower.

EPI is less commonly reported in cats, and no congenital predisposition has been reported for this species. Although the disease is more common in middle-aged to geriatric cats, kittens less than 1 year of age have been reported to develop this disorder and are so diagnosed when TLI concentrations are 8 μg/dl or lower.

Increased Pancreatic Enzyme Activity

Amylase and lipase are most commonly measured in serum to identify pancreatic inflammation in dogs and cats. Although these enzymes are not tissue specific in these species, elevations greater than threefold have been shown to correlate with pancreatitis. Renal disease with decreased glomerular filtration and tubular clearance of amylase and lipase may result in serum elevations of both enzymes. Likewise, trypsin activation peptides may increase in severe renal disease, resulting in elevation of TLI. Gastrointestinal disease has been shown to result in hyperamylasemia and hyperlipasemia, and hepatobiliary disease may also induce hyperamylasemia in serum.

RENAL PARAMETERS

Blood urea nitrogen (BUN) and creatinine are the most commonly assessed indices of glomerular filtration, and thus renal function, in mammals. As these components are freely filtered by the glomerulus, any reduction in the glomerular filtration rate (GFR) results in increases in the concentration of these analytes in serum. However, both BUN and creatinine are affected by other body systems, which may affect their rate of production and their rates of excretion. Age variations have been noted for both parameters.

Urea Nitrogen/Blood Urea Nitrogen

BUN is produced in the liver by breakdown of dietary proteins (see Chapter 37). Therefore BUN may increase in the serum as a result of either decreased renal filtration or increased protein ingestion.

BUN has consistently been shown to be lower in young animals compared with adults. Proposed reasons for lower

BUN concentrations include increased plasma volume after birth, along with immature hepatic production.

BUN is lowest in puppies less than 6 months of age. Initially BUN is high (within adult values) and then decreases between the ages of 2 weeks and 3 months before beginning to increase again to obtain adult values by approximately age 6 months. Proposed reasons for lower BUN in puppies have been attributed to increased protein synthesis as a result of growth hormone influence or possibly increased metabolic state with increased GFR.

Urea nitrogen is initially high in kittens at birth and then decreases to below adult values in kittens less than 8 weeks of age. Adult values are reached shortly thereafter.

Decreased BUN

As urea nitrogen is typically lower than adult values in young animals, interpretation of BUN must be performed in conjunction with clinical signs of disease and in the context of the appropriate reference ranges for each age group. Serum BUN concentrations may be decreased below appropriate reference ranges, either because of decreased intake of protein, which may occur as a result of malnutrition including poor nursing in neonates, or because of decreased hepatic production of urea. In congenital or acquired PSS, intrahepatic or extrahepatic shunting of blood results in tissue hypoxia and functional liver disease. In cases of congenital PSS, liver enzymes are typically within reference range, and decreased urea nitrogen is often the first abnormal parameter to be detected. In patients with acquired PSS (e.g., secondary to infectious disease or toxicity), signs of liver disease typically include detectable abnormalities of liver enzymes.

Common causes for decreased BUN are summarized in Box 30-4.

Increased BUN

An increase in serum BUN is identified as azotemia and may occur as a result of prerenal, renal, or postrenal causes. Prerenal causes of elevated BUN include dehydration with decreased plasma volume and decreased tubular flow rate resulting in increased absorption of urea across the collecting tubules. This typically occurs with a proportional increase in serum creatinine concentration and is recognized by a concurrent elevation in urine-specific gravity in an attempt to increase tubular resorption of water to compensate for the decrease in plasma volume. Increased ingestion of a high-protein meal, including upper gastrointestinal hemorrhage leading to blood ingestion, may also result in an elevation in BUN in animals. This elevation in BUN is independent of elevations in creatinine and typically results in a BUN/creatinine ratio of more than 10:1 and often more than 30:1 in the case of upper gastrointestinal bleeding.

Renal causes of elevated serum BUN occur as a result of decreased glomerular filtration of urea resulting in decreased excretion of urea in urine. Renal azotemia, caused either by congenital defects in function or acquired injury, typically results in a concurrent elevation in serum creatinine and isosthenuria.

| BOX 30-4 | Common causes for abnormal alterations in BUN and creatinine in puppies and kittens |

Blood Urea Nitrogen
Increased BUN
  Dehydration
  Renal disease
  Lower urinary tract obstruction
  Uroabdomen
  High protein meal/upper gastrointestinal hemorrhage
Decreased BUN
  Malnutrition
  Liver dysfunction
  • Infectious disease
  • Toxin
  • Portosystemic shunt

Creatinine
Increased creatinine
  Dehydration
  Renal disease
  Lower urinary tract obstruction
  Uroabdomen
Decreased creatinine
  Decreased muscle mass
  • Disuse
  • Congenital disease (e.g., muscular dystrophy)
  • Starvation
  Portosystemic shunt

Postrenal causes of elevated serum BUN are less common in neonates but may result from renal obstruction or rupture of the urinary bladder, which may occur as a complication during parturition.

Common causes for increased BUN are summarized in Box 30-4.

Creatinine

Creatinine is formed by the spontaneous, irreversible dehydration of muscle creatine and dephosphorylation of creatine phosphate. Creatine and creatinine originate mainly from biosynthesis of the amino acids glycine, arginine, and methionine and partly from alimentary supply as creatine concentration is high in meat. Like BUN, creatinine is freely filtered by glomeruli so that its concentration in plasma is equal to that of the glomerular filtrate. A small amount of creatinine may also be secreted in renal proximal tubules. In young animals, age-associated variations of creatinine have been well recognized, and variations in breed and individual muscle mass have also been shown to occur. The lower creatinine in young animals relative to adults correlates with smaller body size and decreased muscle mass.

In neonatal puppies between 1 and 3 days of age, creatinine levels are high, with wide variation. Then there is a steady decrease until 28 to 33 days of age followed by a slight increase at 7 to 8 weeks of age. Creatinine levels may then increase moderately up to 1 year of age. Breed variations in creatinine have been observed. German Shepherd puppies up to 8 weeks of age have reportedly higher creatinine values than other breeds. Adult Greyhounds have also been shown to have higher creatinine concentrations because of their increased muscle mass relative to other breeds of dogs.

In kittens, similar to puppies, creatinine levels are high at birth and then decrease to equivalent to or less than adult levels through 8 weeks of age. When exactly adult levels are normally reached in cats has not been reported. Concentrations likely remain lower in young kittens as a result of decreased muscle mass, similar to dogs. Therefore abnormal values should be interpreted in conjunction with clinical signs of disease and physical status of the kitten. No breed variations have been reported in cats.

Decreased Creatinine

Creatinine concentrations, lower than the reference range for young animals, are usually caused by decreased muscle mass secondary to muscle atrophy from disuse or starvation. Moderate decreases in plasma creatinine have also been reported in dogs with PSS caused by a disease-associated increase in GFR and renal volume in affected dogs.

Common causes for decreased creatinine are summarized in Box 30-4.

Increased Creatinine

Causes for prerenal, renal, and postrenal azotemia, with subsequent elevations of serum creatinine, are similar to those described for urea nitrogen above. In incidences of urinary tract rupture with postrenal elevation in creatinine, creatinine concentration in peritoneal fluid is higher than in plasma, allowing for identification of the fluid as urine.

Common causes for increased creatinine are summarized in Box 30-4.

MINERALS

The control of calcium, phosphorus, and magnesium is extremely important, not only for proper bone growth in young animals but also for normal cell stability, muscle contraction, and acid-base regulation. These minerals are regulated via three main body systems: the gastrointestinal tract, kidneys, and the parathyroid glands. Therefore any dysfunction in any one of these organ systems may result in severe imbalances of cellular function and growth.

It is well recognized that calcium and phosphorus are higher in young puppies and kittens throughout growth phase because of increased bone growth. Parathyroid hormone–related peptide is present in high amounts in milk throughout lactation and may affect transport of calcium into milk, as well as calcium metabolism in nursing neonates. Growth hormone, which is high in neonates and is also present in high concentrations in milk, also enhances renal phosphate reabsorption.

Calcium

Calcium is necessary for cellular reactions such as nerve conduction, muscle contraction, hormone release, and activation of enzymes. Hormonal control of calcium is maintained by the action of parathyroid hormone (PTH), formed by the parathyroid glands, and by calcitonin, produced by the C cells of the thyroid glands, where the serum concentrations of calcium (and phosphorus) regulate the activity of these hormones by feedback control. The process is complex, and in addition to PTH, calcitonin, and active vitamin D, it requires normal gastrointestinal and renal function. Calcium is obtained by dietary ingestion and absorption by the small intestine in animals. This process is reliant on vitamin D, which cats and dogs primarily obtain by dietary intake of vitamin D_3 (cholecalciferol). After ingestion, vitamin D is stored in the liver in an inactive form, 25-hydroxycholecalciferol ($25[OH]D_3$). Under conditions of low extracellular calcium, it is then transported to the kidney for transformation to its functional form, 1,25-dihydroxycholecalciferol ($1,25[OH]_2D_3$), which is also known as calcitriol. The transport of the storage form of vitamin D to the kidney and its subsequent conversion to calcitriol depends on PTH. In addition to its effect on the production of calcitriol, PTH acts directly on the renal tubules to increase calcium resorption from urine, and it stimulates bone resorption for the subsequent release of calcium and phosphorus. Therefore the major effect of PTH is to increase extracellular calcium by mobilizing calcium stored in bone, increasing renal tubular calcium reabsorption and calcitriol synthesis. When sufficient levels of extracellular calcium (and phosphorus) are achieved, production of calcitonin by the thyroid C cells inhibits PTH secretion and stimulates excess phosphorus excretion by the kidneys.

The majority of calcium is located intracellularly within the skeleton of animals. Only a small amount of calcium is found free in circulation, with approximately 50% being present in the ionized/active form and the remainder being bound to albumin or complexed to other compounds such as citrate and phosphate. Therefore measurement of total calcium reflects not only the active ionized form of this mineral but also the amount bound to protein and complexed to other molecules. Therefore imbalances of calcium should be verified by measurement of the ionized (active) form.

Calcium is highest in puppies less than 8 weeks of age and then decreases to adult levels at about age 1 year.

Like puppies, kittens have higher calcium concentrations, relative to adult levels, before 8 weeks of age. However, concentrations decrease shortly thereafter to reach adult levels by age 3 months.

Hypocalcemia

Renal disease results in decreased renal resorption of calcium and decreased renal production of active vitamin D_3 and thus decreased gastrointestinal absorption of calcium. This progressive hypocalcemia stimulates production and release of

PTH and subsequent bone demineralization. This condition is known as renal secondary hyperparathyroidism and is initially of benefit to the affected animal. Progressive stimulation of PTH excretion later becomes detrimental as bone density is sacrificed for serum calcium homeostasis. Deposition of calcium and phosphorus eventually develops in tissues, including the kidneys, worsening the preexisting renal disease.

Cases of acute renal failure secondary to ethylene glycol toxicosis typically result in profound hypocalcemia caused by the chelation of calcium by oxalate.

Decreased intake of calcium may occur as a result of malnutrition, including poor nursing, and anorexia in young animals.

Pseudohypocalcemia is often seen in animals who are hypoalbuminemic. Total calcium is decreased as approximately 50% of calcium is bound to albumin as previously described. However, ionized concentrations are within normal limits. Calculations for the correction for total calcium based on the levels of albumin in serum have been used for dogs; however, these calculations have been shown to be unreliable in the face of underlying disease. Therefore the use of these calculations to predict ionized calcium concentration is currently discouraged.

Metabolic alkalosis may result in hypocalcemia as a result of decreased availability of hydrogen ions and increased movement of calcium into cells from the extracellular space to maintain electroneutrality.

Common causes for hypocalcemia are provided in Box 30-5.

Hypercalcemia

Most causes for hypercalcemia in young animals are related to nutritional imbalances or renal dysfunction. Vitamin D toxicosis occurs after ingestion of certain cholecalciferol-containing rodenticides that up-regulate intestinal and renal absorption of calcium (and phosphorus). Patients are at risk for mineralization of tissues, particularly the kidney and gastric mucosa, and development of irreversible organ dysfunction.

Acidosis may result in hypercalcemia as calcium ions shift out of the intracellular space as a result of displacement by increased numbers of available hydrogen ions in serum.

Hypercalcemia secondary to renal disease is uncommon in dogs and cats but may be seen in conditions such as hereditary renal dysplasia in Lhasa Apsos (see Table 30-6). Acute renal failure in dogs secondary to ingestion of raisins or grapes has also been shown to occasionally cause hypercalcemia. This finding can help to differentiate renal failure in dogs with grape- or raisin-induced toxicosis from ethylene glycol intoxication, which typically results in a marked depression of serum calcium.

Increases in serum calcium have been described in puppies and kittens secondary to granulomatous disease. The mechanism is suspected to be related to production of $1,25[OH]_2D_3$ by stimulated macrophages in affected animals.

Common causes for hypercalcemia in neonates are summarized in Box 30-5.

Phosphorus

Phosphorus, in the form of inorganic and organic phosphate, functions as an important buffering system in the body. Phosphorus is also an important part of the plasma membrane, nucleic acids, adenosine triphosphate (ATP), and adenosine monophosphate. Absorption of phosphorus by the gastrointestinal system is also under the control of PTH and vitamin D_3 activity on skeletal and gastrointestinal systems. Phosphorus is also actively resorbed by the proximal tubules, and this mechanism is under feedback control of serum phosphorus concentrations, where hyperphosphatemia increases renal excretion of phosphorus, and decreased serum phosphorus stimulates tubular reabsorption.

The majority of phosphorus is located in the intracellular space. Eighty percent to 85% is stored as inorganic hydroxyapatite in bone, and approximately 15% is found in soft tissue, mainly muscle. Therefore, like calcium, less than 1% of total body phosphorus is found in the extracellular fluid. However, most circulates as free ion with only a small amount being protein bound or complexed to calcium, sodium, or magnesium.

In puppies, phosphorus concentrations are lowest at 1 to 3 days of age and then increase above adult levels throughout the growth phase. Adult levels are reached after approximately 1 year of age. However, different breeds of dogs have different growth phases, and this should be taken into consideration when evaluating variations in phosphorus, particularly in giant breeds of dogs.

Serum phosphorus concentrations in young kittens are highest at less than 8 weeks of age and then decrease gradually to reach adult levels after age 1 year.

Hypophosphatemia

The causes for hypophosphatemia in animals primarily involve conditions of decreased oral intake, decreased renal reabsorption, or translocation of phosphorus into the

---

BOX 30-5 Common imbalances of calcium in young animals

Hypocalcemia
Decreased intake
Renal disease
Ethylene glycol toxicosis
Hypoalbuminemia
Alkalosis

Hypercalcemia
Vitamin D toxicosis
Congenital renal disease
Granulomatous disease
Acidosis

intracellular space. Decreased intake of dietary phosphorus is the most common cause of low serum phosphorus in young animals. Anorexia, poor nursing, or poor nutrition of the nursing mother may all contribute to not only decreased phosphorus but also decreased ingestion of vitamin D, which in turn results in decreased absorption of phosphorus. Administration of phosphate binders present in many antacids used for gastrointestinal disorders may also result in decreased gastrointestinal absorption of phosphorus.

Some cases of renal disease such as Fanconi-like syndrome and renal tubular acidosis cause tubular dysfunction, which results in decreased tubular reabsorption of phosphorus and increased excretion into the urine. Likewise, administration of diuretics that work at the level of the proximal tubules affects reabsorption of many minerals and electrolytes, including phosphorus.

Translocation or ion shifting of phosphorus may occur with ingestion of a high carbohydrate diet which stimulates glycolysis resulting in a shift of phosphorus to the intracellular space, after administration of insulin, respiratory alkalosis with stimulation of the glycolytic pathway, and hypothermia.

Decreased production of growth hormone is identified in cases of pituitary dwarfism, an uncommon congenital defect in pituitary development identified in several dog breeds, including German Shepherd Dogs, Spitz, and toy Pinschers (see Table 30-6). Decreased production of growth hormone decreases whole body phosphorus mainly as a result of decreased renal reabsorption of phosphorus (see Chapter 45).

Causes for hypophosphatemia for young animals are summarized in Box 30-6.

BOX 30-6 Common causes for imbalances of phosphorus in young animals

Hypophosphatemia
Anorexia or malnutrition
Renal tubular disease, including Fanconi-like syndrome
Administration of phosphate binders
Administration of some diuretics
High carbohydrate meal
Insulin administration
Respiratory alkalosis
Hypothermia
Pituitary dwarfism (decreased growth hormone)

Hyperphosphatemia
Dehydration
Renal disease
Vitamin D toxicosis
Administration of phosphate enemas
Metabolic acidosis
Hemolysis
Tissue trauma
Uroabdomen

Hyperphosphatemia

Decreased renal excretion of phosphorus caused by decreased glomerular filtration is the most common cause of elevated serum phosphorus. This may result from intense dehydration, shock, or renal disease in animals. In the event of hyperphosphatemia secondary to renal disease, animals are often also initially hypocalcemic. Hypocalcemia increases the risk for development of renal secondary hyperparathyroidism as a result of decreased renal production of vitamin D_3 (previously described) and stimulation of PTH with subsequent bone demineralization.

Hyperphosphatemia caused by increased intake may occur after administration of phosphate enemas or in cases of vitamin D_3 toxicity. Translocation of phosphorus out of the cell into the extracellular space will increase serum phosphorus concentrations. This may result from massive tissue/muscle trauma, hemolytic disease, or metabolic acidosis with ion shifting out of the cell and breakdown of ATP.

Common causes for hyperphosphatemia are listed in Box 30-6.

Magnesium

Serum magnesium concentration depends on dietary intake and is regulated by mineralocorticoids and PTH. Like calcium and phosphorus, the majority of magnesium is located intracellularly with only a small amount (approximately 1%) found in serum. Approximately 60% of serum magnesium is in active/ionized form in dogs, with the remainder being bound to protein or complexed with compounds such as phosphate and citrate. Magnesium is important in the synthesis of nucleic acids and proteins. It also acts as a cofactor for sodium-potassium ATPase, calcium ATPase, and proton pumps. Magnesium is necessary for muscle contraction, membrane stabilization, and metabolism of fats, proteins, and carbohydrates. Therefore imbalances of serum magnesium may have profound impact on numerous body systems, including the cardiovascular, neuromuscular, and dermatologic systems.

Age variations have not been found for serum magnesium concentrations in puppies or kittens, and values are similar to adult reference ranges.

The most common cause for hypomagnesemia in young animals is secondary to decreased dietary intake or loss through malabsorption or diarrhea. Insulin administration in animals with juvenile diabetes mellitus results in intracellular translocation of magnesium. Likewise, translocation of magnesium into the intracellular space results in patients with alkalosis because of decreased availability of hydrogen ions. Renal disease or administration of non–potassium-sparing diuretics often results in decreased tubular resorption of magnesium.

ELECTROLYTES

Maintenance of normal electrolyte balance is tightly regulated by the body and occurs predominately via renal tubular resorption and secretion of these molecules in response to

BOX 30-7   **Potential causes for electrolyte disturbances in puppies and kittens**

Sodium

Hyponatremia
  Diarrhea
  Diabetes mellitus
  Anorexia or dietary deficiency
  Uroabdomen
  Psychogenic polydipsia
  Treatment with hypotonic fluids
  Third space loss
  Whipworms

Hypernatremia
  Dehydration
  Adipsia or hypodipsia
  Diabetes insipidus
  Panting

Potassium

Hypokalemia
  Anorexia or dietary deficiency
  Alkalosis
  Catecholamine release
  Gastrointestinal loss
  • Vomiting
  • Diarrhea
  Third space loss
  Renal disease
  • Chronic renal failure
  • Fanconi-like syndrome
  • Renal tubular acidosis
  Severe burns
  Treatment with hypotonic fluids
  Insulin therapy

Hyperkalemia
  Thrombocytosis
  Hemolysis (Akitas, Jindos, and Shibas)
  Acidosis
  Ischemia and reperfusion injury
  Oliguria or anuria
  Uroabdomen
  Whipworms
  Chylothorax

Chloride

Hypochloridemia
  Renal loss
  Third space loss
  Diarrhea
  GI loss
  • Vomiting
  • Diabetes mellitus
  Psychogenic polydipsia
  Respiratory alkalosis

Hyperchloridemia
  Dehydration
  Adipsia or hypodipsia
  Diabetes insipidus
  Panting
  Respiratory acidosis

variations in hydration status, serum osmolality, and acid-base balance of the individual. In the case of sodium, the most osmotically active particle in the body, variations in hydration status are closely linked to its rate of resorption or loss, and these variations are often coupled to loss of other electrolytes as a result of the body's attempt to maintain electroneutrality. Furthermore, imbalances of electrolytes are useful to predict not only the cause of disease but also response to therapy.

In puppies, serum sodium and chloride concentrations are slightly lower at or before 6 weeks of age relative to adult levels. Serum potassium is low at age 2 to 4 weeks and then peaks at age 6 to 8 weeks before gradually dropping off to values comparable with adult levels. This low serum potassium is presumed to be caused by the presence of sodium/potassium (N/K) pumps in neonatal erythrocytes, resulting in higher concentrations of intracellular potassium (relative to extracellular concentrations) compared with adult dogs. These N/K pumps appear to be lost quickly after birth in most breeds of dogs, with the exception of Akitas, Jindos, and Japanese Shibas (see Table 30-6 and Box 30-7). Thus these latter breeds of dogs have higher concentrations of intracellular potassium than other dog breeds.

Age-associated differences have been identified for potassium and chloride in kittens; however, no differences have been found for sodium. Potassium is slighter lower in kittens less than 3 months of age compared with older kittens. These values increase slightly between 4 and 6 months of age and then gradually decrease again to reach adult levels by 6 months. Chloride is lowest in young kittens less than 3 months of age and then increases to adult parameters by approximately 4 to 6 months of age.

Electrolyte Imbalances

Decreases in one or more electrolytes are extremely variable and depend on the disease process present. Cases of multiple electrolyte imbalances are often caused by decreased intake of electrolytes as a result of anorexia or loss of electrolytes in body fluids through vomiting, diarrhea, third space loss, renal excretion, or renal secretion. These imbalances often result in sequential destabilization of the acid-base status of the patient, ion shifting to maintain electroneutrality, and may often worsen the clinical disease.

Abnormal elevations in electrolytes are typically caused by decreased plasma volume that often occurs with dehydration or electrolyte supplementation in young animals. Causes for electrolyte abnormalities will not be discussed individually in this section, but differential diagnoses for these imbalances are provided in Box 30-7.

SUGGESTED READINGS

Greco DS: Pediatric endocrinology, *Vet Clin North Am Small Anim Pract* 36(3):549-556, 2006.

Grundy SA: Clinically relevant physiology of the neonate, *Vet Clin North Am Small Anim Pract* 36(3):443-459, 2006.

DiBartola SP: *Fluid, electrolyte, and acid-base disorders in small animal practice,* ed 3, St Louis, 2006, Saunders/Elsevier, pp 210-226.

Latimer KS, Mahaffey EA, Prasse KW: *Duncan and Prasse's veterinary laboratory medicine clinical pathology,* ed 4, Ames, IA, 2003, Iowa State Press, pp 270-303.

Troy DB: *Veterinary hematology and clinical chemistry,* Baltimore, 2004, Lippincott, Williams and Wilkins, pp 421-429.

Wellman ML et al: Comparison of the steroid-induced intestinal and hepatic isoenzymes of alkaline phosphatase in the dog, *Am J Vet Res* 43:1204-1207, 1982.

POSTMORTEM EXAMINATION OF THE PUPPY AND KITTEN

CHAPTER 31

Christiane V. Löhr

WHY DO A POSTMORTEM EXAMINATION?

Puppy and kitten losses within the first few months of life are a common but unavoidable problem. Postmortem examinations provide essential information for preventative strategies and should be pursued aggressively. This is particularly important when losses occur in the preweaning period, and contributing factors should be eliminated before the next breeding cycle. Postmortem examinations are also an important part of quality assurance and quality control programs of veterinary clinics and provide great opportunities for continued education when faced with the unexpected or unexplained death of a patient or a patient's death despite diagnosis-based treatment. Postmortem examinations address the owner's concern about littermates and other pets in the household, the future of the breeding program, and the owner's health. Results from a postmortem examination can also provide consolation, particularly after the difficult decision to have a pet euthanized.

WHAT COMPRISES A POSTMORTEM EXAMINATION?

A postmortem examination is actually a series of examinations. The gross examination during the necropsy of the animal is followed by the microscopic examination of fixed tissues (histopathology). Often additional tests on fresh tissues like microbiology (bacteriology, virology, parasitology, mycology, and serology) and/or toxicology (chemical analysis of tissues for toxins, minerals, and heavy metals) are necessary to determine the specific etiology of an identified disease process. These additional tests can be requested at time of necropsy, or samples may be collected and saved for testing at a later time, for example, when histopathology results are available and allow a focused approach to further testing to minimize expenses.

WHO PERFORMS POSTMORTEM EXAMINATIONS?

Ideally, the entire animal is submitted to a diagnostic laboratory for complete postmortem examination. If this is not possible, the necropsy may be performed at the clinic, and collected samples can be sent to a diagnostic laboratory for testing. Some of the advantages and disadvantages of the available approaches are listed in Table 31-1.

PUPPY AND KITTEN LOSSES AND COMMON CAUSES

The pediatric patient poses some unique challenges with respect to postmortem examinations. The quick succession of developmental phases is associated with a rapid change of commonly encountered diseases to which the diagnostic approach has to be tailored. The perinatal puppy or kitten is commonly worked up as an abortion with a simplified gross examination and emphasis on histopathology and microbiological testing. In contrast, animals older than 1 day of age require a thorough and complete necropsy because gross findings determine the menu of additional tests to be performed. Before weaning, health concerns extend to littermates, the dam, and often the breeding program in general. After weaning, the problem is usually viewed as that of an individual animal and rarely of the household.

Very few studies on necropsy findings of the puppy and kitten have been published in the primary literature. In puppies, most deaths occur before rather than after weaning, which amount to more than 20% and less than 5% of all puppy deaths in the first year of life, respectively. More than 50% of the preweaning puppy losses occur during the first week of life. Common causes in this age group are stillbirth (incidence of 2.2% to 4.6%), trauma, failure to thrive, or congenital anomalies resulting in death or euthanasia. In puppies older than 1 week, respiratory and gastrointestinal

---

TABLE 31-1	Pros and cons of postmortem examination at a diagnostic laboratory versus at a clinic	
Examination at	**Advantages**	**Disadvantages**
Diagnostic laboratory	Workup by specialists: gross lesions may be subtle and can be easily missed Coordination of ancillary testing Infrastructure for safe and complete examination Carcass: prearranged disposal or cremation	Transport/shipping: expense and time in transit Additional cost (for gross examination)
Clinic	Immediate sample collection Immediate feedback	Time consuming Biosafety and containment Necropsy equipment and area Disposal of carcass; release to client not recommended Interpretation of findings (more often the challenge is the lack of significant gross lesions)

---

diseases are the most common primary issues identified on postmortem examination, followed by malnutrition. In kittens, 50% of neonatal mortalities are the result of stillbirth (incidence of 4.3% to 10.1%), and an additional 25% occur in kittens less than 1 week of age. Approximately 15% of all litters have at least one kitten with one or more congenital anomalies (nearly 10% of kittens born alive). Based on histopathological examination, more than half of the kitten deaths up to 4 months of age are caused by infectious diseases, with the majority having a viral etiology. Before weaning, feline herpesvirus 1 and feline calicivirus are the main causes; after weaning, it is feline parvovirus followed by feline infectious peritonitis (corona)virus.

Box 31-1 highlights commonly encountered causes of canine and feline mortality by age group.

In a large number of cases, a definitive diagnosis is not established, and the cases are released as idiopathic deaths or abortions. In a retrospective study on kitten losses during the first 4 months of life, this apparent failure to identify a specific cause was significantly associated with submission of tissue samples instead of the entire animal to the diagnostic laboratory for postmortem diagnostics. This underlines the fact that a thorough gross examination and collection of a complete set of samples for histopathology and microbiology are imperative to successful postmortem diagnostics. Gross lesions may be subtle and can be easily missed by an inexperienced examiner. This may result in collection of incomplete sample sets, which in turn will limit the spectrum of available diagnostic tests.

THE POSTMORTEM EXAMINATION

Euthanasia of moribund animals should avoid injection into organs or body cavities that are suspected to be involved in the disease process (e.g., intracardiac, intrapulmonary, and intraabdominal injections are not recommended if the disease/syndrome is suspected to be cardiac, pulmonary, and abdominal, respectively). The remains should be *immediately*

refrigerated at 39° F (4° C). Freezing before collection of samples for histopathology will cause severe artifacts as a result of disruption of the microanatomy by formation of ice crystals and should therefore be avoided. If delays of more than 2 days until a complete postmortem examination are expected, a necropsy at the clinic with collections of a complete set of well-preserved samples is recommended. If in doubt about the appropriate approach, contact a diagnostic pathologist.

Submission to a Diagnostic Laboratory

Shipping of the Entire Animal

The remains should be allowed to completely cool before packaging into plastic bags or containers for transport or shipping. While in transit, the remains should be *chilled* with ice packs placed inside the bag or container. Packages have to be absolutely *leak-proof* and include padding with absorbent material. The remains may be transported to the laboratory by the owner or veterinary practice personnel, or shipped via a carrier service providing same-day or next-day delivery. Shipping of remains late in the week should be avoided as they may end up without adequate cooling over the weekend.

Communication with the Diagnostic Laboratory

Effective communication with the laboratory personnel, especially the pathologist or case coordinator, is central to successful postmortem diagnostics. The importance of a *complete clinical history*, including signalment of the animal and clinical findings and diagnoses, cannot be stressed enough. Important points to cover in the clinical history are provided in Box 31-2. Specific questions from the clinician should be noted on the submission sheet, so that the diagnostician is aware of them at the time of gross examination. Submission sheets should be filled out by the attending veterinarian (not by support personnel) to avoid loss of critical information and miscommunication. If the space on the submission sheet

BOX 31-1   Common causes of mortality by age group

Abortion, Stillbirth, and Perinatal Phase (0 to 1 day)

- Infectious: *Brucella canis/abortus*; canine and feline herpesvirus; *Toxoplasma gondii*; *Escherichia coli*; *Salmonella* and *Mycoplasma* species; *Campylobacter jejuni*; β-hemolytic streptococci; feline leukemia virus (Figure 31-1, *A*)
- Noninfectious
  - Low birth weight (puppies and kittens) and litter size of one (kittens)
  - Congenital anomalies (Figure 31-1, *B* to *D*): in this age group most commonly cleft palate, exencephaly, intestinal agenesis, schistosomas reflexus, limb deformity, atresia ani, diaphragmatic or umbilical hernia, renal hypoplasia or aplasia, and complex cardiovascular or respiratory anomalies
  - Other: intrapartum hypoxia or asphyxiation, trauma in association with dystocia or maternal neglect; hormonal, metabolic, or chromosomal anomalies; drugs and chemicals administered during gestation

Neonatal Phase (Puppies: 1 day to 10 days; Kittens: 1 day to 7 days)

- Malnutrition including primary maternal neglect
- Enteric disease: coronavirus, rotavirus; *Escherichia coli*; cryptosporidia
- Septicemia (Figure 31-2): commonly *Staphylococcus, Streptococcus, Escherichia, Klebsiella, Enterococcus,* or *Salmonella* species

- Other systemic infectious diseases like canine herpesvirus in puppies (Figure 31-3) and toxoplasmosis in kittens (Figure 31-4)
- Omphalitis with or without phlebitis or arteritis as a result of opportunistic bacteria
- Congenital anomalies: in this age group most commonly involving the central nervous, cardiovascular, or respiratory system (e.g., cerebellar hypoplasia because of feline parvovirus, or patent ductus arteriosus Botalli)

Pediatric Phase

- Puppies (older than 10 days)
  - Respiratory disease: infectious tracheobronchitis complex with secondary *Bordetella bronchiseptica* (Figure 31-5) and canine distemper virus
  - Enteric disease: canine parvovirus 2 (Figure 31-6, *A*), canine distemper virus, and coccidia
  - Congenital anomalies with metabolic or systemic consequences like portosystemic shunt and progressive juvenile nephropathy
- Kittens (older than 7 days)
  - Respiratory disease: feline herpesvirus 1 and/or feline calicivirus, and *Bordetella bronchiseptica* as primary or secondary pathogen
  - Enteric disease: feline parvovirus (Figure 31-6, *B*) and feline coronavirus
  - Congenital anomalies with metabolic consequences (less commonly diagnosed than in puppies)

BOX 31-2   Basic components of a clinical history

- Signalment
- History provided by owner
- For abortions: gestation time, due date, type of delivery (normal or cesarean section), duration of labor, breeding history
- Date of onset and duration of illness
- Other animals in the household
- Other animals affected, number, and clinical presentation
- Introductions of new animals
- Husbandry and changes in husbandry
- Results from the clinical examination
- Test results (e.g., clinical pathology and radiology)
- Clinical diagnosis(es) with top differential diagnoses
- Treatment
- Death (euthanasia or natural) and date of death
- Date of postmortem examination and shipping

pathological, or radiographic examinations, can be very helpful and should be included liberally. If additional material is extensive, a brief summary will be welcomed by the diagnostician. Contact information (telephone and fax numbers, e-mail address) will facilitate timely reporting of results. Many laboratories issue preliminary reports, which should be taken as such: preliminary results without final conclusions. Pet owners may be anxious for results, but some tests take a few days to complete or may not be offered daily. For example, the histopathologic examination of a brain can take up to 10 days from the date of necropsy. In this case, sufficient fixation before processing is necessary to ensure high quality and artifact-free microscopic specimens.

Postmortem Examination at the Clinic

Biosafety and containment are major issues associated with postmortem examinations at a clinic. A designated work area and a separate set of instruments for necropsy reduce risk of contamination of clean and sterile areas. Minimal protective equipment includes gloves, a laboratory coat, and goggles. A disposable plastic apron and a surgical mask (3M, St. Paul, MN; filtering >95% of microorganisms) greatly enhance protection. Aerosolization of pathogens can be decreased by wetting down the animal's haircoat and the work surface. Disinfection with household bleach after thorough cleaning provides sufficient decontamination of surfaces.

is too limited, the attending veterinarian should include additional pages.

It may sound trivial, but information needs to be *clearly legible* because text that cannot be deciphered is of no use. Additional information, like results of recent clinical,

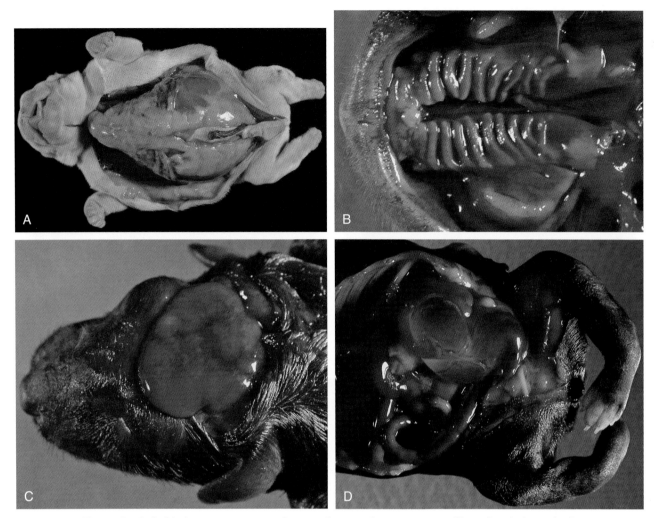

Figure 31-1 A, Moderate anasarca and severe hemoperitoneum, puppy. The subcutis is markedly expanded with edema (anasarca). The abdominal cavity is severely dilated with blood, most likely because of septicemia. Note how the umbilicus has been preserved in this partially skinned puppy. **B,** Cleft palate (palatoschisis), roof of oral cavity, dog fetus. **C,** Exencephaly, dorsal aspect of head and neck, dog fetus. The incomplete closure of the crania with protrusion of the brain through the defect in the bone and skin is often associated with cleft palate and other anomalies of the head. **D,** Bilateral hindlimb deformity and unilateral hydroureter, dog fetus. The abdominal cavity is partially exenterated, and the thoracic cavity is completely exenterated. The left ureter in the upper half of the picture is severely dilated with clear watery fluid (urine).

Setting up for a Necropsy

Getting ready for a necropsy is similar to setting up for surgery. Instruments are set out ahead of time and ideally include the following:

- Sharp knife and steel (a sharp necropsy or meat knife is the ideal tool for most tasks)
- Scissors (blunt/sharp straight work best)
- Forceps (small dissecting forceps minimize crush artifacts of small tissue samples; tissue thumb 1×2 or 2×3 teeth are fine for larger specimens)
- Rib or poultry shears or branch cutters (for cutting ribs)
- Small bone shears, cutting forceps, or rongeurs (to open skull of kittens and small puppies)
- Stryker saw, hacksaw, or meat cleaver (to open larger skulls)
- Scalpel blades and handle
- Measuring tape
- Syringes and needles to collect fluids
- Tongue depressors to scrape intestinal mucosa, collect feces, or fix muscle samples

Scissors will dull quickly when cutting muscle and skin but are the instrument of choice to open hollow organs. For small animals less than 10 lb, a scalpel with a larger blade works better than a necropsy knife.

Sample containers should be kept at hand and ready to use. Please refer to the section on sample collection for further details on appropriate equipment and sampling strategies.

A camera is very helpful to document lesions that are difficult to describe or explain. Printed pictures or digital files

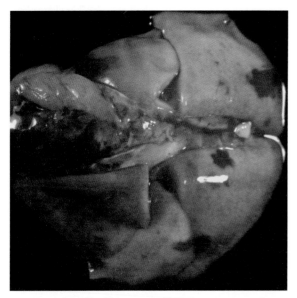

Figure 31-2 Multifocal hemorrhage, lungs, puppy. Compare these normally inflated and pink lungs with the pneumonic lungs depicted in Figures 31-3, *B* and 31-5. Cause of death in this puppy was septicemia.

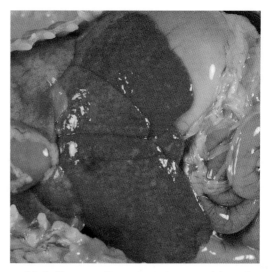

Figure 31-4 Severe disseminated necrotizing hepatitis, abdominal situs, kitten. The liver is severely enlarged and mottled beige-brown. On histopathology, protozoan cysts consistent with *Toxoplasma* sp. were identified in areas of necrotizing hepatitis. The protozoal infection in this kitten involved many other organs, including the brain and lungs.

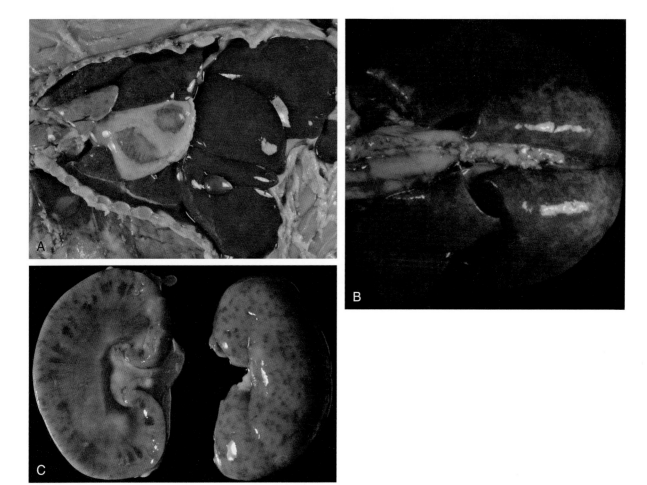

Figure 31-3 Systemic canine herpesvirus 1 infection. All the photographs in this figure show the same puppy. **A,** Severe acute hydrothorax and multifocal acute hepatic necrosis, situs of thoracic and cranial abdominal cavity. Pleural effusion and hepatic necrosis are common findings in herpesvirus infections. Canine herpesvirus infection is commonly diagnosed in puppies that died during the first 2 weeks of life. **B,** Severe acute interstitial pneumonia, lungs. The lungs are poorly collapsed and mottled red-beige. Compare with normally colored and collapsed lungs shown in Figure 31-2. **C,** Multifocal, severe, acute renal necrosis and hemorrhage, sagittal cut, kidney. Petechiation on the cut *(left)* and capsular *(right)* surface in the puppy is characteristic for an infection with canine herpesvirus 1.

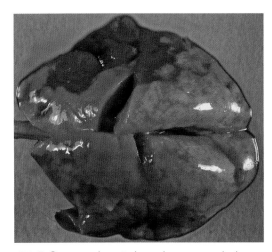

Figure 31-5 Severe subacute bronchopneumonia, lung, puppy. This gross presentation is typical for suppurative bronchopneumonia as a result of aerogenous infection with bacteria. *Bordetella bronchiseptica* was isolated in this case and is the most common bacterial pathogen in feline and canine respiratory disease. Compare with normally inflated and pink lung in Figure 31-2 and interstitial pneumonia depicted in Figure 31-3, *B*.

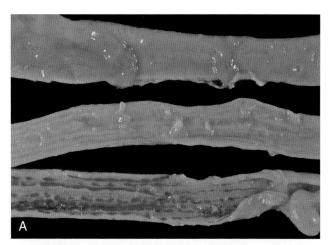
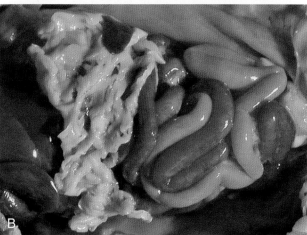

Figure 31-6 A, Necrotizing enteritis, jejunum and ileum, puppy. The Peyer's patches in the affected flaccid segments of small intestine appear sunken because of loss of lymphoid tissue to necrosis. Parvovirus was identified in a mucosal scraping that included the malodorous intestinal contents. **B,** Segmental enteritis, abdominal situs, kitten. The severe hyperemia and dilation of loops of small intestine are typical for parvoviral enteritis (panleukopenia).

of photographs can add tremendous value to a submission— "a picture speaks more than a thousand words." Pictures should be well-labeled, and topographic orientation should be provided.

Complete Necropsy

A complete necropsy is the ideal approach if submission of the remains to a diagnostic laboratory cannot be accomplished in a timely or economical manner. There is no one best necropsy protocol. Regardless of the approach, consistency is what matters most. Recognition of lesions, especially absence or displacement of organs, is greatly facilitated by a standardized approach. Suggestions for necropsy procedures with emphasis on the pediatric patient are provided in Box 31-3.

A necropsy protocol provides a standardized approach to the dissection of animals and should be applied consequently. At times, however, it is essential to deviate from the dissection protocol to preserve a lesion, and technical adjustments have to be made. Congenital anomalies are more commonly encountered in the pediatric patient. Their identification can be challenging and often requires careful examination of organs *before* exenteration.

Partial Necropsy

In any situation other than an abortion or stillbirth, a partial necropsy is not ideal. Most diseases cause lesions in multiple organs, and important changes may be missed by focusing on a single or a few (potentially incorrectly) selected organs or systems. A common scenario is failure to examine and collect the brain from a patient with a history of vague clinical symptoms or even seizures. However, a complete necropsy is not always an option, and a partial necropsy may provide at least some answers.

In case of abortions or stillbirth, the primary concern is the collection of samples without cross-contamination. Sampling is done first and is followed by a close examination of organs and tissues in situ (before exenteration) as it facilitates identification of common anatomic congenital anomalies like aplasia, hypoplasia, and heterotopia.

Sample Collection and Data Recording

Basic sample containers include large and tightly shutting plastic jars filled halfway with formalin for histopathological samples, sterile and sealable plastic bags for fresh samples, red-top Vacutainer tubes (BD, Franklin Lakes, NJ) for safe transport of fluids, and culture swabs. Containers need to be labeled with the owner's name and animal identification. Those containers holding fresh samples should also state the content.

For histopathology, tissue samples are fixed in 10% formalin (3.4% formaldehyde) at a tissue/formalin ratio of

BOX 31-3   **Necropsy technique**

A necropsy entails three basic tasks:
1. External examination
2. Exenteration of organs
3. Examination of internal organs and body parts

   A list with the structures examined during a complete necropsy is given in Figure 31-9. For a more detailed necropsy protocol, see the suggested reading at the end of the chapter.

Laying out the Animal and Opening of Thorax and Abdomen

1. Place body with head facing left and tail facing right, and examine externally. Dorsal recumbency works best.
2. Make a midline skin incision from chin to pubic area (avoid umbilicus and penis), and then partially skin the trunk to expose rib cage and abdominal wall.
3. Transect connections of limbs to trunk in axillary and inguinal regions without cutting limbs off, and disarticulate hip joints.
4. Cut through abdominal wall along midline caudal to sternum, push organs down, and pull body wall up to extend cut to pelvic aperture. Check for *fluid*.
5. Along rib arch, extend cut through body wall bilaterally to the vertebral column. *Check position of diaphragm,* then cut it off along rib arch.
6. Use scissors, poultry shears, or branch cutter to bilaterally cut ribs from renal area to thoracic inlet; lift sternum and ribs off by separating mediastinum from sternum. Check for *fluid*.
7. Take samples for culture; in case of abortion/stillbirth, also for histopathology (see Figures 31-7 and 31-8).

Thoracic Cavity and Plug

1. *Carefully check position of all thoracic organs* for completeness and position, especially for anomalies of the large vessels (once the plug is removed, these are extremely difficult to reconstruct).
2. Cut bilaterally along medial aspect of mandible, and between soft and hard palate, and disarticulate hyoid bones to reflect tongue, pharynx, and larynx.
3. Continue to pull tongue out and to right, and separate trachea and esophagus from neck. Continue to pull on plug to remove it out of the thoracic cavity and transect aorta, vena cava caudalis, and esophagus at the diaphragm.
4. With scissors, open pericardium (leave heart attached to lungs!). Beginning in right ventricle, cut with scissors along septum up into atrium and then pulmonary artery. Start in left ventricle, cut up along septum into left atrium and (under septal leaflet of atrioventricular valve) into aorta transecting pulmonary artery above valves.
5. If heart is less than 3 cm from base to apex, bisect with scalpel along long axis from apex to base perpendicular to septum to open (half) ventricles, and fix heart whole.
6. Open entire length of esophagus with scissors, then larynx and trachea all the way into bronchi.

7. Take samples for histopathology and additional testing (see Figures 31-7 and 31-8).

Abdominal Cavity

1. Before moving anything, carefully check all organs for position and completeness. Carefully examine umbilicus, umbilical arteries, vein (all the way up to liver), and urachus.
2. Separate omentum with spleen from stomach and pancreas.
3. Find distal colon, transect, and separate guts from mesentery as close as possible to its intestinal insertion. This will permit laying out intestines in long straight lines, which facilitates rapid opening along entire length. Be careful at the transverse colon to not cut off cecum and pancreas.
4. Pull liver back from diaphragm, and transect esophagus, aorta, and caudal vena cava; lift out liver, stomach, pancreas, and guts by transecting remaining connections. Secure adrenal glands cranial to kidneys (if they are not there, check dorsal margin of liver).
5. To check patency of bile duct, open duodenum and squeeze gall bladder to extrude bile. Remove liver from other organs.
6. Open stomach along greater curvature from cardia to pylorus and intestines with scissors (as if cutting fabric) along mesenteric insertion to preserve Peyer's patches.
7. Take samples for histopathology and additional testing (see Figures 31-7 and 31-8).

Pelvic Cavity

1. Remove muscles from ventral aspect of pelvis, find obturator foramina, and nip cranial and caudal bony bridges (pubis and ischium).
2. Free pelvic floor and lift off.
3. Using caudal aperture as guideline, cut perineum around external genitalia and anus.
4. Peel kidneys away from body wall.
5. Pull rectum, genital, and lower urinary tract out of pelvic cavity, and lift out with kidneys attached. Open kidneys sagittally from cortex to pelvis, and peel capsule back.
6. With scissors, open urinary bladder and extend cut down urethra (careful: os penis!).
7. Open rectum.
8. Bisect testes and epididymides or ovaries with knife.
9. If large enough open uterus with scissors.
10. Take samples for histopathology (see Figures 31-7 and 31-8).

Bone Marrow

1. Free femur from surrounding muscles, and disarticulate at hip and knee.
2. Scrub remaining muscle off the bone with *back* of knife blade.

BOX 31-3   Necropsy technique—cont'd

3. Place bone perpendicular across edge of table, and smash shaft with *back* of knife. Open induced spiral fracture by breaking shaft.
4. Roll bone marrow cylinder out on glass slide for cytology.
5. Fix in formalin for histopathology by immersing bone half.

Central Nervous System
This is a bit time consuming but essential if the animal showed nervous signs.

Brain:
1. Move head slightly up and down to locate atlantooccipital joint, disarticulate from ventral aspect, and transect spinal cord.
2. Skin head from occiput to cranial of eyes.
3. As long as bones are soft, use scissors to open skull from occipital foramen to a line connecting the caudal canthus of both eyes, and peel off crania. Otherwise, use Stryker saw, hacksaw, or meat cleaver to generate same trapezoid cut, and lift off crania.
4. Cut dura mater with scissors to expose brain, and turn head upside down. Gravity will pull brain away from base of skull.
5. Transect cranial nerves and olfactory bulbs with scissors, and let brain slide out into palm of hand.
6. *Samples for microbiology may include*: small pieces of brainstem, cerebellum, and cerebral cortex; cerebrospinal fluid; swab from ventricle and/or meninges.

7. *Place brain in tenfold volume of formalin* to fix for histopathology.
8. Check tympanic bullae at base of skull by nipping open with bone cutter.
9. Sagittally cut through nose to open nasal cavity, and remove septum. Alternatively, cut nose transversely behind canine teeth.
10. Enucleate eyes if examination is desired, and fix whole.

Spinal Cord:
1. Cut off limbs, rib, and pelvis.
2. Flesh out vertebral column.
3. With bone cutters, cut dorsal arch on each side of vertebrae, and reflect dorsally and back to remove. Once spinal cord is completely exposed, grasp dura mater with forceps, and gently lift out by cutting nerves and attachments as needed with scissors (leave nerve rootlets and ganglia attached).
4. Open dura mater dorsally along entire length, and fix spinal cord (ideally flat) in large tub with formalin.

Tissue Identification (e.g., Left versus Right)
Label paper towel or tongue depressor with pencil or permanent marker, and place tissue (mucosa facing up) on it. Fold paper towel over, and immerse in formalin by squeezing out air. Alternatively, place tissues in separate, labeled containers.

1:10. In cool climates, addition of 10% to 15% methanol will prevent frost damage of fixed tissues. In very cold climates (temperatures well below freezing), tissues may be shipped in 60% ethylene glycol in phosphate-buffered saline and fixed in formalin on arrival at the laboratory as long as cooling is guaranteed during transport. The thickness of tissue sections should not exceed 5 mm (¼ inch) to allow for rapid and complete penetration and fixation. Fresh samples should be collected from areas with visible lesions. Contamination of other tissues or handling of samples with contaminated instruments should be avoided.

Samples for microbiology require immediate refrigeration or cooling (blue ice). Samples for bacteriology, virology, and toxicology may be sent frozen. Freezing of samples for parasitology and mycology should be avoided as it destroys organisms. Swabs for virology and bacteriology have different requirements for transport media (addition or omission of antimicrobials, respectively).

Abortions, stillbirth, and perinatal puppies and kittens up to 24 hours of age

Fetal and perinatal losses warrant aggressive diagnostics to prevent recurrence of problems in subsequent breeding cycles. Some diagnostic laboratories offer discounts on testing in the form of abortion screens, which include but

are not limited to pathology and microbiology. An example of a sampling checklist for abortions is provided in Figure 31-7 (please feel free to photocopy for use in practice). Inclusion of the placenta for both histopathology and microbiological testing is very helpful.

A thorough physical examination of the dam is recommended and may be supplemented with hormonal assays and karyotyping of fetal or placental tissue. The perinatal phase is an extension of gestation and parturition, and neonatal losses within the first 24 hours postpartum should be worked up as an abortion. Nonetheless, a thorough and complete gross examination is recommended for puppies and kittens in this age group.

Neonatal, preweaning, and postweaning puppies and kittens

A datasheet for recording of necropsy findings and a sample checklist are provided in Figures 31-8 and 31-9, respectively (please feel free to photocopy for use in practice). The age and clinical presentation of the animal and the necropsy findings determine the most appropriate panel of samples for a diagnostic workup. The sampling checklist provided covers three scenarios frequently encountered in the pediatric patient: respiratory, gastrointestinal, and systemic (infectious) diseases. Submission of a complete set of tissue

Attach to filled-out submission sheet provided by diagnostic laboratory.

A. History: _____

_____

(continue on back page if needed)

B. Gross examination of abortion

1. Placenta (green discoloration of margins physiologic): _____

2. Fetuses or perinatal puppies and kittens (up to 24h of age)

Gestation Time (Days)	Fetus Identification	Weight	Crown Rump Length	Sex		Placenta
		gram/lb	cm/inch	female	male	present

a. External examination especially umbilicus: _____

b. Internal examination

    i. Congenital Anomalies (e.g., cleft palate, aplasias, anomalies of large vessels)

        1. Anomalies involving one organ: send entire organ fresh.

        2. Complex anomalies: send organ complex or entire body.

        Findings: _____

    ii. Other findings (e.g., fluids, flocculent stomach contents, necrosis, hemorrhage): _____

_____

_____

C. Sample collection *Clearly label all containers with owner name and animal ID*

1. Fresh (unfixed) tissues for Bacteriology and Virology (specify contents on container)

Tissue/Sample	Test	Instructions
Placenta	Bacteriology	Collect all samples into
Lung		**INDIVIDUAL** sealable
Liver		containers (Whirlpack
Kidney (puppy)		or Ziplock bags)
Stomach contents		Red top vacutainer tube
Maternal serum	Serology (*Brucella canis*)	Red top vacutainer tube
Anomalous organ(s)	Gross examination	

2. Formalin-fixed tissues for Histopathology (ideal tissue to formalin ratio = 1:10)

Avoid freezing to prevent artifacts that severely impair histopathologic evaluation!

☐ Placenta (multiple samples)   ☐ Heart   ☐ Thyroid gland

☐ Lung   ☐ Brain   ☐ Adrenal gland

☐ Liver   ☐ Thymus   ☐ Small intestine

☐ Kidney   ☐ Spleen   ☐ *

* Additional organ(s) or organ systems with lesions identified during gross evaluation

All samples need to be collected into leak-proof containers or sealable plastic bags, double bagged, and shipped according to regulations (DOT and carrier service).

Figure 31-7 Abortion screen: data recording and sampling checklist.

samples for histopathology is highly recommended for all disease processes. Many laboratories charge a standard fee for histopathology on necropsies regardless of the number of tissues included; subsequently, the more the better for yielding a diagnosis at no additional expense for the client.

Tissue samples collected for histopathology should be no thicker than 5 mm (¼ inch). Samples of the heart include longitudinal sections taken from the left and right ventricle, ideally the papillary muscles, and a thin cross-section through the septum. In case of organs with multiple

HISTORY + SIGNALMENT
Age: _____   Sex: _____   DOB:__/__/__   Death:__/__/__ ;   died/euthanized?   Weight:_____

_____

A. External
   1. Condition and position of the carcass: _____
   2. Indicators of death (rigor, temperature, eyes, beginning decomposition):_____
   3. Body condition (score): _____
   4. Surface of the body (skin, external genitalia—vulva/prepuce/scrotum; umbilicus): _____

   5. Orifices and mucous membranes: _____
B. Internal
   1. Subcutis:_____
   2. Musculature and tendons:_____
   3. Bones and joints:_____
   4. Lymph nodes:_____
   5. Blood and coagulation:_____
I. Abdominal and Pelvic Cavity
   1. Position of the diaphragm:_____
   2. Position of organs/fluid: _____
   3. Serosal lining: _____
   4. Omentum and spleen:_____
   5. Stomach, intestines, mesentery, mesenteric root, pancreas, lymph nodes:_____
   6. Liver, lymph nodes, bile duct, portal vein, umbilical vein:_____
   7. Abdominal aorta, vena cava:_____
   8. Kidneys, adrenal glands:_____
   9. Ureters, urinary bladder, urethra (to external orifice): _____
   10. Ovaries, salpinx/oviduct, uterus, cervix, vagina:_____
   11. Testes, epididymides, spermatic cord, accessory sex glands, penis: _____
II. Thoracic Cavity
   1. Position of organs/fluid/gas: _____
   2. Pleura, mediastinum, thymus, lymph nodes:_____
   3. Pericardial sac:_____
   4. Lungs, bronchi, pulmonary vasculature, lymph nodes:_____
   5. Heart and main vessels:_____
III. Oral Cavity and Neck
   1. Trachea, larynx:_____
   2. Thyroid gland, parathyroid glands, salivary glands, lymph nodes:_____
   3. Esophagus, pharynx, tonsils, palate, tongue, teeth, gums:_____
IV. Nasal Cavity and Sinuses:
V. Skull and Vertebral Canal:
   1. Brain:_____
   2. Spinal cord:_____
   3. Eyes:_____
   4. Ears:_____
GROSS DIAGNOSES: _____

Figure 31-8 Recording of necropsy findings.

anatomic subunits like the kidney, adrenal gland, or testis, it is important to obtain a sample that includes all components (in the case of the kidney, these are cortex, medulla, and pelvis). Collection of multiple samples is also recommended for multilobar organs like the liver and lungs. In the case of paired organs, a sample from each side is helpful. Hollow organs like the stomach, intestines, and urinary bladder are opened up to expose the mucosa to the fixative. Hollow organs with a diameter of less than 3 mm, like the intestines of neonatal patients or ureters, can be gently filled with

Clearly label all containers with owner name and animal ID

1. **Formalin-fixed tissues for Histopathology** (ideal tissue to formalin ratio = 1:10) *Avoid freezing to prevent artifacts that will severely interfere with histopathologic evaluation*

☐ Lung (multiple samples)   ☐ Colon   ☐ Brain

☐ Liver (multiple samples)   ☐ Thyroid gland   ☐ Pancreas

☐ Heart (multiple samples)   ☐ Adrenal gland   ☐ Lymph node

☐ Kidney (cortex + medulla incl. papilla)   ☐ Spleen   ☐ Bone marrow

☐ Stomach (antrum and pylorus)   ☐ Thymus   ☐ *

☐ Small intestine (duodenum, jejunum, ileum)   ☐ *

* Any other tissues that might be relevant or of interest.

2. **Fresh (chilled unfixed) tissues for Microbiology**

Collect all samples into **INDIVIDUAL** sealable containers to avoid contamination unless stated otherwise and specify contents on container

Example A: **Respiratory disease**

Tissue/Sample	Test	Instructions
Lung	Bacteriology	
Swab (nasal, conjunctival, tracheal)	Virology (FA/VI/PCR)	Transport medium

Example B: **Diarrhea**

Tissue/Sample	Test	Instructions
Small intestine	Bacteriology	
Colon		
Liver		
Kidney		
Lung		
Ileum (mucosal scraping)	Virology (EM)	Collect in plastic vial
Intestinal contents/feces	Parasitology	Collect in vial; avoid freezing

Example C: **Systemic disease**—suspect infectious process (like canine herpesvirus 1)

Tissue/Sample	Test	Instructions
Liver	Bacteriology	
Intestine		
Lung	Bacteriology	
Kidney	Virology	
Serum (0.5 ml)	Serology (FIP, FeLV, FIV)	Red top vacutainer tube
*	#	Depends on requested test: contact laboratory/pathologist

* Any other tissue/sample that might be relevant; # e.g., mycology, parasitology

For toxicology collect fresh (unfixed) liver, kidney, stomach contents, and adipose tissue

All samples need to be collected into leak-proof containers or sealable plastic bags, double bagged, and shipped according to regulations (DOT and carrier service).

Figure 31-9 Necropsy sampling checklist.

formalin using a syringe and needle and left unopened. The nervous system and special senses should be fixed intact. After enucleation, it is best to gently inject formalin into the posterior chamber of the globe to speed up fixation. Bone marrow cores may be fixed in formalin for histopathology and/or rolled out on glass slides and air dried for cytology. Wrapping of samples smaller than 5 mm in diameter in a paper towel reduces the risk of loss during processing. Identification of individual samples can be accomplished by submission in separate, labeled containers or wrapped in a paper towel clearly labeled with pencil, roller ball, or permanent marker and added to the remaining fixed samples.

Packaging and Shipping

Shipping regulations have become increasingly strict and have to be carefully observed. Please check shipping guidelines put forth by the Federal Department of Transportation (DOT) and specific carrier services. Many diagnostic laboratories have websites with helpful information on this topic.

Disposal of Remains

Whether a necropsy is performed, the remains need to be disposed of safely. Release of remains to the owner is not ideal, especially when pets are large or an infectious disease process is suspected. Should there be any potential for a zoonosis release of the remains should be avoided at all cost. Cremation with return of ashes to the owner is popular and generally available both in practice and through diagnostic laboratories. Double bagging with the appropriate strength of tightly closed bags or holding of the carcass in a large leak-proof plastic box with lid in a secured area until pickup is recommended. Ideally, hazardous waste bags are used.

CONCLUSION

Postmortem examinations provide essential information for preventative strategies and should be pursued aggressively. Submission of the whole animal accompanied by a detailed history to a diagnostic laboratory for complete postmortem examination is ideal. If timely transport to a diagnostic laboratory is not feasible, necropsy in the practice is recommended. A thorough gross examination, collection of a complete set of samples, and effective communication of findings are imperative for this approach to be successful. It is in the best interest of the practitioner to maximize the client's benefits. Successful postmortem examinations can only be achieved through proper gross examination, sampling, and close communication with the diagnostic laboratory.

SUGGESTED READINGS

Cave TA et al: Kitten mortality in the United Kingdom: a retrospective analysis of 274 histopathologic examinations (1986-2000), *Vet Rec* 151:496, 2002.

Johnston SD, Raksil S: Fetal loss in the dog and cat, *Vet Clin North Am Small Anim Pract* 17:535, 1987.

King JM et al: *The necropsy book*, ed 4, Gurnee, IL, 2006, Charles Louis Davis, DVM Foundation Publisher.

Lawler DF, Monti KL: Morbidity and mortality in neonatal kittens, *Am J Vet Res* 45:1455, 1984.

McGavin MD, Zachary JF (eds): *Pathologic basis of veterinary disease*, ed 4, St Louis, 2007, Mosby/Elsevier.

Nielen ALJ et al: Investigation of mortality and pathological changes in a 14-month birth cohort of boxer puppies, *Vet Rec* 142:602, 1998.

THE CARDIOVASCULAR SYSTEM

CHAPTER 32

Barret J. Bulmer

Despite decades of advances in cardiac ultrasound and ready access to veterinary cardiologists across the country, the most often used, feasible, and economic means for identifying puppies and kittens with heart disease is by physical examination.

Abnormal or arrested development of the embryologic heart or great vessels is an important cause of morbidity and mortality in young animals. Although congenital heart disease (CHD) is usually considered present at birth, these lesions are not necessarily static from conception through adulthood. Some lesions live in accord with the fetal circulation but undergo profound physiologic modification by the circulatory alterations that occur at birth.

FETAL CIRCULATION

In utero the heart feeds the systemic circulation in parallel, with crossover proximal and distal to the ventricles via the foramen ovale and ductus arteriosus (DA), respectively. Oxygen-rich blood from the ductus venosus and left hepatic vein is preferentially directed across the foramen ovale into the left ventricle.

At birth and through the early neonatal period, circulatory changes occur that transform the circulation into two separate circuits functioning in series. Pulmonary vascular resistance decreases as the fluid medium surrounding the pulmonary vessels is replaced by air, and the pulmonary vasculature dilates following exposure to oxygen. The placental circulation is removed, which increases systemic vascular resistance. Left ventricular systolic pressure in newborn puppies has been measured at 35 to 50 mm Hg, whereas right ventricular systolic pressure was 23 to 40 mm Hg. The decreasing pulmonary resistance and increased systemic resistance prevents right to left shunting through the DA. Increased oxygen tension and presumably prostaglandin inhibition produce muscular constriction of the ductus within the first few hours of life. Closure of the DA and

reduction in pulmonary vascular resistance increase venous return to the left heart. The increased preload increases left atrial pressure and forces the septum primum (or valve of the foramen ovale) against the septum secundum, functionally closing the foramen ovale and producing a circulatory system in series.

DEVELOPMENT OF THE CARDIOVASCULAR SYSTEM

Right ventricular myocardial mass is equal to or greater than left ventricular myocardial mass at birth, presumably because fetal right ventricular blood flow is approximately twice that of the left ventricle. However, as pulmonary vascular resistance decreases and systemic vascular resistance increases, the left ventricular mass/right ventricular mass ratio changes from 0.80 at 1 day of age to approximately 1.0 at day 3. By 3 to 7 days of age left ventricular systolic pressure rapidly increases to 75 to 90 mm Hg, and by 3 to 4 weeks it is 120 mm Hg. Right ventricular systolic pressure remains at 20 to 30 mm Hg throughout. Postnatally the heart grows rapidly, with an average increase in weight of 7.7% daily from 1 to 17 days of age, predominantly as a result of left ventricular growth.

Compared with adults, puppies and kittens have lower blood pressure, stroke volume, and peripheral vascular resistance with greater heart rate, cardiac output, plasma volume, and central venous pressure at birth. These parameters progressively approach adult values during the first 7 months of life. The autonomic innervation of the heart and vessels is also incomplete in newborn animals, providing them with little baroreflex response to changes in homeostasis. In the early neonatal period, ventricular myocytes are different ultrastructurally compared with adults and may explain the significant reduction in the length-tension relationship of neonatal cats compared with adults. This combination of factors seems clinically important wherein young animals may have a limited ability to compensate for circulatory stresses, including hyperthermia, acid-base shifts, and hemorrhage.

PREVALENCE

Congenital cardiac malformations can develop as a consequence of genetic, environmental, chromosomal, infectious, toxicologic, nutritional, or drug-related factors. Although the exact genetics behind cardiac malformations are unknown in most cases, nearly all breeding experiments have yielded positive results, suggesting the common congenital abnormalities have some degree of heritability. Numerous breed predispositions exist for CHD, most of which are identified under the specific lesion.

From 1987 to 1989 the prevalence of CHD in dogs from the Veterinary Medical Data Base at Purdue University was 0.85%. Although regional variations exist, the most common congenital malformations in dogs within the United States continue to be patent ductus arteriosus (PDA), subaortic stenosis (SAS), and pulmonic stenosis (PS). Feline CHD is less common, with a reported overall prevalence of 0.2%. Atrioventricular (AV) valve malformation and ventricular septal defects (VSDs) continue to be the most common defects in cats.

SCREENING FOR HEART DISEASE

History and Physical Examination

CHD is most often identified by auscultation of a heart murmur at the time of immunization in historically asymptomatic animals. Less commonly, puppies and kittens are presented for evaluation of clinical signs, including stunted growth, coughing or tachypnea, abdominal distention, weakness, cyanosis, or syncope that may be attributable to cardiac disease.

A well-performed physical examination begins with an observation period enabling characterization of the pet's general appearance and size, attitude, respiratory rate, and effort. The oral, conjunctival, and genital mucous membranes are inspected for evidence of cyanosis or poor capillary refill time. Cyanosis is seen when the deoxygenated hemoglobin concentration exceeds 5 g/dl and often signifies arterial hypoxemia, as seen with severe pulmonary disease or right-to-left shunting of blood (i.e., tetralogy of Fallot). Differential cyanosis, as occurs in right-to-left shunting PDA, is characterized by normal oral and conjunctival mucous membranes and cyanotic genital mucous membranes. Following examination of the mucous membranes, the jugular veins should be inspected for distention or abnormal pulsation that may accompany right heart abnormalities, like severe tricuspid insufficiency or PS. Normally the jugular veins are flaccid, collapse quickly after manual compression, and pulsations do not traverse greater than one third the height of the neck in a standing animal.

Following inspection of the head and neck, examination of the heart usually begins with localization of the cardiac impulse, or apical beat, and identification of palpable thrills or vibrations. Auscultation of the heart is initiated over the apical beat, and careful attention is given to identification of the heart sounds and the presence or absence of heart murmurs and arrhythmias. Abnormal heart sounds and murmurs are often focal and confined to the heart base or right hemithorax; therefore careful and complete auscultation of all areas of the heart is a necessity. Important considerations for successful auscultation include using a familiar and comfortable stethoscope, auscultating in a quiet environment, having a thorough understanding of the physiologic and pathologic genesis of cardiac sounds, and using a combination of practice and patience.

Heart sounds are brief auditory vibrations that can be defined by their intensity, frequency, and quality. Heart murmurs are prolonged auditory vibrations that occur as blood flows turbulently through stenotic or insufficient cardiac valves or through abnormal communications between the cardiac chambers. Murmurs may also occur subsequent to alterations in blood viscosity (i.e., anemia) or vessel diameter (the larger the vessel, the more likely blood flow is turbulent). The timing, intensity, configuration, location (defined as the point of maximal intensity), and radiation characteristics often provide valuable insight into the pathogenesis and significance of heart murmurs.

Nonpathologic Heart Murmurs

Young, often large and giant breed dogs without underlying cardiac disease may have soft, grade I to III/VI left basilar systolic murmurs. These innocent murmurs are usually midsystolic, high-frequency, and devoid of substantial radiation. Although uncertain, their origin is thought to be increased blood flow velocity and turbulence through the right or left ventricular outflow tract (LVOT). Innocent murmurs are usually nonprogressive and typically disappear in early adulthood. Similar to innocent murmurs, physiologic or functional murmurs are often grade I to III/VI midsystolic left basilar murmurs. Conditions associated with high cardiac output (i.e., fever, sepsis, high sympathetic tone) or decreased blood viscosity (i.e., anemia) may contribute to the development of an audible murmur. These murmurs generally resolve after the underlying disease process is corrected. Unfortunately not all soft murmurs are nonpathologic. Mild SAS, large nonrestrictive VSDs, and atrial septal defects (ASDs) may similarly display soft, systolic murmurs that could be confused with nonpathologic murmurs. Therefore common sense, the patient's clinical status and intended use, and the client's wishes must dictate whether diagnostics to assess the cardiac status are indicated.

Pathologic Heart Murmurs

Compared with innocent and functional murmurs, the murmurs that accompany many CHDs are louder (grade III/VI and beyond), longer in duration, and may obscure the normal heart sounds. Although murmurs of this intensity and duration are invariably indicators of underlying pathology that requires investigation, it is impossible to perfectly correlate the intensity of the murmur with the severity of the disease. Restrictive VSDs and small, restrictive left-to-right shunting PDA may produce minimal hemodynamic burden yet be accompanied by very intense murmurs. Continuous murmurs and diastolic murmurs should always be considered pathologic, no matter their intensity.

Concurrent palpation of the femoral arterial pulses during auscultation may help detect rhythm disturbances or provide useful information for distinguishing conditions with similar auscultatory findings (i.e., PS and SAS). A weak and late-to-rise femoral pulse, combined with a left basilar systolic murmur, suggests moderate to severe SAS. Bounding, or water hammer, pulses are often produced by widening of the pulse pressure subsequent to diastolic runoff in dogs with left-to-right PDA. Other conditions associated with diastolic runoff and bounding pulses include aortic insufficiency and peripheral arteriovenous fistulas.

Electrocardiography

Electrocardiographic evaluation of animals with CHD enables characterization of the cardiac rhythm and identification of conduction abnormalities and patterns of chamber enlargement. With normal right heart dominance at birth, the mean QRS vector is directed cranially, ventrally, and to the right in newborn puppies. Presumably as the left ventricular mass increases over the first 12 weeks of life, the mean electrical axis shifts leftward and caudally as is typically seen in adult dogs. Compared with age-matched normal puppies, animals with severe PS have a pathological right ventricular hypertrophy pattern at birth, and they never develop leftward deviation of the mean electrical axis. Additional cardiac lesions that may contribute to a right ventricular enlargement pattern (right axis deviation; S waves in leads I, II, III, and aV_F; increased S wave amplitude in leads I, II, CV_6LL, and CV_6LU) include tetralogy of Fallot, tricuspid valve dysplasia (TVD), ASD, large VSD, or diseases producing or accompanied by pulmonary hypertension. SAS, left-to-right shunting PDA, mitral valve dysplasia (MVD)/insufficiency, VSDs, and other conditions that result in left ventricular hypertrophy may produce increased amplitude of the R wave (leads II, III, aV_F, CV_6LL, and CV_6LU) and widening of the QRS duration with an otherwise normal mean electrical axis.

Puppies and kittens normally display sinus rhythm without respiratory variations in the heart rate. However, similar to "normalization" of the mean electrical axis over the first several weeks of life, puppies establish vagal reflexes during the first 8 weeks of life that may contribute to sinus arrhythmia, wandering pacemaker, and atropine-responsive second-degree AV block. Pathologic arrhythmias, including supraventricular and ventricular premature contractions (VPCs), often accompany CHD that is capable of producing moderate to severe atrial enlargement (i.e., AV valve dysplasia) or ventricular concentric hypertrophy with compromised myocardial perfusion (i.e., SAS). Life-threatening arrhythmias may also occur as a consequence of accessory pathways (APs) or well-studied, but as of yet unknown, substrates.

Radiography

Radiographs yield valuable insight into pulmonary vascular and parenchymal changes that may accompany CHD. Although radiographs also provide a means to assess the cardiac silhouette, interpretation of specific changes associated with CHD is often inaccurate. Detection of chamber enlargement can be plagued by overinterpretation of normal right heart predominance in young animals or shifting of the cardiac apex in diseased conditions, leading to an erroneous diagnosis. A study assessing normal 3-month-old puppies found the mean ± standard deviation vertebral heart size on a lateral radiograph was 10.0 ± 0.5 vertebral bodies. This value is similar to normal adult dogs, and it did not vary significantly as puppies matured from 3 to 36 months. Although moderate to severe cardiomegaly associated with diseases that produce volume overload is relatively easy to document via radiography, concentric hypertrophy accompanying pressure overload may be difficult to detect without ultrasound.

Assessment of the pulmonary vasculature helps with identification of over- or undercirculation and impending left heart failure. Normally only a small proportion of the pulmonary capillaries are perfused. Left-to-right shunting lesions (i.e., PDA) produce pulmonary vascular overcirculation and recruitment of additional pulmonary capillary beds. Radiographically this may be identified as engorgement of pulmonary arteries and veins with widespread hypervascularity extending to the lung periphery. Right-to-left shunting defects (i.e., tetralogy of Fallot) bypass the pulmonary circulation, yielding small pulmonary arteries and veins with a relatively radiolucent interstitium.

Echocardiography

Advances in ultrasonographic technology have nearly led to the extinction of cardiac catheterization in the routine diagnosis of CHD. Two-dimensional and motion (M) mode echocardiography enable a detailed, noninvasive assessment of cardiac anatomy, chamber dimensions, and ventricular systolic performance. Spectral and color-flow Doppler echocardiography are able to evaluate blood flow and further assess systolic and diastolic cardiac function.

The power of Doppler echocardiography lies in its ability to quickly and accurately evaluate blood flow through cardiac valves and abnormal intracardiac and extracardiac communications.

Accurate estimation of red blood velocity requires the ultrasound beam to be aligned parallel to blood flow. If beam alignment produces an angle of incidence greater than 20 degrees, the peak velocity, and hence the pressure gradient, will be underestimated. Calculation of noninvasive pressure gradients is extremely useful for assessing the severity of stenotic lesions, including SAS and PS. Similarly measurement of pressure gradients associated with pulmonic insufficiency and tricuspid regurgitation allows documentation of pulmonary hypertension. Advanced echocardiographic calculations enable determination of shunt ratios and regurgitant fractions.

CLASSIFICATION OF CONGENITAL HEART DISEASE

The descriptions in the following sections will classify conditions based on the classic location of murmurs associated with the specific congenital lesion. Although exam findings in many animals do not fit the classical descriptions, and complex lesions may further cloud recognition of disease entities, it is believed this classification may prove the most useful to veterinarians examining young dogs and cats on a daily basis.

Lesions Producing Left Basilar Murmurs

An audible systolic murmur with its point of maximal intensity (PMI) over the left heart base is most commonly produced by aortic stenosis, PS, tetralogy of Fallot, or an ASD. Low-grade innocent and physiologic murmurs also frequently display their PMI over the left heart base and will need to be differentiated from their more pathologic counterparts. Auscultation of a variable-intensity, left basilar (axillary), continuous murmur is most consistent with left-to-right shunting PDA.

Aortic Stenosis

SAS has likely replaced PDA as the most common congenital cardiac lesion in areas with a high population of large breed dogs. Although any breed of dog may be affected, evidence suggests Newfoundlands, Rottweilers, Boxers, Golden Retrievers, German Shepherd Dogs, and Bloodhounds have an increased relative risk for SAS. Valvular and supravalvular aortic stenosis are seen infrequently or rarely in dogs, and although uncommon, cats have been described with all three forms of fixed LVOT obstruction. SAS has been most thoroughly investigated in Newfoundlands, for whom breeding studies suggest an autosomal dominant mode of transmission with modifying genes or a polygenic mechanism. These same studies found that SAS may not be present at birth but instead begins to develop during the first 4 to 8 weeks of life. Because SAS lesions may progress as animals grow, it is not uncommon for the severity of the lesion and the associated murmur and cardiac changes to worsen from birth until young adulthood. Detection of mild disease is difficult; therefore ultimately genetic counseling is difficult.

The pathophysiologic consequences of aortic stenosis include left ventricular and in some instances left atrial hypertrophy, myocardial fibrosis, and aortic arch abnormalities. The hypertrophy and fibrosis produce a stiff, noncompliant left ventricle that ultimately necessitates higher atrial pressures to fill. Elevated left atrial, and hence pulmonary venous and pulmonary capillary hydrostatic, pressures may contribute to the development of pulmonary edema.

Puppies with mild to moderate SAS are often reported to be clinically normal at the time of immunization. Owners with severely affected dogs may report exercise intolerance, syncope, or a history consistent with left heart failure. In some cases sudden death occurs without premonitory signs. Auscultatory abnormalities are usually present in cases of moderate to severe SAS because the intensity and duration of the murmur tend to increase and lengthen, respectively, with more severe disease. Obstruction to blood flow through the LVOT produces an ejection, left basilar systolic murmur. The murmur tends to radiate up the carotid arteries and to the right so it can frequently be auscultated in the ventral cervical region, and in some cases the PMI is at the right heart base. Because SAS may progress through early adulthood, the murmur can increase in intensity between sequential physical examinations. Femoral pulse alterations, with palpably reduced and late rising pulse amplitudes, are often found in dogs with moderate to severe obstruction.

Although nonspecific, electrocardiographic changes that may accompany SAS include increased R wave amplitude and QRS duration consistent with left ventricular enlargement, as well as ST segment and T wave alterations suggestive of myocardial ischemia (Figure 32-1). VPCs may be evident on baseline electrocardiography (ECG), and studies of Holter examinations suggest the overall number and grade of VPCs display a modest correlation with pressure gradient. Ventricular tachycardia and ultimately fibrillation are the presumed mechanism for sudden death in dogs with SAS.

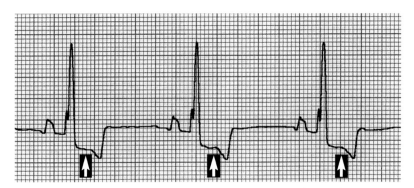

Figure 32-1 Lead II, 10 mm/mV, 50 mm/s. ST segment depression *(arrows)* >0.2 mV may suggest myocardial ischemia in dogs with concentric ventricular hypertrophy and reduced myocardial oxygen delivery.

Radiography is limited in the assessment of ventricular enlargement in dogs with SAS because it produces concentric rather than eccentric hypertrophy. Nonetheless assessment of the cardiac silhouette still proves useful in dogs with moderate to severe SAS for detection of poststenotic dilation of the aorta or left atrial enlargement.

Echocardiography provides a reliable method for identification of moderate to severe SAS. Common findings include left ventricular concentric hypertrophy, a subvalvular fibrous ring or band narrowing the LVOT, and poststenotic dilation of the aorta. Hyperechogenicity of the left ventricular endocardial surface and papillary muscles may be seen in dogs with myocardial ischemia and replacement fibrosis.

Although the exact velocity cutoff to distinguish mild, moderate, and severe SAS is uncertain, it is generally accepted that gradients more than 100 mm Hg represent severe disease with a high likelihood of complications. Currently available diagnostic methods seem incapable of identifying dogs with grade 1 lesions. Even dogs with grade 2 lesions may be difficult to accurately assess purely based on the LVOT velocities because of the likelihood of breed and examination condition variations.

Although many dogs with mild to moderate SAS live normal lifespans devoid of clinical consequences, the natural history and responses to therapy of severe SAS are disappointing. Commonly reported outcomes of dogs with severe SAS include exercise intolerance, syncope, sudden death (most commonly in the first 3 years of life), and the development of congestive heart failure and/or endocarditis. In general, dogs with mild to moderate disease do not require specific therapy and can often exercise normally. Antibiotic prophylaxis is recommended for surgical procedures in all dogs with SAS because they appear to be at increased risk for developing endocarditis; however, the effectiveness of this therapy is uncertain. Exercise restriction is prudent for dogs with moderate to severe SAS, and β-blockers (i.e., atenolol) are frequently administered in an effort to combat arrhythmogenesis, reduce myocardial oxygen demands, and limit tachycardia. Currently the survival benefit imparted by β-blockers is unknown. Additional antiarrhythmic medications may be necessary to treat VPCs, ventricular tachycardia, or atrial fibrillation if they complicate the clinical situation. Similarly standard therapy for left heart failure, including diuretics, angiotensin-converting enzyme inhibitors, and possibly positive inotropic agents, are indicated for animals that develop pulmonary edema.

Pulmonic Stenosis

Valvular PS is the most common congenital right ventricular outflow tract (RVOT) obstruction in dogs and is the third most common congenital cardiac defect encountered. PS is less commonly identified in cats, and both species have been reported to infrequently display sub- and supravalvular forms of RVOT obstruction. Breeds with an increased relative risk for PS include English Bulldogs, Terrier breeds, Miniature Schnauzers, Chihuahuas, and Samoyeds. PS has been identified as hereditary in breeding studies of Beagles with a spectrum of pulmonary valve abnormalities. Grade 1 lesions display mild leaflet thickening with commissural fusion producing a central orifice. More severe cases of PS tend to be grade 2 lesions with moderate to severe thickening of the valve leaflets with fusion or hypoplasia producing RVOT obstruction. Fibrous thickening at the base of the valve may accompany valvular dysplasia. Boxers and Bulldogs have been identified with coronary arterial abnormalities that contribute to a unique form of subvalvular PS that is difficult to address surgically.

Physical examination of animals with PS often reveals a variable-intensity, left basilar, systolic, ejection murmur in a reportedly healthy puppy. Compared with murmurs of SAS, PS murmurs do not radiate as extensively to the right cranial thorax or up the carotid arteries. The femoral arterial pulse is usually normal. Jugular distention or abnormal pulsation should increase suspicion of right heart failure or concurrent cardiac defects (i.e., TVD). Many dogs with PS are reportedly asymptomatic during the first year of life when the murmur is initially detected. However, clinical signs, including exercise intolerance, syncope, and signs consistent with right heart failure often complicate severe cases of PS and have been reported in 34% to 83% of dogs evaluated.

In cases of moderate to severe PS, the ECG almost always displays criteria for right ventricular enlargement (Figure 32-2). The P waves are usually normal. Ventricular arrhythmias appear to be less common than in dogs with SAS.

Radiography usually reveals moderate cardiomegaly with a right heart enlargement pattern (Figure 32-3). Poststenotic dilation of the main pulmonary artery produces loss of the cranial cardiac silhouette on the lateral view and dilation at approximately the 2 o'clock position on the dorsoventral (DV) view.

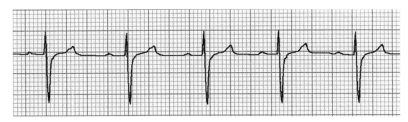

Figure 32-2 Lead II, 5 mm/mV, 50 mm/s. Deep S waves frequently accompany dogs with moderate to severe pulmonic stenosis.

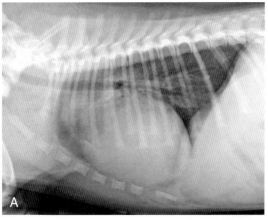

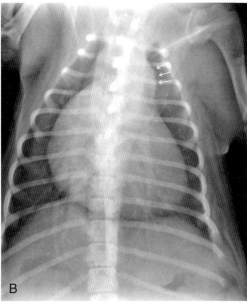

Figure 32-3 Lateral **(A)** and dorsoventral **(B)** radiographs from a dog with severe pulmonic stenosis. The lateral radiograph displays increased sternal contact with lifting of the apex off the sternum and loss of the cranial cardiac silhouette. Right heart enlargement and dilation of the main pulmonary artery *(arrows)* are evident on the dorsoventral view.

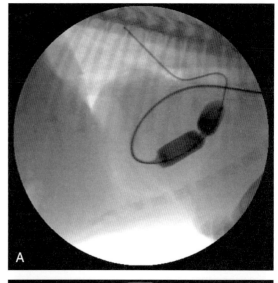

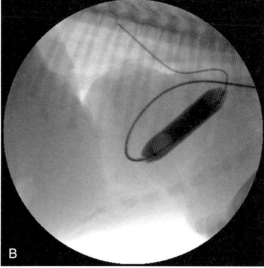

Figure 32-4 Fluoroscopic images obtained during balloon valvuloplasty of pulmonic stenosis. A guidewire is directed through the cranial vena cava, right atrium, and right ventricle into the pulmonary artery. Afterward a balloon dilation catheter is fed across the guidewire and is quickly inflated **(A)** until the stenotic lesion is stretched or torn when the balloon is fully inflated **(B)**.

Echocardiography provides a method for definitive diagnosis and assessment of severity of PS, as well as identification of concurrent cardiac defects. Of the four cardiac valves, the pulmonary valve morphology tends to be the most difficult to clearly assess via transthoracic echocardiography. Therefore in some instances it is challenging to distinguish valvular PS from discrete subvalvular obstruction. Mild PS is usually categorized as a pressure gradient less than 50 mm Hg, whereas the cutoff for severe disease varies with peak gradients described more than 80 or 100 mm Hg. Contrast echocardiography may identify right-to-left shunting at the atrial level as RV diastolic dysfunction, and tricuspid insufficiency contributes to right atrial hypertension.

Although precise criteria for establishing a prognosis for dogs and cats with PS are lacking, it is generally accepted that dogs with uncomplicated mild to moderate PS often

live normal, comfortable lives and do not require specific therapy. Serial echocardiographic examinations should be performed to determine whether the stenosis, right ventricular hypertrophy, tricuspid insufficiency, or right atrial dilation progresses. In animals with severe PS, clinical experience suggests they are more likely to develop exercise intolerance, right heart failure, or die suddenly. Surgical intervention is generally recommended even in asymptomatic dogs with severe PS.

Several techniques have been described and are available for the treatment of PS. Valvular PS with a normally developed pulmonary annulus is most often treated by percutaneous balloon valvuloplasty (Figure 32-4). The goals of intervention include improving survival and resolving clinical signs in symptomatic animals. Surgical success, defined as a reduction of the pressure gradient into the mild category, or in markedly severe cases as a reduction in the pressure gradient of more than 50%, is achievable in up to 80% of dogs. Valvuloplasty has been reported to reduce clinical signs and mortality compared with animals not undergoing surgery.

Tetralogy of Fallot

Tetralogy of Fallot is an uncommon congenital lesion recognized in both dogs and cats. Keeshonds, English Bulldogs, Wire-haired Fox Terriers, and West Highland White Terriers are reportedly overrepresented. Anatomic features of tetralogy of Fallot include RVOT obstruction (i.e., PS), a subaortic VSD, and an overriding or dextropositioned aorta. Right ventricular hypertrophy, constituting the fourth component of tetralogy of Fallot, develops as a compensatory response to the outflow tract obstruction. Extensive pathologic and genetic studies have been accomplished in a Keeshond colony with hereditary conotruncal defects.

The anatomical features of tetralogy of Fallot result in right-to-left shunting of blood, hypoxemia, and decreased hemoglobin oxygen saturation. Increased right ventricular systolic pressure, generated as a consequence of PS, shunts desaturated blood across the VSD and into the lower pressure systemic arterial tree. The magnitude of right-to-left shunting is dynamic and depends on the relative resistances of the pulmonary and systemic circulations. In the case of tetralogy of Fallot, the resistance to right ventricular ejection into the pulmonary circulation is relatively fixed by PS.

The clinical course of tetralogy of Fallot often depends on the severity of the RVOT obstruction. Dogs and cats with relatively balanced pulmonary and systemic arterial resistances are often considered asymptomatic at rest and may live for years. Animals with more severe RVOT obstruction often present for failure to grow, shortness of breath, exertional fatigue, weakness, syncope, or uncommonly right heart failure. Sudden death before 1 year of age is common from hypoxia, hyperviscosity, or cardiac arrhythmias. The most common cardiac auscultatory finding in animals with tetralogy of Fallot is a left basilar, systolic ejection murmur produced by blood flow through the stenotic pulmonary valve.

ECG alterations may include criteria for right ventricular enlargement and ST segment abnormalities in animals with myocardial hypoxia. Cats with tetralogy of Fallot have also been reported with left or cranial mean electrical axis deviation.

Typical radiographic findings in patients with tetralogy of Fallot include a normal-sized heart, rounding of the right ventricular border, pulmonary vascular undercirculation, and hyperlucency of the lung field. The heart in humans with tetralogy of Fallot often displays a distinctive boot-shaped, or *coeur en sabot*, appearance on the DV view.

Common echocardiographic findings in animals with tetralogy of Fallot consist of right ventricular concentric hypertrophy, RVOT obstruction (ranging from PS to pulmonary atresia), small left atrial and left ventricular internal dimensions with pseudohypertrophy of the ventricular walls, a high subaortic VSD, and a variably dextropositioned aorta.

Treatment options for tetralogy of Fallot include both surgical and medical approaches. Open surgical repair of tetralogy of Fallot in two dogs using cardiopulmonary bypass resolved cyanosis and restored normal activity levels and exercise tolerance. Before advances in cardiopulmonary bypass in neonates, palliative creation of a left-to-right shunt distal to the cyanotic defect was commonly performed as a bridge to definitive repair. A systemic-to-pulmonary shunt increases pulmonary perfusion and left heart filling and provides a greater contribution of oxygenated blood to the systemic circulation. The limited availability and expense of cardiac bypass have led to the use of several of these techniques for palliation in dogs and cats with tetralogy of Fallot. Although its efficacy is uncertain in dogs and cats, propranolol may provide symptomatic benefit by increasing peripheral vascular resistance (hence decreasing the right-to-left shunt), decreasing myocardial contractility, preventing tachycardia, and favorably shifting the hemoglobin-oxygen dissociation curve. Steps to target polycythemia in dogs with right-to-left shunting lesions and hyperviscosity syndrome include periodic phlebotomy or administration of myelosuppressive agents. Agents with substantial arterial vasodilating properties should be avoided.

Atrial Septal Defect

An ASD is an uncommonly recognized abnormal communication between the right atrium and left atrium. ASDs, alone or in combination with other congenital lesions, accounted for up to 4.1% of defects in relatively large studies of dogs with CHD. One report found ASDs (including common AV canal) were more common in cats and accounted for approximately 8% of CHD in 287 animals. Boxers, Newfoundlands, Doberman Pinschers, and Samoyeds are reportedly overrepresented with ASDs, and familial patterns have been suggested in a family of Boxer dogs and standard Poodles. Embryologic development of the atrial septum begins with extension of the septum primum from the dorsal atrial wall toward the AV cushions, forming the ostium primum. Fusion of the septum primum with the cushions occludes the ostium primum. Simultaneously, coalescing perforations develop in the dorsal portion of the septum primum, forming the ostium secundum. The septum secundum then arises from the dorsal atrial wall to the right of the septum primum, descends down, and fuses with the AV cushions. An opening, termed the foramen ovale, persists in the septum secundum, although it is normally covered by the septum primum/valve of the foramen ovale. Maldevelopment of the atrial septum can contribute to (1) ostium primum defects (patency of the lower atrial septum due to incomplete fusion of the septum primum and AV cushions), (2) ostium secundum defects (patency located within the fossa ovalis caudal to the intervenous tubercle due to shortening of the valve of the foramen ovale, excessive resorption of the septum primum, or deficient growth of the septum secundum), and (3) sinus venosus defects (patency located high in the atrial septum dorsocranial to the fossa ovalis due to faulty resorption of the sinus venosus). Large ostium primum ASDs can contribute to a more complex and variable lesion, termed atrioventricular septal defect, endocardial cushion defect, or common AV canal. Complete endocardial cushion defects develop when the AV canal never partitions. Consequently all four cardiac chambers share communication through (1) an ostium primum ASD, (2) a high ventricular septal defect, and (3) dysplastic, often cleft and bridging AV valves. Patency of the foramen ovale is not a true ASD in that the structures comprising the atrial septum are formed normally but persistent elevation of right atrial pressure prevents fusion of its valve with the limbus of the fossa ovalis.

The direction and amount of flow across an ASD is dependent on the instantaneous pressure difference between the atrial chambers and the size of the defect. In general, ASDs have predominately left-to-right flow; therefore the pulmonary circulation is overcirculated, and although venous return to the left atrium is increased, the chamber is usually normal size because the blood is shunted immediately to the right heart. The right-sided volume overload and pulmonary overcirculation may contribute to right, left, or biventricular heart failure.

Dogs and cats with small ASDs are often devoid of clinical signs and live normal-length, high quality lives. Even animals with large ASDs may tolerate the lesion for years without developing signs of congestive heart failure. Because ASDs often accompany other forms of CHD, the clinical signs may be reflective of the predominant underlying pathology. The low pressure gradient and flow velocity across uncomplicated ASDs usually do not produce an audible murmur. However, the shunted blood increases the volume of flow across an otherwise normal pulmonary valve and may produce a soft left basilar, systolic murmur. This murmur of "relative" PS can be easily confused with an innocent or physiologic murmur.

Diagnosis of an ASD often requires an astute awareness of the disease and subtle physical examination findings because many dogs remain asymptomatic for long periods. ECG findings in animals with hemodynamically important ASDs usually include right ventricular enlargement. Thoracic radiography reveals right heart and main pulmonary arterial enlargement with pulmonary vascular overcirculation proportional to the severity of the left-to-right shunt. In animals with uncomplicated ASDs, the left atrium is normal to mildly enlarged. ASDs are usually suspected echocardiographically based on the nonspecific changes they produce within the right heart, including right atrial enlargement, right ventricular eccentric hypertrophy, and diastolic interventricular septal flattening associated with severe volume overload. Two-dimensional echocardiography may directly visualize ASDs as a discontinuity or focal dropout in the normal interatrial septum. However, caution should be used in assessing this area because of common false-positive results caused by beam orientation with the atrial septum and some normal dropout in the area of the foramen ovale.

Traditionally repair of ASDs has been limited because of the need for cardiac bypass. Patients that developed clinical signs without access to cardiopulmonary bypass would be treated with standard therapy for heart failure. In recent years, advancements of transcatheter interventional procedures in children have yielded devices suitable for the noninvasive closure of some ostium secundum defects in dogs. Implantation of these self-expanding devices can be performed through jugular or femoral vein access without cardiopulmonary bypass.

Patent Ductus Arteriosus

As described in the section on fetal circulation, the ductus arteriosus (DA) is a normal fetal structure that diverts blood from the pulmonary artery to the descending aorta, away from the collapsed fetal lung. The increase in oxygen tension and inhibition of prostaglandins following parturition stimulate ductal smooth muscle contraction and a dramatic reduction in flow within the first hours of life. Anatomic obliteration of the DA via noninflammatory muscle degeneration begins within 48 hours and is complete within 1 month, leaving remnant adventitial elastic fibers (i.e., ligamentum arteriosum). Abnormal tissue architecture of the DA can lead to residual patency and in most instances left-to-right shunting of blood as aortic pressure increases above pulmonary arterial pressure. PDA is usually reported as the first or second most common congenital lesion in dogs and represents approximately 11% of feline congenital cardiac defects. It appears variations in the genetic pool and breed distribution of dogs in other countries may make PDA less common. Although PDA can be seen in any dog breed, Chihuahuas, Collies, Maltese, toy and miniature Poodles, Pomeranians, English Springer Spaniels, Keeshonds, Bichon Frise, Cavalier King Charles Spaniels, and Shetland Sheepdogs have reportedly been overrepresented. Large breed dogs, including German Shepherd Dogs, Newfoundlands, and Labrador Retrievers, may display regional predisposition to PDA. Female dogs have a higher prevalence of PDA.

The pathophysiologic consequences of PDA depend on the size of the ductus (or more specifically the minimal ductal diameter) (Figure 32-5), the pulmonary vascular resistance, and the adaptive response of the left ventricle to volume overload. Volume overload produces eccentric left ventricular hypertrophy, increases in left ventricular end diastolic (and hence left atrial) pressure, and often contributes to left heart failure and death within 1 year of age if not corrected. The increased left ventricular stroke volume increases systolic aortic pressure, whereas runoff from the systemic to the pulmonary circulation decreases diastolic aortic pressure. The widened pulse pressure creates a hyperkinetic, or water hammer, arterial pulse.

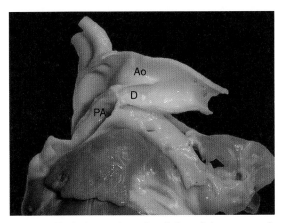

Figure 32-5 Pathology of canine left-to-right patent ductus arteriosus (PDA). In many cases the ductus *(D)* is conical and tapers from its aortic *(Ao)* to pulmonary arterial *(PA)* insertion. The smallest diameter of the PDA and the relative systemic and pulmonary vascular resistances determine the severity and direction of the shunt.

Many dogs and cats are asymptomatic at first examination when a heart murmur is auscultated. Some animals may be small or thin compared with littermates or exhibit signs of left heart failure. Careful physical examination with auscultation of a continuous murmur at the dorsocranial left heart base is nearly pathognomonic for a left-to-right PDA. Auscultation of the left apex (i.e., mitral valve area) in animals with a PDA can usually still detect a murmur, albeit systolic rather than continuous. In animals with left-to-right shunting PDA, the mucous membranes are usually pink because there is no admixture of unoxygenated blood with the systemic circulation. Dogs and cats with documented continuous murmurs should undergo diagnostic testing quickly; there is no reason to wait for the patient to grow larger, and continuous murmurs will not be innocent or functional. Patients may develop left heart failure or in rare instances pulmonary hypertension and right-to-left shunting if a wait-and-reevaluate approach is taken prior to referral.

Criteria for left ventricular enlargement (increased R wave amplitude and QRS duration) are commonly identified by ECG in animals with PDA. Left atrial enlargement may produce widened P waves, and some animals with long-standing volume overload and left atrial enlargement will have supraventricular arrhythmias (i.e., atrial premature complexes or atrial fibrillation).

Radiographic changes associated with left-to-right shunting PDA include left atrial and ventricular enlargement with pulmonary vascular overcirculation on the lateral and DV views (Figure 32-6). A straight DV or ventrodorsal (VD) view usually enables identification of a bulge, or "ductus bump," on the left side of the aortic border, just caudal to the aortic arch and origin of the ductus. The most consistent radiographic features in dogs with PDA include an enlarged cardiac silhouette with aortic and pulmonary arterial aneurysmal dilation. Cats with PDA may

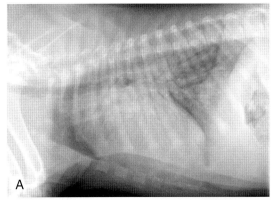

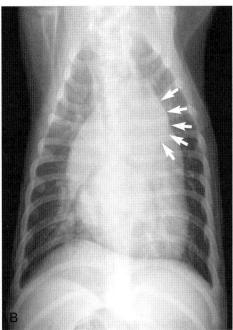

Figure 32-6 Lateral **(A)** and ventrodorsal **(B)** radiographic views from a dog with a large, left-to-right shunting patent ductus arteriosus. The radiographs reveal left ventricular and left atrial enlargement with loss of the cranial cardiac silhouette and a "ductus bump" *(arrows)* on the ventrodorsal view. The pulmonary arteries and veins are overcirculated, and the right caudal lung lobe displays evidence of early congestive heart failure.

have the left apex of the heart displaced into the right hemithorax.

Two-dimensional echocardiography is useful to document the severity of left atrial and left ventricular enlargement, evaluate systolic function, and rule out concurrent congenital cardiac lesions. The PDA can often be visualized from the left cranial parasternal view and may yield valuable insight into the minimal ductal diameter and morphology of the PDA. Spectral and color-flow Doppler reveal continuous, often high-velocity retrograde flow into the pulmonary artery in cases of left-to-right PDA.

Surgical or catheter-based closure is recommended in nearly all young dogs and cats with a left-to-right shunting PDA because early mortality (64% within 1 year of

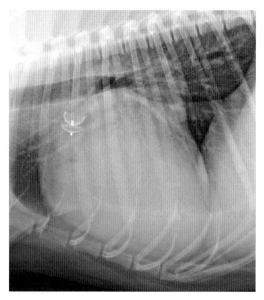

Figure 32-7 A specifically designed canine ductal occluder is now available for transarterial occlusion of left-to-right shunting patent ductus arteriosus.

diagnosis) is very high. Survival time is significantly longer in dogs that undergo PDA closure compared with animals without surgery. The best timing for closure of a PDA is uncertain, but in general it is advisable to close the defect at an early age, usually between 8 and 16 weeks, immediately following diagnosis. Surgical ligation of a left-to-right PDA is usually considered curative, with 1- and 2-year survival rates of 92% and 87%, respectively. A trend for less-invasive closure in humans has led to numerous transvascular techniques for occlusion of PDA in dogs. In a large retrospective study of transarterial coil occlusion, successful coil implantation was achieved in 108 of 125 dogs (86%). Hemodynamic success was maintained during long-term follow-up evaluation, and echocardiographic measurements were similar for dogs with complete ductal closure and all grades of residual ductal flow. The initial success rate was significantly higher with surgical ligation (94% vs. 84%), and there was no significant difference in mortality (5.6% vs. 2.6%) between surgical ligation and transarterial coil occlusion. The recent development of a commercially available, specifically designed Amplatz canine ductal occluder may provide similar or better success rates than coil occlusion (Figure 32-7). Although less common, transarterial PDA occlusion with coils has also been reported in cats.

Right-to-Left Shunting Patent Ductus Arteriosus

In a small percentage of cases the DA is almost completely devoid of smooth muscle, and nearly complete failure of sphincteric contraction produces a nonrestrictive PDA. The aortic and pulmonary arterial pressures are approximately equal at systemic levels; right ventricular afterload is high, and concentric hypertrophy develops; the forward pulmonary flow is reduced, and the left heart is underperfused. Poorly oxygenated blood is shunted into the descending

aorta producing differential (i.e., oxygenated cranial, cyanotic caudal) cyanosis and secondary polycythemia/hyperviscosity.

Animals with right-to-left shunting (or so-called reversed) PDA may present for vague signs of exertional fatigue, hindlimb weakness, shortness of breath, or observed differential cyanosis. Heart failure is an uncommon presentation. Hindlimb weakness may be exacerbated by exercise, as systemic arterial resistance decreases in response to exercise-induced vasodilation, and incorrectly assumed secondary to musculoskeletal or neurologic disease. Cardiac auscultation usually identifies no murmur or only a very soft, systolic left basilar murmur. The most common auscultatory abnormality is an accentuated and split S_2 associated with pulmonary hypertension. Differential cyanosis (pink oral mucous membranes and cyanotic caudal mucous membranes) may be identified at rest or more commonly following exercise.

An ECG almost invariably displays a right ventricular enlargement pattern, and thoracic radiographs reveal right ventricular enlargement, dilation of the main pulmonary artery, and a ductus bump. Echocardiography may identify right ventricular concentric hypertrophy, small left atrial and ventricular dimensions, an enlarged pulmonary artery, and in some instances a PDA with a widely open pulmonic ostium.

Although they are often profoundly exercise intolerant, many dogs with reversed PDA can live for years. Treatment generally consists of enforced rest and limitation of exercise, avoidance of stress, and steps to manage polycythemia and hyperviscosity. Ligation or embolization of a right-to-left PDA is generally contraindicated because removal of the "low" pressure systemic circulation usually leads to late operative or early postoperative acute right heart failure and death.

Lesions Producing Left Apical Murmurs: Mitral Valve Dysplasia

Malformations of the mitral valve complex, hereafter referred to as mitral valve dysplasia (MVD), are a common form of CHD in both dogs and cats. Animals that appear to be overrepresented include cats of all breeds, Great Danes, German Shepherd Dogs, Bull Terriers, Golden Retrievers, Newfoundlands, Dalmatians, and Mastiffs. AV valve malformations may now have surpassed VSDs as the most common congenital cardiac lesion in cats.

The pathophysiologic consequences of MVD depend on whether the principal functional abnormality is systolic regurgitation of blood through an insufficient valve, impaired left ventricular filling through a stenotic valve, or obstruction to left ventricular ejection secondary to systolic anterior motion of the mitral valve.

Similar to many forms of CHD, dogs and cats with MVD are often reportedly asymptomatic at the time of diagnosis. Animals with severe or long-standing disease may have a history of coughing, tachypnea, exercise intolerance, and syncope associated with left heart failure and/or fixed cardiac output. Animals with mitral stenosis may have right heart failure as a consequence of pulmonary hypertension, and on rare occasions animals may die suddenly without premonitory clinical signs. The wide range of valve malformations and functional consequences of MVD produce a variety of abnormal physical examination findings. The most common auscultatory abnormality is a left apical, systolic murmur of mitral valve insufficiency. Gallop sounds (i.e., S₃ or S₄), arrhythmias, and on very rare occasions an opening snap may also be identified during auscultation.

ECG alterations associated with MVD include increased R wave amplitude and prolonged QRS duration suggestive of left ventricular enlargement and a prolonged or widened P wave produced by left atrial enlargement. A right ventricular enlargement pattern may be seen with mitral stenosis and pulmonary hypertension. ST segment and T wave alterations may be seen in animals with myocardial hypoxia secondary to severe left ventricular concentric hypertrophy or pulmonary hypertension. Supraventricular arrhythmias (i.e., atrial premature complexes or atrial fibrillation) are most common with MVD, although VPCs also occur.

Thoracic radiography is useful in the assessment of dogs and cats with MVD and valvular insufficiency to detect heart enlargement and congestive heart failure. Left atrial and ventricular enlargement patterns are common in animals with significant valvular insufficiency and volume overload. The most consistent radiographic finding in patients with mitral valve stenosis is left atrial enlargement.

Echocardiography allows experienced ultrasonographers to noninvasively ascertain the morphologic features of MVD, the principal form (or forms) of valvular dysfunction, the myocardial response to the malfunctioning valve, and the presence or absence of concurrent cardiac anomalies (Figure 32-8).

Clinical experience suggests the overall prognosis depends on the severity and functional consequences of valvular dysfunction and, when required, the response to medical therapy. Animals with mild to moderate MVD often live asymptomatically for prolonged periods without treatment. Periodic follow-up evaluation is indicated to evaluate for the development of arrhythmias, congestive heart failure, and progression of disease. New-onset heart failure has been reported in animals as young as 6 months and as old as 8 years. Therapeutic options for animals with heart failure secondary to MVD include diuretics, angiotensin-converting enzyme inhibitors, and often positive inotropic agents. Arrhythmias may also need to be appropriately addressed. The prognosis following the development of congestive heart failure appears similar to that of dogs with heart failure secondary to acquired degenerative valve disease. Surgical repair or replacement of the mitral valve has also been reported to palliate or resolve clinical signs in dogs with MVD.

Lesions Producing Right-Sided Murmurs
Ventricular Septal Defect

VSDs are caused by malformation of any component of the ventricular septum and allow free communication between the left and right ventricles. VSDs, alone or combined with complex congenital defects, are relatively common in the dog and cat, accounting for 9.8% and 15% of CHD, respectively. Studies suggest Lakeland Terriers, West Highland White Terriers, English Springer Spaniels, Basset Hounds, English Bulldogs, and Keeshonds are at increased risk for VSDs. Most VSDs in dogs and cats are perimembranous, located dorsally in the ventricular septum including a portion of the membranous septum. Viewed from the left ventricle, perimembranous VSDs are located in the LVOT beneath the aortic valve (Figure 32-9). From the right ventricle, perimembranous VSDs are located beneath the septal leaflet of the tricuspid valve or just below the valve on the inlet septum.

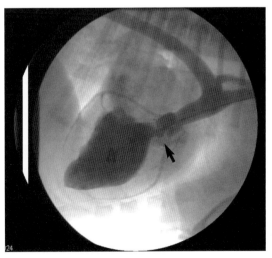

Figure 32-9 Left ventricular angiocardiogram from a dog with a small left-to-right shunting ventricular septal defect. Notice the origin of the shunt *(arrow)* just below the aortic valve. This patient had concurrent severe subaortic stenosis and mild mitral insufficiency accounting for the primary angiocardiographic alterations.

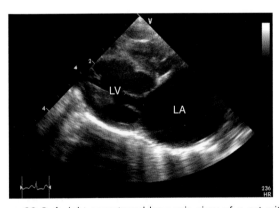

Figure 32-8 A right parasternal long-axis view of a cat with a stenotic and severely insufficient mitral valve. The left atrium *(LA)* is severely dilated, and the left ventricle *(LV)* has undergone eccentric hypertrophy secondary to the valvular insufficiency.

In some cases, the location of these VSDs causes prolapse of the right coronary cusp or the entire aortic root into the defect and may shift the important hemodynamic consequences from shunting through the VSD to severe aortic insufficiency. Defects of the larger muscular septum are uncommon in dogs and cats. In dogs and cats with small- to moderate-sized VSDs with normal pulmonary valve function, pulmonary arterial pressures are normal, and the amount of shunted blood depends on the size and restrictive nature of the defect.

Dogs and cats with small VSDs are usually asymptomatic at diagnosis. The most common auscultatory finding in animals with a small, restrictive left-to-right shunting VSD is a loud, high-frequency, systolic, plateau-shaped murmur with the point of maximal intensity at the right cranial thorax. Femoral arterial pulses are usually normal. Patients with larger VSDs often have softer, right-sided, systolic murmurs, whereas patients with balanced VSDs, because of marked pulmonary hypertension, lack audible murmurs and have a split S_2. Animals with aortic insufficiency caused by aortic root collapse may have a diastolic left basilar murmur with bounding femoral arterial pulses.

ECG findings are usually nonspecific and include left atrial and left ventricular enlargement. Right ventricular enlargement patterns are observed less commonly and often indicate a large defect with equilibration of ventricular pressures, concurrent PS, or pulmonary hypertension.

Radiographic changes will depend on the severity of the volume overload but often include left ventricular and left atrial enlargement patterns with pulmonary vascular overcirculation. The main pulmonary artery is often dilated, and, depending on the size of the lesion and resistance to right ventricular ejection, there may be variable right-sided enlargement.

Two-dimensional and Doppler echocardiography can successfully delineate the VSD in most cases and provide important information regarding the presence or absence of pulmonary hypertension and the significance of left-sided volume overload (Figure 32-10). Doppler interrogation of the aortic valve can confirm incompetence. Echocardiographic findings generally favorable for long-term survival are reportedly (1) maximal defect diameter less than 40% that of the aorta, (2) maximal left-to-right shunting velocity of at least 4.5 m/s, (3) estimated right ventricular systolic pressure less than 45 mm Hg, and (4) absence of significant aortic insufficiency.

The prognosis for animals with small, restrictive left-to-right shunting VSDs is often good for long-term survival. Other potential outcomes often depend on the size of the defect and presence of related complicating factors and may include development of heart failure, partial or complete closure of the VSD, progressive LV volume overload from aortic insufficiency, development of progressive subpulmonic and infundibular outflow obstruction, development of pulmonary hypertension secondary to pulmonary vascular disease, and reversal of shunt with the development of arterial hypoxemia and cyanosis.

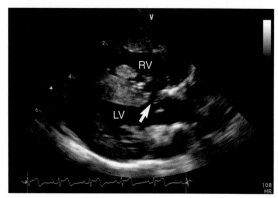

Figure 32-10 Right parasternal long-axis view from a dog with a small perimembranous ventricular septal defect *(arrow)* allowing communication between the right ventricle *(RV)* and left ventricle *(LV)*. The direction and severity of the shunt depend on the size of the lesion and the relative resistance to right and left ventricular ejection. In this case the patient had concurrent pulmonic stenosis with limited left-to-right, or right-to-left, shunting at the ventricular level.

There are several options for management of patients with large left-to-right shunting defects and impending heart failure. Institution of traditional therapy for heart failure, including diuretics, angiotensin-converting enzyme inhibitors, and positive inotropes, may provide symptomatic benefit in animals with heart failure. Furthermore, administration of afterload-reducing agents may reduce the systolic left ventricular pressure and hence the severity of left-to-right shunting. Palliative pulmonary artery banding has been reported to reduce the pressure gradient and flow across the VSD, and definitive surgical correction with cardiopulmonary bypass or catheter-based techniques has been reported.

Tricuspid Valve Dysplasia

Malformation of the tricuspid valve has similar hemodynamic consequences, albeit on the right heart, to MVD. A valve that is primarily insufficient produces right atrial and ventricular volume overload, whereas a stenotic valve impairs right ventricular filling leading to secondarily increased right atrial pressures and dilation. TVD is a relatively common congenital cardiac defect in dogs and cats and has been identified as heritable in Labrador Retrievers. Great Danes, German Shepherd Dogs, Old English Sheepdogs, Great Pyrenees, Borzois, Irish Setters, Boxers, Newfoundlands, Weimaraners, and Shih Tzus are also reported at risk. Many puppies and kittens with TVD, no matter the severity, are reportedly clinically normal at first examination.

Physical examination may identify a variably intense systolic murmur of tricuspid insufficiency at the third to fifth intercostal spaces near the costochondral junction on the right hemithorax with or without a palpable thrill. Some animals with severe TVD, right atrial hypertension, and a large regurgitant orifice will have soft to nearly inaudible murmurs. In these cases it is not uncommon to make a diagnosis of congenital TVD later in life after the animal has developed heart failure. In general the severity of the murmur does not correlate well with the significance of the lesion.

Common ECG abnormalities include prolongation and increased amplitude of the P waves with a right ventricular enlargement pattern, principally in the precordial leads in dogs. Supraventricular arrhythmias may develop as a consequence of severe right atrial enlargement, and dogs and cats with TVD frequently display splintering of the QRS complex. Some Labrador Retrievers with TVD concurrently display ventricular preexcitation (VPE; see Congenital Rhythm Disorders in this section) secondary to an AP.

In severe cases of tricuspid insufficiency, thoracic radiographs reveal marked right atrial and ventricular enlargement, often with a marked apical shift to the left (Figure 32-11). In animals with right heart failure, caudal vena caval distention, hepatomegaly and ascites, and rarely pleural effusion may be identified.

Echocardiography quickly and easily distinguishes the often-confusing radiographic findings in TVD. Two-dimensional imaging allows detection of the degree of right atrial and ventricular enlargement and characterization of the tricuspid valve morphology. Common echocardiographic alterations include adherence of the septal leaflet of the tricuspid valve to the interventricular septum and the presence of a large, fused papillary muscle instead of the small, discrete muscles seen in normal animals.

The natural history of TVD is variable depending on the severity and the type of pathophysiologic alteration (stenosis vs. insufficiency), and the presence or absence of concurrent cardiac lesions that increase right ventricular afterload (i.e., PS) or promote right-to-left shunting (i.e., patent foramen ovale or ASD). Some animals never manifest clinical signs, whereas others develop heart failure from 6 months to many years of age. In most instances, medical therapy is aimed at treating heart failure and includes diuretics, angiotensin-converting enzyme inhibitors, positive inotropes, and periodic abdominocentesis or thoracocentesis.

Congenital Diseases of the Pericardium
Peritoneopericardial Diaphragmatic Hernia

Congenital peritoneopericardial diaphragmatic hernia (PPDH), the most common congenital pericardial defect in dogs and cats, results from faulty development of the dorsolateral septum transversus or failure of the lateral pleuroperitoneal fold and the ventromedial pars sternalis to unite. Acquired PPDH, sometimes seen in people with trauma, is not observed in dogs and cats because of a different anatomic arrangement of the pericardium. PPDH has been reported in cats and dogs, with more than one third of cases diagnosed in animals more than 4 years of age. The liver is the most commonly herniated organ, followed by the small intestine, spleen, and stomach. Therefore gastrointestinal signs, including vomiting, anorexia, and diarrhea, are most frequently reported, followed by respiratory signs. Hepatoencephalopathy may occur in patients with hepatic

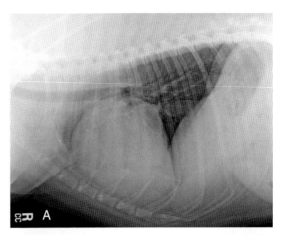

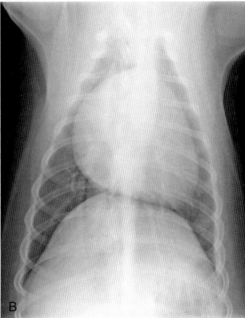

Figure 32-11 Lateral (**A**) and dorsoventral (**B**) radiographic views from a dog with severe tricuspid valve dysplasia. Severe right ventricular and right atrial enlargement is present, although the apical shift to the left on the dorsoventral view often makes interpretation of the cardiac silhouette difficult. Notice the absence of a pulmonary arterial bulge and the modestly distended caudal vena cava.

incarceration and cirrhosis, whereas development of heart failure is rare. It is suggested that Persian cats, Himalayans, domestic longhairs, and Weimaraners may be overrepresented.

Physical examination in affected animals may be normal or reveal muffled heart sounds with displacement or absence of the cardiac impulse. Abdominal palpation may reveal a relative paucity of normal palpable organs. Thoracic radiographs, frequently taken for an unrelated condition, may identify dorsal deviation of the carina, silhouetting of the cardiac and diaphragmatic borders, the presence of gas-filled viscera in an intrapericardial location, and collections of intrapericardial fat (Figure 32-12). The lack of radiographic contrast offered by herniation of solid parenchymal organs

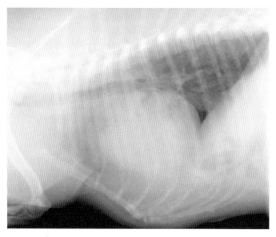

Figure 32-12 Lateral radiographic view from an adult Beagle with a peritoneopericardial diaphragmatic hernia. Notice the differential opacities cranial and caudal to the heart within the pericardium, the silhouetting of the cardiac and diaphragmatic borders, and the missing/deformed sternebrae. This dog had concurrent tetralogy of Fallot.

(i.e., liver or spleen) may make differentiation of PPDH from pericardial effusion, dilated cardiomyopathy, and severe valvular disease difficult. Silhouetting of the cardiac and diaphragmatic surfaces, combined with cranial and ventral displacement of the abdominal organs, supports a diagnosis of PPDH. Echocardiography further facilitates the noninvasive diagnosis of PPDH.

A decision to surgically repair the hernia is often dictated by age at presentation, the presence or absence of clinical signs, and concurrent medical conditions. Subclinically affected animals may only require observation and monitoring for development of clinical signs. A recent study found 2 of 22 conservatively treated cats with PPDH had progression of clinical signs that required surgery or resulted in death. Young animals with clinical signs often require surgery on a nonemergency basis, whereas animals with stomach herniation, intestinal obstruction, or vascular compromise of herniated organs represent surgical emergencies.

Intrapericardial Cysts

Intrapericardial cysts are rare "cystlike" masses reported in dogs and cats that appear to result from congenital herniation and entrapment of omentum or a portion of the falciform ligament into the pericardial sac. Most animals with intrapericardial cysts present in cardiac tamponade as a result of compromised cardiac filling by accumulation of pericardial fluid or direct right heart impingement by the cyst. Therefore physical examination often identifies muffled heart sounds, jugular venous distention, ascites, and weak pulses. ECG may reveal a shift in the mean electrical axis with small amplitude QRS complexes, whereas radiographs display a globoid heart or a protuberance on the right caudal aspect of the cardiac silhouette. Intrapericardial cysts are easily identified via echocardiography. Temporary resolution

of cardiac tamponade can usually be achieved by drainage of the pericardial fluid or the fluid within the cyst. Surgical exploration, usually by a median sternotomy, facilitates cyst removal, subtotal pericardiectomy, and correction of any concurrent defects (i.e., PPDH) to permanently resolve clinical signs.

Congenital Rhythm Disorders
Accessory Atrioventricular Pathways

Normally the only electrical connection across the fibrous barrier that separates the atria and ventricles is the AV node and His bundle. However, during cardiac development as the atrial and ventricular myocardia are continuous, failure of the barrier to completely separate the chambers will produce one or more accessory AV connections. The AP provides a preferential avenue for cardiac conduction (i.e., VPE) from the atrium to the ventricle because transmission occurs at a more rapid rate than across the AV node. Two independent connections may allow the cardiac impulse to traverse to the ventricles down one arm and then conduct retrograde back to the atria, producing AV reciprocating tachycardia (AVRT). VPE can occur without resultant clinical signs throughout the life of the animal if reciprocating tachycardia never develops. When ECG patterns of VPE occur with resultant supraventricular tachycardia (SVT) and related clinical signs, it is termed Wolff-Parkinson-White (WPW) syndrome.

VPE has been described in dogs and cats often with SVT. Numerous reports and further detailed descriptions of APs have been published and suggest Labrador Retrievers may be overrepresented. The ECG hallmarks of VPE (or a WPW pattern) include a short PR interval, wide QRS complex, and a slurred onset of the QRS complex (delta wave) (Figure 32-13). WPW syndrome would display VPE during sinus rhythm combined with demonstrable rapid SVT that usually accompanies clinical signs, including mucous membrane pallor, weak pulses, apprehension, exercise intolerance, weakness, collapse, syncope, or heart failure. The clinical diagnosis of AVRT is more difficult if the AP conducts only intermittently (latent VPE) or when it can only conduct retrograde (concealed AP), meaning there is no evidence of VPE during sinus rhythm. Sustained SVT can produce cardiomegaly and heart failure; therefore radiographs and echocardiography have use in the evaluation of patients with APs. However, radiographic and echocardiographic findings are nonspecific, and in the absence of clear ECG evidence of AVRT, it is difficult to determine whether the cardiac dysfunction precipitated the arrhythmia or if the arrhythmia precipitated the cardiac dysfunction. Therefore diagnosis often requires knowledge of the disease and a high degree of suspicion in young animals with demonstrable SVT. Various antiarrhythmic agents have been proposed to impair conduction or prolong refractoriness in one arm of the reentrant loop, although recent evidence suggests radiofrequency catheter ablation is an effective means to cure animals with APs.

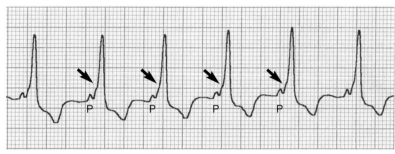

Figure 32-13 Lead I, 10 mm/mV, 50 mm/s. An electrocardiographic image from a cat with an accessory pathway. The PR interval is profoundly shortened, and a prominent delta wave *(arrows)* is observed.

Sudden Death in German Shepherd Dogs

Inherited ventricular arrhythmias with sudden death have been identified and extensively studied in German Shepherd Dogs. Ventricular arrhythmias usually do not develop until after 12 weeks of age, after which their frequency peaks between 24 and 30 weeks of age. Affected animals are asymptomatic until they die suddenly, usually during sleep or at rest, between 4 and 18 months of age. If dogs live beyond 18 to 24 months of age, they typically "outgrow" the ventricular ectopy completely and do not require further therapy.

Physical examination is normal unless an arrhythmia is detected. Arrhythmias in this disease depend on heart rate and behavior, so a routine ECG will only detect abnormalities in the most severely affected animals. Diagnosis and determination of the severity of the disease usually require a 24-hour Holter monitor. Standard ECG measurements, thoracic radiographs, echocardiography, and blood work are normal. Depending on the severity of the arrhythmia, no therapy may be warranted, or owners may consider pacemaker implantation to keep the heart rate greater than 130 beats/min, a combination of mexiletine and sotalol, or implantation of an internal cardiac defibrillator. Several of these therapies may reduce the number of ventricular arrhythmias, but their success at reducing the rate of sudden death is unknown.

Miscellaneous Congenital Cardiac Malformations

Cardiac formation is complex and can produce a large number of anatomical and physiological variants that are beyond detailed discussion in this chapter.

Persistent left cranial vena cava, alone or in combination with other cardiac defects, usually does not impart significant hemodynamic derangements. However, it is important because the vessel may interfere with surgical exposure of the great vessels or a persistent right fourth aortic arch; it also can complicate transvenous pacemaker implantation and may in rare instances impair left atrial filling.

Cor triatriatum dexter (right atrial) and *sinister* (left atrial) are atrial partitioning produced by fibromuscular membranes secondary to persistence or failure of incorporation of fetal structures. The accessory atrial chamber, which collects the

venous drainage, dilates, and venous pressures behind the obstruction increase. The caudal atrial membrane associated with cor triatriatum dexter contributes to hepatic congestion and ascites, whereas the obstructive lesion in cor triatriatum sinister can produce pulmonary edema and pulmonary hypertension complicated by right heart failure. Surgical correction of both lesions has been reported.

Supravalvular mitral stenosis has clinical and pathophysiologic similarities to cor triatriatum sinister.

Double-chambered right ventricle is a partitioning of the right ventricle into a high pressure proximal and normal pressure distal chamber by an anomalous muscle band. The obstruction usually arises from the septal wall, just distal to the tricuspid papillary apparatus, and extends to the parietal right ventricular wall. The lesion has hemodynamic consequences similar to subvalvular PS and has been reported in dogs and cats. Cardiopulmonary bypass seems an effective means for cardiac repair in dogs, and a patch graft technique under total venous in-flow occlusion has been successfully reported in a cat. Balloon valvuloplasty in a symptomatic cat with severe outflow tract obstruction was less rewarding.

Double outlet right ventricle is a rare defect where abnormal ventriculoarterial alignment produces exclusive or predominate origination of both the pulmonary artery and aorta from a morphologic right ventricle. A VSD enables the left ventricle to expel blood into the pulmonary and systemic circulation. The features of the defect, including (1) the connections of the great arteries to the ventricles, (2) the location, size, and relationship of the VSD to the great arteries, and (3) the absence, presence, and degree of pulmonary stenosis, determine whether pulmonary overcirculation or cyanosis will be the predominate clinical manifestation.

Malformation of the pulmonary valve may produce *congenital pulmonic insufficiency*, as opposed to stenosis, imposing volume overload of the right ventricle.

Complete (or D-) transposition of the great arteries is a rare malformation characterized by AV concordance with ventriculoarterial discordance. The right atrial and ventricular and the left atrial and ventricular communications are intact, but they inappropriately connect with the aorta and pulmonary artery, respectively. The malalignment produces two independent circulations that function in parallel and in pure form is lethal. Oxygenation of the systemic circulation, and hence animal survival, depends on the presence or production of shunts (i.e., VSDs, ASDs) between the two circulations to allow admixture of blood.

Truncus arteriosus is produced when the fetal truncus fails to partition into the aorta and pulmonary artery, leaving a single great artery, with a single semilunar/truncal valve, to supply the systemic, pulmonary, and coronary circulations. The truncal septum fails to develop, and the infundibular septum is deficient or absent, giving rise to a nonrestrictive VSD. Although the VSD allows communication between the ventricles and the truncus, its lack of structural support for the great vessel frequently produces truncal valve regurgitation. Classification of the lesion, usually types I, II, and III, depends on the number and location of pulmonary arteries that arise from the truncus. The pathophysiologic consequences and clinical signs manifest, whether they represent left heart volume overload or right-to-left shunting with cyanosis, depend on the size of the pulmonary arteries and the pulmonary vascular resistance.

Aortopulmonary window (or septal defect) is a rare, often nonrestrictive communication between the ascending aorta and pulmonary artery that can be produced by failed fusion of the aorticopulmonary septum and the truncus septum. The clinical features may be similar to a left-to-right shunting PDA, although large lesions and substantial volume overload may contribute to Eisenmenger's physiology with nearly balanced or right-to-left shunting. Surgical management in cases with left-to-right shunting is often difficult without cardiopulmonary bypass because the communication is short and window-like compared with the long and often tubular shape of PDAs. Surgery is contraindicated in aortopulmonary windows with right-to-left shunting, and they are instead managed medically similar to cases of right-to-left PDA.

Coarctation of the aorta is a rare congenital defect composed of a ridge of constricting smooth muscle, fibrous tissue, and elastic tissue similar in composition to the muscular arterial ductus. The ridge, typically located adjacent to the ligamentum arteriosum or PDA, contributes to hypertension proximal to its constriction. Increased afterload may precipitate heart failure, whereas upper extremity hypertension may produce cerebral hemorrhage.

Vascular ring anomalies have been reported in dogs and cats resulting from malformation in the development of the aortic arches. The most common vascular ring anomaly, *persistent right fourth aortic arch* (PRAA), entraps the esophagus with the pulmonary artery to the left, ligamentum arteriosus or PDA to the left and dorsally, right aortic arch to the right, and the heart base and trachea ventrally. Constriction of the esophagus frequently results in regurgitation of solid food in young animals shortly after weaning. German Shepherd Dogs appear overrepresented, but it has been recognized in a variety of breeds and less commonly in cats. Diagnosis of PRAA is usually suspected from the history, and vascular ring compression can often be confirmed by identification of focal leftward deviation of the trachea near the cranial border of the heart in DV or VD radiographs. Surgical correction of PRAA is often an effective means to alleviate the clinical signs of regurgitation.

Endocardial fibroelastosis is a rare disease reported primarily in young Siamese and Burmese cats and some dogs. The left ventricular wall is thin; the left ventricular and atrial chambers are dilated; and heart failure often develops before 6 months of age. There is severe endocardial thickening producing a white, opaque thickening of the luminal left ventricular surface. Histologic changes in cats include diffuse hypocellular, fibroelastic thickening of the endocardium, endocardial edema, and dilation of the lymphatic glands without evidence of myocardial inflammation or necrosis.

SUGGESTED READINGS

Bright JM: The cardiovascular system. In Hoskins JD (ed): *Veterinary pediatrics*, ed 3, Philadelphia, 2001, Saunders, pp 103-134.

MacDonald KA: Congenital heart diseases of puppies and kittens, *Vet Clin North Am Small Anim Pract* 36(3):503, vi, 2006.

Oyama MA et al: Congenital heart disease. In Ettinger SJ, Feldman EC (eds): *Textbook of veterinary internal medicine*, ed 6, St Louis, 2005, Saunders/Elsevier, pp 972-1021.

Sleeper MM, Buchanan JW: Vertebral scale system to measure heart size in growing puppies, *J Am Vet Med Assoc* 219(1):57, 2001.

Trautvetter E, Detweiler DK, Patterson DF: Evolution of the electrocardiogram in young dogs during the first 12 weeks of life, *J Electrocardiol* 14(3):267, 1981.

THE HEMATOLOGIC AND LYMPHOID SYSTEMS

CHAPTER 33

Karyn E. Bird

This chapter is intended to provide information that will aid in the evaluation of the hemogram in normal healthy puppies and kittens, as well as provide information about changes in the hemogram that may be associated with diseases, both inherited and acquired, in these young animals. In addition to the hemogram, the lymphoid system and hemostasis/coagulation in puppies and kittens will be discussed. This discussion will focus on inherited and acquired changes in these systems that affect the ability of the young animal to respond appropriately to challenges. This chapter is not intended to be fully comprehensive for all possible diseases and the hematologic changes that can occur, so suggested readings containing further information about changes in the hemogram associated with disease in puppies and kittens, as well as adult dogs and cats, are included at the end of the chapter.

SAMPLE COLLECTION

Collection of blood samples from neonatal and young animals for hematological and coagulation evaluation can be challenging because of small vessels and relatively small quantities of blood available for testing. Blood collection tubes are available from Becton, Dickinson and Company (Franklin Lakes, NJ; http://www.bd.com/vacutainer/pdfs/VS7629_ProductCat.pdf, BD Microtainer Blood Collection Tubes, BD Microtainer Plastic Clad Micro-Hematocrit Tubes, and 1.8-ml draw BD Vacutainer Citrate Tubes) that will permit collection of sufficient quantities of blood for the various hematological (0.6 ml) and coagulation (<2 ml) testing discussed in the following text.

THE HEMOGRAM

Normal Hematologic Values for the Puppy and the Kitten

Evaluation of the hematologic status of a patient is one of the first procedures used to obtain a baseline status or

diagnostic information helpful in determining the state of health or cause of illness in a pet. When evaluating puppies and kittens, the majority of veterinary practices rely on the normal reference values for adult dogs and cats provided by a reference laboratory. Using these adult values may lead to an erroneous interpretation in very young animals.

Unfortunately, hemogram data have not been reported for mixed-breed puppies and kittens younger than 6 months of age, but some studies have reported data for specific breeds. A recent study reported comparison data for Beagles and Labrador Retrievers. These data were limited but did show some significant differences between these two breeds in the white blood cell (WBC) count, red blood cell (RBC) count, hemoglobin, and hematocrit during the first year, and these differences were particularly prominent during the first 8 weeks of life. The more complete body of data has been obtained on animals from closed colonies of selected breeds, and Tables 33-1 and 33-2 are derived from the values reported in those studies. Although these data represent a more complete dataset, factors such as nutrition, environmental conditions, and health in a closed colony (i.e., research colony) may not adequately reflect the general populations of young animals. If, however, the hematologic values obtained for a puppy or kitten are outside the range of values presented here and the reference values for adult dogs and cats obtained from a reference laboratory, they can be considered abnormal with confidence.

Fetal RBCs predominate in the neonate. The higher mean corpuscular volume (MCV) values indicate that neonates have much larger RBCs than adult animals. As the fetal RBCs are replaced during the first 3 months of life, RBC size, as indicated by the MCV, decreases to within the adult normal range. During the same time that the MCV decreases, the blood volume increases, leading to a decrease in the packed cell volume (PCV). At about 2 months of age, the PCV begins to increase and reaches adult levels between 2 and 6 months of age. During the period of increasing PCV, increased polychromasia and reticulocyte numbers may be seen.

TABLE 33-1 Hematologic values for growing, healthy Beagle dogs

Hematologic parameter	Age (in weeks)														
	Birth*	1*	2*	3*	4*	6*	8	12†	16†	20†	24†	28†	40†	44†	52†
RBC (× 10^6/µl)	4.7-5.6 (5.1)	3.6-5.9 (4.6)	3.4-4.4 (3.9)	3.5-4.3 (3.8)	3.6-4.9 (4.1)	4.3-5.1 (4.7)	4.5-5.9 (4.9)	(6.34)	(6.38)	(6.93)	(7.41)	(8.45)	(8.69)	(8.47)	(7.68)
Hemoglobin (g/dl)	14.0-17.0 (15.2)	10.4-17.5 (12.9)	9.0-11.0 (10.0)	8.6-11.6 (9.7)	8.5-10.3 (9.5)	8.5-11.3 (10.2)	10.3-12.5 (11.2)	(14.3)	(15.0)	(16.0)	(16.7)	(17.7)	(18.2)	(18.8)	(18.1)
PCV (%)	45.0-52.5 (47.5)	33.0-52.0 (40.5)	29.0-34.0 (31.8)	27.0-37.0 (31.7)	27.0-33.5 (29.9)	26.5-35.5 (32.5)	31.0-39.0 (34.8)	(40.9)	(43.0)	(44.9)	(47.6)	(48.8)	(50.8)	(50.2)	(49.3)
MCV (fl)	(93.0)	(89.0)	(81.5)	(83.0)	(73.0)	(69.0)	(72.0)	(64.6)	(67.4)	(64.8)	(64.2)	(57.8)	(58.4)	(59.3)	(63.5)
MCH (pg)	(30.0)	(28.0)	(25.5)	(25.0)	(23.0)	(22.0)	(22.5)	(22.8)	(23.5)	(23.0)	(22.5)	(20.5)	(20.9)	(22.1)	(23.6)
MCHC (%)	(32.0)	(32.0)	(31.5)	(31.0)	(32.0)	(31.5)	(32.0)	(35.3)	(34.8)	(35.6)	(35.1)	(36.1)	(35.9)	(37.3)	(37.1)
nRBC/100 WBC	0-13 (2.3)	0-11 (4.0)	0-6 (2.0)	0-9 (1.6)	0-4 (1.2)	0	0-1 (0.2)								
Reticulocytes (%)	4.5-9.2 (6.5)	3.8-15.2 (6.9)	4.0-8.4 (6.7)	5.0-9.0 (6.9)	4.6-6.6 (5.8)	2.6-6.2 (4.5)	1.0-6.0 (3.6)								
Total WBC (× 10^3/µl)	6.8-18.4 (12.0)	9.0-23.0 (14.1)	8.1-15.1 (11.7)	6.7-15.1 (11.2)	8.5-16.4 (12.9)	12.6-26.7 (16.3)	12.7-17.3 (15.0)	(17.1)	(16.3)	(14.6)	(15.6)	(15.5)	(14.4)	(13.9)	(14.0)
Segmented neutrophils	4.4-15.8 (8.6)	3.8-15.2 (7.4)	3.2-10.4 (5.2)	1.4-9.4 (5.1)	3.7-12.8 (7.2)	4.2-17.6 (9.0)	6.2-11.8 (8.5)	(9.8)	(9.0)	(8.9)	(9.1)	(9.1)	(9.9)	(8.7)	(8.1)
Band neutrophils	0-1.5 (0.23)	0-4.8 (0.50)	0-1.2 (0.21)	0-0.5 (0.09)	0-0.3 (0.06)	0-0.3 (0.05)	0-0.3 (0.08)	(0.08)	(0.1)	(0.02)	(0.02)	(0.08)	(0.02)	(0.02)	(0.04)
Lymphocytes	0.5-4.2 (1.9)	1.3-9.4 (4.3)	1.5-7.4 (3.8)	2.1-10.1 (5.0)	1.0-8.4 (4.5)	2.8-16.6 (5.7)	3.1-6.9 (5.0)	(5.7)	(5.9)	(4.5)	(5.3)	(4.8)	(3.4)	(4.0)	(4.7)
Monocytes	0.2-2.2 (0.9)	0.3-2.5 (1.1)	0.2-1.4 (0.7)	0.1-1.4 (0.7)	0.3-1.5 (0.8)	0.5-2.7 (1.1)	0.4-1.7 (1.0)	(0.9)	(0.9)	(0.8)	(0.7)	(0.7)	(0.5)	(0.6)	(0.5)
Eosinophils	0-1.3 (0.4)	0.2-2.8 (0.8)	0.08-1.8 (0.6)	0.07-0.9 (0.3)	0-0.7 (0.25)	0.1-1.9 (0.5)	0-1.2 (0.4)	(0.4)	(0.4)	(0.3)	(0.5)	(0.8)	(0.6)	(0.5)	(0.5)
Basophils	0-0.2 (0.01)	0-0.2 (0.01)			0-0.15 (0.01)										
Platelets (× 10^3/µl)	178-465 (302)	282-560 (352)	210-352 (290)	203-370 (272)	130-360 (287)	275-570 (371)	240-435 (324)								

RBC, Red blood cells; *PCV*, packed cell volume; *MCV*, mean corpuscular volume; *MCH*, mean corpuscular hemoglobin; *MCHC*, mean corpuscular hemoglobin concentration; *nRBC/100 WBC*, number of nucleated red blood cells per 100 white blood cells; *total WBC*, total white blood cell count.

Values in parentheses are mean values.

*Normal ranges and/or mean values from Earl Fl, Melveger BA, Wilson RL: The hemogram and bone marrow profile of normal neonatal and weanling beagle dogs, *Lab Anim Sci* 23:690-695, 1973.

†Mean values from Anderson AC, Gee W: Normal blood values in the beagle, *Vet Med* 53:135-138, 156, 1958.

TABLE 33-2 Hematologic values for growing, healthy cats

Hematologic parameter	Age (in weeks)										
	0-2*	2-4*	4-6†	6-8*	8-9*	12-13*	16-17*	20†	30†	44†	52†
RBC ($\times 10^6$/µl)	5.29 ± 0.24	4.67 ± 0.10	5.89 ± 0.23	6.57 ± 0.26	6.95 ± 0.09	7.43 ± 0.23	8.14 ± 0.27	7.4 ± 0.7	8.0 ± 0.5	7.9 ± 0.8	7.7 ± 0.8
Hemoglobin (g/dl)	12.1 ± 0.6	8.7 ± 0.2	8.6 ± 0.3	9.1 ± 0.3	9.8 ± 0.2	10.1 ± 0.3	11.0 ± 0.4	10.7 ± 1.2	12.1 ± 1.8	13.0 ± 2.1	13.3 ± 1.8
PCV (%)	35.3 ± 1.7	26.5 ± 0.8	27.1 ± 0.8	29.8 ± 1.3	33.3 ± 0.7	33.1 ± 1.6	34.9 ± 1.1	33.4 ± 3.3	37.1 ± 3.4	37.3 ± 3.5	36.6 ± 3.6
MCV (fl)	67.4 ± 1.9	53.9 ± 1.2	45.6 ± 1.3	45.6 ± 1.0	47.8 ± 0.9	44.5 ± 1.8	43.1 ± 1.5	45 ± 5.2	46 ± 3.5	47 ± 3.4	47 ± 3.9
MCH (pg)	23.0 ± 0.6	18.8 ± 0.8	14.8 ± 0.6	13.9 ± 0.3	14.1 ± 0.2	13.7 ± 0.4	13.5 ± 0.4				
MCHC (%)	34.5 ± 0.8	33.0 ± 0.5	31.9 ± 0.6	30.9 ± 0.5	29.5 ± 0.4	31.3 ± 0.9	31.6 ± 0.8	32 ± 2.0	33 ± 3.3	34 ± 3.0	36 ± 3.1
Total WBC ($\times 10^3$/µl)	9.67 ± 0.57	15.31 ± 1.21	17.45 ± 1.37	18.07 ± 1.94	23.68 ± 1.89	23.20 ± 3.36	19.70 ± 1.12	15.9 ± 6.0	21.9 ± 6.8	18.3 ± 7.8	24.0 ± 12.5
Segmented neutrophils	5.96 ± 0.68	6.92 ± 0.77	9.57 ± 1.65	6.75 ± 1.03	11.00 ± 1.41	11.00 ± 1.77	9.74 ± 0.92				
Band neutrophils	0.06 ± 0.02	0.11 ± 0.04	0.20 ± 0.06	0.22 ± 0.08	0.12 ± 0.09	0.15 ± 0.07	0.16 ± 0.07				
Lymphocytes	3.73 ± 0.52	6.56 ± 0.59	6.41 ± 0.77	9.59 ± 1.57	10.17 ± 1.71	10.46 ± 2.61	8.78 ± 1.06	6.2 ± 2.1	5.3 ± 1.2	6.1 ± 2.0	5.5 ± 2.7
Monocytes	0.01 ± 0.01	0.02 ± 0.02	0	0.01 ± 0.01	0.11 ± 0.06	0	0.02 ± 0.02				
Eosinophils	0.96 ± 0.43	1.40 ± 0.16	1.47 ± 0.25	1.08 ± 0.20	2.28 ± 0.31	1.55 ± 0.35	1.00 ± 0.19				
Basophils	0.02 ± 0.01	0	0	0.02 ± 0.02	0	0.03 ± 0.03	0				

RBC, Red blood cells; *PCV*, packed cell volume; *MCV*, mean corpuscular volume; *MCH*, mean corpuscular hemoglobin; *MCHC*, mean corpuscular hemoglobin concentration; *nRBC/100 WBC*, number of nucleated red blood cells per 100 white blood cells; *total WBC*, total white blood cell count.

Values in parentheses are mean values.

*Normal ranges ± one standard deviation from Meyers-Wallen VN, Haskins ME, Patterson DF: Hematologic values in healthy neonatal, weanling, and juvenile kittens, *Am J Vet Res* 45:1322-1327, 1984.

†Normal ranges from Anderson L, Wilson R, Hay D: Haematological values in normal cats from four weeks to one year of age, *Res Vet Sci* 12:579-583, 1971.

At birth, plasma protein in both puppies and kittens is low as a consequence of low levels of immunoglobulins, even in the face of adequate passive transfer of immunoglobulin G. In normal animals, with the maturation of the lymphoid/immune system, immunoglobulins increase after birth. Plasma protein concentration usually will be within the normal adult reference interval by 2 to 4 months of age.

Generally WBC counts for kittens and puppies are within the normal adult reference intervals from birth to about 6 to 8 weeks of age and vary only slightly during that period. For the dog, the WBC, segmented neutrophils, and lymphocytes are usually within the adult normal reference interval at birth, although lymphocytes may be low in some animals. These values increase between 1 and 3 months of age and may be greater than the normal adult reference interval during this time. These values will then decrease gradually over the next several months (see Table 33-1). Band neutrophils have been reported in one study to be increased at about 1 week of age and then decreased to within the adult normal reference interval thereafter. Like the dog, the WBC, segmented neutrophil, and lymphocyte counts for kittens are within the normal adult reference intervals at birth, but the WBC and lymphocyte counts increase above the normal adult reference interval between 2 and 4 months of age. These values then return to within the normal adult reference interval by about 5 to 6 months of age (see Table 33-2). It has been proposed that this increase in WBC and lymphocyte counts in kittens is associated with excitement caused during blood collection, although an increase in mature neutrophils was not documented during this period.

Erythrogram Evaluation

The complete blood count (CBC) and a blood film evaluation will provide most of the information necessary to evaluate the circulating RBC mass for changes related to disease. By far the most common and diagnostically significant hematologic change in puppies and kittens, as well as adult dogs and cats, is anemia. Anemia is not a primary disease, but determining the type of anemia along with the associated potential differential diagnoses will aid in diagnosis of the primary disease. For this discussion, anemia will be classified pathophysiologically as regenerative, iron deficiency, or nonregenerative anemia. Box 33-1 lists some possible causes of anemia in puppies and kittens.

Regenerative anemia can be further classified as being caused by hemorrhage (blood loss) or hemolysis and results in a characteristic increase in RBC *polychromasia* and *reticulocytes* in circulation. Polychromasia, seen on a Romanowsky-type (Wright's, Wright's-Giemsa, or DifQuik) stained blood film, and reticulocytes, seen on a new methylene blue or brilliant cresyl blue-stained blood film, can be observed as early as 2 days following the onset of blood loss or hemolysis but usually require 5 to 7 days to reach a maximum response (Figure 33-1). Polychromasia is only semiquantitative and can be difficult to determine on some preparations, depending on the quality of the blood film and the stain used. A

BOX 33-1   **Causes of anemia in the puppy and kitten**

Regenerative
Blood loss
   Trauma or surgery
   Flea or tick infestation
   Hookworms (*Ancylostoma* spp., *A. caninum*, *A. braziliense*, and *A. tubaeforme* in the cat)
   Feline panleukopenia
   Coagulopathies (acquired or hereditary)
   Lead toxicity*
Hemolysis
   Neonatal isoerythrolysis (immune-mediated)
   Immune-mediated hemolytic anemia
   • Idiopathic
   • Drugs (e.g., penicillin, cephalosporins, trimethoprim-sulfamethoxazole, levamisole)
   • Infectious agents
   • Vaccination with modified live virus
   • Bee stings
   • Neoplasia
   Oxidative injury with Heinz body formation (e.g., onion, various drugs)
   Hemoparasite infection
   • *Babesia*
   • *Mycoplasma* spp. (formerly *Hemobartonella*): *M. haemocanis, M. haemofelis, M. haemominutum*
   • *Cytauxzoon*
   Microangiopathy (e.g., vasculitis, FIP)
   Zinc-induced
   Hereditary RBC enzyme deficiencies
   • Pyruvate kinase (PK) deficiency
   • Phosphofructokinase (PFK) deficiency

Iron Deficiency
Chronic blood loss
   Flea and tick infestation
   Hookworms (*Ancylostoma* spp.)
Nutritional (milk only diet)

Nonregenerative†
Shortened RBC lifespan
Low erythropoietin activity‡
Low iron availability
Bone marrow suppression
Dyserythropoiesis (English Springer Spaniels)

*Anemia, when present, is usually mild.
†Usually associated with primary diseases, such as renal failure, endocrinopathies, inflammation, infection (especially viruses), and neoplastic disease.
‡Especially with renal disease or abnormal kidney development.
Note: Lists serve only as examples of possible causes.

---

reticulocyte count, which is quantitative, is a more accurate technique for assessing the regenerative response. Nucleated RBCs (nRBCs) are not specific for a regenerative response but may be present in a regenerative response. The presence of nRBCs should not be used as the sole indicator of a regenerative response. Other indicators of an adequate bone

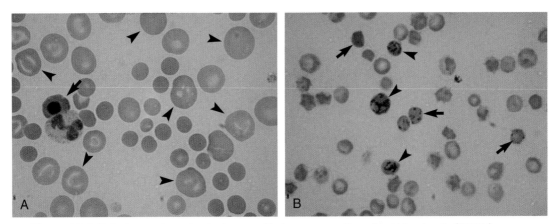

Figure 33-1 Polychromasia and reticulocytes. During regeneration of red blood cells (RBCs), young RBCs will be seen in the peripheral blood. These may be seen as polychromasia in RBCs *(arrowheads)* from a Wright's-stained smear **(A)**. Nucleated RBCs *(arrow)* may also be seen, but must accompany polychromasia to be used as a sign of a regenerative response. **B,** Reticulocytes *(arrowheads)* are seen in a new methylene blue (NMB)-stained smear. A reticulum stain, such as NMB, must be used to visualize reticulocytes. In cats, punctate reticulocytes *(arrows)* may also be seen but are not counted as reticulocytes; these are transitional cells that are not seen in dogs during a regenerative response. **A,** Dog; **B,** Cat, 1000×.

TABLE 33-3	Regenerative response in puppies and kittens				
	Puppies			**Kittens**	
PCV (%)	**Polychromasia**	**Reticulocytes***		**Polychromasia**	**Reticulocytes***
>25	1-2+	>80,000/µl		1-2+	>60,000/µl
15-25	2-3+			2-3+	
<15	4+			4+	

*These values represent the minimum absolute numbers of reticulocytes required for an interpretation of a regenerative response. If the PCV is lower, the absolute number of reticulocytes should increase proportionately.

marrow response, such as polychromasia and reticulocytes in proportion to the level of anemia, must also be present.

The number of reticulocytes, or polychromatophilic RBCs, necessary to determine a regenerative response depends on the PCV; the lower the PCV, the more reticulocytes (or polychromatophils) are necessary to support an interpretation of a regenerative response. The criteria used to determine adequate regeneration for adult dogs and cats can probably be used for puppies and kittens more than 4 months of age (Table 33-3), but young animals less than 4 months of age should mount a more vigorous response than the older animals. Ideally, an absolute reticulocyte concentration (Abs RC) should be used to determine regeneration (Abs RC = RBC/µl × % reticulocytes = retics/µl). For most puppies and kittens, a regenerative response can also be assessed using a corrected reticulocyte percentage (cRP = RP × patient Hct/avg Hct). Normal canine values for corrected reticulocyte counts during the first year of life can be found in Table 33-1.

Once it has been determined that the patient has a regenerative anemia, the total plasma (or serum) protein can be used to aid in differentiating between *blood loss* and *hemolysis*. Because plasma will be lost from the body with hemorrhage, the total plasma protein usually will be low. In contrast, for hemolytic anemia, the plasma remains in the body, and total plasma protein will be normal to increased. The magnitude of the decrease in total plasma protein associated with hemorrhage will be associated with the severity and duration of the hemorrhage. Some causes of hemorrhagic regenerative anemia are shown in Box 33-1. With continued hemorrhage, iron stores are lost, leading to decreased hemoglobin synthesis in developing erythrocytes. Because hemoglobin concentration determines the end of the division phase of erythrocyte development, decreased iron stores will lead to increased cell division resulting in microcytic RBCs with decreased concentrations of hemoglobin (hypochromasia). Hypochromasia is a hallmark of iron deficiency. Even if RBCs do not look smaller, the hypochromasia will be evident as cells with larger pale centers with a thin ring of hemoglobin at the periphery of the cells.

In both kittens and puppies, hemolytic anemia can have a number of causes (see Box 33-1). To date, there is no evidence that kittens and puppies are more prone to hemolytic anemia than adult animals. Although not common, *neonatal isoerythrolysis* is the most common type of immune-mediated hemolytic anemia in newborn kittens and is related to their blood type (types A, B, AB). Neonatal isoerythrolysis is covered in greater detail in Chapter 2. Briefly, hemolysis does not manifest itself during gestation or at birth, but results when a blood type A kitten receives colostrum containing anti-type A alloantibodies from the blood type B queen. Affected kittens may exhibit lethargy progressing to depression, lost suckle reflex, anemia, icterus, and hemoglobinuria followed by death in 2 to 3 days if not treated. Not all type A kittens born to type B queens will necessarily be affected, however. Specific blood types are associated with specific breeds and specific areas of the world. Neonatal isoerythrolysis is most common in Cornish and Devon Rex, Exotic, British Shorthair, and Persian cats, but has also been reported in Himalayan and in domestic shorthair and longhair cats. Neonatal isoerythrolysis is rare in puppies.

RBC morphology observed on a stained blood film is valuable in determining possible causes of hemolytic anemia. A summary of some of the most common RBC changes in association with the causes of hemolytic anemia are given in Table 33-4. In dogs, *immune-mediated hemolytic anemia* (IMHA) is suspected when *spherocytes* are seen on the blood film of dogs. Because cat RBCs do not show a consistent central pallor and are smaller than dog RBCs, spherocytes are more difficult to identify on blood films from cats. In addition to the intravascular and extravascular hemolysis that occurs in cases of IMHA, RBC agglutination and/or a positive direct Coombs test are often detected.

Oxidation of hemoglobin caused by some foods (e.g., onions), food additives (e.g., propylene glycol), drugs, and plant derivatives leads to hemoglobin denaturation and *Heinz body* formation. Heinz bodies (Figure 33-2) appear as small, sometimes clear, spherical protrusions (Romanowsky type-stained blood films) or blue spheres (new methylene blue-stained blood films) at the surface of RBCs. Heinz

bodies also have been strongly correlated to some diseases, such as diabetes mellitus, hyperthyroidism, and lymphoma in cats, but these diseases are uncommon in kittens. Depending on the extent of hemoglobin denaturation, and thus the numbers of Heinz bodies, the resulting hemolytic anemia may be mild to severe. Heinz bodies are removed by the spleen, which may result in spherocytosis, especially apparent in dogs.

Some diseases cause *microangiopathies*, which may be characterized by fibrin strands or vascular sclerosis. When RBCs pass through these areas of the vessel, they are damaged and appear as *blister cells, keratocytes* (helmet cells), or *schistocytes* in circulation. The damaged RBCs are removed from circulation by macrophages in the spleen, leading to an extravascular hemolytic anemia.

Hemoparasite infections often result in extravascular hemolytic anemia. When the infection is primary, the immune system acts to remove the parasite from the RBCs, leading to a regenerative hemolytic anemia. If, however, the hemoparasite infection is recrudescent secondary to other disease processes, the anemia may become nonregenerative. Because hemoparasite carrier states are unusual in puppies and kittens, this type of secondary hemoparasite infection leading to a nonregenerative anemia is unusual in animals less than 1 year of age.

Iron deficiency anemia in young puppies and kittens most often within a short period after birth when maternal milk, which is very low in iron, is the sole diet. RBC numbers, hemoglobin concentration, and PCV begin to increase when maternal milk is supplemented with solid foods or other sources of iron. Chronic blood loss also may lead to iron deficiency anemia, related to the loss of iron used for hemoglobin synthesis. Common etiologies associated with chronic blood loss are flea and tick infestation and hookworms

TABLE 33-4	Morphologic features of RBCs useful for diagnosis of hemolytic anemias	
Cause of hemolysis	**RBC feature**	**Description of RBC abnormality**
Immune-mediated	Agglutination	Small to large clumps of RBCs that are not dispersed with an equal volume of normal saline
	Spherocytes	Small RBCs with no central pallor (may be difficult to distinguish from normal RBCs in the cat)
Hemoglobin oxidation	Heinz bodies	One to several spherical structures within or protruding from the RBC membrane; nonstaining and refractile with DifQuik, nonstaining to pale staining to normal hemoglobin staining with Wright's stain, blue with new methylene blue stain
Microangiopathies	Schistocytes	Irregular fragments of RBCs
	Helmet cells (keratocytes)	Football helmet-shaped RBCs with strap-like extensions of RBC membrane from each side
	Blister cells	RBCs with eccentric vacuoles, often at the periphery of the cell
Hemoparasites	*Mycoplasma* spp.	Dark staining, very small, round to ring-shaped to rod-shaped organisms, usually dotted epicellularly along the periphery or across the surface of the RBC
	Babesia	Large pear-shaped (piriform) structures, present singly, in pairs, or tetrads in the RBC
	Cytauxzoon	Tiny, densely stained to piriplasm-type organisms within the RBC; usually single, but tetrads have been reported

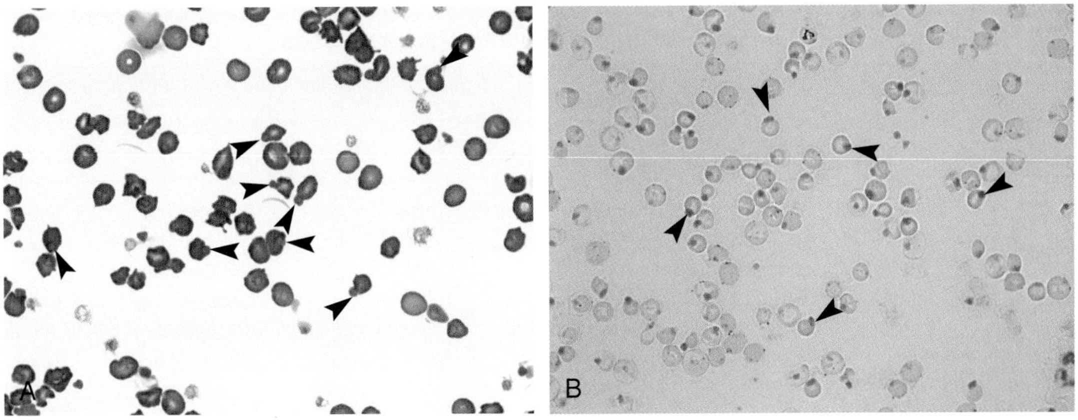

Figure 33-2 Heinz bodies *(arrowheads)* may be seen on a Wright's stained smear **(A)**, but are more readily visualized using a stain such as new methylene blue (NMB) **(B)**. Heinz bodies are formed by various substances, such as onions, that lead to oxidation of hemoglobin and formation of round, refractile (on a Wright's stain) or blue (on an NMB stain) inclusions often attached to the red blood cell (RBC) membrane. Heinz bodies also may separate from the RBC and be found in the background. Cat, 1000×. (Courtesy Marlyn S. Whitney, University of Missouri, Columbia, MO.)

(*Ancylostoma* spp.). The severity and duration of the blood loss, as well as the age of the puppy or kitten, will determine the characteristics of the anemia, which may vary from a mildly regenerative to a markedly regenerative to a microcytic, hypochromic iron deficiency anemia.

Nonregenerative anemia is rare in young animals. Nonregenerative anemia is usually associated with chronic disease processes (e.g., chronic renal failure, endocrinopathies, inflammatory diseases, neoplastic diseases, some viral diseases) that are uncommon in animals less than 1 year of age. Anemia of chronic disease is the most common type of nonregenerative anemia and is characterized by normal cell size and hemoglobin concentration (as determined by the MCV and mean corpuscular hemoglobin concentration, respectively) and a poor reticulocyte response. Nonregenerative anemia usually develops over long periods, although some cases have developed in just a few days. Some congenital diseases (e.g., congenital renal failure in small breed dogs) do occur, but anemia in these cases may not be seen before 6 months of age.

Leukogram Evaluation

Changes in the leukogram generally consist of patterns indicative of a disease process or physiologic response in a puppy or kitten. Even though a disease process may exist, the leukogram may not necessarily reflect expected changes, and a single blood sample may not always reflect the changes occurring in the tissues. Although the presence of a specific leukogram pattern is helpful clinically, the absence of changes in the leukogram does not necessarily rule out a physiologic or pathologic process. Changes in the leukogram in response to inflammation, fear/anxiety, and stress (Table 33-5) are similar to those seen in adult animals, so these changes will be discussed only briefly here.

Physiologic and stress leukograms primarily result from physiologic processes, so it is important to differentiate the changes associated with the response to normal physiologic processes from those associated with clinically important inflammatory disease processes. *Physiologic leukocytosis*, consisting of a mature neutrophilia, lymphocytosis, and occasionally monocytosis, is the most common leukogram pattern seen in puppies and kittens but is more commonly seen in kittens. The lymphocytosis seen in the leukogram of a physiologic response may be confused with lymphocytic leukemia, especially if reactive or atypical lymphocytes are present on the blood film. Reactive lymphocytes associated with a physiologic response are caused by stimulation of the immune system and are commonly present in recently vaccinated young animals. A clinical pathologist can help to determine whether these atypical lymphocytes are reactive or neoplastic. The *stress* leukogram, consisting of neutrophilia, lymphopenia, and occasionally monocytopenia and eosinopenia, is a response to endogenous or exogenous corticosteroids. The total WBC count in a stress leukogram is usually moderate (30 to 35,000 cells/μl) but may be superimposed on an inflammatory response, which will result in WBC counts greater than 35,000/μl.

The *inflammatory* leukogram provides clinically significant information about inflammatory processes within the body, and the type of response may provide additional information about the quality and severity of the inflammatory process (see Table 33-5). In normal puppies and kittens with adequate bone marrow reserves, the most common response to inflammation is a *regenerative* response, characterized by a mature neutrophilia and a mild increase in band neutrophils *(regenerative left shift)*. As a general rule, the bone marrow is functioning normally if a mature neutrophilia or a regenerative left shift is detected. In the presence of an overwhelming inflammatory process (e.g., a highly virulent infectious agent), the bone marrow may be unable to respond adequately, either because the bone marrow has been compromised or because of overwhelming destruction of cells in the tissues; this response is categorized as a *leukopenic degenerative left shift*. If the bone marrow has sufficient time to

TABLE 33-5	Leukogram patterns in physiologic and pathologic processes					
Pattern	**Physiologic**	**Stress**	**Leukocytosis and regenerative left shift**	**Leukopenia and degenerative left shift**	**Leukocytosis and degenerative left shift**	**Mature neutrophilia**
Cause	Fear Anxiety	Pain Restraint Illness/surgery	Acute inflammation	Acute, overwhelming inflammation	Prolonged, overwhelming inflammation	Prolonged inflammation
Mechanism	Epinephrine	Corticosteroids	Inflammatory mediators	Inflammatory mediators	Inflammatory mediators	Inflammatory mediators
Characteristic features	Neutrophilia	Neutrophilia, mature	Neutrophilia, mature	Neutropenia	Neutrophilia*	Neutrophilia, mature
	Lymphocytosis	Lymphopenia	Bands >500/µl	Bands ≥10% of leukocytes[†]	Immature neutrophils ≥ mature neutrophils	Bands within normal reference interval
	Monocytosis[‡]	Monocytosis[‡] Eosinopenia[‡]				

*Normal neutrophil count seen occasionally.
[†]Another common definition for a degenerative left shift is that nonsegmented neutrophils are equal or greater than the number of segmented neutrophils.
[‡]Seen occasionally.

respond, increased numbers of mature neutrophils may be seen on the blood film, but cells representing immature stages of neutrophil maturation (typically bands, metamyelocytes, and myelocytes) are still in numbers equal to or greater than those of the mature cells seen; this is termed a *leukocytic degenerative left shift*. Both leukopenic and leukocytic degenerative left shifts alert the clinician to the severity of the patient's condition and the need to take urgent action—identification of the inciting cause and initiation of treatment as soon as possible are critical.

Inflammatory mediators in the bone marrow affect the maturation of neutrophils and lead to the *toxic changes* (i.e., cytoplasmic basophilia, vacuolization, *Döhle bodies* [except in cats], and/or toxic granulation) in neutrophils seen on blood films. Detection of toxic changes in neutrophils on a blood film indicates a significant inflammatory response. Toxic changes seen in the absence of an inflammatory leukogram alerts the clinician to the presence of an inflammatory process in the puppy or kitten. Toxic changes in neutrophils can be caused secondary to viral or bacterial infections, noninfectious inflammatory conditions (e.g., pancreatitis), or neoplasia, but a bacterial etiology is more likely the more severe the toxic changes. *Degenerative changes*, characterized by cytoplasmic vacuolization and nuclear swelling with loss of the chromatin pattern and light staining that may progress to nuclear lysis (karyolysis), in neutrophils usually occur at local sites of bacterial infection outside the blood circulation, but rarely they may be seen in circulation in cases of septicemia.

Many texts present information regarding normal and abnormal features of the various leukocytes (neutrophils, lymphocytes, monocytes, eosinophils, and basophils) seen on a blood film. The changes seen in the cells in response to numerous diseases do not differ from the responses seen in adult animals and so will not be covered in detail here. To aid the clinician in generating differential diagnoses, Boxes 33-2 to 33-5 are provided as quick references for causes of neutrophilia/neutropenia, monocytosis, eosinophilia, and basophilia, respectively. A similar table will be provided for lymphocytes in a later section of this chapter.

Heritable Diseases of Puppies and Kittens Resulting in Hemogram Changes

Although some diseases that cause changes in the hemogram have been discussed previously, a number of heritable diseases are primarily characterized by anemia and/or changes in leukocyte morphology or function. Most of the heritable defects in leukocytes and RBCs are relatively uncommon to rare and are confined to specific breeds of cats and dogs.

Pelger-Huët anomaly is an autosomal dominant disorder characterized by hyposegmentation of the nuclei of neutrophils, basophils, and eosinophils (Figure 33-3). Hyposegmented neutrophils often resemble bands or even metamyelocytes and myelocytes but have coarse mature chromatin and normal neutrophil function. Affected animals are usually healthy, and the anomaly is discovered incidentally when evaluating blood films; however, homozygous animals may be stillborn. Pelger-Huët anomaly has been reported in domestic shorthaired cats and various dog breeds (Australian Shepherd, Australian Blue Heeler, Basenji, Boston Terrier, Coonhounds, Cocker Spaniel, English-American Foxhound, German Shepherd Dog, Samoyed, and cross-breed dogs).

Chédiak-Higashi syndrome, an inherited autosomal recessive disorder, is found primarily in "blue smoke" Persian cats. The syndrome is characterized by abnormally large primary granules in granulocytes (Figure 33-4), large lysosomes in

---

BOX 33-2   **Causes of neutrophilia and neutropenia**

Neutrophilia

Inflammatory
- Infections: bacterial, viral, fungal, protozoan
- Immune-mediated hemolytic anemia
- Necrosis
- Sterile foreign body

Stress
- Pain
- Injury
- Surgery

Physiologic
- Fight or flight response that includes excitement, pain, exercise, fright/anxiety
- Catecholamines

Neoplasia
- Paraneoplastic syndrome
- Leukemia (granulocytic)

Other
- Granulocyte colony-stimulating factor (G-CSF) administration
- Deficiency of leukocyte adhesion molecules leading to an apparent neutrophilia

Neutropenia

Inflammation
- Overwhelming bacterial infections
- Some viral infections: canine and feline parvovirus
- Endotoxemia

Granulocytic hypoplasia
- Infectious: canine and feline parvovirus, FeLV, *Toxoplasma*, *Ehrlichia*
- Toxic: chemotherapeutic drugs, chloramphenicol (cats), idiosyncratic phenylbutazone, and griseofulvin toxicity
- Bone marrow necrosis
- Myelofibrosis

Ineffective production
- Immune mediated
- Phenylbutazone toxicity
- Colony-stimulating factor deficiency (G-CSF) leading to chronic idiopathic neutropenia

Cyclic hematopoiesis
- Grey Collies and grey Collie-crosses
- FeLV-infected cats

Note: This list serves only to provide examples of possible causes.

BOX 33-3   **Causes of monocytosis***

Inflammation
- Infections: bacterial, fungal, protozoal
- Necrosis

Stress (physical or neurogenic)

Excitement (physiological leukocytosis)

Immune neutropenia, secondary

Cyclic hematopoiesis in Grey Collies and Grey Collie-crosses

Colony-stimulating factor (G-CSF) administration

Neoplasia (monocytic leukemia)

*Monocytopenia is difficult to document and is not considered to be clinically relevant.
Note: The list serves only to provide examples of possible causes.

BOX 33-4   **Causes of eosinophilia***

Hypersensitivity (Allergy)
Fleas (e.g., flea bite dermatitis)
Asthma and eosinophilic respiratory disorders
Hypersensitivity to *Staphylococcus* and *Streptococcus*

Parasites
Fleas
Heartworms
Tissues (including lung and gastrointestinal)
- Puppies: coccidia (*Cryptosporidium*, *Isospora*, *Toxoplasma*), *Dirofilaria*, *Dipetalonema*, hookworm (*Ancylostoma*, *Uncinaria*), and roundworm (*Toxocara*, *Toxocaris*) larval migration, *Paragonimus*, *Spirocerca*, *Strongyloides*, tapeworms (*Dipylidium*, *Taenia*), whipworms (*Trichuris*)
- Kittens: lungworms (*Aelurostrongylus),* coccidia (*Toxoplasma*, *Isospora*), hookworms (*Ancylostoma*, *Uncinaria*), *Paragonimus*, tapeworms (*Dipylidium*)

Idiopathic Eosinophilic Syndromes

Hypoadrenocorticism (Caused by Maldevelopment of the Adrenal Cortex)

Neoplasia (Rare)

*Eosinopenia is difficult to document, especially in the cat, which limits its clinical usefulness.
Note: The list serves only to provide examples of possible causes.

---

lymphocytes and other cell types (e.g., liver and kidney), large melanin granules in melanocytes, an increased susceptibility to infection, especially in the upper respiratory tract, and septicemia. In addition to coat color changes, affected cats have light-colored irises and red fundic light reflections, which cause them to be photophobic. Cataracts also form at an early age. Although coagulation screening tests are normal and platelet numbers are normal, platelet function may be abnormal, resulting in hematomas at venipuncture sites and bleeding following even minor surgery. Treatment involves supportive and symptomatic care, but allogenic bone marrow transplants have successfully corrected the neutrophil migration defect and platelet storage pool deficiency associated with Chédiak-Higashi syndrome.

Several inherited storage diseases have been reported in dogs and cats. *Mucopolysaccharidosis* is a group of rare inherited lysosomal storage disorders documented in dogs and cats. Lack of specific enzymes needed for catabolism of

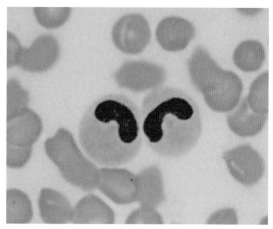

Figure 33-3 Pelger-Huët anomaly is an autosomal dominant disorder characterized by hyposegmentation of the nuclei of normally segmented cells, such as the neutrophils shown here, basophils, and eosinophils. Although cells may appear as bands with horseshoe-shaped nuclei, as seen here, or with round nuclei, the chromatin of the nucleus will appear mature, containing more dark, condensed chromatin (heterochromatin) than seen in immature cells. Australian Shepherd Dog. Wright's-Giemsa stain, 1000×. (Courtesy Kenneth Latimer, Covance Laboratories, Inc., Vienna, VA.)

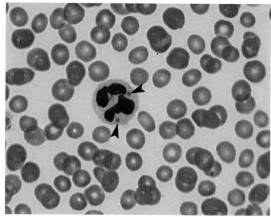

Figure 33-4 Chédiak-Higashi syndrome is an autosomal recessive disorder found primarily in "blue smoke" Persian cats. The syndrome is characterized by abnormally large primary granules *(arrowheads)* in granulocytes, as seen in the neutrophils shown here. Similar abnormally large granules may also be seen in other cell types that contain granules, such as some lymphocytes, melanocytes, and hepatocytes. In granulocytes, these granules are lysosomes, and their dysfunction may result in increased susceptibility to infection. Cat, Wright's-Giemsa stain, 1000×. (Courtesy Kenneth Latimer, Covance Laboratories, Inc., Vienna, VA.)

BOX 33-5	Causes of basophilia in puppies and kittens*

Allergy
    Drugs, food, fleas, other insect bites/stings
Parasites
    Fleas
    Heartworms (*Dirofilaria*) and *Dipetalonema*
    Gastrointestinal parasites
    Migrating parasites (lung and other tissues)
Neoplasia (rare)

*Basopenia is difficult to document and is not considered to be clinically relevant.

Note: This list is not meant to be complete and serves only to provide examples of possible causes.

---

mucopolysaccharides leads to accumulation of metachromatic granules in most mature neutrophils, as well as some lymphocytes and large cells that resemble macrophages. The numbers of neutrophils are not abnormal, and most animals are presented with various abnormalities, such as skeletal abnormalities and deformities (e.g., dwarfism, degenerative joint disease), central nervous system defects, and/or signs related to enzyme deficiencies in the catabolism of mucopolysaccharides (dark purple to magenta granules in neutrophils and granules and vacuoles in lymphocytes). Bone marrow transplants have been used experimentally to treat some forms of mucopolysaccharidosis in cats. An autosomal recessive lipid storage disorder, *cholesteryl ester storage disease,* has been reported in two Siamese kittens. Hematologic changes included anemia, vacuolated lymphocytes in the

peripheral blood, and vacuolated, sea blue macrophages in the bone marrow. Clinical signs included corneal clouding, vomiting, diarrhea, hepatomegaly, lymphadenopathy, and muscle wasting. An autosomal recessive anomaly characterized by fine intracytoplasmic granules in neutrophils has been reported in an inbred family of Birman cats. Affected cats are healthy and have normal neutrophil function. The neutrophil changes seen in this anomaly must be differentiated from toxic granulation (rare in cats) and mucopolysaccharidosis.

Canine cyclic hematopoiesis (also called Grey Collie syndrome) is an uncommon autosomal recessive disorder of Grey Collies. Affected puppies are smaller and weaker than their littermates, and, in addition to the haircoat changes, have regular, cyclic fluctuations in all of the cellular blood elements, including platelets. Typical 11- to 12-day cycles begin as early as the second week of life. Young puppies have episodes of anorexia, malaise, fever, painful joints, severe bilateral keratitis, and infection 1 to 2 days following neutropenia. Therapy includes antibiotics, but most affected puppies die from moderate to severe secondary infections by 6 months of age.

Inherited deficiencies of enzymes associated with the glycolytic pathways in RBCs (e.g., phosphofructokinase and pyruvate kinase) have been reported in dogs and cats. These enzyme deficiencies result in a mild to severe regenerative anemia. The regenerative response as shown by polychromasia and reticulocytosis sometimes may be excessive in relation to the level of anemia. Deficiencies in these RBC enzymes in affected animals can be detected before the age of 6 months. *Phosphofructokinase (PFK) deficiency* has been reported in English Springer Spaniels and American Cocker Spaniels and is characterized by a persistent mild anemia with periodic episodes of hemolytic anemia often initiated by hyperventilation and the resulting alkalosis. During periods of hemolytic crisis, clinical signs are referable to intravascular hemolysis: weakness, pale or icteric mucous membranes, hepatosplenomegaly, hemoglobinuria, and fever. Affected puppies can be diagnosed by their low serum PFK levels. *Pyruvate kinase (PK) deficiency* has been reported in several breeds of dogs (Beagle, Basenji, West Highland White Terrier, Cairn Terrier, and American Eskimo dog) and an Abyssinian cat. In dogs, signs of PK deficiency are seen before 1 year of age, and are characterized by a persistent, severe, highly regenerative anemia that becomes less responsive as the dog ages and some musculoskeletal abnormalities. Affected puppies usually die by 3 to 4 years of age because of bone marrow failure and hepatic insufficiency. Diagnosis of PK deficiency is complex and requires specialized laboratory techniques.

A syndrome consisting of a nonregenerative anemia and polysystemic disorders (polymyopathy, megaesophagus, and cardiomyopathy) has been reported in English Springer Spaniels. The nonregenerative anemia is characterized by dyserythropoiesis resulting in abnormal RBCs with arrested or abnormal stages of mitosis in the bone marrow and nRBCs without evidence of reticulocytes, schistocytes, spherocytes, microcytes, and other poikilocytes on a blood film.

Acquired Diseases Resulting in Hemogram Changes in Puppies and Kittens

Acquired diseases are the most common causes of hemogram changes in puppies and kittens. Most acquired diseases in puppies and kittens are associated with infections (e.g., viral, rickettsial, protozoal, fungal, and bacterial) or heavy metal toxicity.

Young animals, especially those that are unvaccinated, are particularly susceptible to viral infections that can cause leukopenia or leukocytosis and anemia. *Feline panleukopenia virus* primarily affects kittens less than 1 year of age and is characterized by profound leukopenia with an absolute neutropenia without a regenerative response (no increase in bands) and lymphopenia. Although bloody diarrhea is a common clinical sign, anemia is not usually observed. During recovery, the leukogram may show a degenerative left shift or occasionally a regenerative left shift. *Canine parvovirus* is usually seen in puppies 6 to 20 weeks of age. At first presentation, puppies may not exhibit leukopenia, but leukopenia will be detected on subsequent days. Leukopenia is often less than 6000 cell/μl, and the severity often parallels the severity of the clinical signs. A mild anemia and panhypoproteinemia may occur within the first week after presentation, whereas a rebound leukocytosis may occur during the recovery period. *Canine distemper virus* is most common in puppies less than 2 years of age. Hematologic changes in canine distemper are extremely variable, ranging from mild anemia to polycythemia (from hemoconcentration) and from leukopenia to leukocytosis. Lymphopenia, attributed to

viral-induced lymphoid atrophy or necrosis, is also a common feature of canine distemper. The variability in the leukogram associated with canine distemper may reflect the variable clinical course of the disease and secondary bacterial infections. During the viremic stage, small round to irregularly shaped red- to blue-staining viral inclusions (on a Romanowsky-type stain) have been reported in RBCs, neutrophils, and lymphocytes.

Hemoparasite infections are relatively common in dogs and cats of all ages, but because of young animals' maturing immune systems, they are particularly susceptible to hemoparasite infections. Infection with hemotrophic mycoplasma (hemoplasma) organisms, although occasionally seen in dogs, is primarily a disease of domestic cats. *Mycoplasma haemofelis* and the less pathogenic *Mycoplasma haemominutum* (together formerly classified as *Hemobartonella felis*) are the most common hemoplasma organisms in cats, whereas *Mycoplasma haemocanis* (formerly *Hemobartonella canis*) is the most common in dogs. *M. haemofelis* is a small, highly pleomorphic organism that appears as cocci, ring forms, or rods arranged singly or in short chains on the surface of RBCs. *M. haemocanis* is similar, but arrangements of organisms into short chains are more common. By the time cats or dogs are presented with signs of infection, a regenerative anemia, usually related to the duration of the anemia, is evident. Hemoplasma organisms are easily dislodged from the surface of RBCs, so blood films for microscopic identification should be prepared with fresh blood. The diagnostic method preferred for *M. haemofelis* and *M. haemominutum* in cats is polymerase chain reaction (PCR). The direct Coombs test is commonly positive during early stages of the disease, whether or not the infected animals are parasitemic. In cats, mycoplasma infection also has been associated with feline leukemia virus (FeLV) and feline immunodeficiency virus (FIV), two organisms that often lead to immunocompromise. Several antibiotics (e.g., tetracycline, doxycycline) can effectively control the acute disease, but to date no antibiotics have been found to effectively eliminate the infection completely.

Babesiosis is caused by a tickborne hematozoon organism that results in anemia in dogs and to a lesser degree in cats. At presentation, the primary finding is progressive anemia. Three organisms have been associated with clinical disease in the dog: two strains of *Babesia canis* (*B. canis canis* and *B. canis vogeli*) and *Babesia gibsoni*. Puppies less than 4 months of age are more susceptible to infection with these organisms and may have more severe infections than adult dogs. Organisms are seen as "tear drop" or pear-shaped structures within RBCs; the *B. canis* strains are most often found in pairs, whereas a single *B. gibsoni* organism is usually seen. In cats, babesiosis (*B. cati, B. felis, B. herpailuri,* and *B. pantherae*) is primarily seen in animals less than 2 years of age but is a disease primarily found outside the United States. The organisms in cat RBCs are similar in appearance to those of *B. gibsoni. Babesia* spp. in puppies and kittens induce a parasitemia that results in both intravascular and extravascular hemolysis, although early in the disease intravascular hemolysis predominates. Generally the severity of the anemia (usually normocytic, normochromic) parallels the severity of the parasitemia. The PCV is often less than 10%, and nRBCs may be evident late in the disease. Laboratory findings that may accompany infection are hemoglobinuria, bilirubinemia, bilirubinuria, azotemia, urinary casts, and thrombocytopenia. Metabolic acidosis and/or disseminated intravascular coagulation (DIC) also may develop as complications of infection. *Babesia* organisms may not be detected in infected, asymptomatic carriers because few organisms will be in circulation at any one time. Young Greyhounds have been reported to be particularly susceptible to babesiosis. In addition to visual identification of *Babesia* organisms in RBCs on a blood film, an indirect immunofluorescent antibody (IFA) assay and an enzyme-linked immunosorbent assay (ELISA) for *B. canis* are used to diagnose a patent or occult parasitemia. A PCR assay has been used in a research setting but is not available at this time for clinical diagnosis of disease. Treatment is difficult, and a veterinary internist or pharmacologist should be consulted regarding appropriate therapy.

Ehrlichiosis is a relatively common tickborne rickettsial infection of dogs but is relatively uncommon in cats. Various *Ehrlichia* spp. infect mononuclear cells (*E. canis*, *E. risticii*, and *E. chaffeensis*), granulocytes (*E. ewingii*, *E. phagocytophila*), platelets (*E. platys*), or, rarely, multiple cell types (*E. chaffeensis*, *E. risticii*, and *E. phagocytophilia*). Hematology commonly reveals thrombocytopenia and nonregenerative anemia. In severe, chronic ehrlichiosis, a pancytopenia, which is more common in German Shepherd Dogs, may be evident. Low numbers of *Ehrlichia* morulae may be seen transiently in infected cells on Wright's-Giemsa–stained blood films, buffy coats, or bone marrow aspirates. The IFA test using acute and convalescent serum also has been used to diagnose ehrlichiosis, but immunoblotting and PCR techniques are not yet available commercially. Ehrlichiosis has been diagnosed in naturally infected cats, but the actual species has not been determined. Morulae also have been observed in mononuclear cells and neutrophils on blood films from infected cats.

Cytauxzoonosis is a tickborne, usually fatal, disease of cats. The etiologic agent, *Cytauxzoon felis*, has an erythrocyte phase and a leukocytic, or tissue, phase that consist of large schizonts in macrophages. Diagnosis of *C. felis* is made during the erythrocyte phase, when round "signet ring"–shaped, "safety pin"–shaped, round "dot," or tetrad forms are seen in up to 4% of RBCs on a Wright's-Giemsa–stained blood film. The results of treatment in young cats have been poor; however, supportive therapy with fluids and broad-spectrum antibiotics may extend the course of the illness but does not effect a cure.

Hepatozoonosis is primarily a tickborne disease of dogs, although *Hepatozoon* organisms also have been identified in some domestic and exotic cats. Low numbers of *Hepatozoon* spp. gametocytes can been seen as light blue intracytoplasmic inclusions in neutrophils and monocytes on Wright's-Giemsa–stained blood films and buffy coat smears. Because organisms will exit the monocytes, leaving only empty, nonstaining capsules, blood films must be made with fresh blood. Hepatozoon infection may be inapparent or may cause severe disease characterized by mild anemia and a marked leukocytosis with or without a left shift. Even with antiprotozoal therapy, few dogs recover completely. Most dogs will show temporary improvement with relapses and death within 2 years of diagnosis.

Histoplasma capsulatum is a systemic, dimorphic yeast that in cases of disseminated disease (histoplasmosis) may be seen in neutrophils and monocytes on a Wright's-Giemsa–stained blood film, buffy coat, or bone marrow aspirate. Disseminated disease is often associated with compromise of the immune system, so may occur more frequently in kittens and puppies with maturing immune systems. The organisms appear as small (2 to 4 μm), oval, basophilic cytoplasmic inclusions surrounded by clear halos. Clinical signs are generally nonspecific. *Leishmania* is a diphasic protozoan organism, transmitted by sand flies, that affects dogs and cats to a lesser degree. *Leishmania* amastigotes appear as round structures with dark blue nuclei and kinetoplasts within the cytoplasm of monocytes on Wright's-Giemsa–stained blood films or bone marrow aspirates. A range of immunodiagnostic tests (e.g., complement fixation, IFA, and ELISA) have been used to monitor therapy, but results are not consistent and relapses occur frequently even when tests are negative. Relapses occur even with treatment, but treatment may prolong survival for up to 4 years. Cats are rarely clinically affected.

Although heavy metal (e.g., lead and zinc) toxicity occurs in dogs and cats of all ages, puppies and kittens are more susceptible because of their tendency to chew on and ingest foreign objects, such as lead-based painted objects and surfaces and zinc-containing coins and nuts often found on pet carriers. In puppies and kittens affected with *lead poisoning*, hematologic changes (increased nRBCs, basophilic stippling in RBCs, and polychromasia) are observed at the time patients exhibit either gastrointestinal or neurologic signs. Usually no or only mild anemia is seen. Definitive diagnosis of lead poisoning can be made by evaluating serum and urine lead levels. Clinical signs of *zinc toxicity* include diarrhea, vomiting, depression, anemia, hemoglobinemia, and hemoglobinuria. Because gastric secretions rapidly dissolve zinc-containing objects, radiographs may or may not reveal foreign bodies within the stomach. The anemia is usually regenerative (increased reticulocytes, polychromasia, and normal plasma protein), and morphology changes in RBCs include Heinz bodies, ghost cells, nRBCs, spherocytes, and basophilic stippling. Other laboratory findings include regenerative left shift, hyperbilirubinemia, and azotemia. Diagnosis of zinc toxicity can be confirmed by increased plasma, urine, and tissue zinc levels.

LYMPHOCYTES AND THE LYMPHOID SYSTEM

The lymphoid system is composed of both primary (bone marrow and thymus) and secondary lymphoid organs (spleen, lymph nodes, and other diffuse or dense lymphoid tissues often scattered along mucosal surfaces). Lymphocytes are the second most common WBCs in the circulating blood of cats and dogs. Produced in the primary lymphoid organs, lymphocytes use the circulatory system to migrate to secondary lymphoid organs within tissues where they serve as sentinels in the immune system.

Lymphocytes in Circulation

The lymphocytes seen in circulation are usually small, mature lymphocytes, primarily composed of T cells and B cells. Although T cells predominate in circulation (45% to 70% of lymphocytes in dogs and 30% to 90% of lymphocytes in cats), B cells and T cells or their subsets cannot be differentiated microscopically and are similar in appearance and function to those seen in adult animals. Several studies in young kittens have reported that the ratios of T-lymphocyte subsets, as determined by the presence or absence of surface markers (i.e., CD4+ or CD4$^-$ and CD8+ or CD8$^-$), may be different in very young animals. Reactive lymphocytes also may be seen in circulation when animals respond to a strong antigenic stimulus (e.g., following vaccination of puppies and kittens).

Lymphocytes in circulation increase dramatically during the first 4 to 6 weeks of life in both puppies and kittens, but in kittens the initial lymphocyte count at birth has been reported to be higher than in puppies (see Tables 33-1 and 33-2). After birth, studies in kittens have shown that as the overall lymphocyte count increases, both the CD4+ subset (T-helper cells) and the CD8+ subset (T-suppressor cells and cytotoxic T cells) increase; however, the CD4/CD8 ratio decreases during the first 2 months. At birth, the T cells in circulation have not been exposed to antigens, so few T cells are capable of responding to specific antigens. In circulation, both the proportion and the number of B lymphocytes (those lymphocytes capable of producing immunoglobulins) increase dramatically during the first month after birth. Small numbers of larger, granular lymphocytes, known as natural killer (NK) cells, also are present in circulation. Because they do not have surface immunoglobulins (Ig) or T-cell receptors, NK cells are classified as neither T cells nor B cells. NK cells differentiate normal from abnormal cells in tissues through a different combination of surface receptors and markers than those used by T or B cells. Therefore NK cells are able to kill cells directly without using the normal antigen-presenting mechanisms requiring major histocompatibility antigen recognition used by T cells with surface CD4+ or CD8+ antigens.

Etiologies resulting in increased (lymphocytosis) or decreased (lymphopenia) numbers of circulating lymphocytes in kittens and puppies are similar to those for adult cats and dogs. Box 33-6 lists some causes of lymphocytosis and lymphopenia in the cat and dog.

The most clinically significant lymphocyte abnormality caused by an inherited disorder is vacuolization associated with lysosomal storage diseases. Inherited disorders associated with cytoplasmic vacuolization in lymphocytes include G_{M1} and G_{M2} gangliosidosis, α-mannosidosis,

---

BOX 33-6	Causes of lymphocytosis and lymphopenia

Lymphocytosis
Chronic inflammation
- Bacterial infections, especially *Rickettsia*
- Systemic fungal infections
- Viral infections, FeLV
- Protozoal infections, especially *Babesia* and *Theileria*

Physiologic
- Fight or flight response, including excitement, pain, exercise, fright/anxiety
- Catecholamines

Hypoadrenocorticism
- Associated with hypoplasia, dysplasia, or aplasia of the adrenal cortex

Neoplasia
- Lymphoma (FeLV), leukemic phase
- Leukemia, lymphocytic

Lymphopenia
Acute inflammation
- Acute bacterial infections
- Acute viral infections
- Endotoxemia

Stress (physical or neurogenic)
Depletion
- Lymphoid effusion (e.g., cardiomyopathy, chylothorax)
- Loss of afferent lymph (e.g., protein-losing enteropathy, ulcerative or granulomatous enteritis, lymphangiectasia)

Lymphoid hypoplasia or aplasia
- Drugs, especially immunosuppressive drugs
- Destruction of lymphoid tissues (e.g., generalized lymphadenitis, multicentric lymphoma)
- Combined immunodeficiency (Basset Hound, Cardigan Welsh Corgi, Jack Russell Terrier)
- Irradiation
- Viral infections

Note: The list serves only to provide examples of possible causes.

Niemann-Pick disease, fucosidosis, acid-lipase deficiency, and mucopolysaccharidosis. All of these disorders, except mucopolysaccharidosis and acid-lipase deficiency, lead to progressive neurological disease that results in death.

Bone Marrow and Thymus

Both B and T cells arise from bone marrow precursors, but B cells further develop in the bone marrow and Peyer's patches (in the dog) and T cells develop in the thymus. The *bone marrow* is a very vascular organ found in the central cavities of all bones in young animals. In healthy, older animals, the functional marrow can be found in the epiphysis of long bones (e.g., head of the femur) or in flat bones of the skull, pelvis, ribs, or sternum. Development of B cells within the bone marrow does not occur in any specific location, although it has been suggested that the lymphoid precursor cells are located at the margins of the bone marrow, and the early pre-B cells then migrate centrally as they mature and multiply. Before their release from the bone marrow to migrate to and populate secondary lymphoid organs, most of the pre-B cells are selected for their ability to respond only against non–self-antigens; thus a majority of the B lymphocytes formed in the bone marrow are destroyed.

The *thymus* is a large organ located in the thorax, extending from the thoracic inlet down over the heart. At puberty, the thymus reaches its largest absolute size and then begins to involute until it is extremely small (and difficult to find) in adults. Although there is only a small amount of thymus tissue remaining in the adult, there is strong evidence that this small thymic remnant is still functional. The thymus consists of lobules of loosely packed epithelial cells divided into a medulla and cortex covered by a connective tissue capsule. T cells must be able to recognize foreign antigens without responding inappropriately to normal, self-antigens. Within the thymic medulla, T lymphocytes go through a negative selection process in which they are destroyed if they recognize self-antigens or cannot bind major histocompatibility class II (MHC II) molecules. The T lymphocytes that "pass the test" in the medulla are then allowed to enter the thymic cortex where the capillaries are surrounded by a thick barrier to prevent exposure of the naive T lymphocytes to circulating antigens. While in the cortex, T lymphocytes undergo a positive selection to determine their affinity for the MHC II–antigen complexes. Those cells with at least a moderate affinity are allowed to grow. No lymphatic vessels leave the thymus, so these newly "trained" T cells leave the thymus via the blood capillaries, enter the blood circulation, and then populate the various secondary lymphoid organs.

Thymectomy in young animals has shown that the thymus is critical to normal cell-mediated immune response. Because T cells assist in antigen presentation to B cells and their stimulation to produce immunoglobulins, the humoral immune response (antibody production by B cells) will also be affected by reduced numbers of T cells. Developmental disorders of the thymus have been reported in puppies and kittens but are rare. Occasional cases of fading puppy and kitten syndrome have been associated with thymic dysfunction. Most often, animals with congenital or heritable diseases of the thymus will present with immunodeficiency, sometimes accompanied with such abnormalities as dwarfism, hairlessness, and/or dermatitis. Congenital abnormalities of the thymus have been reported in Basset Hounds, Weimaraners, Mexican Hairless Dogs, Bull Terriers, and Birman cats. Benign congenital cysts may occur uncommonly in the thymus of puppies and kittens but are asymptomatic and are usually discovered as an incidental finding on thoracic radiographs. A cystic thymic lymphangioma has been diagnosed and successfully surgically resected in an 8-week-old dog.

Infectious agents, toxins, malnutrition, or neoplasia may damage the thymus sufficiently to cause immunodeficiency.

Some infectious agents that have been associated with thymic lymphoid atrophy, apoptosis, or necrosis are FeLV, FIV, feline infectious peritonitis (FIP) virus, canine distemper virus, canine parvovirus, and feline panleukopenia virus. Toxic insults to the thymus may accelerate thymic involution resulting in impaired T-cell production and cell-mediated immune responses. Lymphoma and thymoma have been identified in the thymus, but lymphoma has a higher incidence in puppies and kittens. Lymphoma in kittens is often associated with FeLV.

Cellular function within the thymus is regulated by thymic hormones consisting of cytokines and small peptides. One of the major thymic hormones, thymulin, is a zinc-containing hormone that can at least partially restore thymic function in thymectomized animals. Therefore, zinc is an essential element for the normal development of the thymus. Zinc-deficient animals will have an impaired cell-mediated immune response. Protein malnutrition in puppies and kittens may lead to decreased immunoglobulin synthesis and decreased thymic function.

Lymph Nodes and Tonsils

Lymph nodes are small- to moderate-sized masses of encapsulated lymphoid tissue scattered throughout the body. Although lymph nodes are readily apparent at birth, they are not fully populated by lymphocytes, and only limited organization is apparent. Organization into a cortex with typical cortical nodules and a medulla occurs rapidly during the first weeks of life. The primary function of lymph nodes is to filter lymph and recirculate lymphocytes. Tissues are drained by lymph vessels that lead into nearby lymph nodes, thus providing a mechanism for the immune system to respond to antigens that gain entrance into these tissues. When the lymphocytes within the nodules in lymph nodes are exposed to "foreign" antigens, they become *reactive*. Although all lymph nodes can become reactive when exposed to sufficient antigen, those lymph nodes adjacent to portals into the body (mesenteric and mandibular lymph nodes) normally are more reactive than other lymph nodes located at a distance.

Enlargement of lymph nodes *(lymphadenopathy)* may be palpated in young animals and is an expected response as young animals are exposed to large numbers of new antigens (Box 33-7). As puppies and kittens age and exposure to new antigens decreases, lymph nodes and tonsils will decrease in size. In young animals, lymph nodes draining vaccination sites may be easily palpated. Neoplasia may also be the cause of lymphadenopathy but is a rare cause of lymph node enlargement in kittens and puppies. Distribution of the lymphadenopathy may help in determining an etiology. If one or several localized lymph nodes are enlarged, the areas drained by these lymph nodes should be carefully examined for wounds, infection, inflammation, and possible neoplasia. If the patient shows generalized lymphadenopathy, a disease that causes systemic antigenic stimulation or primary lymphoid neoplasia then should be high on the list of differentials.

BOX 33-7   Diseases and disorders associated with lymphadenopathy

Reactive Hyperplasia
Noninfectious
- Vaccination
- Immune-mediated disorders
- Allergy (especially associated with the skin)
- Eosinophilic granuloma complex
- Inflammation (localized)
- Tumor related
- Extramedullary hematopoiesis

Infectious
- Bacterial (numerous)
  - Localized infection
  - Septicemia
- Fungal
  - Systemic (*Histoplasma capsulatum, Blastomyces dermatitidis, Cryptococcus neoformans, Coccidioides immitis, Sporothrix schenckii*)
  - *Aspergillus*
  - Zygomycetes (a group of environmental fungi usually infecting immunocompromised patients)
- Rickettsial (*Ehrlichia canis, Rickettsia rickettsii, Neorickettsia helminthoeca*)
- Viral (FeLV, FIV, FIP, ICH, canine distemper virus)
- Protozoal (*Toxoplasma gondii*, especially in cats; *Leishmania* spp. in dogs, *Hepatozoon americanum* or *H. canis*)
- Algal (*Prototheca* spp., *P. zopfii* or *P. wickerhamii* in the United States)

Neoplasia
Primary lymphoid neoplasia (rare in young animals)
- Lymphoma
- Leukemias

Metastatic neoplasia (rare in young animals)
- Mast cell tumors or systemic mast cell disease
- Carcinomas
- Malignant melanoma
- Transmissible venereal disease (dogs)

FeLV, Feline leukemia virus; *FIV*, feline immunodeficiency virus; *FIP*, feline infectious peritonitis; *ICH*, infectious canine hepatitis.
Note: This list serves only to provide examples of possible causes.

Aspiration cytology, biopsy, bacterial culture, serology, radiographs, and ultrasonography are useful for determining an etiology for lymphadenopathy. Aspiration cytology is the most cost-effective diagnostic procedure, but it is critical to aspirate an appropriate lymph node. The largest lymph node may have a necrotic center. Also, because mandibular lymph nodes are more reactive than other nodes because of their location, they should not be primary aspiration sites in most circumstances. Reactive changes, including plasma cells, reactive lymphocytes, mast cells, neutrophils, eosinophils, and/or macrophages seen on an aspiration cytology, can support a diagnosis of inflammation and reaction to antigenic stimuli. Cytology may also provide a definitive diagnosis in the case of infection, when microorganisms are observed, or neoplasia. However, cytology or biopsy of lymph nodes should be carefully evaluated in light of possible marked responses to "new" antigens by young animals. A lymph node cytology showing a high degree of reactivity from a puppy or kitten may be mistakenly interpreted as neoplasia if not interpreted in light of the patient's age and possible antigenic exposure (e.g., vaccination).

Reactive lymphoid hyperplasia is a relatively common cytologic interpretation in puppies and kittens, as well as adult dogs and cats. In young cats, reactive lymphoid hyperplasia is often a transient reaction in response to an initial infection and viremia associated with many viruses, including FeLV and FIV. Although reactive lymphoid hyperplasia has numerous etiologies in young animals, a cause may not be determined, and the reactivity and lymphadenopathy, especially in kittens, may regress without treatment over a matter of several weeks.

Mandibular lymphadenopathy accompanied by granulomatous inflammation and pustules progressing to ulceration on the face and ears (*canine juvenile cellulitis* or puppy strangles) may be seen in puppies 3 to 16 weeks of age. The patient also may show pyrexia, anorexia, lethargy, and sometimes joint pain, but microorganisms have not been identified in association with this syndrome. The granulomatous inflammation in the mandibular lymph nodes and skin resolve with corticosteroid therapy.

Neoplasia in puppies and kittens less than 1 year of age is uncommon, and lymphoma is considered rare. When present, the multicentric form of lymphoma is more common in puppies, and either the mediastinal or multicentric form is more common in kittens. Kittens diagnosed with lymphoma should be tested for FeLV and FIP. Chemotherapy regimens are commonly used for treatment of lymphoma in dogs and cats, but an oncologist should be consulted regarding the best protocol to use in a specific patient.

Abnormalities in the lymph vessels lead to *lymphedema*. A congenital form of lymphedema may be evident at birth or soon afterward. The edema develops slowly, often beginning in the distal limbs and progressing proximally. Usually the patient exhibits pitting edema without pain, unless massive swelling occurs. Differential diagnoses include arteriovenous fistula, venous stasis, congestive heart failure, and hypoproteinemia. Trauma and some major surgical procedures may lead to lymph vessel damage and local areas of lymphedema.

Tonsils consist of dense, unencapsulated small to large solitary or aggregated lymphoid nodules located in the oral pharynx. Unlike lymph nodes, tonsils do not have afferent lymph vessels but react to antigens on the oral mucosa. Efferent lymph vessels lead from the tonsil into the lymphatic drainage system. In some tonsils, blind, sometimes branched, invaginations of the tonsil surface form *crypts*. In tonsils without crypts, the pharyngeal surface of a tonsil may be smooth or slightly folded to create more surface area. Like lymph nodes found at the body's portals, the lymph nodules within tonsils are often reactive. The location of tonsils, along with the surface folds or invaginations, makes tonsils susceptible to inflammation and infection. Neoplasia (e.g., lymphoma and squamous cell carcinoma) associated with tonsils is not common and would be rare in young kittens and puppies.

Spleen

The spleen is a major hematopoietic organ during fetal development, but this function decreases at or immediately after birth. However, the ability of the spleen to initiate extramedullary hematopoiesis is maintained even into adulthood. Although the spleen performs multiple functions, including phagocytosis, destruction of abnormal RBCs, hemoglobin and iron metabolism, blood storage, hematopoiesis, and immune response, blood filtration is the major function. Although the normal spleen is the largest tissue mass of lymphocytes in the body, it may be difficult to palpate in puppies and kittens. The spleen becomes more easily palpated when enlarged *(splenomegaly)* by various inflammatory and noninflammatory etiologies (Box 33-8). Diagnostic evaluation of puppies and kittens with a splenic disorder or disease is similar to that used for adult animals and would consist of a history, physical exam, hematology, imaging, serology, and possibly aspiration cytology and/or biopsy.

The unique vascular structure of the spleen places the blood in close contact with macrophages. The splenic lymphoid tissue is composed of both T cells and B cells. As a result, the spleen also is a major site for antibody and effector T-cell production. The spleen also filters particles, including blood-borne bacteria, creating a potential for septicemia following splenectomy or hyposplenism.

PLATELETS AND DISORDERS OF HEMOSTASIS

Normal hemostasis is achieved through a complicated balance of antithrombotic and fibrinolytic proteins, the blood vasculature, plasma coagulation, and platelets. Following an injury, a reflex constriction of the vasculature slows blood flow, thus reducing blood loss and promoting platelet adhesion to the exposed subendothelium. Platelet adhesion is an important early step in the normal hemostatic process and is mediated by subendothelial collagen and von Willebrand factor (vWF), an endothelial-derived adhesive plasma and subendothelial protein. On release of platelet secretory granule components, such as adenosine 5′-diphosphate (ADP) and serotonin, additional platelets are recruited to the site of injury. Platelets also secrete potent platelet agonists, such as thromboxane A_2 and platelet-activating factor (PAF), that potentiate platelet aggregation and vasoconstriction.

When tissues are injured, tissue factor released by damaged cells, particularly vascular smooth muscle and fibroblasts, initiates the sequential activation of coagulation proteins, ultimately leading to formation and stabilization of a fibrin network that stabilizes the clot formed at the site of

---

BOX 33-8 — Diseases and disorders associated with splenomegaly

Inflammatory

Infectious
- Bacteria (*Brucella canis* or various other etiologies leading to systemic disease)
- Erythroparasites (*Mycoplasma haemocanis, M. haemofelis*)
- Fungi (systemic: *Histoplasma capsulatum, Blastomyces dermatitidis, Sporothrix schenckii*)
- Rickettsia (*Ehrlichia canis*)
- Virus (FIP, ICH)
- Protozoa (*Toxoplasma gondii*, especially in cats; *Leishmania* spp. in dogs)

Noninfectious
- Hemolytic disorders
- Hypereosinophilic syndrome
- Eosinophilic gastritis

Other
- Splenic torsion
- Abdominal wounds
- Foreign body migration

Noninflammatory

Congestive
- Splenic torsion
- Portal hypertension (intrahepatic obstruction, right-sided congestive heart failure)
- Drugs (anticonvulsants, tranquilizers)

Infiltrative
- Extramedullary hematopoiesis
- Neoplasia (lymphoma, leukemia, mastocytosis)

Other
- Hematoma
- Trauma leading to splenic rupture

FIP, Feline infectious peritonitis; *ICH,* infectious canine hepatitis.
Note: This list serves only to provide examples of possible causes.

---

injury (Figure 33-5). The activities of many of the enzymes involved in coagulation depend on phospholipids provided by the surface of activated platelets, which increases the efficiency of activation and limits the scope of the clot formation to the area of injury. Thrombin, an enzyme that cleaves fibrinogen to form fibrin, acts both to intensify coagulation and to inhibit it. At relatively low to moderate concentrations, thrombin promotes coagulation. However, when thrombin is in excess, it binds to thrombomodulin, a receptor on endothelial cells, which activates protein C. Along with protein S, protein C acts to inactivate coagulation factors Va and VIIIa, which helps to localize the coagulation response to the area of injury. Lysis of the fibrin-rich clot is activated simultaneously with initiation of coagulation, and serves to remove the clot once healing has begun. The conversion of plasminogen to plasmin is the core component of clot dissolution. Tissue plasminogen activator converts plasminogen

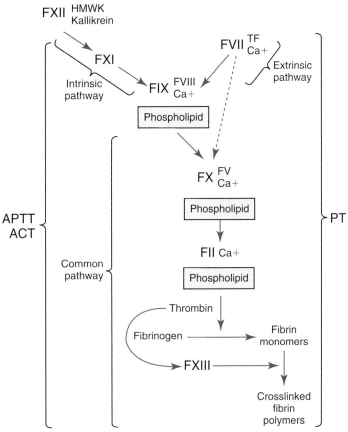

Figure 33-5 Classic coagulation cascade. A sequence of enzymes and cofactors ultimately convert prothrombin to thrombin, which in turn cleaves fibrinogen and activates FXIII in the formation of a stable, cross-linked fibrin network. *APTT,* Activated partial thromboplastin time; *ACT,* activated clotting time; *HMWK,* high-molecular-weight kininogen; *PT,* partial thromboplastin time.

to plasmin only in the presence of fibrin, which restricts the action of plasmin to the site of the clot.

Platelets

As mentioned previously, platelets quickly adhere to sites of injury. In mammals, platelets are small, anucleate cell fragments derived from megakaryocytes in the bone marrow and then released into the blood (Figure 33-6). The small pink to reddish granules seen within platelets on blood films are composed of *dense* granules and α-*granules,* named based on their appearance on transmission electron microscopy. Dense granules and α-granules contain different mixtures of substances that together are composed of divalent ions, platelet agonists, cofactors, fibrinogen, vWF, growth factors, adhesive proteins, and protease inhibitors. Platelets can easily adhere to surfaces and may aggregate in a blood sample even in the presence of an anticoagulant, such as ethylenediaminetetraacetic acid (EDTA) or trisodium citrate. This is especially true in cats; therefore care should be taken when obtaining a blood sample for hematologic evaluation to minimize platelet clumping.

Whole blood (EDTA or citrate) should not be shipped to a reference lab for platelet function tests. The delay created by shipping will adversely impact the quality of the testing.

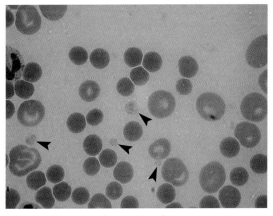

Figure 33-6 Platelets *(arrowheads)* are small nonnucleated cytoplasmic fragments *(arrowheads)* about 1 to 2 μm in diameter found in peripheral blood. Proper function of platelets is critical to proper clot formation and wound healing. Dog, Wright's-Giemsa stain, 1000×.

These tests must be run within 3 to 4 hours of sample collection to ensure that the results will be accurate. Also, care should be taken in interpreting the platelet count results obtained from anticoagulated (EDTA or citrate) whole blood samples shipped to a reference laboratory because an extended delay can result in an underrepresentation of the patient's platelet count.

Platelet Counts

Commonly the number of platelets and *mean platelet volume* (MPV) are obtained when performing an automated hematological evaluation of EDTA anticoagulated blood. In many private veterinary practices where automated counters are not available, the platelet count is performed using a Unopette system (Becton, Dickinson and Company), a hemocytometer, and a microscope. Platelets usually are further evaluated on a blood film for size, shape, and clumping. A crude estimate of platelet numbers also can be made from the blood film. Increases in MPV in the face of decreased platelet numbers *(thrombocytopenia)* indicate an adequate bone marrow response. However, a low MPV suggests an insufficient response, which may be caused by decreased numbers or poorly functional megakaryocytes.

Although platelet counts are most often performed on EDTA-anticoagulated whole blood, counts also can be performed on citrated whole blood. Normal platelet counts in cats and dogs usually exceed 200,000 platelets/µl. Although information is scarce, platelet numbers and function in puppies and kittens are considered to be similar to that measured in adult cats and dogs. However, predictions of whether a patient will be prone to bleeding episodes or will bleed spontaneously cannot be made based on platelet numbers. For unknown reasons, spontaneous bleeding may not occur in some individuals with platelet counts of less than 10,000/µl, whereas other animals may bleed spontaneously when platelet counts are 100,000/µl. Such variables as platelet size, platelet function, and vascular integrity may result in the variability seen among patients.

Platelet Function Testing

Adequate platelet numbers are important, but assessment of platelet function adds another level to the evaluation of platelets. Primary hemostasis, initial adherence of platelets to a site of injury, can be easily assessed using a technique to determine the bleeding time. Bleeding times are used often in human medicine, but the technique has not gained widespread use in veterinary medicine. *Buccal mucosa bleeding times* have been shown to be good indicators of primary hemostasis in dogs and cats, but buccal mucosa bleeding times have the best utility in those animals with adequate platelet numbers but questionable platelet function. The buccal mucosa bleeding time is a very useful tool for screening animals, such as Doberman Pinschers, before ear cropping and/or tail docking. *Clot retraction* is associated with an interaction among platelet receptors, thrombin, and fibrinogen. A measurement of clot retraction in those animals with adequate platelet numbers but questionable platelet function provides valuable information regarding these interactions. However, not all animals with a platelet function defect will show abnormal clot retraction.

Platelet aggregation is the definitive method for evaluating platelet function. Platelet aggregation requires specialized equipment and expertise in the technique; because the testing must be done within 4 hours of blood collection, the patient must be in close proximity to the testing laboratory. Therefore this technique can be used only by a small number of specialized laboratories.

Platelet Disorders

Platelet disorders can be divided into congenital and acquired platelet function defects and congenital and acquired thrombocytopenias (Boxes 33-9 and 33-10). Congenital platelet function defects can be further classified according to effects on adhesion, aggregation, or secretion, and may be intrinsic or extrinsic to the platelet. Because of the previously discussed difficulties associated with testing platelet function, the prevalence of intrinsic platelet function defects is not known. Acquired platelet function disorders are often accompanied by thrombocytopenia. Congenital thrombocytopenia has not been reported in animals.

Chédiak-Higashi syndrome, also mentioned in a previous section, is an autosomal recessive disorder in which granulated cells (leukocytes, melanocytes, and platelets) show abnormal granulation. Platelets in affected individuals lack dense granules and are deficient in serotonin, adenine nucleotides, and divalent cations. Affected individuals develop hematomas after venipuncture and experience prolonged bleeding at surgical sites or following trauma. This platelet function disorder has been reported in a line of "blue smoke" Persian cats that also showed ocular abnormalities.

Canine thrombopathy is an intrinsic platelet function disorder characterized by signs typical of quantitative and qualitative platelet defects: gingival bleeding, epistaxis, and petechia. Although the mode of inheritance has not been definitively determined, inheritance is thought to be autosomal dominant with variable penetrance. The fibrinogen receptor on platelets of patients with canine thrombopathy is abnormal, so dense granule release is impaired. Canine thrombopathy has only been described in Basset Hounds and Spitz dogs. Because diagnosis requires specialized facilities with highly trained personnel, a Basset Hound with signs typical for a platelet function defect, no thrombocytopenia, and normal vWF may be considered to have canine thrombopathy until appropriate testing can be performed. The clot retraction test will be normal in this disorder.

Glanzmann's thrombasthenia and Bernard-Soulier syndrome are platelet receptor defects that result in abnormal platelet adhesion and/or aggregation. *Glanzmann's thrombasthenia* is characterized by a severe (type I) or mild to moderate (type II) reduction of the glycoprotein $\alpha_{IIb}\beta_3$ (also termed GPIIb-IIIa) receptor on platelets. The type I defect has been described in Great Pyrenees dogs and Otterhounds. Platelets fail to aggregate in the presence of ADP, collagen, PAF, or thrombin, and clot retraction is markedly impaired. Young dogs with the type I disorder usually exhibit excessive bleeding during teething and may have chronic epistaxis. Although episodes of spontaneous bleeding usually subside as puppies get older, excessive bleeding still may occur during surgical procedures or following trauma. *Bernard-Soulier syndrome* is

---

BOX 33-9   **Causes of thrombocytopenia and thrombocytosis**

Thrombocytopenia
Decreased production
- Drugs: known or idiosyncratic
- Immune mediated
- Infections (e.g., *Ehrlichia canis*, *E. platys*, FeLV, endotoxemia)
- Necrosis affecting the bone marrow (may be caused by infection, neoplasia)
- Decreased thrombopoietin or erythropoietin
- Idiopathic (likely immune mediated)
Sequestration
- Spleen
Consumption/destruction
- Platelet activation leading to consumption (DIC, vasculitis, thrombosis, severe injury)
- Blood loss
- Drugs
- Immune mediated (idiopathic, drugs, infection, neoplasia, transfusion)
- Vaccine induced (likely immune mediated)
- Infection (may also lead to decreased production): canine distemper, parvovirus, Cytauxzoonosis, *Ehrlichia* spp., endotoxemia, FeLV, FIP, leptospirosis, leishmaniasis, Rocky Mountain spotted fever, canine herpesvirus
- DIC
- Idiopathic (likely immune mediated)
Hemodilution
Pseudothrombocytopenia
- Platelet clumping (especially in cats and some dog breeds)
- Lower platelet numbers (normal) in Greyhound dogs

Thrombocytosis
Increased production
- Iron deficiency
- Inflammation
- Blood loss
- Rebound from thrombocytopenia
Redistribution
- Physiologic (exercise, fear/anxiety, epinephrine)
- After splenectomy
Hemic neoplasia and myeloproliferative diseases

DIC, Disseminated intravascular coagulation; *FeLV*, feline leukemia virus; *FIP*, feline infectious peritonitis.
Note: The list serves only to provide examples of possible causes.

BOX 33-10   **Causes of decreased platelet function**

Hereditary Defects (Uncommon and Usually Limited to Specific Breeds)
Intrinsic
- Canine thrombopathia (Basset Hound, Spitz)
- Cyclic hematopoiesis (Grey Collie and Grey Collie-crosses)
- Chédiak-Higashi syndrome (blue smoke Persian cats)
- Glanzmann's thrombasthenia, defect in the platelet receptor $\alpha_{IIb}\beta_3$ (Great Pyrenees, Otterhounds)
- Bernard-Soulier syndrome (also called giant platelet syndrome), defect in the platelet receptor GPIb (Cavalier King Charles Spaniels)
Extrinsic
- von Willebrand disease

Acquired Disorders
Drugs (aspirin, NSAIDs, antibiotics, anesthetics, antihistamines)
FDPs, byproducts of fibrin breakdown (DIC, fibrinolysis)
Uremia (renal failure)
Liver disease
Infections (FeLV, FIP, panleukopenia, *Toxoplasma* in the cat)
Hyperglobulinemia (*Ehrlichia* spp.)

NSAIDs, Nonsteroidal antiinflammatory drugs; *FDPs*, fibrin degradation products; *DIC*, disseminated intravascular coagulation; *FeLV*, feline leukemia virus; *FIP*, feline infectious peritonitis.
Note: The list serves only to provide examples of possible causes.

---

been detected in about 30% to 50% of Cavalier King Charles Spaniels.

von Willebrand disease (vWD), an inherited *extrinsic* platelet function disorder caused by defective or deficient vWF, is the most common inherited bleeding disorder in dogs. Platelets are normal, but because platelet adhesion at sites of injury in high sheer rate vessels requires vWF, the disorder mimics thrombocytopenia or an intrinsic platelet function defect. There are three main types (types I, II, and III) and a number of subtypes of vWD. Depending on the type, the mode of inheritance may be autosomal dominant with variable penetrance or autosomal recessive. More than 50 dog breeds and some mixed breeds have been diagnosed with vWD, and several breeds have been designated as high-risk candidates: Doberman Pinscher, Scottish Terrier, Miniature Schnauzer, Rottweiler, Basset Hound, Golden Retriever, Shetland Sheepdog, standard Poodle, German Shepherd Dog, German Shorthaired Pointer, Pembroke Welsh Corgi, Keeshond, Dachshund, and Manchester Terrier. vWD has also been reported in a Himalayan cat. The Doberman Pinscher has the highest prevalence of vWD (>70%), with up to 16% of dogs in the breed clinically affected. In Doberman Pinschers, the mode of inheritance is autosomal dominant with variable penetrance. Puppies showing signs of epistaxis, gingival bleeding, prolonged

associated with a defect in the platelet surface glycoprotein Ib/IX/V (GPIb/IX/V) complex, so that platelet binding to vWF is defective. The characteristic clinical presentation consists of thrombocytopenia, giant platelets (macroplatelets), and decreased platelet aggregation in response to ADP. *Giant platelet syndrome*, an autosomal recessive trait that has clinical characteristics of Bernard-Soulier syndrome, has bleeding after ear cropping, tail docking, or dew claw removal but having normal coagulation screening tests and no thrombocytopenia should be tested for vWD. Citrated plasma, frozen immediately after collection, is the appropriate sample for testing for vWD and should be sent to a diagnostic lab for testing within 2 weeks of sample collection. A quantitative ELISA test is most commonly used for diagnosis, but the ristocetin assay and gel electrophoresis is still used by some laboratories to differentiate the different types of vWD. Animals in hemorrhagic crisis are treated with whole blood or, preferably, plasma or cryoprecipitate transfusions. Desmopressin acetate also has been used to augment plasma transfusion therapy.

Acquired platelet function disorders have been related to infection, primarily FeLV in cats, myeloproliferative disease, and certain drugs, such as penicillin, lidocaine, aspirin, acetaminophen, phenylbutazone, and pentobarbital. Impaired platelet function should be suspected in a patient when hemorrhage occurs in the presence of normal or elevated platelet numbers and a normal coagulation profile. Various drugs impair platelet function by blocking or inhibiting platelet receptor binding to platelet agonists, by inhibiting message transduction from the platelet surface, and/or by inhibiting platelet response mechanisms, such as aggregation, secretion, or generation of thromboxane A_2. The acquired platelet defect will usually not be clinically significant unless there is an underlying platelet function defect. Also, because platelets are continuously renewed, the acquired defect usually will resolve in 3 to 11 days after the drug is discontinued.

Acquired thrombocytopenias are commonly associated with infections (e.g., *Ehrlichia* spp.), many drugs, vaccine administration, immune-mediated disease, or are idiopathic. *Ehrlichia* infection, especially with *E. canis*, often leads to increased platelet consumption and decreased platelet survival associated with vasculitis and immune-mediated mechanisms. *Ehrlichia* infection may result in epistaxis, gingival bleeding, retinal hemorrhage, melena, petechia, ecchymoses, and prolonged bleeding from sites of surgical incision or venipuncture. In some affected individuals, thrombocytopenia may not be seen, but platelet function may be impaired.

Many drugs induce platelet destruction or suppression of bone marrow production of platelets, leading to thrombocytopenia. Thrombocytopenia may be the result of a toxic effect of the drug or may be immune mediated. Immune-mediated destruction of platelets occurs when the drug binds to or is adsorbed to the surface of the platelet, resulting in antibody formation. Drug-induced thrombocytopenia may be idiosyncratic, which makes it difficult to predict the action of a drug in a certain individual. Drug-induced bone marrow suppression occurs at the stem cell level and in addition to the thrombocytopenia will often result in a pancytopenia. Usually the thrombocytopenia will resolve when the drug is discontinued, but in some cases, the thrombocytopenia may persist.

Although not documented, *idiopathic thrombocytopenia purpura* is probably an immune-mediated disease. Depending on the target of the immune response, megakaryocytes

may also be reduced. Corticosteroids are commonly used to treat this type of thrombocytopenia, but danazol has been used in some cases of corticosteroid-resistant thrombocytopenia. In cases of recurrent immune-mediated thrombocytopenia, splenectomy also has been recommended as a management tool.

Coagulopathies

Coagulopathies may result from inherited or acquired defects in the coagulation proteins (see Figure 33-5; Box 33-11). Inherited defects in coagulation proteins usually manifest by the age of 6 months. During this time, young animals have an immature coagulation system, which is related to a still-developing liver, the site of synthesis of most of the coagulation proteins. Puppies and kittens with severe coagulopathies, usually associated with extremely low levels (<1%) of factor VIII (FVIII), factor IX (FIX), prothrombin (FII), or fibrinogen (FI), are stillborn or die shortly after birth. Less severely affected animals (1% to 5% of normal levels) will present with coagulopathies between 1 and 6 months of age, a time when puppies and kittens experience such procedures and physiologic changes as vaccination, ear cropping, tail docking, dew claw removal, declawing, loss of deciduous teeth, and

---

BOX 33-11 **Coagulation and vascular disorders in puppies and kittens**

Hereditary Defects
FXII deficiency: Cats, German Shorthaired Pointer, standard Poodle, miniature Poodle
FXI deficiency: Springer Spaniel, Great Pyrenees, Weimaraner, Kerry Blue Terrier
FX deficiency: American Cocker Spaniel
FIX deficiency: Mixed breed and purebred dogs; British Shorthair and Siamese-cross cats
FVIII: Many purebred and mixed breed dogs and cats
FVII deficiency: Beagle, Miniature Schnauzer, Alaskan Malamute, Boxer, Bulldog
Prothrombin (FII)
　Dysprothrombinemia: English Cocker Spaniel, Boxer
Fibrinogen (FI)
　Dysfibrinogenemia: Russian Wolfhound
　Hypofibrinogenemia: Saint Bernard, Vizsla
Defective γ-glutamylcarboxylase (vitamin K multifactor coagulopathy): Devon Rex cats
Cutaneous asthenia or Ehlers-Danlos Syndrome (connective tissue disorder): Various breeds of dogs and cats

Acquired Disorders
Anticoagulant rodenticide toxicity: coumarin, brodifacoum, indanedione
DIC
Liver disease
Infections (RMSF, canine herpesvirus)

DIC, Disseminated intravascular coagulation; *RMSF,* Rocky Mountain spotted fever.
Note: The list serves only to provide examples of possible causes.

initial estrus. Animals with more than 5% of the normal levels may not show any signs of spontaneous bleeding. Small dogs and cats also are less likely to bleed spontaneously than large dogs, even with coagulation protein levels less than 5%. Acquired coagulopathies are more common than inherited coagulopathies and occur at any age. In very young animals, it may be difficult to determine whether a coagulopathy is inherited or acquired.

Coagulation Screening Tests

Several in vitro tests have been developed to evaluate the various stages of the coagulation cascade. Most coagulation screening tests require citrated plasma (typically 3.2% to 3.8% trisodium citrate at an anticoagulant/blood ratio of 1:9). The exceptions are tests for fibrinogen and fibrin degradation products, for which serum is used. The most commonly used coagulation screening tests are *activated coagulation, or clotting, time* (ACT), *activated partial thromboplastin time* (APTT), *prothrombin time* (PT), *thrombin time* (TT), *fibrinogen* and *fibrin degradation products* (FDP), and *antithrombin* (AT or ATIII).

The ACT and APTT are used to evaluate the intrinsic and common pathways of the coagulation cascade (see Figure 33-5). The *ACT* test is usually performed on 2 ml of whole blood added to an ACT tube containing diatomaceous earth, incubated at body temperature and agitated at specific intervals while observing for clotting. This test has some dependence on platelets for phospholipids; therefore platelet counts less than 10,000/μl may result in a prolonged ACT test. It is often difficult to obtain enough blood for this test in addition to other tests that may need to be run for diagnostics. Veterinary point-of-care coagulation analyzers (CoagDx, IDEXX, Westbrook, ME: http://www.idexx.com/animalhealth/analyzers/coag/index.jsp; i-STAT, Heska Corporation, Boulder, CO: http://www.heska.com/istat/index.asp) are available for performing not only ACT but also PT and APTT on small volumes (50 μl) of whole blood. For the *APTT*, phospholipids, calcium, and a negatively charged activator are added to citrated plasma, and the time to clot is recorded. Specific factor activities must be less than 30% before a prolonged APTT will be observed. Detection of a prolonged APTT may not always be clinically significant (e.g., prolonged APTT will be observed for deficiencies in FXII or kallikrein but is not usually associated with hemorrhage), but evaluation of specific coagulation factors is warranted when a prolonged APTT in the presence of bleeding and a normal PT is observed. The lower coagulation factor levels in very young puppies and kittens may result in slightly prolonged APTTs (usually less than 3 seconds longer than normal) compared with APTTs in adult dogs and cats, but APTTs should be at adult levels by 6 months of age.

The *PT* assay evaluates the extrinsic and common pathways of the coagulation cascade. For the PT test, tissue factor and calcium are added to citrated plasma, and the time to clot is recorded. The PT test is very sensitive for warfarin (an inhibitor of the vitamin K–dependent mechanism of synthesis of factors II, VII, IX, and X) toxicity because the

vitamin K–dependent factor VII (FVII) has the shortest half-life. A FVII deficiency alone may not be accompanied by spontaneous hemorrhage. Like the ACT and APTT, normal ranges for very young animals should be used rather than the reference ranges for adults. Ideally reference ranges for normal puppies and kittens should be determined in the veterinary facility where the test is performed. For animals less than 2 months of age, this cannot usually be accomplished. A recommended alternative is to run an age-matched, normal animal (if available, a normal sibling from the same litter) along with the affected individual.

The *thrombin time* is performed by adding thrombin to citrated plasma and recording the time to clot. The rate of clot formation is directly related to the amount of functional fibrinogen present in the plasma; therefore it is very useful in evaluation of DIC, as well as less common to rare conditions associated with hypofibrinogenemia or dysfibrinogenemia. The test for increased levels of *fibrinogen and/or fibrin degradation products* (FDP) in serum is also used to evaluate a patient for DIC, but the test also may be elevated in animals with inflammation, hemorrhage, and thromboses (e.g., around a catheter). The serum sample must be collected in a special FDP tube containing thrombin and a trypsin inhibitor.

Antithrombin is a circulating protein inhibitor of the activated serine proteases in the coagulation cascade: thrombin (FIIa), FIXa, FXa, FXIIa, and FXIa. The activity of AT is greatly enhanced in the presence of heparin. AT is a 62,000-dalton α_2-globulin produced in the liver; thus liver failure may lead to decreased AT synthesis. Because of its relatively low molecular mass, AT levels also may be reduced as a result of a protein-losing enteropathy or a glomerulopathy. AT levels are also reduced in DIC; therefore testing for AT is useful in evaluations of cases of suspected DIC. However, the AT test is not useful for cats with DIC. As with the previous tests, age-matched normal controls are highly recommended.

Inherited Coagulation and Vascular Disorders

The most common inherited coagulopathy in cats and dogs is *hemophilia* caused by a *FVIII deficiency* (hemophilia A). Factor VIII deficiency is an X-linked disorder; therefore males are usually affected, and females are asymptomatic carriers (30% to 60% of normal FVIII activity). Affected puppies will show prolonged bleeding from the umbilicus at birth, from gingiva during tooth eruption, and from routine surgical procedures, such as tail docking, ear cropping, or dew claw removal. More severe manifestations of the disorder, such as spontaneous hematomas, hemarthroses, and hemorrhagic effusions, also are common. Patients with less than 5% of the normal FVIII activity experience the most severe manifestations of the disorder. *Factor IX deficiency* (hemophilia B) is less common than FVIII deficiency but has been reported in dogs and cats (British Shorthair cats, Siamese-cross cats, and a single domestic medium-haired cat). Puppies or kittens with severe FIX deficiency (<1%) may die at or soon after birth. Clinical signs in cases of severe

FIX deficiency are similar to those seen in FVIII-deficient young animals. Patients with more than 5% of the normal FVIII or FIX activity generally do not show spontaneous bleeding; therefore these young, affected animals may not be identified until after trauma or surgery. For unknown reasons, small dogs and cats with FVIII or FIX deficiency may not show prolonged bleeding even after trauma or surgery. Like FVIII deficiency, FIX deficiency is an X-linked disorder; thus males are more commonly affected, and females are asymptomatic carriers (30% to 60% of normal), except in some inbred families where females may also be affected. Prolonged ACT and APTT are seen with both FVIII and FIX deficiency. Care should be taken when interpreting decreased FVIII or FIX carrier states in young animals because young animals may normally have lower levels of FVIII and FIX. Also, in vWD in which there are decreased levels of vWF, FVIII levels may also be decreased because vWF is the carrier protein for FVIII in circulation. When following a patient with FIX or FVIII deficiency, be aware of the consequences of unseen or undetected hemorrhage into body cavities, the brain, muscle, and along facial planes—episodes of bleeding in these areas may lead to necrosis, paralysis, seizures, and/or hypovolemic shock. Multiple transfusions of fresh or frozen plasma are used to treat both FVIII and FIX deficiencies.

Prekallikrein deficiency is a rare disorder in domestic animals and has been reported in a dog (Poodle) but not in cats. The disorder usually is not associated with bleeding, but affected animals will have prolonged ACT and APTT and a normal PT. Like prekallikrein deficiency, a *deficiency in FXII* (Hageman factor) is not associated with spontaneous bleeding. However, because of its role in complement activation and fibrinolysis, FXII deficiency may be associated with a predisposition for infection and thrombosis. Factor XII deficiency has been reported in a German Shorthaired Pointer, a standard Poodle, a family of miniature Poodles, and cats. Affected animals will have prolonged ACT and APTT and a normal PT. *Factor XI deficiency* is relative rare and has been reported in Springer Spaniels, Great Pyrenees, Weimaraners, and Kerry Blue Terriers. A case of a circulating coagulation factor XI (FXI) inhibitor, which results in clinical signs similar to FXI deficiency, such as epistaxis, has been reported in an adult cat. The mode of inheritance of FXI deficiency is autosomal, but it has not been determined whether it is recessive or dominant. Patients with FXI levels less than 30% to 40% will have prolonged ACT and APTT. When they occur, bleeding episodes associated with FXI deficiency can be treated with autologous fresh or frozen plasma.

Factor X deficiency is a rare autosomal recessive hemostatic disorder with variable penetrance. To date, it has only been described in a family of American Cocker Spaniels. Puppies homozygous for the gene are usually stillborn or die shortly after birth with massive hemorrhage into the abdominal and thoracic cavities. Animals heterozygous for the gene have intermediate levels of FX activity and have tendencies for mild to severe bleeding. Individuals with less than 30%

of normal FX levels will have prolonged ACT, APTT, and PT. Factor X deficiency is treated with fresh or frozen plasma.

Patients affected with *FVII deficiency* may show evidence of bruising or prolonged bleeding after surgery or parturition, but overt bleeding is not usually seen. Inheritance of FVII deficiency is autosomal dominant with incomplete penetrance and has been detected in Beagles, Miniature Schnauzers, Alaskan Malamutes, Boxers, and Bulldogs. Animals with a FVII deficiency will have a prolonged PT.

Prothrombin (FII) abnormalities are extremely rare and have only been described in the English Cocker Spaniel and Boxer. In the Boxer, the prothrombin defect has an autosomal recessive mode of inheritance. A prothrombin deficiency has not been documented in either the Boxer or the Cocker Spaniel, and in Boxers the disorder has been characterized as a dysprothrombinemia. Affected puppies exhibit gingival bleeding and epistaxis, which decrease with age. Coagulation screening studies show prolonged ACT, APTT, and PT but a normal TT. Preferred treatment is with transfusions of fresh or frozen plasma.

A *congenital fibrinogen (FI) deficiency* has not been reported in dogs or cats, but inherited dysfibrinogenemia has been reported in one family of Russian Wolfhounds. Coagulation screening tests show prolonged ACT, APTT, PT, and TT. In affected Russian Wolfhounds, fibrinogen could be detected by quantitative but not qualitative methods. The affected animals showed signs of epistaxis and lameness, as well as life-threatening bleeding with trauma or surgery. Severe bleeding associated with hypofibrinogenemia has been reported in the St. Bernard and Vizsla. The coagulation screening tests are similar to those reportedly used for dysfibrinogenemia (e.g., PT, APTT, TT, reptilase time, fibrinogen activity/antigen ratio), but decreased levels of fibrinogen are detected using quantitative methods. Treatment to stop bleeding episodes consists of transfusions of fresh or frozen plasma or plasma cryoprecipitate.

A *multifactor congenital coagulopathy* characterized by hemorrhage into conjunctiva, joints, and body cavities has been described in Devon Rex cats. The defect is in the synthetic pathway for vitamin K–dependent coagulation factors (prothrombin, FVII, FIX, FX); therefore affected cats have prolonged APTT and PT. Vitamin K_1 treatment can be used to control hemorrhage.

A defect in synthesis or maturation of type I collagen (cutaneous asthenia or Ehlers-Danlos syndrome) leads to decreased vascular support and formation of subcutaneous hematomas. This disorder, characterized by loose, hyperextensible skin and possibly a platelet function defect, has been reported in dogs and cats. There is no treatment.

Acquired Coagulation and Vascular Disorders

Acquired coagulopathies are far more common than inherited disorders in the dog and cat. The most common causes of acquired coagulopathies are toxic chemicals (e.g., rodenticides), infection, liver disease, and DIC associated with multiple etiologies. *Anticoagulant rodenticides* (e.g., coumarin, brodifacoum, indanedione) interfere with carboxylation of the vitamin K–dependent coagulation factors (prothrombin, FVII, FIX, FX, protein C, and protein S) and the recycling mechanism that maintains body stores of vitamin K. Signs of a rodenticide-associated coagulopathy are lethargy, respiratory distress, lameness, epistaxis, hemoptysis, and petechial and ecchymotic hemorrhages. In contrast to the older anticoagulant rodenticides containing first-generation anticoagulants (e.g., coumarin compounds, such as warfarin) that have anticoagulation effects for 7 to 10 days, the second generation of compounds (e.g., brodifacoum compounds) and indanedione compounds may have anticoagulant effects for 20 to 120 days. Although the rodenticide coagulopathies are characterized by prolonged ACT, APTT, and PT, the PT may be the best test for early detection because FVII has the shortest half-life (1 to 6 hours) of the vitamin K–dependent coagulation factors. Hemorrhage may not be present in early stages, although there may be a history of rodenticide consumption within the previous 24 hours. The preferred treatment is vitamin K₁, but therapy should be closely monitored for possible development of Heinz body anemia, an adverse reaction to vitamin K₁ therapy previously reported in a dog. Long-term (up to 6 weeks) vitamin K₁ treatment is recommended in those cases of indanedione toxicity.

Infections with *Rickettsia rickettsii*, the causative agent for *Rocky Mountain spotted fever* (RMSF), and *canine herpesvirus* have been associated with coagulopathies in dogs (significance of RMSF in cats is not known). The rickettsial organism and canine herpesvirus cause vasculitis characterized by cell necrosis and increased vascular permeability that results in perivascular hemorrhage and edema. In RMSF, early signs may include petechial and ecchymotic hemorrhages of the skin and mucous membranes, epistaxis, hematuria, and melena. Canine herpesvirus-associated disease is associated with multiple hemorrhages in various tissues, including the liver, kidneys, brain, gastrointestinal tract, and lung. RMSF can be diagnosed using an immunofluorescence assay on paired acute and convalescent serums. Evaluation of IgM levels may also help in the determination of the course of the disease. Antibiotic treatment for RMSF includes tetracycline, doxycycline, chloramphenicol, and fluoroquinolones (enrofloxacin). However, enrofloxacin is not recommended for use in young animals. In the case of canine herpesvirus, puppies often die within 24 hours, leaving little time for diagnostic procedures. Additional information about canine herpesvirus can be found in Chapter 16. Synthesis of most of the coagulation, antithrombotic, and fibrinolytic proteins, as well as clearance of activated coagulation factors and products of fibrinolysis, occurs in the liver. Because coagulation proteins have relatively short half-lives, liver disease may lead to a rapid decrease in factor activity. Levels of coagulation factors must decrease to less than 30% of normal values to affect the coagulation screening tests. However, it has been reported that APTT and PT were abnormal in up to two thirds of dogs with liver disease. Coagulation screening tests are not specific for a particular liver pathology and cannot be used as predictive tests. Paradoxically, vWF and fibrinogen may be increased in liver disease, as fibrinogen is an acute phase reactant and vWF is synthesized primarily by endothelial cells.

Disseminated intravascular coagulation is an overwhelming activation of coagulation proteins and platelets, often accompanied by enhanced fibrinolysis. DIC occurs secondarily to various diseases or events: viral, bacterial, protozoal, and rickettsial infections, parasite migration, trauma, heat stroke, burns, and shock. In the acute phases of disease, disseminated microclots are quickly formed and lysed throughout the body, which leads to consumption of many of the coagulation and antithrombotic proteins, as well as consumption of platelets. As a result, DIC is characterized by prolonged ACT, PT, APTT, and TT, elevated FDPs, decreased levels of AT, and thrombocytopenia. Young animals are more at risk for DIC because of immature clotting mechanisms and reduced levels of AT and protein C. Chronic DIC may be more difficult to detect because the bone marrow and liver compensate for loss of coagulation factors and platelets. This compensation may result in a normalization of the screening tests or even a hypercoagulable state. The key to control DIC is identification and treatment of the underlying disease, but supportive fluid therapy to maintain fluid volume and organ perfusion is critical to the patient's recovery. Plasma transfusions also may be used to increase levels of AT and coagulation factors.

Although obtaining appropriate samples, whether it is blood or tissue aspirates, from neonates and young cats and dogs can be challenging, it is an essential component of diagnosing the various diseases and conditions that can affect these young animals. Additionally, although information is available regarding reference values for some hematology parameters, one should remember that to obtain usable, interpretable data from the small samples available from very young, sick animals, sample(s) from an age-matched animal, usually a normal littermate, should be obtained for comparison.

SUGGESTED READINGS

Ettinger SJ, Feldman EC (eds): *Textbook of veterinary internal medicine*, ed 7, St Louis, 2010, Saunders/Elsevier.

Feldman BF, Zinkl JG, Jain NC (eds): *Schalm's veterinary hematology*, ed 5, Philadelphia, 2000, Lippincott Williams & Wilkins.

Jain NC: *Essentials of veterinary hematology*, Philadelphia, 1993, Lea & Febiger.

Merck Veterinary Manual: www.merckvetmanual.com: Circulatory System, Immune System, Clinical Pathology Procedures/Diagnostic Procedures for the Private Practice Laboratory/Hematology.

Tizard IR: *Veterinary immunology: an introduction*, ed 8, St Louis, 2009, Saunders/Elsevier.

THE RESPIRATORY SYSTEM

CHAPTER 34

Craig Ruaux

Diseases of the respiratory system are common reasons for presentation of neonatal and immature dogs and cats. The respiratory system represents a large percentage of the total surface area of the body exposed to the external environment. With extensive mucosal surfaces in the nasal passage and trachea, as well as the very large surface area of the respiratory bronchioles and alveoli, the respiratory system is a frequent site of entry for the major viral and bacterial pathogens likely to affect puppies and kittens. Respiratory diseases in the puppy and kitten can rapidly proceed to severe, life-threatening disorders if they are not recognized early.

NORMAL RESPIRATORY SYSTEM DEVELOPMENT

The embryology of the respiratory system, including the nasal passages, larynx, trachea, bronchi, and alveolar tissue of the lungs, is highly complex. The primordial respiratory system arises as an outpouching of the embryonic foregut. This outpouching subsequently develops via elongation into the respiratory diverticulum. The respiratory diverticulum remains contiguous with the embryonic foregut during development, with the connection forming the pharynx. As the embryo develops, the respiratory diverticulum elongates and bifurcates at the blind end of the pouch, forming bronchial buds, the primordia of the lungs. The trachea subsequently develops from the section of the respiratory diverticulum cranial to the bronchial buds. The bronchial buds undergo extensive bifurcation to form the bronchial tree. Each bronchial bud bifurcates between 14 and 18 times, eventually resulting in the extensive system of terminal bronchioles. Each terminal bronchiole will then subdivide another two to three times to yield the respiratory bronchioles. Respiratory bronchioles represent a transitional zone between the air-conducting structures of the upper airways and the alveolar tissue, in which gas exchange takes place. At birth, the lungs are not fully developed. Alveolar growth and formation of additional respiratory bronchioles continue for some period after birth. In the puppy, almost all the alveolar stage (the final stage of lung development) occurs in the initial postnatal period.

During fetal life the lungs are not inflated and are not functional from a respiratory perspective. The fetal lung tissue is filled with fluid secreted by the pulmonary epithelial cells and mucosal glands. The presence of a normal quantity of this fluid within the developing lung is an important stimulus for ongoing expansion of the alveolar tissue. Insufficient production of this fluid is associated with pulmonary hypoplasia. During the later stages of fetal life, respiratory muscle activity commences. The fetus "breathes" fluid secretions from the pulmonary epithelium and a small amount of amniotic fluid. This breathing action prepares the respiratory muscles for activity in the postnatal period. In the last stages of fetal development, the pulmonary epithelium commences the synthesis of surfactant. This fluid forms a phospholipid layer over the alveolar surface, dramatically reducing the surface tension of the alveoli. Adequate surfactant formation is critical to the early stages of postnatal life. Inadequate surfactant production may be associated with acute respiratory distress in the newborn and in fading puppy or kitten syndromes.

In some scenarios when assisted mating and elective cesarean section delivery are planned, there may be uncertainty regarding adequate development of surfactant. Inadequate surfactant in the neonate will complicate peripartum management. While the puppies are still fetal and before delivery, the presence of surfactant can be indirectly documented using the "foam stability test." This technique was originally used in human obstetric medicine as a rapid test to determine the timing of a cesarean section. One milliliter of amniotic fluid is collected (via ultrasound-guided centesis or laparotomy) and is mixed with 1 ml of 100% ethanol in a glass tube. The solution is then vigorously shaken for 15 seconds. If surfactant is present, a ring of bubbles will form

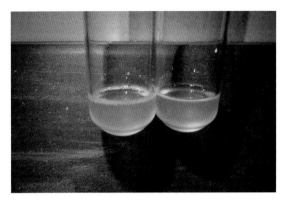

Figure 34-1 Foam stability test. Equal volumes (1 ml) of amniotic fluid and ethanol are added to a glass tube and shaken vigorously for 15 seconds. The ring of foam (bubbles) around the glass tube at the air-fluid interface indicates that surfactant is present in the sample on the left but not in the sample on the right. (Courtesy Dr. M. Kutzler.)

TABLE 34-1	Characteristics of obstructive and restrictive breathing patterns	
Pattern	**Obstructive**	**Restrictive**
Respiratory depth	Increased	Shallow
Respiratory rate	Normal to mild increase	Markedly increased
Inspiratory dyspnea	Extrathoracic airways	Not typically distinguished
Expiratory dyspnea	Intrathoracic airways	Not typically distinguished

at the fluid-air interface and remain for at least 15 minutes (Figure 34-1). In human obstetrics, this method was used as a surgery room test to indicate fetal readiness for delivery. Results of this test in elective cesarean section delivery of canine fetuses have indicated that adequate surfactant production is not present until 62 days past the luteinizing hormone (LH) surge for female canine fetuses and 63 days past the LH surge for male canine fetuses. This sex difference is consistent with observations in human obstetrics, as female fetuses begin surfactant production earlier than males.

CLINICAL EXAMINATION OF THE RESPIRATORY SYSTEM

It is important to remember that some aspects of respiratory system development continue to occur in the postnatal period. Thus physical examination findings of neonatal puppies and kittens are expected to differ from older puppies and kittens and the young adult animal. Typically puppies and kittens have more rapid breathing rates and shallower respiratory excursions than adults. The cardinal sign of respiratory disease is dyspnea or respiratory distress. Respiratory distress may manifest as increased respiratory rate, increased respiratory effort, decreased exercise tolerance, increased respiratory sounds, or acute collapse. The initial physical examination of an animal presented in respiratory distress should be brisk, thorough enough to provide initial diagnostic information, and carried out in a manner that causes minimal distress to the patient. In some circumstances, it may be appropriate to conduct the initial examination and triage without the animal's owner present in the room to reduce the stress on both the patient and the owner.

Panting in dogs is a normal response to increased heat load and is not normally considered pathological. In the kitten or young cat, however, panting is almost always a sign of significant respiratory distress. Open-mouth breathing in both puppies and kittens is considered a strong indicator of respiratory distress. Animals presented in severe respiratory distress should receive supplemental oxygen therapy. This may be necessary before detailed examination can take place. Supply of supplemental oxygen using an oxygen cage is usually less stressful than via a mask and is more effective than flow-by oxygen delivery. If an oxygen cage is not available, however, all efforts should be made to supply supplemental oxygen in a minimally stressful manner. Some patients with dyspnea are panicked and struggle excessively. In these patients, sedation may be helpful and, in some cases, lifesaving.

Respiratory Patterns

Definition of the phase of the respiratory cycle showing the greatest alteration in respiratory effort can be helpful in defining an initial list of differential diagnoses and formulating a diagnostic plan. The general characteristics of the two main pathological respiratory patterns, obstructive and restrictive, are summarized in Table 34-1. Respiratory diseases that lead to restriction of the airway diameter typically present with an *obstructive* breathing pattern. In a patient presenting with a typical obstructive breathing pattern, respiratory rate is mildly to moderately increased, and the depth of respiratory excursions is usually increased. Obstructive breathing patterns may be seen with conditions affecting either the extrathoracic or intrathoracic airways. With obstructive lesions in the upper airways, inhalation tends to cause worsening obstruction as a result of decreasing airway diameter. Therefore patients with upper airway obstruction tend to show increased respiratory effort on inhalation. The reverse applies in lower airway obstructive diseases, as the diseased airways are more likely to collapse during exhalation, leading to increased expiratory effort. Respiratory diseases that limit the ability of the lungs and airways to expand lead to a *restrictive* breathing pattern. Inability to expand the lung parenchyma leads to a reduction in respiratory excursions. Patients presenting with restrictive breathing patterns show a shallow depth of respiration and increased respiratory rate in an attempt to maintain adequate ventilation. Restrictive breathing patterns may be seen with diseases

---

BOX 34-1   Common differential diagnoses of obstructive and restrictive breathing patterns and tachypnea in puppies, kittens, and young dogs and cats

Obstructive	**Tachypnea**	**Restrictive**
Brachycephalic airway syndrome	Metabolic acidosis	Congenital emphysema
Cleft palate	Anemia	Pulmonary edema
Everted laryngeal saccules	Heat stress and heat stroke	Electrocution injury
Feline asthma	Exercise	Cardiac disease
Foreign body inhalation (acute onset)	Metabolic acidosis	Pleural effusions
Lymphadenopathy	Anemia	Pyothorax
Severe inflammation, lymphosarcoma (thymic)	Heat stress	Hemorrhage
Nasopharyngeal polyp	Heat stroke	Transudative effusions
Severe inflammation	Exercise	Pneumothorax
Bacterial, viral, fungal, or allergic etiologies		Traumatic wounds
Stenotic nares		Flail chest
Tracheal collapse		Rib fractures
Tracheal hypoplasia		Diaphragmatic hernia
		Pleuroperitoneal hernia
		Peritoneopericardial hernia

---

affecting either the lung parenchyma or the pleural space. In particular, space-occupying lesions of the pleural cavity (e.g., pleural effusion, diaphragmatic hernia, pneumothorax, and pleuroperitoneal or peritoneopericardial hernias) may severely restrict the ability of the lungs to expand during inflation.

Thoracic auscultation is an integral part of the physical examination of animals with respiratory disease. The thorax of the neonate and very young puppy and kitten is much smaller than in adults. Auscultation with specific neonatal and pediatric stethoscopes is recommended to increase accuracy when attempting to localize respiratory sounds. The neonatal puppy has a normal respiratory rate at rest between 25 and 35 breaths/min for the first 2 weeks of life. Between 3 and 4 weeks of age, the normal respiratory rate decreases to between 15 and 25 breaths/min. After 4 weeks, most puppies show respiratory rates appropriate for adult dogs, including the onset of panting for thermoregulation. In theory, animals with upper airway obstructive disease have louder respiratory sounds on inhalation. Lower airway obstructive diseases (e.g., feline asthma) will tend to have louder respiratory noise on exhalation. In practice, it is often difficult to localize respiratory pathology with this degree of certainty. Even when signs of the respiratory pathology are localized to one area, this does not rule out the presence of disease in other regions. Animals with restrictive pulmonary diseases tend to have an overall reduction in the volume of breath sounds. Pleural effusions tend to settle to the ventral pleural cavity; therefore lung sounds may be muffled ventrally and prominent dorsally. In patients with pneumothorax, on the other hand, the lungs may settle ventrally, leading to muffled lung sounds dorsally. Although the lung sounds overall are decreased with restrictive diseases, auscultation directly over the partially collapsed lung tissue may reveal

harsh respiratory sounds and pleural friction rubs. Common differential diagnoses of obstructive and restrictive breathing patterns are summarized in Box 34-1.

Diagnostic Imaging

Radiography of the thorax is indicated in the assessment of animals with lower airway, pulmonary parenchymal, and pleural space diseases. Radiographic examination should be delayed until the patient is stable. Sedation and supplemental oxygen delivery via mask are often necessary to achieve diagnostic quality radiographs. The radiographic signs of respiratory disease (e.g., presence of air bronchograms with an alveolar pattern or peribronchial cuffing with bronchial disease) are common between the young animal and adults. In the young animal, the thymus is often prominent, and there may be significant brown fat deposits in the cranial mediastinum. Care should be taken to avoid overinterpretation of these findings. Advanced imaging methods (e.g., computed tomography, magnetic resonance imaging) are becoming increasingly available. These imaging modalities allow selective reconstruction of three-dimensional data and may be very useful for the assessment of cranial mediastinal structures, peribronchial lymph nodes, and congenital anomalies (e.g., peritoneopericardial hernias). Computed tomography is the imaging modality of choice for assessment of the nasal cavity and sinuses in most cases of chronic nasal disease.

Endoscopic Examination

Endoscopic examination of the airways, particularly with flexible endoscopic equipment, is a valuable method for assessing the respiratory system. This method is particularly appropriate to assess the nasopharynx, chronic lower airway diseases, and for detection of upper airway obstructive lesions. Collapsing trachea, tracheal hypoplasia, bronchial collapse, and abnormalities of laryngeal function may all be readily detected. Cytological samples may be obtained via brushing the upper airways or bronchoalveolar lavage of the lower airways. Laryngoscopic and bronchoscopic examination technique is the same in puppies and kittens as in older dogs and cats and carries similar risks. The smaller size of the airways in younger animals requires the use of endoscopic equipment with a finer diameter than in adult animals. Care must be taken to ensure adequate oxygen delivery as the endoscope will often occupy a large proportion of the airway. In puppies and kittens, rhinoscopic examination is a relatively low-yield procedure because the very narrow nasal passages often prevent thorough examination. Chronic nasal passage disease in puppies and kittens is better assessed through computed tomographic examination of the nasal cavity and sinuses.

CONGENITAL ANOMALIES OF THE RESPIRATORY SYSTEM

Brachycephalic Airway Syndrome

The brachycephalic airway syndrome is a common cause of respiratory distress in affected brachycephalic breeds. This condition is frequently identified in English Bulldogs, French Bulldogs, Pugs, Boston Terriers, Shih-Tzus, and Boxers. Although this condition is generally held to be heritable, the mode of inheritance has not been identified in any affected breed. Brachycephalic airway syndrome is much less commonly observed in brachycephalic cat breeds, but feline cases have been reported. Affected animals will display increased inspiratory effort and disordered respiration during sleep. Clinical signs are common from an early age in affected breeds. Essentially all British Bulldog puppies show abnormal respiration during sleep from the age of 2 weeks onward.

Primary lesions of brachycephalic airway syndrome are stenotic nares and soft palate elongation. Eversion of the laryngeal saccules is a common secondary condition. Tracheal hypoplasia, tracheal collapse, and laryngeal collapse, if present, are associated with more severe presentations. Development of the brachycephalic airway syndrome is related to the anatomical narrowing of the nasal passages and upper airways common to these breeds. Prolonged exposure of the airways to marked negative intraairway pressure leads to dynamic collapse of these airways, further decreasing the airway lumen and requiring greater respiratory effort. The soft palate further elongates, while the soft tissue of the pharynx swells and becomes redundant. Increased turbulence of airflow in the pharynx and upper airways acts as an inflammatory stimulus, exacerbating the soft tissue swelling. Soft tissue swelling and turbulent airflow are responsible for the characteristic marked stridor exhibited by these breeds.

A diagnosis of brachycephalic airway syndrome should be suspected in any brachycephalic animal presented for respiratory distress. Diagnosis of the component disorders of this syndrome typically requires a combination of clinical

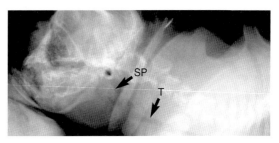

Figure 34-2 Lateral radiograph of skull and upper airways from a 6-month-old British Bulldog with severe brachycephalic airway syndrome. Note the dramatically compressed nasal cavity architecture and elongated, thickened soft palate *(SP)* overlying the epiglottis. The tracheal diameter *(T)* is also reduced.

examination, upper airway examination via laryngoscopy, and diagnostic imaging. Stenotic nares are readily visible during physical examination. Elongation of the soft palate can be documented via visual examination of the distal pharynx or radiographic examination of the upper airways (Figure 34-2). The normal soft palate should just overlap the epiglottis, whereas in brachycephalic airway syndrome the soft palate extends more than 3 mm caudal to the tip of the epiglottis and may completely occlude the epiglottic opening. In symptomatic individuals, early resection of the elongated soft palate is associated with a better long-term prognosis. Although the technique for surgical resection of an elongated palate is relatively simple, these patients represent a significant anesthetic risk and must be managed aggressively in the perioperative period to avoid swelling of the surgical site and acute upper airway obstruction. Placement of a temporary tracheostomy may be required in some patients.

Everted laryngeal saccules, when present, are readily visible as smooth swellings at the ventral aspect of the opening of the glottis. These structures are readily removed via surgical resection. Removal of everted laryngeal saccules is often combined with correction of stenotic nares and soft palate resection during the one anesthetic procedure. Everted laryngeal saccules are the first stage of laryngeal collapse. Their presence implies significant upper airway pathology and indicates a need for surgical intervention before more severe laryngeal collapse occurs.

Stenotic Nares

Stenotic nares is a common congenital condition of brachycephalic breeds in both dogs and cats. On external examination, the dorsolateral nasal cartilages are medially displaced, impinging on the external nasal opening and dramatically decreasing the available lumen. Stertorous and stridorous inspiratory noise, coughing, reduced exercise tolerance, and sleep disturbances are common in affected animals. The presence of stenotic nares is thought to be a predisposing factor for development of the other changes present in the brachycephalic airway syndrome as previously described. Early intervention may reduce the likelihood or severity of these secondary changes and is recommended in most young animals with stenotic nares. Weight control and exercise restriction may be beneficial. The most direct approach to management of this condition is via surgical resection of the affected dorsolateral nasal cartilages. This technique is described in detail in most textbooks of small animal surgery. Given the greater difficulty of managing patients with more advanced brachycephalic airway syndrome, early surgical correction of the stenotic nares is recommended, particularly if the puppy or kitten is symptomatic.

Laryngeal Collapse

Laryngeal collapse is a severe complication of brachycephalic airway syndrome. As laryngeal collapse is caused by chronic upper airway obstruction, this condition is usually not diagnosed until after the animal is 6 months of age. Laryngeal collapse begins with eversion of the laryngeal saccules as discussed previously. Stage II laryngeal collapse occurs when one or both of the aryepiglottic folds deviates medially, obstructing the ventral glottis. Stage III laryngeal collapse is present when the corniculate processes of the arytenoid cartilages are displaced medially and fail to be abducted during respiration. Stage II and stage III laryngeal collapses usually occur in animals older than 2 years but may be present in younger animals with severe upper respiratory tract obstructive disease. Medical management for severe respiratory distress and weight loss programs are indicated in management of these patients. Surgical correction of the upper airways is the treatment of choice. Patients with stage II or stage III laryngeal collapse are very high-risk anesthesia candidates, and aggressive postsurgical management with preemptive placement of a tracheostomy may be necessary.

Hypoplastic Trachea

Hypoplastic trachea is a congenital anomaly of tracheal development that is common in the British Bulldog and Boston Terrier and is occasionally diagnosed in the Boxer. This condition is commonly diagnosed in association with the brachycephalic airway syndrome but represents a distinct entity. In animals with a hypoplastic trachea, the free ends of the tracheal cartilage rings occur in apposition or overlap. This dramatically reduces the tracheal cross-sectional diameter. Clinical signs of tracheal hypoplasia are often apparent within the first 6 months of life and may include decreased exercise tolerance, syncope, coughing, and respiratory distress. In many cases, brachycephalic airway syndrome is present. Therapeutic interventions are directed toward other causes of upper airway obstruction and therapy for chronic upper airway infection, if present. The diagnosis of hypoplastic trachea is typically made radiographically either by dividing the tracheal diameter by the thoracic inlet diameter (TD/TI) or by comparing the width of the trachea to the third rib where they cross. The normal TD/TI is 0.16 or greater, and the trachea should be at least 2 times the diameter of the third rib. Although a TD/TI of 0.16 or greater is considered normal for most breeds of dogs, British Bulldogs are considered to be normal with a TD/TI greater than 0.09 (Figure 34-3).

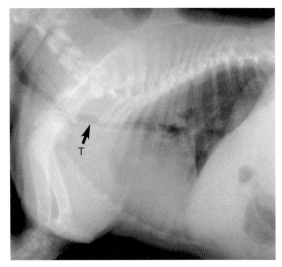

Figure 34-3 Lateral radiograph of the thorax from a 6-month-old British Bulldog with hypoplastic trachea. Note the decreased diameter of the intrathoracic trachea *(T)* when compared with the thoracic inlet. The TD/TI ratio in this dog is 9%. This dog also shows fat deposits and residual thymus visible as a soft tissue density in the cranial mediastinum. This is a normal finding in dogs of this age.

Cleft Palate

Congenital abnormalities of the lips, hard palate, and soft palate are relatively common in puppies and kittens. There is a predisposition for development of this condition in brachycephalic breeds. Beagles, Cocker Spaniels, Dachshunds, German Shepherd Dogs, Labrador Retrievers, Schnauzers, Shetland Sheepdogs, and Siamese cats also show increased incidence. In most cases, cleft palate is a genetic disorder with varying modes of inheritance in differing breeds. In the Brittany Spaniel, cleft palate is thought to be autosomal recessive. However, in the West Highland White Terrier, the condition is polygenic and does not display a single gene mode of inheritance. Exposure of the bitch to teratogenic compounds may also lead to cleft palate in the offspring. Primidone, griseofulvin, and sulfa-based antibiotics should be avoided in the pregnant bitch to reduce the likelihood of cleft palate. Despite the teratogenic potential, most cases of cleft palate in puppies and kittens are genetic in origin.

Affected animals often present with upper respiratory disease. Common presenting complaints include sneezing, gagging, coughing, and discharge of milk or soft food from the nares. Growth of affected animals is often slower than littermates. These patients are predisposed to aspiration pneumonia, laryngotracheitis, and chronic rhinitis. Depending on the size and location of the lesion, surgical closure of the cleft may be possible. Surgical techniques for palate closure typically rely on the creation of sliding pedicles of the existing oral mucosa and underlying hard palate bone. Surgery is usually delayed until the puppy or kitten is more than 16 weeks of age to allow maturation of the oral mucosae.

More detailed descriptions of surgical techniques for cleft palate reconstruction can be found in most textbooks of small animal surgery. Frequently more than one surgical procedure will be necessary to achieve complete repair of the cleft palate.

Diaphragmatic Hernia

Defects of the diaphragm, allowing abdominal viscera to enter the thoracic cavity, may dramatically reduce the potential space within the thoracic cavity and lead to respiratory distress. The most common presentation of diaphragmatic hernia is a traumatic pleuroperitoneal hernia. Patients presenting with this condition will typically have acute onset of respiratory distress. The respiratory distress is commonly restrictive in character. Breath sounds may be reduced in the region of the thorax occupied by the displaced viscera. If recent, other signs of trauma (e.g., shredded nails, bruising, oral lesions) may be noted. Diaphragmatic hernias are usually readily diagnosed radiographically (Figure 34-4). Following immediate stabilization with sedation, pain control, and supplemental oxygen, traumatic diaphragmatic hernias are best managed by surgical repair.

Peritoneopericardial Hernia

Peritoneopericardial hernia is the most common of the congenital diaphragmatic defects in dogs and cats. These hernias may be simultaneously present in several members of a litter, implying a genetic basis for this disorder. The mode of inheritance is not known for any breed. A ventral defect in the diaphragm communicating with the caudal mediastinum allows access of abdominal viscera into the pericardial sac. The clinical signs of peritoneopericardial hernia are variable and depend on the abdominal organ(s) entrapped within the pericardium. Gastrointestinal, cardiovascular, or respiratory signs may dominate. With marked pericardial sac enlargement, restrictive respiratory signs may be noted. Incarceration of stomach or intestines, particularly if the blood supply to the affected organ is compromised, may lead to rapid deterioration in the clinical state of the patient. Radiographically, the cardiac silhouette is typically enlarged and rounded. In many cases with cardiovascular or respiratory signs, primary cardiac disease may be suspected. Pericardial ultrasonography reveals the presence of abdominal organs within the pericardial sac. Management of symptomatic peritoneopericardial hernia is via corrective surgery.

Congenital Pleuroperitoneal Hernia

Congenital pleuroperitoneal hernias are much less commonly diagnosed than peritoneopericardial hernias. The genetic basis and mode of inheritance of this condition are unknown. Many puppies and kittens with congenital pleuroperitoneal hernia are either stillborn or die soon after birth, as the presence of abdominal viscera within the thorax restricts the ability of the neonatal lungs to expand. The defect in congenital pleuroperitoneal hernias is often dorsolateral in the diaphragm.

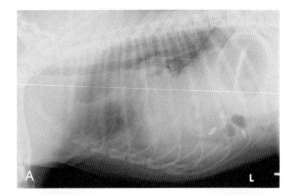

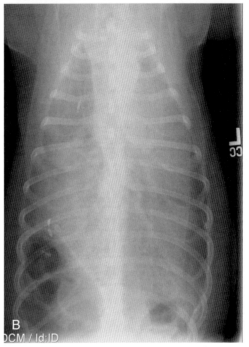

Figure 34-4 Lateral **(A)** and dorsoventral **(B)** radiographic views of the thorax from a young dog with traumatic diaphragmatic hernia. Note the presence of gas-filled bowel loops, radiodense material, and soft tissue densities within the thoracic cavity and occluding the cardiac silhouette.

Laryngeal Hypoplasia

Congenital hypoplasia of the larynx has been reported in brachycephalic dog breeds and the Skye terrier. In the Skye Terrier, the condition is inherited as a simple autosomal recessive. The laryngeal cartilages fail to develop correctly, and the larynx is excessively flexible and prone to dynamic collapse. The epiglottic opening is narrow, and the vocal folds fail to abduct during respiration. Clinical signs are of chronic upper airway obstructive disease and are present from an early age. Surgical intervention carries a high risk of laryngeal stricture and further upper airway collapse. The prognosis for animals with congenital laryngeal collapse is guarded to poor.

Laryngeal Paralysis

Congenital laryngeal paralysis is recognized in Bouvier des Flandres, Dalmatians, Siberian Huskies, and Husky-crosses. In the Bouvier des Flandres, this condition occurs as a discrete disorder and shows an autosomal dominant mode of inheritance. In the Dalmatian, this condition shows an autosomal recessive mode of inheritance. The condition is typically associated with a generalized distal neuropathy. The mode of inheritance in Huskies and Husky-crosses has not been defined.

Clinical signs of congenital laryngeal paralysis usually appear at 4 to 6 months of age and include obstructive respiratory pattern, reduced exercise tolerance, changes in phonation, dyspnea, and gagging or coughing while eating or drinking. These clinical signs are similar to those seen in adult dogs with idiopathic laryngeal paralysis. Congenital laryngeal paralysis in the Bouvier des Flandres may be managed surgically via arytenoid lateralization. Management of Dalmatians with congenital laryngeal paralysis is typically complicated by concurrent neuropathy.

Pectus Excavatum

Pectus excavatum is the result of a sternal malformation, with the sternum impinging into the thoracic cavity and the ventral rib ends turned medially to meet the displaced sternum. This condition is commonly diagnosed in kittens and puppies and may be obvious from an early age. Severe displacement of the sternum may lead to reduced compliance of the thoracic cage and respiratory distress. Many cases of pectus excavatum are mild, cause no appreciable respiratory distress, and require no specific treatment. Severely affected individuals may require surgical management.

Primary Ciliary Dyskinesia

Primary ciliary dyskinesia, also called "immotile cilia syndrome," is a relatively uncommon diagnosis in companion animals. Originating from a congenital absence or defect in the ciliary protein dynein, primary ciliary dyskinesia results in defective mucociliary clearance from the upper airways. Disturbed mucociliary clearance predisposes the animal to recurrent, chronic rhinitis, sinusitis, and bronchopneumonia. Clinical signs may be obvious from birth. Definitive diagnosis of this condition may be challenging and relies on demonstration of decreased mucociliary clearance. Decreased clearance is documented by timing the movement through the upper airways of a drop of macroaggregated albumin labeled with Technetium[99]. Management revolves around the control of upper airway infections, possibly requiring continuous antibiotic therapy. Supportive care with mucolytic agents may be beneficial. Primary ciliary dyskinesia is one component of Kartagener syndrome. This syndrome also includes situs inversus, bronchiectasis, and chronic sinusitis. Affected males with Kartagener syndrome are usually sterile because of decreased motility of the sperm.

ACQUIRED CONDITIONS OF THE RESPIRATORY SYSTEM

Acute Respiratory Distress Syndrome

Acute respiratory distress syndrome is a descriptive term for severe deterioration in respiratory function that may occur in patients with other, often critical, systemic illnesses. Acute respiratory distress syndrome is not a specific disease process but is a common terminal event in patients with sepsis, severe systemic inflammatory response syndrome, inhalation injuries (e.g., smoke, aspiration pneumonia, and meconium aspiration), pancreatitis, and severe trauma. Inflammatory change in the pulmonary parenchyma leads to increased pulmonary capillary permeability and alveolar dysfunction. Severe, noncardiogenic pulmonary edema may develop rapidly. Acute respiratory distress syndrome may occur in puppies or kittens in association with septicemic illnesses or trauma. Affected animals may be found dead. If onset of clinical signs is noted, affected puppies or kittens may die within hours. Acute respiratory distress syndrome may be the terminal event in fading puppy or fading kitten syndromes.

Management of acute respiratory distress syndrome is extremely challenging, particularly in the neonate or young individual. Artificial ventilation via mechanical means is often necessary; for greatest benefit, positive end-expiratory pressure ventilation is usually indicated. These highly critical and fragile patients should be transferred to a dedicated critical care facility where possible. Prognosis is guarded to grave. Most patients will succumb to either the primary disease process or progressive loss of respiratory function.

Aspiration Pneumonia

Aspiration pneumonia is more commonly diagnosed in puppies than kittens, but both species are susceptible. In many cases, aspiration pneumonia occurs secondary to esophageal or pharyngeal dysfunction, particularly congenital megaesophagus, persistent right aortic arch, or cricopharyngeal achalasia. These conditions often manifest around the time of weaning and the transition to solid food. Aspiration pneumonia may also occur in bottle-reared puppies and kittens following inhalation of milk replacement formulas or with misplacement of a gastric feeding tube. Aspiration pneumonia is also a risk following anesthesia if the patient regurgitates.

The clinical signs of aspiration pneumonia are essentially the same as infectious pneumonia (e.g., increased respiratory rate, fever, productive cough) and typically develop rapidly following aspiration. Radiographic signs of aspiration pneumonia may not be present until 12 to 24 hours after aspiration (Figure 34-5). Right cranial and medial lung lobes are most commonly affected in animals who aspirate while in sternal recumbency or upright; other lobes may be affected if the animal aspirates under anesthesia, depending on positioning at the time of regurgitation. Aspiration pneumonia is managed using the same principles as infectious pneumonia. Treatment is described in the section on infectious pneumonia below.

Meconium Aspiration

In human neonates, meconium aspiration syndrome is recognized as a severe, potentially life-threatening condition occurring during the perinatal period. Risk factors for

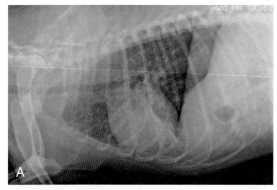

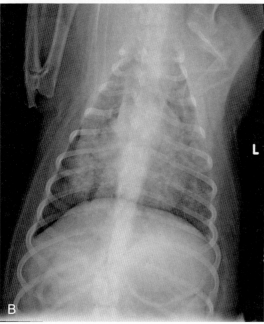

Figure 34-5 Left lateral **(A)** and dorsoventral **(B)** radiographic views of the thorax from a 5-month-old dog with aspiration pneumonia. Note the heavy alveolar pattern and air bronchograms, particularly visible in the dorsoventral projection and overlaying the cardiac silhouette in the left lateral view.

aspiration of meconium in human infants include perinatal fetal stress, prolonged delivery, fetal hypoxia, and fetal acidosis. Aspiration of meconium leads to severe pneumonitis and aspiration pneumonia. Although puppies are used as models for human meconium aspiration syndrome, the occurrence of this condition under natural circumstances is rare. Induction of meconium aspiration syndrome in puppies requires instillation of acid solution and meconium into the upper airways, a scenario that is unlikely to occur during natural whelping.

Infectious Tracheobronchitis

Canine infectious tracheobronchitis, also commonly known as "kennel cough" or canine cough, is a highly contagious upper respiratory disease. This condition results from infection with a complex of infectious organisms. *Bordetella bronchiseptica*, canine parainfluenza virus, and *Mycoplasma* spp. are the most frequent causative agents. However, canine

distemper virus, canine herpesvirus, adenoviruses, and reoviruses 1 to 3 may all be involved. More information pertaining to viral diseases can be found in Chapter 16. In adult dogs, this condition is typically self-limiting. In puppies and young adult dogs, more serious disease may be seen. Affected dogs typically have a history of recent exposure to other dogs and acute onset of a harsh, paroxysmal "goose honk" cough. Gentle pressure on the cervical trachea will typically trigger a bout of paroxysmal coughing in these patients. Other clinical signs commonly noted include fever, depression, oculonasal discharge, and conjunctivitis.

The diagnosis of infectious tracheobronchitis is typically made from the characteristic clinical signs and history of recent exposure to other dogs. The recently recognized canine influenza (see next section) is an important differential diagnosis. In uncomplicated cases, additional diagnostics (e.g., thoracic radiography, culture of airway fluids) are usually not indicated. In more severely ill individuals, particularly when secondary bronchopneumonia is suspected, thoracic radiographs should be obtained.

Antimicrobial therapy is indicated in systemically ill patients, especially those with secondary bronchopneumonia. Ideally antibiotic selection should be guided by culture and sensitivity results from airway lavage fluids. Amoxicillin with clavulanic acid or chloramphenicol are both reasonable empiric choices, as most isolates of *B. bronchiseptica* and *Mycoplasma* spp. from affected dogs are susceptible. Antitussive therapy may be used in cases where there is no evidence of bronchopneumonia.

Infectious tracheobronchitis is less common in kittens but may be caused by any of the viruses that lead to upper respiratory tract infections. Typically signs of more upper respiratory tract disease (e.g., sneezing, oculonasal discharge) will predominate. *B. bronchiseptica* may play a role in some cases of feline infectious tracheobronchitis. This organism has been isolated as part of fatal respiratory infections in kittens.

Patients hospitalized with infectious tracheobronchitis should be isolated from other patients and barrier nursed. Isolation protocols should be defined and rigorously followed for patients showing signs of respiratory disease. All equipment and facilities used for hospitalization of infectious tracheobronchitis cases must be rigorously cleaned and disinfected after use. Clothing that becomes contaminated during handling of infected dogs must be changed before other patients are handled, and disposable gowns and gloves should be worn while handling infectious tracheobronchitis patients. Stethoscopes and other diagnostic equipment should be thoroughly cleaned and disinfected after use on patients with infectious tracheobronchitis. The use of dedicated diagnostic equipment such as stethoscopes and thermometers that remain within the isolation area is preferable to staff using their own equipment that will subsequently be used with uninfected patients. Ideally these patients should be housed in a dedicated isolation ward or room with separate ventilation from the remainder of the hospital. Maintenance of slight negative pressure within the isolation facility while animals are present will reduce the likelihood of airborne spread of pathogens.

Canine Influenza

A member of the type A Orthomyxovirus family, in common with equine, avian, and human influenza, canine influenza is a highly contagious viral disease affecting dogs. Dogs of all ages are susceptible. As the canine population becomes exposed to this organism and older animals develop effective immunity, cases are more likely to be seen in puppies and young adult dogs. Canine influenza arose as a result of cross-species transfer of a strain of equine influenza to dogs. At the time of writing, canine influenza is endemic within the states of Florida, Colorado, and New Jersey, as well as the New York City region. Sporadic cases and seropositive dogs have been detected in many eastern U.S. states.

Canine influenza is spread by aerosol transmission in respiratory secretions and via fomites. The virus is enveloped and is apparently highly susceptible to killing by routine disinfectants (e.g., quaternary ammonium compounds) used in veterinary and boarding facilities. Isolation protocols should be defined for each individual practice; these protocols must be rigorously followed for patients showing signs of contagious respiratory disease. All equipment and facilities used for hospitalization of canine influenza cases must be rigorously cleaned and disinfected after use. Clothing that becomes contaminated during handling of infected dogs must be changed before other patients are handled, and disposable gowns and gloves should be worn while handling canine influenza patients. Stethoscopes and other diagnostic equipment should be thoroughly cleaned and disinfected after use on patients with canine influenza. The use of dedicated diagnostic equipment such as stethoscopes and thermometers that remain within the isolation area is preferable to staff using their own equipment that will subsequently be used with uninfected patients. Ideally these patients should be housed in a dedicated isolation ward or room with separate ventilation from the remainder of the hospital. Maintenance of slight negative pressure within the isolation facility while animals are present will reduce the likelihood of airborne spread of pathogens.

Canine influenza virus causes clinical disease mimicking infections caused by the *B. bronchiseptica*/parainfluenza virus complex; a consequence of this is that canine influenza is commonly mistaken for kennel cough. Clinical presentations of canine influenza may vary from mild to severe and life threatening. Essentially all dogs that are exposed to the virus become infected. Most dogs (about 80%) show a mild form of the disease, developing a persistent cough that is unresponsive to antibiotics or cough suppressants. Clinical signs typically persist for up to 21 days and are of similar severity in puppies and adult dogs. Infected dogs shed viral particles for 7 to 10 days after the onset of clinical signs. Some dogs will be more severely affected and show high fever and increased respiratory rate and respiratory effort. Thoracic radiographs may show severe consolidation of lung lobes, particularly if secondary bacterial bronchopneumonia is present.

Treatment for this condition is largely supportive in the majority of dogs with more mild clinical signs. Intravenous fluids, airway humidification, and nursing care may be necessary. In more severe cases, particularly those with severe pulmonary consolidation and secondary bacterial bronchopneumonia, broad-spectrum bactericidal antibiotic therapy becomes necessary. In addition, nutritional support, intravenous fluid therapy, airway humidification, mucolytic agents (e.g., *N*-acetylcysteine either via nebulization or orally at 50 mg/kg three times daily), and intensive nursing care are necessary. Patients hospitalized with severe disease should be isolated from other patients and barrier nursed. At the time of writing, there is no effective vaccine against canine influenza. There is no readily available, rapid diagnostic test for canine influenza. Serological detection of antibodies to the canine influenza virus and polymerase chain reaction methods to detect influenza virus infections are available via the Animal Health Diagnostic Center at Cornell University. To demonstrate recent infection via serology, paired serum samples collected at least 2 weeks apart are compared. A fourfold increase in titer in the convalescent sample is considered diagnostic for canine influenza. If an acute sample is not present, high titer against canine influenza only indicates previous infection at some time. This is not a strong diagnostic finding for recent respiratory disease.

Infectious Pneumonia

Infectious pneumonia in puppies and kittens usually represents a secondary process to some other underlying respiratory disease. Opportunist infections may develop secondary to aspiration pneumonia, meconium aspiration, following systemic spread of another infectious disease, or via extension from tracheobronchial diseases (e.g., infectious tracheobronchitis, canine influenza). Primary bacterial pneumonia is more commonly diagnosed in puppies than kittens. Any of several infectious agents (Box 34-2) may be present, either as mixed infections or a single agent. In kittens, *B. bronchiseptica* and *Pasteurella* spp. infections are more likely to result in primary bacterial pneumonia. Although kittens are less frequently affected than puppies, they are often more severely affected and may present critically ill. Secondary bacterial pneumonias following aspiration or foreign body inhalation may involve a broad variety of organisms, including oral or enteric flora. In endemic regions, fungal causes of pneumonia (e.g., *Coccidioides immitis*, *Blastomyces dermatitidis*) should be considered.

Puppies and kittens with pneumonia will typically present with increased respiratory rate, fever, and a productive cough. Respiratory sounds may be harsh. Crackles may be auscultated over the affected regions of the thorax. Wheezing is less common but may be heard if there is significant bronchial involvement. The combination of fever, productive cough, and tachypnea should lead the clinician to a strong suspicion of pneumonia. Radiographic findings with pneumonia are variable. Bacterial pneumonia typically shows a

BOX 34-2   Infectious organisms associated with pneumonia in puppies and kittens less than 12 months of age

Bacterial
Bordetella bronchiseptica
Streptococcus zooepidemicus
Pasteurella spp.

Fungal
Aspergillus spp. (disseminated)
Blastomyces dermatitidis
Coccidioides immitis
Candida albicans
Cryptococcus neoformans

Protozoal
Toxoplasma gondii
Pneumocystis carinii

Helminth
Aelurostrongylus abstrusus
Paragonimus kellicotti
Filaroides hirthi

BOX 34-3   Infectious organisms associated with infectious rhinitis and laryngitis in puppies and kittens

Viral (Kittens)
Feline rhinotracheitis virus (herpes)
Feline calicivirus
Feline reoviruses

Viral (Puppies)
Canine parainfluenza virus
Canine adenovirus 2
Canine distemper
Canine herpesvirus
Canine influenza

Bacterial
Staphylococcus intermedius
Chlamydia psittaci
Opportunist aerobes and anaerobes

Fungal
Cryptococcus neoformans (kittens)
Blastomyces dermatitidis
Aspergillus spp. (puppies)

cranioventral distribution of interstitial to alveolar patterns; viral pneumonias tend to show a more diffuse, interstitial pattern. Antibacterial therapy is critical to the management of bacterial pneumonia. Ideally antibiotic selection is based on the results of culture and sensitivity from lower airway lavage fluids or lung aspirates. However, the collection of these samples may represent a severe anesthetic risk in compromised patients. Awaiting results of these cultures may also unduly delay therapy in critical patients. Thus empirical use of broad-spectrum bactericidal antibiotics is usually recommended. In puppies, amoxicillin with clavulanic acid or trimethoprim with sulfonamide combinations are reasonable first-line choices for antibiotic therapy. In the kitten, both amoxicillin with clavulanic acid or a first-generation cephalosporin are reasonable options. Fluoroquinolones should be avoided because of the potential for cartilage damage in growing animals. Relatively long-term antibiotic therapy is required, for either 4 weeks or until 10 days after radiographic resolution.

Severely ill animals should be hospitalized and receive intravenous fluid therapy to maintain hydration. Clearance of inflammatory mucus and exudates is improved when the airways remain well hydrated. Local support of airway hydration by saline nebulization is beneficial. In addition, mucolytic agents (e.g., N-acetylcysteine), postural drainage maneuvers, and thoracic coupage should all be used to assist in removal of exudates. Cough suppression is contraindicated in these cases. Provision of additional oxygen, either via nasal oxygen cannula or use of a humidified oxygen environment cage, is beneficial. Patients hospitalized with pneumonia usually require intensive monitoring and nursing in a 24-hour care facility. Many patients with pneumonia are

inappetent. Particularly in the neonate, hypoglycemia and inadequate thermoregulation may complicate case management (see Chapter 2).

Infectious Rhinitis and Laryngitis

A broad variety of infectious agents potentially lead to rhinitis and laryngitis in the young dog and cat (Box 34-3). Viral upper respiratory disease is more common in the young cat than the dog, owing to extensive population vaccination against canine distemper virus. In the cat, viral upper respiratory disease is usually caused by the feline herpesvirus (type 1) and calicivirus. All young cats are susceptible before vaccination. Kittens in multi-cat households and cattery environments are at the greatest risk. Severe upper respiratory viral disease in young cats can be life threatening. Primary bacterial rhinitis is rare in both kittens and puppies. Bacterial involvement is usually secondary to an underlying disorder (e.g., viral rhinitis).

Viral upper respiratory disease in kittens is presumptively diagnosed based on age, history, and clinical signs. In individual patients, virus isolation is of little clinical value, as the therapy remains the same regardless of the causative organism. Virus isolation may be of benefit in a cattery with endemic disease for development of vaccination and quarantine protocols aimed at eliminating the infection. In the majority of kittens with viral upper respiratory disease, the condition is self-limiting. Outpatient therapy with broad-spectrum antibiotics to prevent secondary bacterial complications is appropriate. In more severely affected individuals, hospitalization for fluid support, parenteral antibiotic therapy, airway nebulization, nutritional support, and diligent nursing care may be necessary.

Fungal rhinitis is most commonly diagnosed in dolicho-cephalic dog breeds. It is unusual to diagnose fungal rhinitis in dogs less than 6 months of age. Most cases are caused by local infection with *Aspergillus* spp. The diagnosis is typically made on rhinoscopy, with observation of characteristic plaque lesions on the nasal mucosa or within the frontal sinuses. Fungal rhinitis caused by *Aspergillus* infection is most effectively treated via topical application or enilcon-azole or clotrimazole.

Infectious laryngitis is occasionally recognized as a discrete disorder without accompanying rhinitis. The major infectious organisms causing laryngitis in the puppy and kitten are the same as those that cause rhinitis. In puppies with acute laryngitis, there is typically an acute change of voice, paroxysmal coughing, gagging, and harsh respiratory sounds. With laryngitis as a discrete disease in the young dog, palpation of the trachea usually does not trigger paroxysmal coughing. Therapy for laryngitis in the dog is symptomatic and supportive. Some dogs require sedation to decrease anxiety and allow the laryngeal mucosa to heal. Antitussive medications provide symptomatic relief in many cases. Kittens and young cats with viral laryngitis typically develop laryngeal mucosal edema, voice changes, and stridor, rather than coughing.

Nasopharyngeal Polyp

Nasopharyngeal polyps are relatively common inflammatory mass lesions in young cats. These polyps originate from the epithelium of the tympanic membrane or auditory tube, usually following upper respiratory tract viral infection. The common isolation of feline calicivirus from these lesions suggests a role for this agent in initiation of the disease. Cats with nasopharyngeal polyps commonly present with stertorous respiration, even if the polyp is small. Nasopharyngeal polyps can usually be visualized in the nasopharynx under general anesthesia. Cranial retraction of the soft palate with a spay hook may aid in visualization of masses. Polyps in the nasopharynx can often be successfully removed via gentle traction under general anesthesia (Figure 34-6). When polyps are treated by removal with traction, removal should be followed by treatment with oral glucocorticoids at 1 to 2 mg/kg for 14 days with an additional tapering dose over 14 days. There is approximately 10% local recurrence. Cats with recurrent nasopharyngeal polyps may require middle ear surgery (bulla osteotomy) to resolve.

Pleural Effusion

The most common etiologies for pleural effusion in the puppy and kitten are pyothorax and the effusive form of feline infectious peritonitis, respectively. Patients presenting with pleural effusion will typically demonstrate a restrictive breathing pattern with shallow and rapid respiration. These patients often show respiratory distress at rest. Particularly in the kitten, respiratory distress at rest implies a severe disease process. These patients are at high risk for respiratory arrest if stressed during handling for radiography or sample collection. Sedation and the provision of supplemental

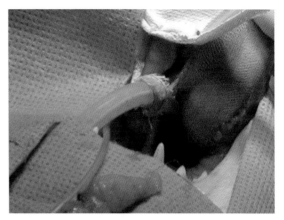

Figure 34-6 An inflammatory polyp following removal by traction from the nasopharynx of a cat. Note the tapering shape of the polyp, following the contour of the eustachian tube. (Courtesy Dr. B. Séguin.)

oxygen should be considered. Materials for resuscitation (e.g., endotracheal tubes, ambu-bag ventilators) should be readily available.

Radiographic examination of the thorax may reveal lung lobe retraction, rounding of the lung lobe tips, prominent interlobar fissures, widening of the pleural space with fluid density, and loss of the cardiac silhouette (Figure 34-7). On suspicion of pleural effusion, collection of a pleural fluid sample is indicated. Often a diagnostic sample can be obtained in a minimally invasive manner with a butterfly-type catheter or side-fenestrated intravenous catheter. Adequate drainage of pleural fluid usually cannot be achieved via a small-bore catheter, and the placement of larger-bore chest drains is indicated. Therapy will depend on findings of fluid analysis, culture, and sensitivity. Medical management of pyothorax can be attempted via regular thoracic lavage and antibiotic therapy. However, the prognosis for full recovery is usually better if exploratory thoracotomy surgery and pleural cavity lavage are carried out.

Pneumothorax

The most common cause of pneumothorax in both young dogs and cats is thoracic trauma. Bite wounds, projectile injuries, thoracic trauma after being hit by motor vehicles, tracheal laceration or rupture following fight wounds, and rupture of congenital pulmonary cystic lesions can all lead to pneumothorax. The presenting clinical signs can range from mild dyspnea or tachypnea to severe respiratory distress, cyanosis, and cardiovascular collapse. Animals with tension pneumothorax will often have a barrel-chested appearance and tympanic resonance on thoracic percussion. With gas in the pleural space, the ability to inflate the lungs is dramatically reduced, leading to a restrictive respiratory pattern. Tension pneumothorax can rapidly lead to cardiovascular failure, as increasing pressure in the thorax leads to diastolic dysfunction of the ventricles and reduced cardiac output. Prompt recognition of tension pneumothorax and relief of the pleural pressure via thoracocentesis may be

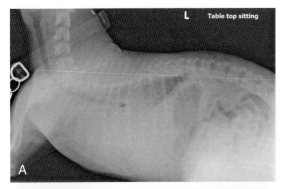

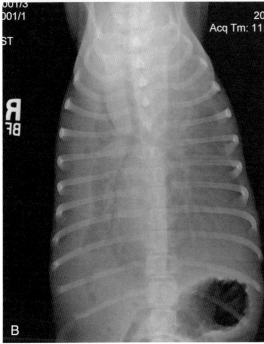

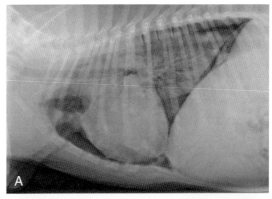

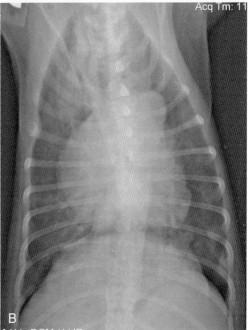

Figure 34-7 Lateral (horizontal beam, **A**) and ventrodorsal (**B**) radiographic views of the thorax from a 3-month-old dog with severe pyothorax. Note the dramatic loss of pleural space, presence of interlobar fissures, and blunting of the lung borders. The dog was successfully managed via thoracotomy, thoracic lavage and resection of necrotic lung, and placement of chest tubes.

Figure 34-8 Lateral (**A**) and dorsoventral (**B**) radiographic views of the thorax from a young dog with pneumomediastinum and pneumothorax following thoracic trauma. Note the loss of cardiac shadow sternal contact on the lateral view, retraction of the lung margins in the dorsocaudal thorax, and increased detail within the cranial mediastinum.

lifesaving. If necessary, needle thoracocentesis should be performed before diagnostic imaging.

Pneumothorax is readily diagnosed radiographically (Figure 34-8), with retraction of the lung lobes toward the hilus and dorsal separation of the heart from the sternum on lateral views. Management of pneumothorax in the young dog and cat is essentially as for adult animals, including placement of pleural drains and either continuous evacuation or regular intermittent evacuation until the defect heals. Many patients will require long periods of continuous suction drainage to allow healing. There is a moderately high risk of recurrence. In most cases where aspiration of gas is required for greater than 24 hours after presentation, it is more cost-effective and overall prognosis is improved if exploratory thoracotomy and reparative intent surgery are performed.

SUGGESTED READINGS

Anonymous: Backgrounder: canine influenza, AVMA Public Health Press Release, 2007. Accessible at Http://Www.Avma.Org/Public_Health/Influenza/Canine_Bgnd.Asp. (Last accessed February 17, 2008.)

Billet JPHG, Sharpe A: Surgical treatment of congenital lobar emphysema in a puppy, *J Small Anim Pract* 43(2):84, 2002.

Fossum TW: Surgery of the lower respiratory system. In Fossum TW (ed): *Small animal surgery*, ed 3, St Louis, 2007, Mosby/Elsevier, pp 867-929.

Hedlund CS: Surgery of the upper respiratory system. In Fossum TW (ed): *Small animal surgery*, ed 3, St Louis, 2007, Mosby/Elsevier, pp 817-866.

Radlinsky MA, Fossum TW: Tracheal collapse in a young boxer, *J Am Anim Hosp Assoc* 36(4):313, 2000.

DENTAL AND ORAL CAVITY

CHAPTER 35

Andrea Van de Wetering

Many of the common dental conditions found in puppies and kittens carry a favorable prognosis if addressed and treated correctly. Providing a pain-free functional bite is the primary goal of a dental treatment plan. It is important to evaluate when treatment should be provided by a general practitioner or if referral to a dental specialist is appropriate.

NORMAL ANATOMY AND DEVELOPMENT

Knowledge of the normal deciduous dental formulas and eruption times for the dog and cat will help determine whether pathology exists (Table 35-1 and Box 35-1). The deciduous dentition in the canine and feline contains no molar teeth. In addition to no molar teeth, there is no deciduous counterpart to the first premolar tooth in the dog. Mixed dentition is the term applied to the mouth when both deciduous and permanent teeth are present. This is a normal condition between 4 and 6 months of age.

The number of roots a particular tooth has is important when an extraction is indicated or if a particular tooth has an abnormal number of roots. Often teeth with abnormal numbers of roots or shapes have other structural defects, such as communication through the dentin and pulp to the outside environment. This may lead to endodontic disease. For normal tooth root numbers, see Box 35-2.

NOMENCLATURE

Use of the modified Triadan system of tooth numbering has become common in veterinary nomenclature. A dental chart should be used in the patient's permanent record to document any abnormalities and subsequent treatment performed. There are numerous charts available from various sources. For the general practitioner, the dental labels made by DentaLabels (Kensington, CA) are useful as they are user friendly and self-adhesive for easy placement in the

permanent record. The American Animal Hospital Association provides a very complete dental chart for its members. Most paperless computer programs have dental chart capability as well. See Figures 35-1 and 35-2 for sample dental charts demonstrating the modified Triadan system of tooth numbering.

NORMAL OCCLUSION

The cat and the dog have an anisognathic jaw relationship, meaning the jaw lengths are not equal, with the lower jaw slightly shorter than the upper jaw. The incisor relationship in the canine is defined as a "scissor" bite. The upper incisors overlap the lower incisors with 1 to 2 mm of space between the upper and lower teeth, and the lower incisor cusps rest on the cingula of the upper incisors. In the feline, the incisor cusps may meet in a level bite. In both species the premolars should interdigitate in a "pinking shears" type of relationship with the lower premolars occluding rostrally to the upper premolars. The large cusp tip of the lower fourth premolar should be centered between the upper third and fourth premolar. The upper premolars should occlude buccally (toward the cheek) to the lower premolars and first molar.

CONGENITAL AND HEREDITARY PROBLEMS

Persistent Deciduous Teeth

When deciduous teeth exfoliate improperly or incompletely, the deciduous tooth and the permanent tooth are present in the mouth at the same time. No tooth of the same type should be present in the mouth at the same time. If this occurs, the deciduous tooth should be extracted immediately. Persistent deciduous teeth are never normal and should be extracted as soon as a diagnosis is made. Persistent deciduous teeth are also a common cause of malocclusion because they can cause the permanent teeth to erupt in an abnormal

TABLE 35-1	Approximate eruption times for the deciduous feline and canine dentition

Tooth	Deciduous dentition (wk)
Canine	
Incisors	3-5
Canines	3-6
Premolars	4-10
Molars	Not present
Feline	
Incisors	2-3
Canines	3-4
Premolars	3-6
Molars	Not present

BOX 35-1	Dental formulas for the canine and feline

Canine Formula*
Deciduous: 2 (i 3/3, c 1/1, pm 3/3) = 28
Permanent: 2 (I 3/3, C 1/1, PM 4/4, M 2/3) = 42

Feline Formula*
Deciduous: 2 (i 3/3, c 1/1, pm 3/2) = 26
Permanent: 2 (I 3/3, C 1/1, PM 3/2, M 1/1) = 30

*Lowercase letters indicate deciduous or temporary teeth, whereas uppercase letters indicate permanent dentition.

BOX 35-2	Tooth root numbers*

Canine
1 root: I1-3, C, PM1, Lower M3
3 roots: Upper PM4, Upper M1-2
2 roots: All others

Feline*
1 root: I1-3, Upper PM2, Upper M1
3 roots: Upper PM
2 roots: All others

*Compared with the canine, cats are missing the upper PM1 and M2 and the lower PM1-2 and M2-3.
Data from Holmstrom SE, Fitch PF, Eisner ER: *Veterinary dental techniques for the small animal practitioner*, ed 3, Philadelphia, 2004, Saunders.

location. The permanent premolar teeth generally erupt to the inside (lingually or palatally) of the deciduous counterpart. The exception to this is the upper canine teeth, which erupt in front (mesial) of the deciduous teeth. Figure 35-3 shows an example of a dog with a persistent deciduous left upper canine tooth. The permanent tooth has erupted in an abnormal position because of the failure of the deciduous

tooth to exfoliate. This abnormal mesioversion (the tooth is angled toward the front of the mouth) of the canine tooth has also been termed a "lance canine" tooth.

Treatment for persistent deciduous teeth consists of complete extraction of the deciduous tooth. Preoperative intraoral dental radiographs identify location and shape of the tooth to be extracted. A gingival flap may be appropriate to allow adequate visualization and minimize chance of root fracture. Extraction techniques are covered in detail in other texts (see Suggested Reading list); however, it is important to note that deciduous teeth have deceptively long roots compared with crown size, very thin enamel walls, and break easily with overzealous extraction technique (Figure 35-4). It is essential to remove the entire deciduous tooth root when extraction is performed. Incomplete extraction may lead to infection, pain, or malocclusion. Postoperative dental radiographs should be obtained to ensure complete extraction. When performing deciduous tooth extractions, special care should be exercised to avoid trauma to the permanent tooth bud as this can cause damage to the permanent tooth enamel (Figure 35-5).

Missing and Impacted Teeth

Normal tooth eruption occurs in two stages: the intraosseous stage and the supraosseous stage. In the first stage, the overlying bone and the deciduous tooth root (if present) are resorbed. In the second stage, the permanent tooth erupts through the soft tissues. This process can be delayed or interrupted by a number of local and systemic causes, including genetic and congenital problems, trauma, persistent deciduous teeth, thickened fibrous tissue (operculum) covering the unerupted tooth, and failure of bone resorption. It is important to note there are no deciduous precursors to the permanent first premolar teeth in the canine or the molar teeth in both the canine and feline. Knowledge of normal permanent tooth eruption times in addition to dental radiography can differentiate between congenital absence of teeth (oligodontia or anodontia) and impaction. Impaction occurs when a tooth is covered by a tough gingival tissue called the operculum that prevents eruption. When a tooth is embedded, the tooth is not only covered by the operculum but also is covered by bone (Figures 35-6 and 35-7). It is not uncommon to see lower first premolar teeth that are impacted or in an abnormal position, particularly in brachycephalic breeds. Unerupted teeth are prone to developing destructive cystic lesions. These cysts can cause significant damage to the soft and hard tissues surrounding them, including loss of surrounding permanent teeth (Figure 35-8). Because impacted lower first premolar teeth are often in an abnormal position, extraction is usually appropriate.

Breeders may request preeruption dental radiographs to determine whether a particular dog has a full complement of permanent teeth. In some breeds, such as the Doberman Pinscher, Rottweiler, and German Shepherd Dog, absence of teeth may be grounds for elimination in the show ring because of the hereditary component of this problem.

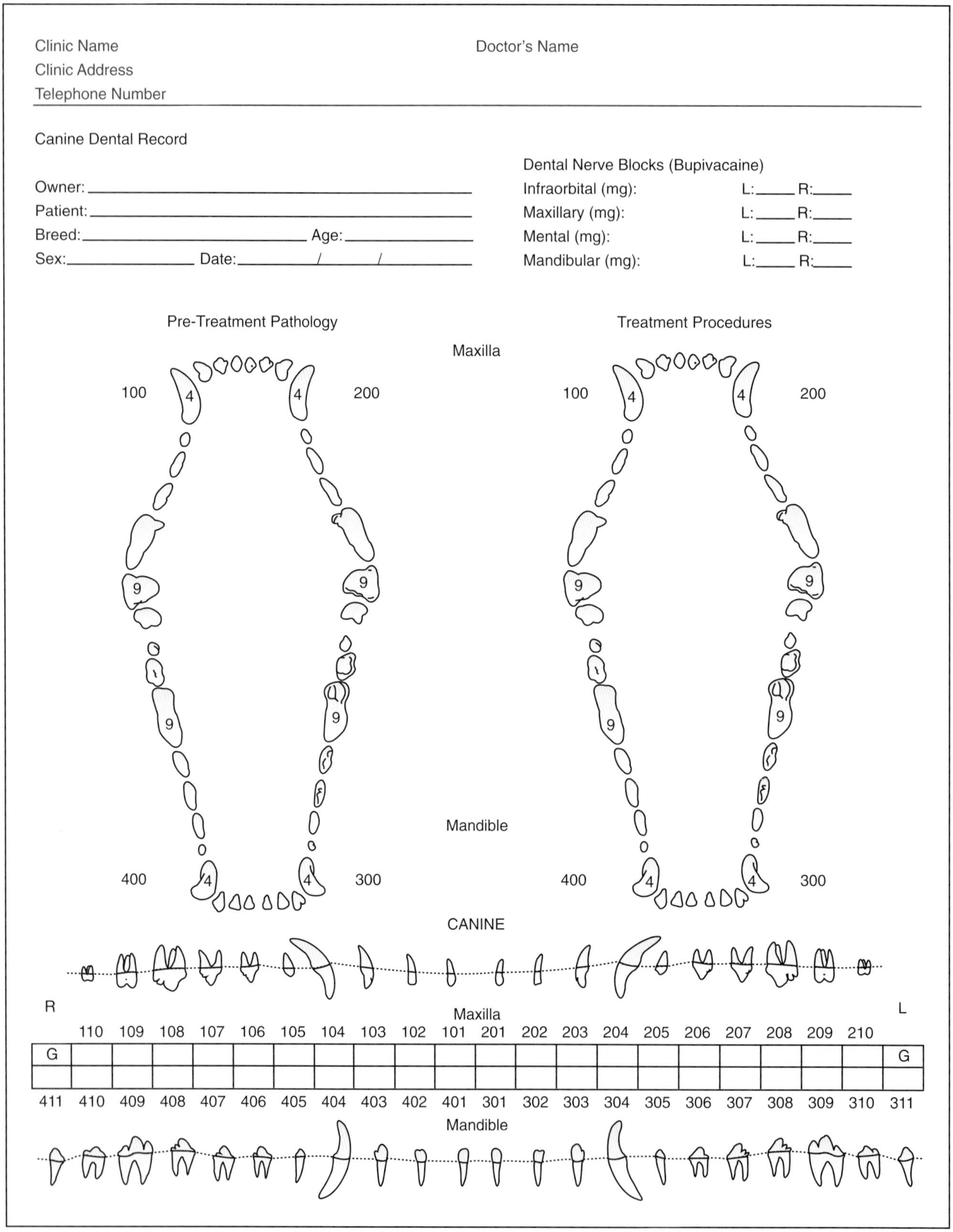
Clinic Name
Clinic Address
Telephone Number
Doctor's Name
Canine Dental Record
Owner:
Patient:
Breed:
Age:
Sex:
Date: / /
Dental Nerve Blocks (Bupivacaine)
Infraorbital (mg): L: R:
Maxillary (mg): L: R:
Mental (mg): L: R:
Mandibular (mg): L: R:
Pre-Treatment Pathology
Treatment Procedures
Maxilla
100
200
Mandible
400
300
CANINE
R
L
Maxilla
110 109 108 107 106 105 104 103 102 101 201 202 203 204 205 206 207 208 209 210
G
G
411 410 409 408 407 406 405 404 403 402 401 301 302 303 304 305 306 307 308 309 310 311
Mandible

Figure 35-1 Canine dental record. (Courtesy Allen Matson, Eastside Veterinary Dentistry, Woodinville, WA.)

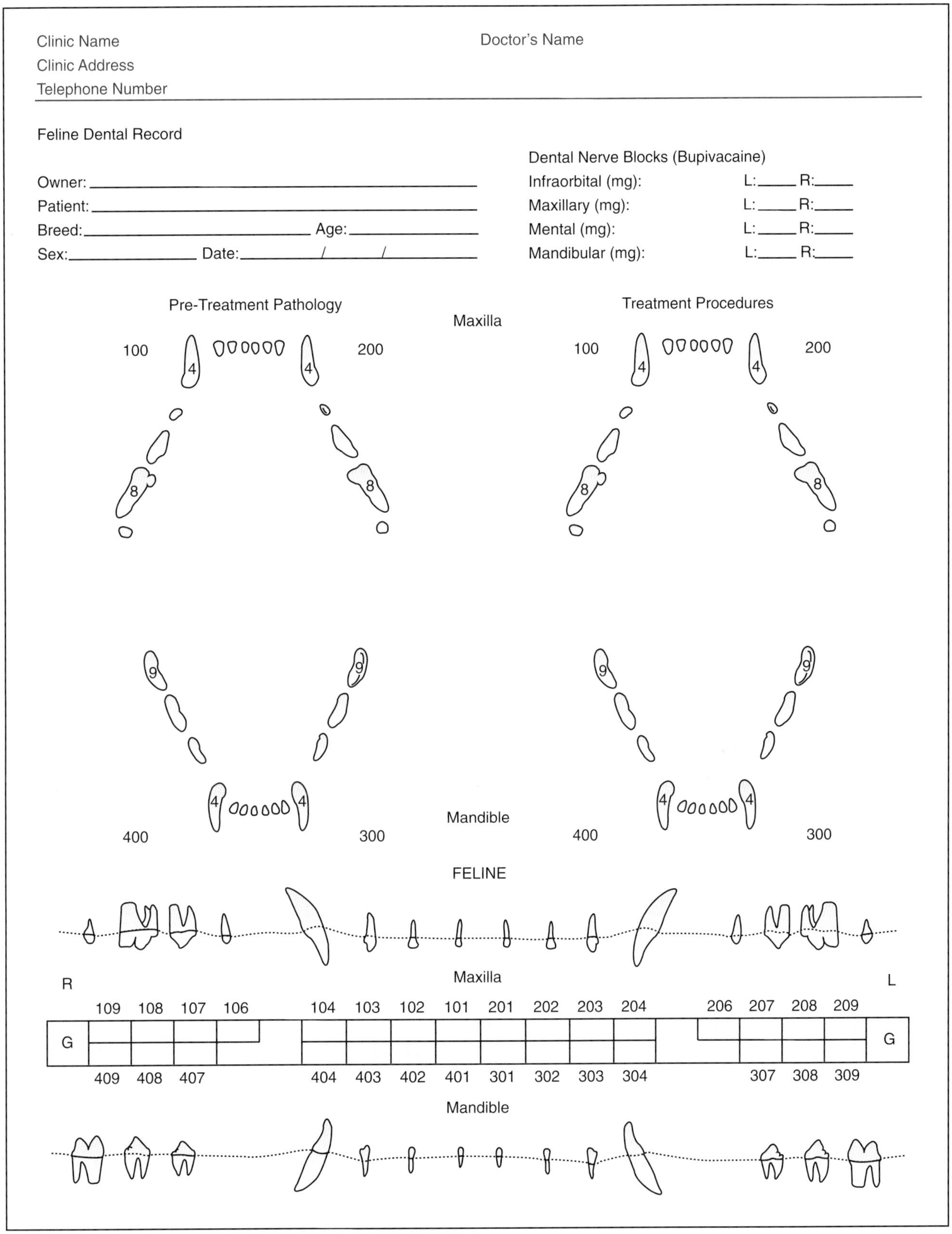

Clinic Name   Doctor's Name
Clinic Address
Telephone Number

Feline Dental Record

Owner: _____
Patient: _____
Breed: _____ Age: _____
Sex: _____ Date: _____ / _____ / _____

Dental Nerve Blocks (Bupivacaine)
Infraorbital (mg):   L:_____ R:_____
Maxillary (mg):   L:_____ R:_____
Mental (mg):   L:_____ R:_____
Mandibular (mg):   L:_____ R:_____

Pre-Treatment Pathology   Treatment Procedures

Maxilla

100   200   100   200

Mandible

400   300   400   300

FELINE

R   Maxilla   L

	109	108	107	106		104	103	102	101	201	202	203	204		206	207	208	209	
G																			G
	409	408	407			404	403	402	401	301	302	303	304			307	308	309	

Mandible

Figure 35-2 Feline dental record. (Courtesy Allen Matson, Eastside Veterinary Dentistry, Woodinville, WA.)

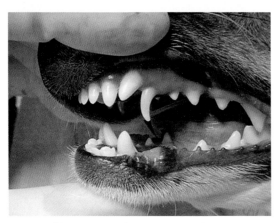

Figure 35-3 Photos of the left upper arcade in a Beagle dog showing a persistent deciduous canine that has caused the permanent canine tooth to erupt mesially. This is also called a lance canine tooth. Left untreated, these teeth develop severe periodontal problems over time, which can result in oronasal fistulas.

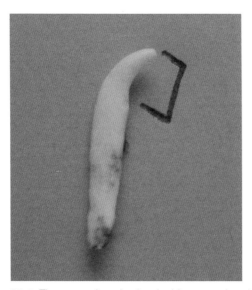

Figure 35-4 The crown length of a deciduous canine demonstrates the deceptively short crown compared with root length. The bracket is outlining the crown. The remainder of the tooth is root. It is imperative to extract the root entirely. This may require creating a gingival flap for increased exposure and visualization. Complete extraction should always be verified radiographically.

Preeruption radiographs are most diagnostic after 8 to 10 weeks of age.

It is simple to diagnose these abnormalities at the time of routine well puppy exams or spay and neuter appointments. At this time, any missing teeth should be noted in the medical record, and dental radiographs should be obtained. Treatment of impacted or embedded teeth involves making mesial and distal releasing incisions on both the buccal and lingual or palatal surfaces, and then elevating a full-thickness mucoperiosteal flap on both surfaces. The fibrous tissue (operculum) covering the crown is excised with a No. 15 blade, and any overlying bone is gently removed

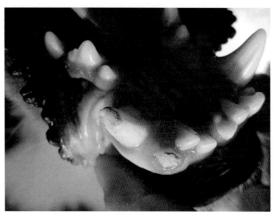

Figure 35-5 Enamel dysplasia of the permanent teeth after extraction of the deciduous teeth in a dog. If the permanent tooth bud is traumatized during the extraction procedure, dysplasia will occur. Dysplasia exposes the dentin tubules to the environment and may weaken the tooth, possibly requiring composite or crown restoration to avoid further damage to the teeth. Enamel dysplasia may also result from a puppyhood illness or facial trauma while the permanent tooth is still developing.

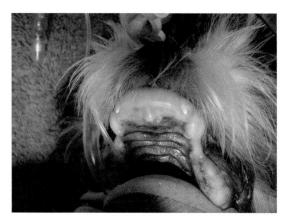

Figure 35-6 Intraoral photo of missing teeth in a 14-week-old puppy. Dental radiographs must be obtained to ascertain whether the teeth are truly missing or are impacted.

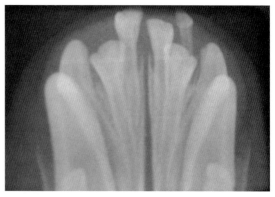

Figure 35-7 Intraoral radiographs of the puppy in Figure 35-6. This radiograph demonstrates that although the teeth are missing clinically, they are present under the gingiva. Left untreated, dentigerous cysts are likely to follow.

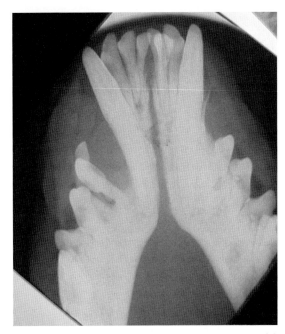

Figure 35-8 Radiograph of a dentigerous cyst caused by an impacted right lower first premolar in a 5-year-old Japanese Chin. Timely diagnosis and treatment early in life could have prevented the extensive damage and tooth loss caused by this pathology. All puppies and kittens should be monitored for full dentition by 6 months of age, and abnormalities should be investigated radiographically.

with rongeurs. A high-speed dental bur should not be used to remove bone as it may cause trauma to the underlying tooth. The releasing incisions are closed using 4-0 or 5-0 absorbable suture, leaving the coronal aspect of the flap open.

Supernumerary, Fusion, and Gemination Teeth

Abnormalities of the developing tooth bud can result in abnormal numbers of roots or crowns or entire teeth in the dog and the cat. Supernumerary teeth occur when two of the same tooth are present in the mouth. It is not uncommon to see supernumerary incisors in breeds such as the Boxer and Mastiff. Supernumerary first premolar teeth are common in many dog breeds as well. Cats can have supernumerary premolars. These teeth should be extracted if they cause crowding or impingement on adjacent teeth.

Fusion and gemination teeth are seen in many breeds of dogs and cats. A fusion tooth typically has two fused crowns, a common pulp chamber, and separate root canal systems. In contrast, gemination teeth have two crowns and pulp chambers but a single root canal system. Intraoral dental radiographs can differentiate the two. These teeth are often extracted because of the frequency of enamel, dentin, and root canal system abnormalities that may lead to endodontic disease.

Malocclusions

No controlled studies have been conducted to evaluate the hereditary component of malocclusion; however, abnormal bites are generally considered to have at least some genetic component (see Box 35-3 for classes of malocclusions). The use of an occlusal evaluation table (Table 35-2) is useful as a means to help determine the genetic influence on a particular malocclusion. Each area of the mouth is assigned a numeric value and then added together for a total point score. The total point score helps determine whether a particular malocclusion is likely to be genetic in origin and aids discussions with breeders.

Common malocclusions include anterior cross-bite, posterior cross-bite, lance canine teeth, and base narrow canine teeth. Jaw length discrepancies that lead to more severe malocclusions can be noted very early in life. It is interesting to note that the mandibles and maxillae grow at different rates. That is, the right mandible may grow separately from the left mandible, and discrepancies may or may not persist once growth is complete. Traumatic malocclusions cause extreme discomfort for the puppy or kitten and must be addressed without delay. Puppies and kittens with painful malocclusions may become head shy or have significant behavior problems because of oral pain. Often the permanent occlusion (or malocclusion) will be the same or very similar to the deciduous.

Common Malocclusions
Anterior cross-bite ("reverse scissor bite")

An anterior cross-bite exists when one or two of the upper incisors are located to the inside of the lower incisor teeth. This problem needs correction if the gingiva becomes traumatized, if the bite will excessively wear the opposing teeth, or if overcrowding will cause periodontal disease in the future. Correction involves selective extraction or referral to a dental specialist for orthodontic movement (e.g., braces). The benefit of orthodontic movement for any malocclusion is retention of teeth. Retention of strategically important teeth keeps normal tooth alignment, allows a nonpainful bite, and in many cases gives good cosmetic results. If all the lower incisors occlude mesially to the upper incisors, the malocclusion is due to discrepancy in jaw lengths and is termed a class III malocclusion.

Lance canine teeth (mesioversion of the upper canine teeth)

Lance canine teeth are most common in the Shetland Sheepdog, the Dachshund, and the Persian cat but can occur in any breed (see Figure 35-3). This problem is often precipitated by persistent deciduous teeth; however, its origin may also be idiopathic. Persistent deciduous teeth cause mesioversion of the upper canine teeth. The lower canine teeth are then prevented from erupting into normal position. This is typically a bilateral problem. Neglecting to address this malocclusion ensures severe problems later in life. If untreated, painful occlusions, severe periodontal disease, tooth loss, and oronasal fistulas may occur. Correction involves referral for orthodontic movement to retain a strategically important tooth or extraction.

BOX 35-3 Classes of Malocclusion

Type 0: Normal Occlusion

The upper and lower canines and upper third incisors are evenly spaced in a "scissor" relationship. The upper incisors overlap the lower incisors with approximately 1 to 2 mm of space between them, and the lower incisor occlusal cusps rest on the cingula of the upper incisors. The lower canine teeth should occlude in the center of the space (diastema) between the upper third incisor and the upper canine tooth. The upper premolars interdigitate in a "pinking shears" manner, with the lower first premolar occluding rostral to the upper first premolar. The upper fourth premolar and lower first molar teeth occlude to create a shearing function, with the upper fourth premolar located buccally to the lower first molar tooth. The crowns of the molar teeth occlusal surfaces meet to allow a grinding action.

Class I Malocclusion

The overall dental relationship is normal with one or two malpositioned teeth. Examples include but are not limited to any single tooth in an abnormal position, such as rotated or tipped, or an open bite.

Class II Malocclusion

The maxillary relationship to the mandible is such that either the maxillae are too long or the mandibles are too short. This is evident when evaluating either the relationship between the incisors or the relationship between the premolars. Often this is termed a "parrot" mouth, mandibular brachygnathism, or maxillary prognathism. A common abnormality associated with a Class II malocclusion is base narrow mandibular canine teeth. This may manifest as interference of the lower canine teeth with the upper canine teeth or the palate. If the malocclusion is severe, the lower canine teeth may occlude distally to the upper canine teeth.

Class III Malocclusion

The maxillary relationship to the mandible is such that either the maxillae are too short or the mandibles are too long. This is often called an "underbite," "sow mouth," maxillary brachygnathism, or mandibular prognathism, depending on which jaw the abnormality is present. This occlusal relationship may be considered normal for some breeds.

Severe examples of this malocclusion may include lower incisors and canines that occlude so rostrally to the upper incisors that the cusp tips of the upper incisors cause trauma to the lower mandibular soft tissues distal to the incisors. It is not uncommon to see the lower canine teeth interfering on the distal aspect of the upper third incisors, necessitating extraction of the upper third incisors.

Class IV Malocclusion

This classification is reserved for the extremely severe malocclusions, including wry bites or other severe skeletal discrepancies as the etiology for the malocclusion.

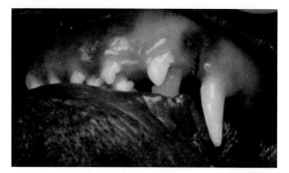

Figure 35-9 Palatal trauma in a 12-week-old puppy as a result of lower canine teeth that have erupted lingually. Treatment at this point is extraction of both deciduous lower canine teeth. This condition should be monitored closely as the permanent dentition appears, and if the same condition occurs, referral to a veterinary dentist or extraction is appropriate.

Mandibular canine tooth (linguoversion of the lower canine teeth, with "base narrow canine teeth" being the lay term)

Base narrow mandibular canine teeth are tipped or bodily displaced lingually. Persistent deciduous teeth and mandibular brachygnathism (foreshortened mandible) are the most common etiologies. When the lower canine teeth are base narrow, trauma to the hard palate and gingival tissues occurs (Figure 35-9). If left untreated, pain, infection, or oronasal fistulas follow. Many treatment options are available for this problem. When the deciduous teeth cause trauma to the palate, they should be extracted. If the permanent dentition erupts abnormally because of persistent deciduous teeth, the deciduous teeth should be extracted immediately. No tooth of the same kind can be in the mouth at the same time. If the permanent dentition continues to be abnormal, treatment consists of extraction or referral to a veterinary dentist for crown height reduction and vital pulp therapy or orthodontic movement.

Breeders have been known to "clip" the crowns of the offending deciduous teeth to prevent palatal trauma. This is cruel to the puppy as the procedure leads to extreme pain, severe pulpitis, infection, and potential damage to the permanent tooth bud.

Class II malocclusion (overbite or "parrot mouth")

Class II malocclusions are considered discrepancies of mandibular length when compared with the maxilla in which the upper jaw exceeds the normal relationship with the lower jaw, also called a parrot mouth. This is caused by either mandibular brachygnathism (foreshortened mandible) or maxillary prognathism (excessively long maxilla). This malocclusion is not normal in any breed, is grounds for elimination in the show ring, and is thought to have a strong hereditary component. This malocclusion causes severe problems and is usually noted very early in life, as soon as the deciduous teeth begin to erupt. As the teeth erupt they become entrapped in the soft tissues of the palate or behind

TABLE 35-2 Occlusal evaluation table	Point value

Incisor Relationship (5 Points Possible)

A. If lower incisors hit the cingula of the uppers (normal scissor bite)	5
B. If lower incisors hit the cusp tips of the uppers or hit the gingival tissue behind the uppers	4
C. If lower incisors are in front of the uppers or are behind the uppers with space between the upper and lower incisors (in a rostral-caudal plane)	3
D. Marked space between the upper and lower incisors (rostral-caudal plane)	2
E. Extreme differences in jaw lengths	1

Canine Tooth Relationship (5 Points Possible)

A. Lower canines are centered between the upper third incisor and the upper canine tooth and not touching either (normal)	5
B. The lower canine (one or both) is touching either upper premolar or upper canine	4
C. Canine teeth are causing wear on upper teeth or downward angulation of incisors so that the lower canine tip touches upper canine and its base hits upper third incisor	3
D. The lower canine tooth is positioned inside (lingually) or outside (labially) of the upper canine tooth or upper incisor	2
E. The lower canine tooth is behind the upper canine or ahead of the upper third incisor tooth	1

Lower Fourth Premolar Relationship (5 Points)

A. The large cusp is centered between the upper third and fourth premolar (normal)	5
B. Lower cusp tip shifts mesially (forward) to the small third developmental groove in the upper third premolar or distally (backward) to the front edge of the upper fourth premolar	4
C. Lower cusp tip shifts mesially to the middle developmental groove in the upper third premolar or distally to the mesial aspect of the upper fourth premolar	3
D. Lower cusp tip shifts mesially to the large first groove in the upper third premolar or distally half the distance to cusp tip of the upper fourth premolar	2
E. Lower cusp tip shifts mesially or distally to meet the cusp tip of either the upper third or fourth premolar	1

Premolar Horizontal Alignment (5 Points)

A. Interdigitation with cusp tips as far forward as the lower second premolar with the upper second premolar (normal)	5
B. Lower third premolar with the upper third	4
C. Lower fourth premolar with the upper third	3
D. Space between tips of lower fourth and upper third	2

Temporomandibular Angle of Mandible Relationship (5 Points)

A. Angle directly below posterior border of coronoid process or within 3 mm of that point	5
B. Angle displaced by 4-6 mm from point below posterior border of coronoid process	4
C. Angle displaced by 7-10 mm from point below posterior border of the coronoid process	3
D. More than 10-mm displacement from point below posterior border of the coronoid process	2

Head Symmetry (5 Points)

A. Perfect midline of head and dentition alignment	5
B. Subtract 1 point for:	4
1. Rotated teeth (either premolars or incisors)	
2. Midline of upper and lower arches off center by less than width of upper incisor	
3. Missing one tooth	
C. Subtract two points for:	3
1. Rotated teeth in premolar and incisor areas	
2. Midline off by width of one tooth	
3. Missing two teeth	
D. Subtract three points for:	2
1. Midline off by more than width of one tooth	
2. More than two missing teeth	
3. Noticeable deviation of muzzle to left or right of midline of rest of skull	

Continued

TABLE 35-2	Occlusal evaluation table—cont'd	
		Point value

Area scores and reasons (30 points possible)
A. Incisors _____
B. Canines _____
C. Fourth premolar _____
D. Horizontal alignment _____
E. Angle of mandible _____
F. Oral symmetry _____
Total points: _____

Grade Scale:

Excellent (27-30 points): No apparent genetic defects.
Near normal (21-26 points): Mild genetic problems; select mates with equal or better oral evaluation scores.
Genetic defect (16-20 points): Careful use if other body traits warrant use in breeding program.
Severe defect (0-15 points): Not suitable for breeding purposes.

Adapted from Ross DL: Orthodontics for the dog: bite evaluation, basic concepts, and equipment, *Vet Clin North Am Small Anim Pract* 16(5):955, 1986.

the upper teeth, creating a dental interlock that further inhibits mandibular growth. When recognized early (by 6 to 8 weeks of age for best prognosis), extraction of the lower deciduous incisors and canine teeth is indicated to remove the dental interlock. This procedure eliminates the painful condition for the puppy and possibly allows the lower jaw to catch up in growth. If the jaw length discrepancy is not severe, the growth of the mandible may catch up to the maxilla; however, if the mandible is more than a few millimeters too short, it is very unlikely to normalize. Treatment consists of extraction or referral.

Class III malocclusion (underbite, undershot jaw, or "sow mouth")

A Class III malocclusion presents as abnormal positioning of the lower dentition in a more mesial (rostral) position in relation to the upper dentition. This occurs either as a result of maxillary brachygnathism or mandibular prognathism, although the occlusion may be considered normal in some breeds with brachycephalic anatomy such as the English Bulldog. The common manifestation of this malocclusion is interference of the lower canines with the palatal or distal aspect of the upper third incisor teeth and trauma to the lingual mucosa from the upper incisors (Figure 35-10). Providing a functional bite can be as simple as extraction of the upper third incisor teeth.

Wry bite (Class IV malocclusions)

This classification involves wry bites in which one side of the mandible and/or maxilla is displaced forward or backward of its counterpart. These conditions are typically treated with selective extractions to eliminate a painful bite.

Other Congenital and Hereditary Conditions

Crowded and Rotated Teeth

Crowded teeth are common problems in small breed dogs. Rotated teeth seen frequently in brachycephalic breeds as a

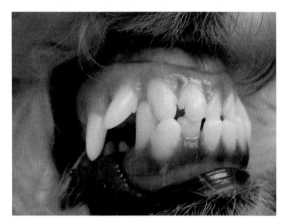

Figure 35-10 Lower canine interference with the upper third incisors caused by a Class III malocclusion. Treatment consists of extraction of the involved incisor teeth to create space for the lower canine teeth. This dog also has a reverse scissor bite involving the right lower first and second incisor and the left lower first incisor.

result of extreme crowding are prone to periodontal disease. To maintain periodontal health, each tooth must have a complete collar of attached gingiva. When teeth are crowded or rotated, the normal gingival attachments are compromised, thus predisposing the animal to periodontal disease. Selective extraction is the treatment of choice.

Cleft Lip/Palate

Clefts may be classified as primary or secondary. Primary clefts present as a cleft lip and are cosmetic only. These can be repaired surgically as soon as the puppy or kitten is old enough for surgery. Secondary clefts involve the hard and/ or the soft palate (Figure 35-11). Communication between the oral and nasal cavity makes nursing impossible. Animals with this condition have milk in the nasal passages during nursing. Affected animals sneeze, gag, cough, have nasal

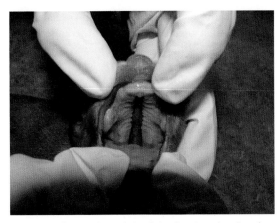

Figure 35-11 Secondary cleft of the hard and soft palate in a newborn English Bulldog.

discharge, and commonly develop aspiration pneumonia. This condition is extremely rare in cats.

Tight Lip Syndrome

A genetic abnormality found primarily in the Shar-Pei dog (but may occur in other breeds) presents with the lower lip curled up over the lower incisors. This prevents forward growth of the mandible, thus causing mandibular insufficiency, trauma to the lip from the upper incisors, and distocclusion of the lower incisors. Surgical correction, recommended at about 3 months of age, carries the best prognosis. Surgical techniques are described elsewhere.

Craniomandibular Osteopathy (Lion Jaw, Westie Jaw, Scottie Jaw)

This disease is most often recognized in West Highland White Terrier puppies between 4 and 7 months of age; however, it has been recognized rarely in other breeds.

A simple autosomal recessive mode of inheritance has been identified in the West Highland White Terrier. Clinically dogs present showing signs of pain on opening the mouth, lethargy, and inappetence. Radiographically new bone production and periosteal proliferation are noted on the ramus of the mandible and occasionally extending to the temporomandibular joint and other regions of the skull (see Figure 42-3). This syndrome most commonly presents bilaterally. Treatment encompasses pain control, antiinflammatory medications, and time. This disease usually regresses spontaneously between 11 and 13 months of age when the growth plates close. However, long-term sequela involving fusion of the temporomandibular joint has been reported, which, if it occurs, carries a very poor prognosis.

ACQUIRED PROBLEMS

Immune-Mediated and Viral Diseases

The common immune-mediated diseases in the dog and cat often manifest with oral lesions. The most common viruses include feline leukemia (FeLV), feline immunodeficiency viruses (FIV), and calicivirus and rhinotracheitis virus. In the dog, autoimmune disorders include pemphigus and pemphigoid-like diseases.

Viral Papillomatosis

These benign oral wartlike lesions are caused by a papovavirus. They typically spontaneously regress and require no treatment. Transmission is thought to be horizontal from animal to animal.

Feline Juvenile Gingivitis

Feline juvenile gingivitis is characterized by gingival hyperplasia. Treatment includes dental prophylaxis and gingivectomy, followed by excellent home care during the first 2 years of life to prevent recurrence. Cats usually outgrow this problem with good oral hygiene. Differential diagnosis includes gingival fibropapillomatosis, which presents as excessive gingival growth (proliferation) covering the crown of the tooth. Treatment for this syndrome involves gingivectomy and it does not usually recur.

Feline Juvenile-Onset Periodontitis

This syndrome is found typically in cats less than 9 months of age. Clinical signs include weight loss, pain, halitosis, and ptyalism. Abundant plaque and calculus formation causes destruction of bone and soft tissues. Gingival recession, formation of pockets, furcation (the space between tooth roots) exposure, and severe gingivitis characterize the changes seen with this disease. In extreme cases, the gingivitis can extend to include the caudal buccal folds, fauces, and pharynx. Various reports in the literature suggest that the more common breeds affected include Siamese, Burmese, Maine Coon, and Abyssinian cats; however, this syndrome has been seen in other breeds as well. The etiology may be idiopathic but can include FIV, FeLV, feline calicivirus, and other underlying immune disorders. The role of *Bartonella henselae* as an etiology has yet to be shown definitively. Treatment is directed at combining frequent professional dental prophylaxis, analgesics, antibiotics, oral antiseptics, meticulous home care, and selective extractions.

Enamel Defects

Enamel dysplasia can be caused by enamel hypoplasia (thin enamel) or hypocalcification (inadequate mineralization). Enamel hypocalcification presents as areas of the enamel that are pitted, brown or yellow, and flake away easily. The enamel usually appears roughened. Enamel defects may be congenital abnormalities or result from puppy and kitten illnesses or trauma. When the normal enamel covering of the tooth is absent, the underlying dentin is exposed. Microscopically, dentin appears porous. This can allow invasion of bacteria into the pulp of the tooth and subsequent endodontic disease. Severe defects should be treated with composite restoration or crown therapy.

Discolored Teeth

Normal teeth are white or slightly yellow colored. Yellowed permanent teeth in the juvenile animal are typically caused by tetracycline staining. This occurs if tetracycline is given to an animal during permanent tooth development and is a cosmetic problem only. Teeth that are pink, purple, tan, brown, or gray are abnormal, and trauma is the most common cause of this discolorization. Acute trauma or bleeding disorders such as von Willebrand disease (factor VIII deficiency) will often cause hemorrhage into the dentin from the pulp cavity, resulting in acute pulpitis (inflammation of the dental pulp). Acute pulpitis is a very painful condition. As the pulp of the tooth dies and the hemorrhagic areas mature, the tooth will change to a dull gray, purple, or brown coloration. Reports in the literature have shown that the majority of discolored teeth have some degree of pulp necrosis. These teeth should be treated with extraction or referral to a specialist for root canal therapy.

Oral Trauma

Craniofacial trauma is common in the young dog and cat and usually is caused by vehicular accidents, falling from heights (high-rise syndrome), aggression from other animals, electrical and chemical burns, foreign bodies, and lacerations. Mandibular symphyseal fracture and separation, lip avulsion, maxillary and mandibular fractures, and temporomandibular fractures occur frequently, as well as tooth injuries.

Repair of these problems must take occlusion into account first and foremost. It is unimportant how well a fracture site heals if the animal can no longer close its mouth, is left with a painful occlusion, or sustains damage to the permanent dentition. Although detailed discussion of fracture repair techniques is beyond the scope of this text, oral fracture repair techniques include tape muzzles for minor injuries, external fixators, internal fixators, or, preferably, intraoral acrylic splints. Internal fixators (pins and plates) often damage vital tooth and anatomic structures and are not commonly recommended by the veterinary dental community.

Tooth Trauma

Fractures involving pulp exposure are one of the few true dental emergencies. Pulp exposure of the primary teeth should be treated with either extraction or referral to a dental specialist for vital pulp therapy. Failure to treat fractured deciduous teeth can lead to infection of the permanent tooth bud.

Fractures of the permanent dentition involving pulp exposure in the young dog and cat require treatment in the form of extraction or referral to a dental specialist for vital pulp or root canal therapy. Vital pulp therapy can only be performed within 72 hours of tooth injury in dogs after 11 months of age. Prior to 11 months of age, the root apex has not closed and vital pulp therapy can be performed up to 2 weeks after injury. Often the duration of tooth injury is unknown and referral to a dental specialist should be offered. In this case vital pulp therapy is not a treatment option. Failure to treat fractures involving pulp exposure leads to severe pain, root end infection, inflammation, root abscessation, resorption, and possibly osteomyelitis.

In the feline it is often difficult to determine whether pulp exposure has occurred because of the small size of the pulp chamber. Typically if more than 1 to 2 mm of crown has fractured off the feline canine tooth, one can assume pulp exposure. Treatment recommendations are the same as for the dog.

Tooth Luxation/Avulsion

Luxation (partial displacement of a tooth from its alveolus) and avulsion (the loss of a tooth from the alveolus) are considered dental emergencies. Both conditions carry a guarded prognosis in terms of salvaging a vital tooth. If a tooth has been avulsed, it should be packaged and transported in the correct media, such as Hanks balanced salt solution, milk, or saline (in that order of preference). If the owners desire treatment to salvage the tooth, the animal should be referred to a dental specialist immediately for treatment. Otherwise, removal of the luxated or avulsed tooth and closure of the soft tissues are appropriate.

SUGGESTED READINGS

DeForge DH, Colmery BH: *An atlas of veterinary dental radiology,* Ames, Iowa, 2002, Iowa State University Press.

Hale FA: Juvenile veterinary dentistry, *Vet Clin North Am Small Anim Pract Dent* 35(4):789-818, 2005.

Holmstrom SE, Fitch PF, Eisner ER: *Veterinary dental techniques for the small animal practitioner,* ed 3, Philadelphia, 2004, Saunders.

McCoy DE: Surgical management of the tight lip syndrome in the Shar-Pei dog, *J Vet Dent* 14(3):95-96, 1997.

Step by Step Compendium: Compilation of veterinary dental techniques. Available through the *Journal of Veterinary Dentistry,* www.jvdonline.org/step-by-step.html. (Last accessed March 2, 2009.)

Wiggs RB, Lobprise HB: *Veterinary dentistry. Principles and practice,* Philadelphia, 1997, Lippincott-Raven.

THE DIGESTIVE SYSTEM*

Michael E. Peterson

PRENATAL AND NEONATAL DEVELOPMENT

The signals that regulate the differentiation and development of the fetal gastrointestinal tract (GIT) are not well understood. It is likely that factors exist in the amniotic fluid that may play a role in this process. Gut peptides are found in the fetal human GIT within the first trimester and in the amniotic fluid by the second trimester. In porcine and ovine fetuses, GIT development was impaired when the swallowing of amniotic fluid was prevented. Compared with controls, these animals showed a decrease in the weight of their small intestine, pancreas, and liver and a generalized thinning of the gut wall throughout the length of the GIT. Other factors, including cortisol, insulin, and numerous other hormones, present in both the fetal and maternal circulation also may have significant effects on GIT development. Although there have been very few studies examining the prenatal development of the GIT in dogs and cats, some brush-border enzymatic activity and nutrient transport activity are developed by parturition.

At birth, the GIT undergoes perhaps the most drastic change in function of any organ system except the lungs. During the first 24 hours, the canine small intestine nearly doubles in weight. At this time, the GIT must take over from the placenta the huge task of transferring nutrients from the outside world to the neonatal circulation. However, the intestinal wall of kittens grows little during the first week after birth. Because neonatal puppies and kittens have very small energy and glucose reserves, failure to make this accommodation becomes a serious if not fatal problem in a matter of hours.

The normal neonatal GIT is fully capable of digestion and absorption of its primary substrate, mother's milk. Many of the brush-border enzymes found in the mature GIT are present to facilitate the final stages of digestion and thus absorption. The activity of these enzymes increases markedly just before parturition; therefore premature animals may experience digestive difficulties.

The neonatal GIT is not well suited for ingesta other than milk. Newborn puppies lack certain pancreatic enzymes, and the muscularis layer of their small intestine is about 50% thinner than that found in adult dogs. Some of the brush-border enzymes, particularly the α-glycosidases, are not well developed, and this can cause problems if sugars such as sucrose or maltose are used in homemade milk replacers. Brush-border enzymes of the mature GIT are present, but their activity increases as the puppy ages. Suckling induces hypertrophic and hyperplastic mucosal cells in the neonatal dog.

Although the neonatal GIT may have difficulty handling foods other than milk, it is highly specialized for milk digestion and absorption. Not surprisingly, the changes that occur in the developing GIT are well matched to changes in the composition and volume of the milk with which it is presented. The first milk, colostrum, is rich in protein, immunoglobulins, hormones, and other factors that promote hypertrophy and hyperplasia of the neonatal GIT. Puppies fed milk replacer instead of colostrum experience a much smaller increase in intestinal mass during the first 24 hours of life.

The ability to internalize large molecules such as proteins persists up to 2 weeks after birth in many species. In puppies, this may help compensate for inadequate activities of pancreatic proteases that are secreted in only small amounts during the first 1 to 2 weeks of life. Neonatal puppies also secrete very little pancreatic lipase, but this is compensated for by secretion of gastric lipase. As the concentration of fat in milk increases over time, the secretion of pancreatic lipase also increases.

Gastric capacity can be approximated as 100 to 250 ml/ kg body weight in adult dogs with puppies having a greater

*Adapted from Hoskins JD: The digestive system. In Hoskins JD (ed): *Veterinary pediatrics: dogs and cats from birth to six months*, ed 3, Philadelphia, 2001, WB Saunders, p 147.

range in relative size. The entire neonatal GIT is colonized with bacteria at day 1; subsequentially the relative proportions of various groups of bacteria change, with anaerobic groups increasing in numbers.

From the second week to the seventh week of life, there is a multifold decrease in milk intake as a percentage of body weight. Similarly there is a threefold increase in solid food intake as a percentage of body weight from the third week to the seventh week. By 3 weeks of age, the puppy's GIT will have undergone considerable changes. The thickness of the gut wall will have nearly doubled primarily because of hypertrophy of the tunica muscularis. This will facilitate the passage of solid ingesta along the lumen of the gut. The pancreas will have developed adequate capacity to produce digestive enzymes and antibacterial factors. The introduction of solid food provides both a source and a substrate for bacterial growth, and these factors take over from those found in milk to help establish normal GI microflora.

In later life, the ability to change digestive function varies among species in accordance with natural variation in the diet. The cat, which is an obligate predator, is less able to vary its pancreatic and GIT enzyme activity than is the more omnivorous dog. Dogs also possess a tremendous capacity to adapt their GIT function over an enormous range of energy requirements. For most dogs, the largest demand on the GIT for processing nutrients occurs during growth. A weaned puppy may require 2 to 3 times the energy per unit body weight of a sedentary adult dog.*

THE ORAL CAVITY

Examination of the oral cavity should be consistent and systematic and include inspection and palpation of the gingiva, teeth, tongue, lingual frenulum, floor of the mouth, buccal surface, and hard and soft palates. Gentle opening and palpation of the oral cavity should not be painful or cause prompt withdrawal of the head. The breath of a growing, healthy dog or cat is not unpleasant. Alterations in the odor of the breath usually indicate a disease state, food the animal has eaten, or medication it has received. Offensive, foul-smelling breath may be caused by oral lesions, necrotic respiratory disease, or alimentary tract disease associated with belching.

The ingestive and masticatory functions of the oral cavity depend largely on the ability of the oral cavity to form a closed, hollow compartment, requiring labial and palatal competence. Cleft palate, cleft lip, or other causes of altered competence of the oral cavity should be identified during the oral examination.

Stomatitis

Any infectious, physical, or chemical agent or traumatic insult that significantly alters the replication, maturation, or exfoliation of the healthy mucosa favors the occurrence of stomatitis.

Feline rhinotracheitis virus (FRV) and feline calicivirus (FCV) cause most of the oral lesions seen in young cats. Buccal, lingual, and nasal ulcers frequently accompany these viral respiratory infections, although ulcers are generally more severe in FCV than in FRV infections. Feline leukemia virus and feline immunodeficiency virus may also be associated with oral lesions as a persistent glossitis, periodontitis, palatitis, and/or gingivitis, presumably because of virus-induced immunosuppression.

Foreign objects frequently cause traumatic insult to the oral mucosa of young dogs and cats, probably owing to the animals' curious natures and normal developmental chewing habits. The animal generally presents in varying phases of recovery, with secondary bacterial infection and scar tissue often camouflaging the foreign object(s). Removal of the foreign object(s) usually effects a cure. Intermittent problems from migrating grass awns or porcupine quills may be eliminated only by thorough dissection of irritated tissue. Traumatic injury to the tongue, palate, or lips is common, and the original wound is often aggravated by secondary bacterial infections. Oral burns from electrical cords are especially common in young dogs and cats that chew through the insulation of the cords. Pulmonary edema, seizures, and cardiac arrhythmias frequently accompany these electrical shock injuries.

In the immune-mediated diseases (i.e., pemphigus diseases, bullous pemphigoid, and lupus erythematosus), it is unusual in either the dog or cat for oral lesions to occur without skin involvement, especially at other mucocutaneous junctions, such as eyelids, nostrils, anus, vagina, and prepuce. Pemphigus foliaceus, the most common of the pemphigus diseases, rarely affects the oral cavity. Any of these immune-mediated diseases may first appear in the dog or cat at 4 to 6 months of age and typically follow the same lesion(s) development and patterns as seen in the adult. Their treatment follows the same regimen as used for the adult.

Lymphoplasmacytic stomatitis commonly affects young to middle-aged cats, but a cat as young as 4 months of age may be affected. Calicivirus has been isolated from some affected cats. The definitive cause of the oral lesions is unknown, but an immunologic basis has been suspected. Abyssinian and Somali are commonly affected cat breeds. Lymphoplasmacytic stomatitis typically follows the same lesion(s) development (i.e., small erythemic papules to severe mucosal proliferation of gingiva and/or palatal arches) as seen in the adult cat. Oral lesion(s) treatment follows the same regimen as used for the adult.

Mineral and vitamin deficiencies, heavy-metal poisoning, and coagulation abnormalities may also cause oral lesions. Although rarely seen, deficiencies in many of the B-complex vitamins and possibly in zinc may contribute to the appearance of oral lesions in growing, malnourished dogs or cats. Silver-gray Collies affected with cyclic hematopoiesis often develop a recurrent stomatitis that coincides with absolute neutropenia. Proliferative eosinophilic granulomas have

---

*Adapted from Reynolds AJ: Nutritional considerations in the pediatric dog: dietary and developmental relationships, Purina Research Report, Spring 2000.

been seen in the oral cavity of Siberian Huskies and in many breeds of young cats (i.e., in kittens as young as 8 weeks of age).

The definitive cause of a stomatitis cannot always be determined by history, physical examination, cytologic examination, bacterial and fungal culture, or tissue biopsy. In many cases, bacterial cultures reveal the normal mixed flora of the oral cavity, often making antimicrobial etiologies unreliable. In these cases, therapy to treat the symptoms is often efficacious. Daily flushing of the mouth with chlorhexidine (diluted to 0.1% to 0.2% solution in tepid water) followed by rinsing the mouth with copious amounts of fresh water will help cleanse the affected areas. Soft, palatable food may need to be provided for several days during the initial healing phase. Ampicillin, amoxicillin, or cephalosporins may be administered daily in an oral liquid form for both a local antimicrobial effect and subsequent systemic effect after absorption. Antimicrobial therapy may be indicated for up to 3 weeks.

Tumors of the Oral Cavity

Oral papillomas are caused by papillomavirus, commonly occur in dogs younger than 1 year of age, and may spread through a kennel in 2 to 4 weeks. The cauliflower-like growths begin as smooth, cream-colored elevations, which later become rough and gray. The oral mucosa and commissures of the lips are most commonly affected. The number and size of lesions are variable. In most cases, therapy is usually unnecessary because the lesions regress spontaneously in 6 to 12 weeks. Surgical excision may be a means of stimulating regression and eliminating confluent pedunculated masses, which may impair the prehension and mastication of food. Lifetime immunity generally follows recovery.

Tonsillitis

Small-breed young dogs are most commonly affected with primary tonsillitis. Anorexia, lethargy, dysphagia, coughing, gagging, and fever are the usual complaints. The absence of tonsillar swelling does not necessarily preclude the diagnosis of tonsillitis, especially in cats. Improvement of the animal, observed with antimicrobial therapy, generally precedes resolution of the inflammation, although tonsillar swelling may continue to be present. Recurrence is common, with exacerbations lasting several days. Tonsillectomy is rarely required in recurrent tonsillitis unless the tonsillar enlargement obstructs the pharynx. Most dogs can be effectively treated medically and appear to "outgrow" the problem. Medical treatment of tonsillitis includes using broad-spectrum antimicrobial agents and supportive care as discussed for stomatitis. Bacterial culture of inflamed tonsillar tissue usually produces β-hemolytic streptococci, coliforms, or other bacteria of the normal oral flora; therefore identification of antimicrobial etiologies may be unreliable.

Secondary tonsillitis may be associated with systemic disease or local predisposing anatomic or pathologic factors. The presence of tonsillitis does not indicate the site of primary disease. Any persistent irritation or inflammatory process of the oral cavity or pharynx (e.g., abscesses, gingivitis, lodged foreign object(s), or persistent vomiting or regurgitation) may induce a secondary tonsillitis. The gagging, regurgitation, and vomiting of foam in cases of tonsillitis necessitate differentiation from megaesophagus, pyloric disorders, cricopharyngeal achalasia, productive cough, retropharyngeal abscesses, and lodged foreign object(s) in the pharynx, larynx, or esophagus. Treatment should be directed toward eliminating the underlying secondary cause of the tonsillitis.

THE SALIVARY GLANDS

Congenital enlargement of the parotid salivary glands has been reported in dogs. The dogs typically present with hypersalivation (drooling) and are treated effectively with parotid duct ligation.

Sialadenitis may be caused by bite wounds, lacerations, blunt trauma, or extension from cellulitis and abscesses of the head and neck. Sudden swelling in the region of a salivary gland, fever, inappetence, and pain on opening the mouth are usually evident on physical examination. Diagnosis of sialadenitis is usually obvious, but cytologic examination confirms salivary tissue involvement. Treatment should be aimed at the underlying cause. Ways of providing symptomatic relief include the administration of antimicrobial agents, application of warm compresses, replacement fluid therapy, drainage if abscess is present, and frequent feeding of small amounts of a nutritionally complete, soft, palatable food.

A sialocele is a collection of saliva in tissue. Any age, sex, and breed of dog or cat can be affected. Sialocele formation most commonly involves the sublingual and mandibular salivary glands, where blockage of a duct or rupture of the gland causes extravasation of saliva into the surrounding connective tissue. The saliva may gravitate to the sublingual area (often referred to as a *ranula*), intermandibular space, mediastinum, or pharyngeal area (Figure 36-1). Swelling may develop suddenly but is more likely to be in the form of a slowly developing, fluctuant sac. Diagnosis of sialocele is based on physical appearance of the cervical swelling and on cytologic evaluation. Needle aspiration of the swelling yields a viscous, mucoid fluid that is usually clear or brown. Total excision of the affected gland, which is usually the sublingual or mandibular gland, and drainage of the sialocele provide the only long-term therapy. Removal of an elliptic portion of the wall of a ranula allows direct drainage of saliva into the oral cavity. The surgical techniques for the management of salivary gland disorders are described elsewhere.

THE OROPHARYNX

The events of swallowing can be divided into oral, pharyngeal, and cricopharyngeal stages. Dysphagia is uncommon in dogs and rare in cats. Dysphagia is usually recognized in puppies and kittens shortly after weaning.

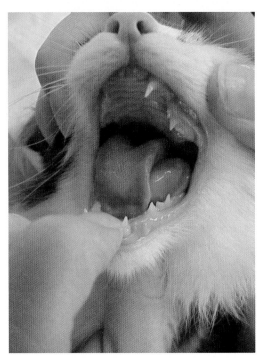

Figure 36-1 Ranula under the tongue of young cat. (Courtesy Bethany Grobson, DVM, Veterinary Information Network.)

Oral dysphagias may result from disturbances to various motor and sensory tracts and peripheral nerves. Branches of cranial nerves V, IX, and X provide sensory innervation for swallowing, and cranial nerves V, VII, IX, X, XI, and XII deliver motor innervation via the nucleus ambiguus and the respiratory centers. Signs of oral dysphagia may include difficulty in prehension of food and lapping water, excessive chewing or chomping, hypersalivation, and diminished or absent gag reflex. Evidence of denervation of the tongue may exist, and food may drop from the animal's mouth or be retained in the buccal cavity.

Pharyngeal dysphagias are less consistent, and related signs are more difficult to localize. The most common signs are coughing with repeated unsuccessful attempts at swallowing and laryngotracheal aspiration of swallowed material. Often the puppy or kitten will regurgitate masticated food several hours after ingestion, or food or liquid material will be misdirected into the nasopharynx, leading to nasal discharge.

Cricopharyngeal dysphagias typically manifest as problems of asynchrony (i.e., incoordination of pharyngeal contraction and cricopharyngeal sphincter relaxation) or as achalasia (i.e., failure of cricopharyngeal sphincter relaxation). Signs of cricopharyngeal dysphagias can vary, depending on whether there is an achalasia or asynchrony.

Differentiation of oral, pharyngeal, and cricopharyngeal dysphagias is important. Myotomy of the muscles of the cricopharyngeal sphincter gives dramatic improvement in cricopharyngeal achalasia. However, oral and pharyngeal dysphagias are generally made worse by the myotomy procedures. Oral and pharyngeal dysphagias are best managed by treating any underlying medical illness, changing the consistency of the animal's usual diet, and feeding the animal in an elevated position. If conservative therapy is not helpful and the owner does not wish to continue feeding by one of the enteral methods, cricopharyngeal myotomy may be considered. The owner should be aware that cricopharyngeal myotomy may make the animal's condition worse.

THE ESOPHAGUS

An important species difference between the dog and cat is in the musculature of the esophageal body. The entire length of the canine esophageal body is composed of striated muscle, whereas the distal one third to one half of the feline esophagus is composed of smooth muscle.

Vascular ring anomalies are congenital malformations of the great vessel system that interfere with esophageal function. These anomalies produce an extramural obstruction of the esophagus at the base of the heart and rarely affect the trachea or cardiovascular system. The most frequently encountered vascular ring anomaly in the young dog or cat is persistent right aortic arch. The incidence of vascular ring anomalies is higher in young dogs than in young cats. Irish Setters, Boston Terriers, and German Shepherd Dogs are the most commonly affected dog breeds.

Signs caused by the vascular ring anomalies result from esophageal entrapment and obstruction, with subsequent precordial megaesophagus. When weaning to solid food, puppies and kittens will repeatedly regurgitate. Although regurgitation is usually associated with eating when solid food is first fed, it will occur at variable times after eating as the precordial megaesophagus worsens. Occasionally signs in the puppy or kitten are associated with ingestion of maternal milk. Affected animals are obviously malnourished and underweight. The diagnosis of a vascular ring anomaly-induced megaesophagus can usually be confirmed by a positive contrast esophagogram (Figure 36-2).

Treatment is early surgical correction by ligation and transection of the stricturing ligament or vessel and complete mobilization of the esophagus from the connective tissue in the area of entrapment. Prognosis is guarded pending complete postoperative recovery because of frequent complicating factors (e.g., existing malnourishment, weakened state of the animal, aspiration pneumonia, and persistent megaesophagus despite surgical correction). Most animals show substantial improvement if they survive the immediate postoperative period. Persistent megaesophagus occurs if the esophagus develops sacculations, an extensive dilation that fills the anterior region of the mediastinum, or dilation of the esophagus caudal to the vascular ring anomaly.

Esophagitis is unusual in the young dog and cat and usually occurs because of traumatic insult, ingestion of a chemical or thermal irritant, or gastric acid reflux. Thermal injuries may occur when eager eaters bolt hot food or when puppies or kittens are fed hot gruel. Gastric acid reflux is uncommon as a primary event but can occur any time the

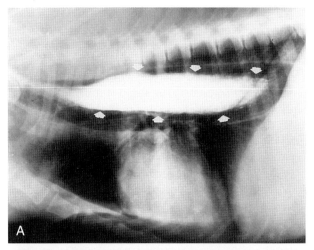

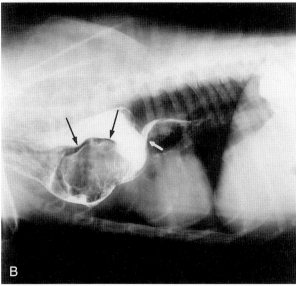

Figure 36-2 A, Lateral thoracic contrast-enhanced esophagram from a dog with generalized esophageal weakness. Note that barium is retained throughout the length of the esophagus (arrows). **B,** Lateral thoracic contrast-enhanced radiograph of a dog with an esophageal obstruction caused by a vascular ring anomaly. The column of barium stops abruptly (short arrow) in front of the heart, a finding characteristic of a persistent fourth aortic arch. A filling defect is also displacing barium in the dilated portion of the esophagus (long arrows). (From Nelson RW: *Small animal internal medicine*, ed 4, St Louis, 2009, Mosby. Courtesy Dr. Phillip F. Steyn, Colorado State University, Fort Collins, CO.)

lower esophageal sphincter pressure is compromised, such as during anesthesia or severe blunt trauma directly to the thorax or abdomen. Esophagitis can be limited to mucosal damage or may extend into the submucosa and musculature. If only the mucosa is involved, the esophagitis is usually mild and self-limiting. However, esophagitis with submucosal and musculature involvement often leads to severe ulceration with subsequent perforation, fibrotic stricture formation, persistence of inflammation, and/or disturbed motor activity (acquired megaesophagus).

Signs of esophagitis are regurgitation and dysphagia. Esophagoscopy may be required to make a definitive diagnosis by visualization of mucosal changes; questionable cases may be confirmed by histopathology. Treatment of esophagitis is aimed at eliminating the underlying cause and symptomatic management of the esophagus and the systemic effects that the esophagitis created. Means of providing symptomatic relief include esophageal rest by feeding through a gastrostomy tube or by frequent small feedings of nutritionally complete, soft, bland food and administration of antimicrobial agents, H_2-receptor antagonists, metoclopramide, and sucralfate slurry (crush 1 gm of sucralfate and mix with 10 ml of water; give 5 ml of slurry 4 to 6 times daily).

Idiopathic megaesophagus is characterized by motor disturbances of the esophagus that result in abnormal or unsuccessful transport of ingesta between the pharynx and stomach.

Both congenital and acquired forms of idiopathic megaesophagus occur in young dogs and cats. There is evidence that congenital idiopathic megaesophagus is inherited in both the dog (e.g., Wire Fox Terrier and Miniature Schnauzer) and cat. The incidence is highest in Great Danes, German Shepherd Dogs, Irish Setters, Labrador Retrievers, and Chinese Shar-Peis. Esophageal dysfunction in Chinese Shar-Peis may result from segmental hypomotility and esophageal redundancy. In the cat, Siamese and Siamese-related breeds have the highest incidence.

Acquired idiopathic megaesophagus may occur spontaneously in any young dog or cat. In most instances, the underlying cause is undetermined; however, megaesophagus may occur in several systemic diseases that affect the nervous system or skeletal muscles. These diseases include myasthenia gravis, polymyositis, toxoplasmosis, canine distemper, hypothyroidism, hypoadrenocorticism, and myotonia with myopathy. Other potential diseases that could contribute to megaesophagus are systemic lupus erythematosus, tick paralysis, botulism, tetanus, lead poisoning, ganglioradiculitis, dysautonomia, anticholinesterase compounds, and polyneuritis. Megaesophagus has also been associated in cats with pyloric dysfunction and feline dysautonomia, often referred to as the Key-Gaskell syndrome. Canine or feline dysautonomia, the main features of which are dilated pupils, dry mucous membranes, megaesophagus, constipation, and dysuria and urinary incontinence with urinary bladder distention, is a dysfunction of the autonomic nervous system. The cause of dysautonomia is currently unknown.

The onset of signs associated with congenital idiopathic megaesophagus usually begins around the time of weaning. Signs may include effortless regurgitation of esophageal contents, weight loss, polyphagia, weakness, dehydration, impaired skeletal mineralization, ballooning of the cervical esophagus that is synchronized with respiration, and recurrent laryngotracheal aspiration that often leads to recurrent pneumonia. Oral fetor may be present owing to stagnation of fermenting ingesta retained in the dilated esophagus. Regurgitation may be seen immediately on feeding or up to

12 or more hours later. The time interval between eating and regurgitation can be related to the degree of dilation or to the general activity of the animal. Usually both liquids and solids are poorly tolerated.

Survey thoracic radiographs consistently reveal a dilated esophagus (Figure 36-3). Evidence of aspiration pneumonia is frequently present and consistent with the signs of dysphagia and regurgitation.

When the esophagus is not observed visually on survey radiographs, a contrast esophagogram is required. A barium contrast study better defines the degree of esophageal dilation, lack of function, and extent of involvement (Figure 36-4). The study helps rule out congenital vascular ring anomalies or other causes of localized obstruction that might contribute to megaesophagus and outlines the funnel shape of the caudal region of the esophagus to rule out invasive processes that may cause irregular or asymmetric narrowing.

Treatment of congenital idiopathic megaesophagus consisting of proper dietary management in terms of frequent, elevated feedings with foods of appropriate consistency for the particular animal (some handle bulky foods well; others better tolerate gruels) generally results in spontaneous improvement in a number of animals. This had led investigators to believe that congenital idiopathic megaesophagus may be caused by delayed neurologic development of esophageal innervation. With elevated feedings and

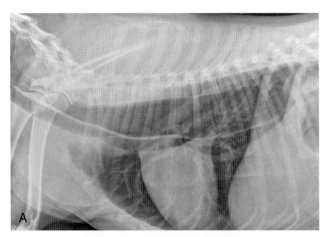

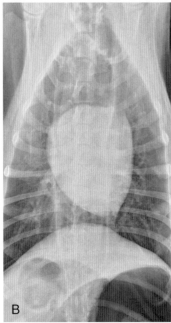

Figure 36-3 Lateral **(A)** and ventrodorsal **(B)** radiographs of a dog with generalized megaesophagus; the esophagus is filled with gas. **A,** Note the sharp demarcation between the esophagus and longus coli muscles, the ventral depression of the trachea, the long tracheal stripe sign, and the visibility of the esophageal walls in the caudal aspect of the thorax. A dilated esophagus is more difficult to see in the ventrodorsal view, but in this patient note the radiopaque lines paralleling the spine on each side of the thorax and how these lines converge caudally as they approach the stomach **(B)**. (From Thrall DE: *Textbook of veterinary diagnostic radiology*, ed 5, St Louis, 2007, Saunders.)

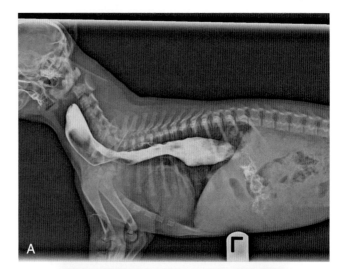

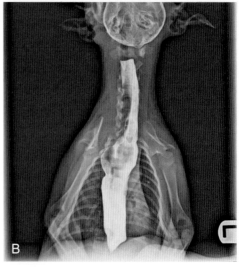

Figure 36-4 Megaesophagus in a puppy. **A** and **B,** A two-view contrast study demonstrating the extent of the dilation. (Courtesy John Feleciano.)

minimal distention of the esophagus, normal esophageal motor function may develop. If stasis of esophageal contents is allowed, however, gradual overdistention and atony result, contributing to persistent megaesophagus. The earlier the dysfunction is recognized and the dietary management instituted, the better the prognosis. Puppies and kittens diagnosed at weaning and managed appropriately have a better prognosis than those whose condition is recognized later, at around 4 to 6 months of age. Once severe megaesophagus occurs, complete recovery is unlikely. Aspiration pneumonia and malnourishment limit the longevity of these animals.

Disorders of the Gastroesophageal Junction

Disorders affecting the function of the gastroesophageal junction are uncommon. The disorders more commonly associated with its altered function are hiatal hernia with reflux esophagitis and gastroesophageal intussusception. Hiatal hernia is the result of a congenital or acquired defect of the phrenoesophageal ligament that allows displacement of the gastroesophageal junction forward into the thoracic cavity. Hiatal hernia may also be associated with an upper respiratory obstruction, especially common in young Chinese Shar-Peis. Gastric contents reflux through the incompetent junction into the caudal region of the esophagus, where they produce varying degrees of irritation to the esophageal mucosa. Signs may include regurgitation with possible hematemesis, dysphagia, altered breathing pattern, and weight loss. Diagnosis requires a high index of suspicion followed by a barium contrast study performed under fluoroscopic observation.

Gastroesophageal intussusception or invagination involves the telescoping of all or part of the stomach into the esophageal lumen (Figure 36-5). Occasionally the spleen and pancreas are also included. The cause of this condition is not understood, but an incompetent gastroesophageal junction must be suspected. Gastroesophageal intussusception generally occurs in puppies of large breeds and in kittens, particularly those with congenital megaesophagus. A puppy or kitten will be presented to the veterinarian with sudden onset of difficulty in breathing, impending shock, and a history of vomiting. The sudden onset of signs and radiographic appearance of the mass are the keys to the diagnosis. Treatment is surgical reduction of the intussusception and a gastropexy.

THE STOMACH

Gastritis, inflammation, and mucosal damage that have occurred in response to an insult to the gastric mucosa frequently occur in dogs and cats from weaning through adulthood. Vomiting is typically the primary sign. Vomiting as an event first appears in puppies and kittens with a full stomach at 3 days and 10 days of age, respectively.

Observation of the amount, color, and consistency of vomitus is useful for obtaining insight into the origin of a gastric disorder and the degree of mucosal damage. If the vomitus consists of food, the degree of digestion indicates

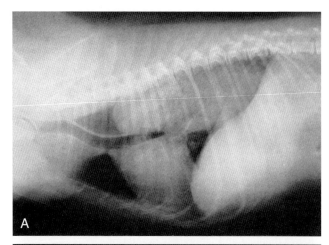
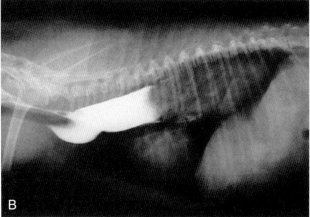

Figure 36-5 Survey **(A)** and contrast **(B)** radiographic appearance of gastroesophageal intussusception in a 12-month-old mixed-breed dog. (From Ettinger SJ: *Textbook veterinary internal medicine*, ed 5, Philadelphia, 2000, WB Saunders.)

the length of time food has remained in the stomach. Vomitus containing feces usually indicates intestinal stasis or possibly intestinal obstruction. Fresh blood from gastric bleeding may be present as small red flecks or as large blood clots. Blood that has been retained in the stomach soon becomes partially digested and has a brown "coffee grounds" appearance. The presence of blood in vomitus usually signifies a more serious gastric disorder.

Gastritis can be associated with a multitude of factors but more commonly results from dietary indiscretions, infectious diseases, and possibly endoparasites. It is often associated with ingestion of rancid or contaminated foodstuffs that leads to food intoxication. The incidence of ingested foreign material is much higher in young dogs and cats, possibly owing to their developmental chewing habits and curious natures. Many drugs (e.g., antimicrobial agents, nonsteroidal antiinflammatory drugs, anthelmintics, and corticosteroids) and chemicals (e.g., heavy metals, cleaning agents, fertilizers, and herbicides) may also contribute to gastritis in the young animal.

The incidence of bacteria-induced gastritis is extremely low because the acidic gastric lumen does not favor the growth and colonization of bacteria. A gastric chlamydial infection has been identified in young cats. Other conditions, including renal failure, liver disease, neurologic disease, shock, sepsis, and possibly altered behavior, may also play a role in the cause of gastritis in the young dog and cat.

Gastritis is generally diagnosed and treated based on the animal's history, signs, and physical findings. Symptomatic treatment of most cases of gastritis and vomiting is begun without extensive diagnostic procedures. Most animals show improvement within 12 to 24 hours after little or no therapy and usually are treated on an outpatient basis. Those animals with persistent vomiting, evidence of dehydration, abdominal pain, organomegaly or palpable abdominal mass, or failure to respond to previous symptomatic treatment require further medical and laboratory evaluation.

Dietary restriction is the initial management for gastritis. An animal with gastritis should be withheld food for 24 to 48 hours and water for 12 to 24 hours. If no vomiting occurs during this period of management, over the next 2 to 5 days the animal is gradually returned to full feed and water. Water is offered initially in small, frequent amounts or provided in ice cubes, enough to keep the mouth moist and to supply a modest fluid replacement. Until vomiting is well controlled, small amounts (3 to 6 times daily) of a highly digestible, low-fiber diet are fed frequently, including cooked rice or cooked cereals supplemented in a 50:50 ratio with boiled chicken, lean boiled ground beef, or commercial baby foods (without garlic or onion). Commercial diets formulated for gastrointestinal disease may also be prescribed. One can expect most cases of vomiting in young dogs and cats to respond to just dietary and water intake management.

Administration of parenteral fluids is initiated when electrolyte or acid-base imbalances or dehydration occurs. The quantity of fluids given should be enough to supply daily maintenance needs (approximately 40 to 60 ml/kg/day), to correct existing dehydration, and to replace fluid losses caused by continued vomiting.

Antiemetic drugs may be given to control refractory vomiting in dogs and cats older than 3 months and when the presence of a pyloric dysfunction or a gastric foreign object has been ruled out. These drugs inhibit vomiting but do little for primary treatment of gastritis. Antiemetic drugs act centrally by suppressing either the chemoreceptor trigger zone (CRTZ), the emetic center, or the vestibular apparatus. The phenothiazine tranquilizers (chlorpromazine) have a broad-spectrum pharmacologic effect in blocking the emetic center and the CRTZ and some anticholinergic action. Anticholinergic drugs reduce gastric motility and smooth muscle spasms. In addition to blocking the parasympathetic stimulation of smooth muscles, these drugs block the cephalic and gastric phases of gastric acid secretion, but they do not block histamine or gastrin-stimulated acid secretion. These drugs have the adverse effect of slowing gastric emptying, which results in gastric distention and further gastric acid secretion. Overuse of the anticholinergic drugs can cause gastric atony and a pharmacologic gastric outflow obstruction, resulting in further vomiting. Anticholinergic drugs used in the

therapy of gastric disorders include atropine and propantheline. These drugs often are combined with an antiemetic for veterinary use.

Oral protectants, such as kaolin and pectin, and antimicrobial agents are usually not indicated for the treatment of gastritis in the young dog or cat. Protectants may bind certain bacteria or toxins, but they do not coat or protect the irritated gastric mucosa. Any potential benefit is frequently outweighed by difficulty in owner administration and vomiting that occurs because of gastric distention. However, sucralfate in tablet form or given as a slurry (crush 1 gm of sucralfate and mix with 10 ml of water; give 5 ml of slurry 4 to 6 times daily) may be protective when the gastric mucosa is irritated or ulcerated. Antimicrobial agents are not required unless a bacterial infection is suspected.

Secretory blockers (H_2-receptor antagonists), such as cimetidine, ranitidine, and famotidine, are effective in reducing gastric acid production by blocking the H_2 receptors of the parietal cells. Use of these drugs has been recommended in the symptomatic treatment of gastric and duodenal ulcers and in syndromes resulting in gastric acid hypersecretion. They may be useful as adjunctive therapy in some types of gastritis; however, they probably should not be administered to dogs or cats younger than 2 months of age.

Gastric retention and paresis are most often associated with pyloric dysfunction, motility disturbances of the stomach, or both. Pyloric dysfunction in the young dog or cat usually results from congenital pyloric stenosis or from an intraluminal foreign object obstructing the gastric outflow area. Traumatic injury and inflammatory disease can reduce motility throughout the GIT, resulting in the retention of gastric contents. Drugs, hypokalemia, recurring gastric dilation, and long-term obstruction of the pylorus may also contribute to altered gastric motility and gastric retention.

Congenital pyloric stenosis is recognized most often in the Boxer and Boston Terrier dog breeds. It rarely occurs in the young cat, although Siamese cats have the highest reported incidence. Congenital pyloric stenosis probably is caused by excessive secretion of gastrointestinal hormones. Gastrin, produced by the G cells in the stomach wall, has a potent trophic effect on pyloric circular smooth muscle, as well as on the mucosa. With altered gastric motility and antral distention, the G cells are stimulated to release gastrin, ultimately leading to an increase in gastric acid production and pyloric stenosis from hypertrophy of the circular smooth muscle.

Gastric retention either is present at birth or develops with advancing age. Vomiting at variable intervals after ingestion of solid food, with accompanying gastric distention, is the primary sign of gastric retention. The vomitus is usually undigested food and is rarely bile stained. Animals with gastric retention may exhibit projectile vomiting; the vomiting occurs abruptly and without the warning of hypersalivation and retching. In most instances, the vomitus is propelled a considerable distance and readily empties the stomach. After vomiting, the animal will usually resume feeding, only to vomit again at variable intervals.

On survey abdominal radiographs, the presence of gastric distention with food or air, long after the ingesta should be in the intestine (within 6 to 8 hours after eating), is suggestive of gastric retention. Contrast medium studies are useful for assessing the rate of gastric emptying of liquids in those animals suspected of having abnormal gastric retention. Less than 30 minutes is generally considered to be a normal gastric emptying time for a quiet, well-behaved animal. The presence of contrast medium or food in the stomach for longer than 12 to 24 hours is definitely abnormal and should be considered evidence of gastric retention. Chemical or manual restraint of the young animal will slow gastric emptying for a variable length of time.

Congenital pyloric stenosis is generally managed surgically with pyloroplasty. Medical therapy has been generally directed toward the control of signs, mainly through the use of dietary management and antiemetic drugs. Gastric stimulation with metoclopramide is helpful in animals with functional, but not anatomical, gastric retention. Metoclopramide increases gastric antral contractions, promotes relaxation of the pylorus, and increases smooth muscle contraction in the proximal small intestine. Metoclopramide is contraindicated whenever increased gastrointestinal motility might be harmful. It should not be administered to animals with central nervous system disease, given in conjunction with phenothiazines or narcotic analgesics, or administered to animals younger than 2 months of age.

Gastric dilation-volvulus (GDV) syndrome is most frequently seen in dogs between the ages of 2 and 10 years and seldom in cats or dogs younger than 6 months. However, owners of deep-chested breeds at high risk for development of GDV may elect preventive gastropexy at the time of spay or neuter. Several surgical techniques have been described to prevent GDV.

THE INTESTINE

Congenital disorders of the intestinal tract are rarely encountered in puppies and kittens, probably because most such affected animals die at birth or become fading puppies or kittens. The congenital disorders that have been reported include atresia of intestinal segment and duplication of intestinal segment. These disorders in the newborn puppy or kitten are usually incompatible with life unless corrected surgically.

Enterocolitis frequently occurs in dogs and cats from weaning through adulthood. Enterocolitis is inflammation and mucosal damage that has occurred in response to an insult to the small and large intestine. Diarrhea is the primary sign of enterocolitis and often occurs secondary to many nonintestinal diseases. Diarrhea of young dogs and cats typically is of abrupt onset and has a short course that ranges from transient and self-limiting to fulminating and explosive. With the aid of history, physical examination, and stool characteristics (i.e., frequency, volume, consistency, color, odor, and composition), diarrhea can be localized to the

small intestine, large intestine, or both (Table 36-1), and a search for the cause and treatment can be undertaken.

Enterocolitis is associated with many factors but more commonly results from dietary indiscretions, infectious diseases, and endoparasitism. Dietary causes may include intestinal overload from overeating; ingestion of rancid or spoiled foodstuffs from scavenging of decomposing garbage or

TABLE 36-1	Differentiation of small intestinal diarrhea from large intestinal diarrhea	
Signs	Small intestine	Large intestine
Feces		
Volume	Always increased	Normal or increased (small quantities)
Mucus	Absent	Invariably present
Blood	Dark black (digested)	Red (fresh)
Fat droplets	Present with maldigestive or malabsorptive disease	Absent
Undigested food	May be present with maldigestion	Absent
Color	Color variations occur; lighter colored (e.g., creamy brown), orange, green, or gray	May appear bloody
Defecation		
Frequency	Normal or slightly increased	Very frequent
Urgency	Absent	Usually present
Tenesmus	Absent	Usually present
Associated Signs		
Vomiting	May be present	Uncommon
Generalized malaise	May be present	Uncommon
Flatulence and borborygmus	May be present	Absent
Belching	May be present	Uncommon
Altered breath odor in the absence of stomatitis	May be present	Absent
Weight loss or failure to gain weight	May be present	Uncommon

carrion; ingestion of indigestible and abrasive foreign material, such as bones, rocks, plants, wood, cloth, thread and sewing needles, and plastic objects; intolerance of lactose ingested as milk; and intolerance of miscellaneous types of food, such as fatty or spicy food. Trichobezoars (hairballs) are frequently encountered in the diarrheic stools of long-haired cats and some dogs. Care should be taken to mix the first couple of days of milk replacer with a balanced electrolyte solution instead of water to prevent an osmotic diarrhea from occurring. Many drugs (e.g., corticosteroids, nonsteroidal antiinflammatory drugs, antimicrobial agents, and anthelmintics) and chemicals (e.g., heavy metals, cleaning agents, fertilizers, and herbicides) may cause enterocolitis. Many ingested plants and plant toxins may cause diarrhea and an associated enterocolitis.

Many infectious agents are generally associated with varying degrees of enterocolitis. Bacteria reside in, and may contribute to severe mucosal damage in, the small and/or large intestine. Viruses are important causes of enterocolitis in young dogs and cats. In refractory diarrheal problems, feline leukemia virus, feline immunodeficiency virus, and feline infectious peritonitis virus should be considered in the diagnosis.

Endoparasites generally do not produce intestinal lesions but contribute importantly to generalized unthriftiness, diarrhea, and weight loss or failure to gain adequate body weight. The younger the animal, the more frequently endoparasites are present and the more severe the consequences. Endoparasitism often complicates other existing intestinal disorders such as virus- or bacteria-induced enterocolitis.

The diagnosis of acute enterocolitis is usually made based on an animal's history, signs, and physical findings, often without detailed diagnostic procedures. A review of the animal's vaccination status, diet, current medications, and possible exposure to chemicals or infectious diseases is warranted. Diagnostic evaluations considered for short-term diarrhea are fecal identification of endoparasites, virologic tests, fecal cultures for bacteria, and survey abdominal radiographs for detection of intestinal foreign material or an obstruction.

Symptomatic treatment is given initially for most cases of enterocolitis and diarrhea without extensive diagnostic procedures. Most animals with enterocolitis show improvement within 24 to 48 hours with little or no therapy and usually are treated on an outpatient basis. The basic principles in the treatment of enterocolitis include removing the inciting cause; providing proper conditions to promote mucosal repair; correcting fluid, electrolyte, and acid-base abnormalities; and alleviating secondary complications of enterocolitis, such as vomiting, abdominal pain, and infection.

Dietary restriction is the initial step in the management of enterocolitis. Animals with severe intestinal disturbances should be deprived of food for 24 to 48 hours or longer. Water may be offered in small amounts during the first 24 hours. If the animal is vomiting, however, water should be restricted. Restriction of food and possibly water allows for restoration of mucosal integrity and a more rapid return of

gastrointestinal function. In most cases, fasting reduces or eliminates diarrhea by removing the osmotic or irritating effects of undigested or unabsorbed nutrients. If no diarrhea has occurred during the 24- to 48-hour fast, small amounts of a highly digestible, low-fiber, moderately low-fat diet are fed 3 to 6 times daily, such as cooked rice or cooked cereals supplemented in a 4:1 ratio with lean boiled ground beef or chicken or commercial baby foods. Commercial diets formulated for gastrointestinal disease may also be prescribed. With the commercial diets, the animal is first fed one third the amount needed to meet normal maintenance caloric needs. Over the next several days, the amount of food is gradually increased to meet the animal's needs to maintain body weight.

Parenteral fluids are initiated when electrolyte or acid-base imbalances or dehydration occurs. Diarrhea in enterocolitis generally results in volume depletion and losses of sodium, chloride, bicarbonate, and potassium with metabolic acidosis. An isotonic, balanced electrolyte solution such as lactated Ringer's solution is usually recommended. Potassium levels are often depleted, particularly if inappetence has accompanied profuse diarrhea, and additional potassium chloride should be added to the fluids. The amount of potassium chloride added is based on the existing serum potassium levels.

Protectants are used frequently in the general treatment of diarrhea, although they are probably not beneficial in animals. However, there is some evidence that pectin plus salicylates can absorb and inactivate enterotoxins, such as those produced by *Escherichia coli*. Of the salicylates, bismuth subsalicylate appears to be more effective as an oral antidiarrheal compound. The dose is about 0.25 ml/kg body weight divided into 4 to 6 equal daily doses (liquid, not tablets). Bismuth subsalicylate probably should be administered with caution in cats because of their increased sensitivity to aspirin and should not be administered to cats younger than 3 months of age.

The use of narcotic analgesics as antimotility drugs is warranted in the treatment of some diarrheas. The rationale behind their use is based on their direct action on the smooth muscle of the small intestine and colon, causing increasing tone and segmentation. This produces increased resistance to luminal transit of ingesta. These drugs effectively relieve abdominal pain and tenesmus and reduce the frequency of stools. The narcotic analgesics, such as diphenoxylate hydrochloride and loperamide hydrochloride (this is a compound cleared by P-glycoprotein and should not be used in animals deficient [e.g., herding breeds]), are the preferred motility modifiers to be used in the symptomatic treatment of diarrhea. If the diarrhea is caused by an infectious agent such as *Salmonella*, the narcotic analgesics may be detrimental because they may trap organisms and their toxins within the intestine, and the infection may persist longer.

The use of antimicrobial agents in the treatment of diarrhea is controversial. In diarrhea, antimicrobial therapy is warranted only when there is evidence of inflammation in the GIT (numerous inflammatory cells in the feces), damaged intestinal mucosa (blood in the stool), a systemic inflammatory reaction (fever and leukocytosis), and/or abnormal fecal culture results.

Protein-Losing Enteropathy

Protein-losing enteropathies are characterized by the loss of protein into the intestinal lumen. Causes of protein-losing enteropathies in young dogs and cats include congenital lymphangiectasia, congestive heart failure, and infectious inflammatory and ulcerative enteric diseases. Congenital lymphangiectasia results from malformation of the lymphatic system; it rarely occurs in puppies and kittens. Two breeds of dogs are reported to be predisposed to a form of lymphangiectasia and protein-losing enteropathy, that is, the Norwegian Lundehund and the Basenji. In the Norwegian Lundehund, the disorder appears to have a hereditary basis and is characterized by intermittent diarrhea, vomiting, weight loss, anorexia, hypoalbuminemia, ascites, and edema.

In the Basenji, the lymphangiectasia occurs secondary to a unique intestinal disease that has been referred to as immunoproliferative enteropathy of Basenjis. This disorder appears to have a hereditary basis and is characterized by bouts of intermittent diarrhea, weight loss, hypoalbuminemia, hyperglobulinemia (an unusual finding in protein-losing enteropathy), and widespread lymphocytic-plasmacytic infiltration of the GIT. In puppies, swelling of buccal lymph nodes, adverse effects from routine vaccinations, and transient neurologic signs are additional features of the disorder. Neurologic signs may include incoordination, paresis, seizures, and contracture of the facial musculature.

The diagnosis of protein-losing enteropathy and lymphangiectasia is established by the animal's history, signs, physical findings, and histologic confirmation of the characteristic lesions in intestinal biopsy specimens. Biopsy specimens may be obtained via laparotomy or less invasively by endoscopy or peroral suction biopsy capsule. Surgery in dogs with severe hypoalbuminemia or emaciation is not without risk. Full-thickness surgical biopsy tissue from the intestine often leads to dehiscence of the enterotomy incisions and postoperative peritonitis; serosal patching at incisional sites may be needed. Thus when possible, biopsies performed via endoscopy or suction biopsy capsule are preferred over full-thickness biopsies.

With congenital protein-losing enteropathy and lymphangiectasia, carrier dogs may be subclinically affected well into breeding age. A developed fecal enzyme-linked immunosorbent assay (ELISA) can be used in early screening of potential breeding animals and for puppies as young as 3 months of age. In testing progeny of affected dogs, results of the fecal ELISA become abnormal well before identifiable hypoalbuminemia occurs.

The primary therapy for protein-losing enteropathies is to decrease the intestinal loss of plasma proteins so that normal serum protein levels can be restored and edema and effusions controlled. Dietary manipulation and elimination of the underlying cause of the protein-losing enteropathy are the primary methods used in its treatment. The preferred diet for young dogs and cats with protein-losing enteropathy should contain minimal fat and provide an ample amount of high-quality protein. Commercial diets formulated for gastrointestinal diseases or commercial diets formulated for weight reduction may be prescribed. These diets should be supplemented with the fat-soluble vitamins and be divided into three or more feedings daily.

Low-fat diets are inherently low in calories; however, another part of therapy is to reverse the weight loss and malnourishment that usually accompany protein-losing enteropathies. As an immediate caloric source, medium-chain triglycerides can be added to the diet to replace the calories lost by removal of fat from the diet. Commercially available medium-chain triglycerides are derived from coconut oil and can be added to the daily diet as an oil (e.g., MCT, Mead Johnson Nutritionals, Glenview, IL; 8.3 kcal/g; 1 tbsp weighs 14 gm and contains 115 kcal, to be given at a dosage of 1 to 2 ml/kg body weight) or as a powdered elemental diet mixture (e.g., Portagen, Mead Johnson Nutritionals; 1.5 cups added to water to make 1 quart of mixture with 30 kcal/fl oz). Excessive intake of these medium-chain triglyceride products may contribute to vomiting or aggravate diarrhea.

In addition to dietary manipulation, protein-losing enteropathies often improve with antiinflammatory doses of corticosteroids, such as oral prednisolone at an initial dosage of 2 to 3 mg/kg/day. Once remission has been achieved, this dosage is adjusted to a lower maintenance level.

Wheat-Sensitive Enteropathy in Irish Setters

A wheat-sensitive enteropathy has been identified in Irish Setter dogs that is characterized by poor weight gain or weight loss and bouts of intermittent diarrhea, with an onset of signs typically between 4 and 7 months of age. In this disorder, morphologic changes in the mucosa of the small intestine, as determined by mucosal biopsies, are variable; changes appear patchy within individual animals and consist of partial villous atrophy with no remarkable alterations in the cellular components of the lamina propria. Specific activities of important brush-border enzymes of the villus are selectively decreased, and this is probably responsible for hypersensitivity to various components in dietary wheat. Thus the diarrheal disorder is attributed more to brush-border enzyme abnormalities than to specific morphologic changes in the small intestinal mucosa. Dietary management is the most practical approach to its diagnosis and treatment. A wheat-sensitive enteropathy can usually be determined by a positive response to removal of wheat from the diet and return of signs when wheat is reintroduced.

Selective Cobalamin Malabsorption in Giant Schnauzers and Border Collie Dogs

A selective cobalamin malabsorption disorder has been identified in Giant Schnauzer and Border Collie dogs that is characterized by poor weight gain or weight loss and bouts of lethargy and inappetence, with an onset of signs typically between 3 and 6 months of age. There is a defect in transport of intrinsic factor/cobalamin complex receptor to the ileal brush-border membrane. All other nutrients are absorbed normally. In addition, a moderate nonregenerative anemia with marked anisocytosis, occasional megaloblasts, and moderate poikilocytosis, as well as a neutropenia with occasional hypersegmented neutrophils, are noted. Serum cobalamin levels are low, and urine samples contain large amounts of methylmalonic acid. Parenteral, but not oral, administration of vitamin B_{12} (0.25 to 1 mg weekly for 1 month, then every 3 to 6 months) reverses all hematologic and clinical abnormalities. Serum cobalamin levels should be monitored every 6 to 12 months or if signs occur. Affected animals should not be bred.

Enteropathy of Chinese Shar-Peis

Enteropathy has been identified in Chinese Shar-Pei dogs that is characterized by poor weight gain or weight loss and bouts of intermittent diarrhea, with an onset of signs typically between 2 and 6 months of age. Small intestinal biopsy samples are necessary for diagnosis; most severe cases show eosinophilic and lymphocytic-plasmacytic infiltrates of the intestine. Determination of serum cobalamin and folate concentrations may also be helpful in identifying bacterial overgrowth problems. Elimination diets and immunosuppressive therapy are the most practical approach to treatment. A guarded prognosis is always warranted.

Intestinal Obstruction

Partial and complete luminal obstructions of the intestine, particularly of the small intestine, are frequently seen in dogs and cats younger than 6 months. Ingested foreign object(s) and intussusception are the most frequent causes of these luminal obstructions.

Ingested Foreign Objects

Foreign objects ingested by a dog or cat may pass through the pylorus but have difficulty in passing aborally through the intestinal tract, commonly lodging in the jejunum. Foreign objects that are likely to be ingested include stones, coins, pecans, plastic and rubber objects, and jewelry. Whether partial or complete luminal obstruction occurs depends on the shape and size of the foreign object and on whether the object is stationary or is slowly progressing aborally. Once an object is able to pass through the ileocolic junction into the large intestine, signs of obstruction usually abate, and the object passes without complication.

Gastrointestinal foreign bodies are managed as in the adult dog and cat, keeping in mind the anesthesia and surgical requirements of the neonatal and pediatric patients (see Chapters 23 and 24).

Intussusception is commonly seen as a cause of intestinal obstruction in the young dog and occasionally in the young cat. The ileocolic junction is the most common site of intussusception, which also occurs in decreasing frequency in the ileum, jejunum, cecum, and duodenum.

Abnormal intestinal motility is thought to lead to the development of an intussusception. Irritation of the intestinal mucosa resulting from disorders such as intestinal parasitism, virus- or bacteria-induced enteritis, and acute inflammatory disorders or from orally administered drugs and anthelmintics may contribute to abnormal intestinal motility and the intussusception.

The presence of a palpable cylindric mass together with abdominal pain, vomiting, and passage of mucus and/or blood in the stool are usually diagnostic. Tenesmus may also occur with the diarrhea. If the intussusception has prolapsed through the anus, it must be differentiated from a rectal prolapse; this is done by passing a finger or blunt probe into the rectum between the mass and rectal wall. If the mass is a prolapsed intussusception, the probe or finger may be inserted a considerable distance. An intussusception is confirmed with abdominal radiographs. Results of survey radiographs depend on whether the intussusception is causing a complete or a partial obstruction. If the obstruction is complete, dilated gas- and fluid-filled loops of intestine are seen cranial to the intussusception, and the colon is void of feces. If the obstruction is partial, there is little, if any, distention of the intestine, and feces are usually present in the colon. The intussusception itself may not be seen owing to its fluid density and to the overlapping density of fluid-filled intestine. Probably the better method of demonstrating a nonopaque intussusception is via barium enema (Figure 36-6) or abdominal ultrasonography.

When an intussusception is diagnosed, surgical intervention is warranted. It is also important to determine the inciting cause of the intussusception and to eliminate it if possible. If the intussusception is caused by altered motility secondary to parasite-induced enteritis, the appropriate anthelmintic should be administered. The ability to manually reduce an intussusception at surgery depends on its duration. One hand is used to hold the ensheathing layer (intussuscipiens), while the other hand pushes the apex of the invaginating layer (intussusceptum) cranially and exerts gentle traction on the intestine cranial to the intussusception. After manual reduction of the intussusception, the intestine and mesentery are carefully checked for viability. If the involved segment is nonviable, then that segment should be resected and the remaining ends anastomosed. In intussusceptions of longer duration, manual reduction may be impossible. Adhesions often develop as a result of vascular damage, and production of a fibrinous exudate from the serosal surfaces. With time, the compromised circulation causes an ischemic necrosis and often a localized peritonitis. In those cases in which manual reduction is impossible because of adhesions or if the segment of intestine is no longer viable, resection and anastomosis are warranted.

The most frequent postoperative complication, barring intestinal dehiscence and peritonitis, is the recurrence of the intussusception because of existing intestinal irritation and/or altered motility. This may occur whether manual reduction or intestinal resection was performed. If the intussusception recurs, it may be helpful to double the intestine on itself so that the portion causing the problem lies at the turn of a U-shaped segment. The serosa of the segments cranial and

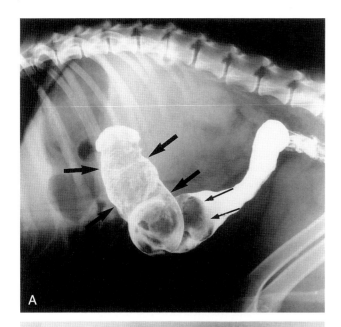

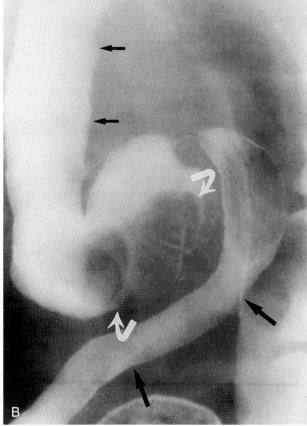

Figure 36-6   A, Lateral radiograph taken during a barium enema of a dog. Contrast medium outlines the end of a large ileocolic intussusception *(thin arrows).* Note that barium does not fill up the normally positioned colonic lumen because of a long filling defect *(large arrows).* **B,** Spot radiograph taken during a barium enema of a dog. The colon is descending on the left *(short arrows),* and the ileum *(long arrows)* is entering the colon. There is an area in which barium is displaced, representing an intussuscepted cecum *(curved arrows).* (From Nelson RW: *Small animal internal medicine,* ed 4, St Louis, 2009, Mosby. **A,** Courtesy Dr. Alice Wolf, Texas A&M University.)

caudal to the site of the intussusception is sutured together at the antimesenteric border with absorbable suture material. Three loops of plicated bowel should be used cranial and caudal to the intussusception.

Fecal impactions resulting from a mixture of feces and nondigestible hair or bones are the most common cause of infrequent defecation in dogs and cats younger than 6 months. Other causes of fecal impaction may include ingested foreign objects, narrowed pelvic canal after traumatically induced fractured pelvis, collapsed pelvic canal associated with pathologic fractures caused by nutritional imbalances, and congenital defects and inflammatory disease of the rectum and anus. Of these, foreign objects and fractured pelvis are the more likely causes of fecal impaction.

Animals with fecal impaction usually have a history of failure to defecate for days. The owner may have observed the animal making frequent, unsuccessful attempts to defecate and, in some cases, straining to pass small amounts of liquid feces, often containing blood or mucus. Some animals have the misleading complaint of diarrhea. The disruption and irritation of the intestinal mucosa promote secretion and accumulation of fluid that cannot penetrate the densely packed fecal materials and thus produce diarrhea. If defecation has not been observed, the animal may be brought to the veterinarian because it is depressed, listless, inappetent or anorexic, and vomiting intermittently.

Animals presenting with fecal impaction are generally dehydrated. Cats may assume a crouching, hunched attitude indicative of abdominal pain, and obvious abdominal distention is observed occasionally. Abdominal palpation typically reveals hard fecal mass(es) that may fill the entire length of the large intestine. Rectal examination combined with abdominal palpation is useful in determining the amount of feces retained and compressibility of the material present and possibly in identifying the underlying cause of the fecal impaction, such as foreign object(s) or a narrowed pelvic canal. Survey abdominal radiographs confirm the presence of fecal impaction and any opaque foreign object(s).

The treatment of fecal impaction consists of gentle removal of impacted fecal material and, if possible, identification and removal of the underlying cause. The animal with mild to moderate fecal impaction can generally be treated with oral laxatives and frequent small-volume enemas. The animal with more severe fecal impaction is often dehydrated and requires fluid replacement therapy for dehydration and electrolyte imbalances before correction of the fecal impaction is attempted. Breakdown and removal of the impacted fecal mass(es) should be accomplished as slowly and gently as possible. It is less traumatic for the young animal if the fecal mass(es) are softened and removed over 2 or 3 days than if removal of all the fecal impaction is attempted at one time. In dogs and cats older than 4 months of age with mild to moderate fecal impaction, after fluid replacement therapy has been accomplished, oral administration of a colon electrolyte lavage preparation such as Colyte (Reed & Carnrick, Pewaukee, WI) or NuLytely (Braintree Laboratories,

Braintree, MA), about 20 to 30 ml/kg body weight every 12 hours, can be used for completing the removal of residual feces. Sodium phosphate enema solutions should not generally be used as they can cause severe electrolyte disturbances in small animals.

Laxatives are mild in their effects and usually cause elimination of formed feces. Their effects depend on dosage; major drugs and dosages are presented in Table 36-2. The dioctyl sodium sulfosuccinate and dioctyl calcium sulfosuccinate laxatives act as detergents to alter the surface tension of liquids and promote emulsification and softening of the feces by facilitating the mixture of water and fat. The animal should be well hydrated before compounds containing these substances are administered. They should not be administered in conjunction with mineral oil because they aid in the absorption of the mineral oil.

Mineral oil (liquid petrolatum) and white petrolatum are nondigestible and poorly absorbed laxatives. They soften feces by coating them to prevent colonic absorption of fecal water and promote easy evacuation. A small amount of oil absorption does occur, but the primary danger of giving mineral oil is laryngotracheal aspiration. Bulk-forming laxatives such as psyllium and bran increase the frequency of evacuation of the upper large intestine via stimulation produced by added bulk or volume. They soften feces by the retention of water. Metamucil, which contains natural psyllium and generic bran, is best given with moistened food to ensure a high degree of water intake.

Another useful laxative is bisacodyl; this compound exerts its action on colonic mucosa and intramural nerve plexuses. It should be given only to well-hydrated animals older than 4 months of age and is contraindicated when obstruction is present. Lactulose, a synthetic disaccharide of galactose and fructose, may be used for its laxative effects in the young dog and cat. After oral administration, lactulose is metabolized to organic acids by intestinal bacteria and promotes an osmotic catharsis of feces. The dose is individualized based on the stool consistency and is titrated until a semiformed stool is obtained, two to three soft bowel movements per day. Overdosage may induce intestinal cramping (colic signs), profuse diarrhea, flatulence, dehydration, and acidosis.

Enemas act by softening feces in the distal region of the large intestine, stimulating colonic motility and the urge to defecate. The enema fluid used should be at room

TABLE 36-2   Summary of therapeutic products available for management of constipation

Therapeutic agent	Dosage and route*	Comments
Bisacodyl	5 mg sid PO	Available in 5-mg tablet and 5-mg suppository; takes 6-12 hours for tablets to take effect; animal should be well hydrated and feces softened before its use
Bran	1-2 tbsp mixed in 400 g of canned food and given sid or bid	Available in powder form; takes 12-24 hours to take effect
Dioctyl sodium sulfosuccinate	1-4 capsules (50 mg) sid PO (dogs) 1 capsule (50 mg) sid PO (cats)	Available in 50- and 100-mg capsules, 1% liquid, 4 mg/ml syrup; takes 12-72 hours to take effect; animal should be well hydrated before its use
Dioctyl calcium sulfosuccinate	2-3 tablets (50 mg) sid PO (dogs) 1-2 tablets (50 mg) sid PO (cats)	Available in 50- and 240-mg tablets; similar activity and precautions as for dioctyl sodium sulfosuccinate
Lactulose	1 ml/4.5 kg tid PO for dogs to start; then adjust dosage to stool consistency and 2-3 soft bowel movements per day 0.25-1 ml for cats sid–bid PO to start; then adjust dosage to stool consistency and 2-3 soft bowel movements per day Retention enema procedure: 5-10 ml of lactulose diluted 1:3 in water tid–qid (this procedure is only used for management of hepatoencephalopathy)	Overdosage may cause diarrhea, flatulence, intestinal cramping (colic), dehydration, and acidosis
Psyllium (natural)	1-3 tsp mixed with food and given sid or bid	Available in powder form; takes 12-24 hours to take effect
White petrolatum	1-5 ml sid PO initially; then 2-3 days/week	Available in paste form; should be given only between meals; takes 12-24 hours to take effect

*PO, Oral administration; *sid*, once daily; *bid*, twice daily; *tid*, three times daily; *qid*, four times daily.

temperature or tepid. Tap water, normal saline solution, and sodium biphosphate solution add bulk; petrolatum oils soften, lubricate, and promote the evacuation of hardened fecal material; and soap-sud solutions promote defecation by their irritant action. Tepid normal saline solution and tap water (about 5 ml/kg body weight) are generally preferred for enemas in animals younger than 6 months of age. If these are ineffective, a soapy water solution can be used after ensuring that the animal is well hydrated. About 5 ml/kg body weight of a mild soap solution is slowly instilled through a lubricated enema tube. In general, better results with normal saline solution, tap water, or soapy water enemas are obtained if the enema is repeated several times using small volumes. Small volumes are retained for longer periods, allowing time to soften and break down fecal impactions. Sodium phosphate retention enemas are convenient preparations for the relief of fecal impaction. However, their use in young dogs and cats is absolutely contraindicated because they cause marked hyperphosphatemia, hypernatremia, and hypocalcemia.

After the successful relief of fecal impaction, attention is directed to the prevention of recurrence. If possible, nondigestible materials should be eliminated from the diet, regular grooming instituted, and the opportunity for regular defecation provided. In all instances, the goal should be to have the animal pass soft, formed feces and to defecate regularly. Commercial veterinary laxatives containing petrolatum as their active ingredient are useful for preventing minor hair impaction in cats.

Rectal Prolapse

Rectal prolapse is the protrusion of one or more layers of the rectum from the anal orifice. The degree of rectal prolapse can vary, from protrusion of the mucosal layer at the anal orifice to full-thickness extrusion of several centimeters of the rectum through the anal orifice. Rectal prolapse commonly occurs in dogs and cats that are experiencing habitual or continual straining; therefore obvious causes of straining to void feces or urine should be evaluated. Any defect in the supporting structures of the anorectum or disturbance of the anal sphincters such as innervation disorders will predispose the dog or cat to a rectal prolapse. In dogs and cats younger than 6 months of age, rectal prolapses of only the mucosal layer are most often associated with severe diarrhea. Soiling of the perianal area and diarrhea may create considerable straining to void feces and result in a rectal prolapse of the mucosa. Foreign objects, such as needles or bones, that lodge in the rectum may also contribute to severe straining, leading to rectal prolapse of the mucosa. If the underlying cause of a rectal prolapse is not eliminated, the prolapsed mucosa may quickly convert into a full-thickness extrusion of the rectum.

A rectal prolapse of only the mucosal layer assumes a swollen donut shape as it protrudes from the anal orifice. If all the layers are involved, the prolapsed rectum takes on a more cylindric shape. A rectal prolapse can be mistaken for a rare intussusception of a more cranial section of the intestine that has prolapsed through the anal orifice. Differentiation between rectal prolapse and intussusception is made by attempting to insert a finger or blunt probe between the mucocutaneous junction of the anus and protruding bowel. If the finger or blunt probe is easily passed, an intussusception is present; if resistance is met, a rectal prolapse has occurred.

A rectal prolapse does not occur without cause. Failure to identify and treat the underlying cause of rectal prolapse often results in its unsuccessful treatment. The initial treatment should include fluid replacement therapy for dehydration and electrolyte disturbances, symptomatic control of diarrhea, and administration of appropriate medication in the case of parasitic or bacterial enterocolitis. The rectal prolapse itself can be managed by several methods, including reduction and purse-string suture, amputation, and colopexy. The method selected depends on the viability of the prolapsed tissue, the size and reducibility of the prolapse, and recurrence after a previous method has failed. Edematous but viable prolapsed tissue appears moist and varies from pink to dark red. Mucosa that is irreversibly damaged or necrotic appears leather-like and may be purple or black. With the animal under general anesthesia, a minor rectal prolapse of viable mucosa may be reduced manually and maintained by a purse-string suture in the anus for about 7 days, leaving a small orifice for stool passage. The small orifice is created by drawing the purse-string suture closed around a 4-inch rectal thermometer or another object of similar diameter. Desiccants such as hypertonic solutions of glucose or granulated sugar can be applied on the prolapsed tissue to reduce the edema before reduction and placement of the purse-string suture. Topical anesthetic ointment with 1% dibucaine can be instilled in the rectum postoperatively and continued for 2 or 3 days after removal of the purse-string suture.

A nonreducible rectal prolapse with necrosis of the mucosa is best managed by full-thickness amputation and anastomosis. A nonreducible viable prolapse or a recurrent rectal prolapse that fails to respond to more conservative treatment may be treated by celiotomy and colopexy. For the colopexy, scarified surfaces of the descending colon and the sublumbar body wall are sutured together with several interrupted mattress stitches of nonabsorbable suture material, attaching the submucosal layer of the colon to the muscles of the abdominal wall. Topical anesthetic ointment is instilled rectally after colopexy and continued for 5 or 6 days postoperatively.

THE ANUS

Congenital anorectal anomalies that are infrequently identified in the young dog and cat include imperforate anus, segmental aplasia, rectovaginal fistula, rectovestibular fistula, anovaginal cleft, and rectal urethral fistula. Of these anomalies, imperforate anus, although rarely seen, is the most common. Puppies or kittens with congenital anorectal anomalies usually are presented to a veterinarian because of an absence of defecation, obvious defect in the anatomy of the perineal structures, or voiding of urine or feces through an inappropriate orifice. A distended abdomen often accompanies these anomalies if obstruction is present. The anorectal anomalies occasionally go unnoticed until the animal is several weeks of age and may not be readily apparent from the appearance of the perineum.

Often with the imperforate anus, an anal dimple is present ventral to the base of the tail, showing where the anal orifice should have been. The colon is distended with feces and gas if any degree of obstruction is present, and fecal impaction may be severe enough to cause abdominal distention. The presence or absence of voluntary bladder function and an external anal sphincter should be evaluated in the animal presenting with imperforate anus. The presence and function of the external anal sphincter muscle can be evaluated by pinching the bulb of the penis or vulva and watching carefully for an anal wink (bulbourethral reflex). If the sphincter is present and functional, the prognosis for surgical correction is much better.

Imperforate anus encompasses several types of congenital deformity. Imperforate anus type 1 results from a failure of perforation of the anal membrane. Treatment consists of simply rupturing the membrane and trimming the excess tissue. A 4-inch rectal thermometer is used to ensure that the anal opening is adequate. Imperforate anus type 2 (also referred to as *atresia ani*) results from failure of the cloacal membrane to rupture, leaving a relatively thick membrane covering the anal orifice (Figure 36-7). The anal sphincter is usually intact and functional. Treatment is directed at locating the anal dimple, dissecting the membrane to the level of the rectal mucosa, and suturing the mucosa to the subcutaneous tissue and skin. A convenient way of excising the anal membrane and exposing the underlying rectum is to make two incisions at right angles to each other, forming a "+" centered on the anal dimple. Thus the four angled skin flaps formed are undermined and excised. The subcutaneous tissue is bluntly separated, and the blind-ended rectum is isolated and gently pulled toward the anus with forceps or stay sutures. The end of the rectum is then incised, and the mucosa is apposed to the skin with simple, interrupted stitches of absorbable suture material.

Imperforate anus type 3 (also referred to as *rectal agenesis*) results when the rectum ends blindly at a variable distance from the anal membrane. A lateral abdominal radiograph with the animal's hindquarters slightly elevated will allow visual observation of gas in the termination of the rectum. The distance from the rectum to the anal membrane allows differentiation between imperforate anus types 2 and 3. Treatment requires a combined abdominal and perineal surgical approach. The distal region of the rectum is exposed abdominally and then delivered through the pelvic canal to an opening made in the anal dimple. Rectal mucosa is then sutured to the subcutaneous tissue and skin in the perianal

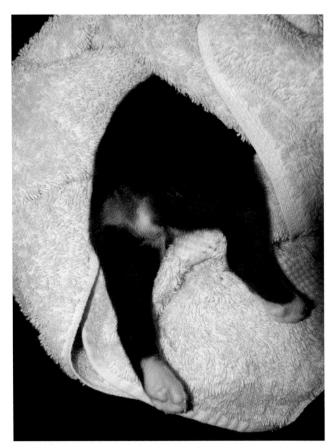

Figure 36-7 Atresia ani in a newborn Bernese Mountain Dog. (Note this puppy has no tail.) (Courtesy Sherri Schoorl.)

region. Animals may remain fecal incontinent after surgical correction.

Imperforate anus may be associated with other anorectal anomalies, especially of the genitourinary tract, with the rectum opening into the vagina, urinary bladder, or urethra. The age and size of a dog or cat with imperforate anus or its combination of concurrent anorectal anomalies make surgical correction difficult because of the complications that may occur postoperatively. The prognosis is good if the animal survives the immediate postoperative period.

Correction of anovaginal and rectovaginal fistulas that are predominately cosmetic problems should be delayed until the puppy or kitten is 12 to 16 weeks of age. Contrast radiography is needed to establish the presence and position of fistulas between the anorectum and urogenital tract before surgical correction is attempted. Fistulas require lengthy dissection procedures and general anesthesia. Most of these fistulas can be isolated through a vertical midline perineal incision from the ventral region of the anus to the vulva. Gentle blunt dissection is used to separate the supporting tissue between the rectum and urogenital tract. Once isolated, the fistula is excised, and the lumina of the anorectum and urogenital tract are closed separately with simple interrupted stitches of 4-0 or 5-0 synthetic absorbable suture material. If the anorectum is malpositioned, it is relocated in the center of the external anal sphincter muscle, and the mucosa is sutured to the skin circumferentially with simple interrupted stitches of the same suture material. The fecal impaction is relieved manually and with judicious use of enemas. The large intestine often is atonic and may require intermittent evacuation until normal defecation is established.

SUGGESTED READINGS

Davidson AP (ed): Pediatrics, *Vet Clin North Am Small Anim Pract* 36(3):533, 2006.

Dressman JB: Comparison of canine and human gastrointestinal physiology, *Pharm Res* 3(3):123, 1986.

THE LIVER, BILIARY TRACT, AND EXOCRINE PANCREAS

CHAPTER 37

Sharon A. Center

DEVELOPMENT OF THE HEPATOBILIARY SYSTEM AND PANCREAS

Development of the Hepatic Circulation

In the developed fetus, blood from the umbilical vein flows directly to the caudal vena cava through the ductus venosus, thereby bypassing the liver. By passively responding to changes in the systemic or hepatic circulation, this conduit stabilizes venous return to the fetal heart as the umbilical venous return fluctuates. Functional and morphologic closure of the ductus venosus does not occur simultaneously. In most dogs, functional closure of the ductus gradually occurs during the second and third days after birth. Morphologic closure occurs as the ductus atrophies, leaving behind a thin fibrous band (ligamentum venosum) within the liver. Ductus closure reflects the physiologic response to changes in pressure and resistance across the hepatic vasculature after postnatal obliteration of the umbilical circulation. Normally complete morphologic closure of the ductus is established by 1 to 3 months after birth. Congenital malformations of the intrahepatic and extrahepatic portal circulation and persistence of a functional ductus venosus are well documented in the dog and cat. Anomalous portal circulatory circuits in small breed dogs most commonly involve a single extrahepatic portosystemic vascular anomaly or malformation of the intrahepatic microscopic vasculature (microvascular dysplasia). A persistent or patent ductus venosus is more common in large breed dogs, being particularly notable as a family-associated defect in Irish Wolfhounds and Scottish Deerhounds. Delayed functional closure of the ductus venosus likely explains finding hyperammonemia in some Irish Wolfhound pups (up to 4 to 8 weeks of age) that resolves within several months of age.

Metabolic Functions

Despite early embryogenic differentiation of the liver, many of its metabolic functions are incompletely developed at birth. The fetal liver has reduced capabilities for gluconeogenesis, glycogenolysis, bile acid metabolism, and other biotransformation, detoxification, and elimination processes. Consequently the fetus is susceptible to transplacental and postnatal toxic and infectious challenges that may be inconsequential in adults. During gestation, the functional immaturity of the hepatobiliary system is masked by the maternal placental circulation. However, when maternal support is abruptly severed at birth, certain aspects of hepatobiliary insufficiency may become evident when the neonate is inappetent and exposed to infectious or toxic agents.

Biochemical indicators of hepatic disorders

Normal values for routinely used biochemical indicators reflecting the status of the hepatobiliary system in newborn and growing puppies and kittens are given in Table 37-1.

Blood glucose

Hepatic gluconeogenesis and glycogen storage are the mainstays of blood glucose regulation. Newborns depend on their hepatic glycogen reserves during the first 24 hours, with minimal glucose derivation from gluconeogenic branched chain amino acids. Although the ability to synthesize glycogen develops early, stores of hepatic glycogen accumulate only near term. Hepatic glycogen stores may be low at birth subsequent to intrauterine malnutrition (i.e., multiple pregnancies) or maternal malnutrition. Within 12 hours of birth, hepatic glycogenolysis consumes most glycogen stores, necessitating nutritional intake and gluconeogenesis to maintain euglycemia. It is during this interval that newborns are most susceptible to hypoglycemia. Generally initial blood glucose concentrations in newborn dogs are lower than in adults, although values exceeding 200 mg/dl have been documented. However, puppies deprived of food, especially toy breeds, may develop symptomatic hypoglycemia within 48 hours in contrast to adults, which can fast for days or weeks without becoming hypoglycemic. Comparatively,

TABLE 37-1   Normal values for routine biochemical indicators of hepatobiliary disorders in young dogs and cats (median [unless otherwise stated] and range)

Test	Puppy age						Normal adult reference range
	1-3 days (n = 30)	2 weeks (n = 14)	4 weeks (n = 7)	8 weeks (n = 8)	8.1-16 weeks (n = 78)*	16 weeks-1 year (n = 78)*	
BSP% 30 min	<5	<5	<5	<5	<5	<5	(0-5)
Total serum	<15	<15	<15	<15	<15	<15	(0-15)
Bile Acids (βM/L)							
Total bilirubin (mg/dl)	0.5 (0.2-1.0)	0.3 (0.1-0.5)	0 (0-0.1)	0.1 (0.1-0.2)	0.1 (0-0.1)	0.1 (0-0.1)	(0-0.4)
ALT (U/L)	69 (17-337)	15 (10-21)	21 (20-22)	21 (9-24)	31 (22-48)	37 (29-46)	(12-94)
AST (U/L)	108 (45-194)	20 (10-40)	18 (14-23)	22 (10-32)	27* (15-83)	27* (15-83)	(13-56), (15-83)*
ALP (U/L)	3845 (618-8760)	236 (176-541)	144 (235-301)	158 (144-177)	169 (27-416)	108 (19-285)	(4-107)
GGT (U/L)	1111 (163-3558)	24 (4-77)	3 (2-7)	1 (0-7)	<12 (0-12)	<12 (0-12)	(0-12)
Total protein (g/dl)	4.1 (3.4-5.2)	3.9 (3.6-4.4)	4.1 (3.9-4.2)	4.6 (3.9-4.8)	5.5* (4.4-7.3)	5.63* (4.8-6.7)	(4.0-5.2), (4.4-7.3)*
Albumin (g/dl)	2.1 (1.5-2.8)	1.8 (1.7-2.0)	1.8 (1.0-2.0)	2.5 (2.1-2.7)	2.8* (2.6-4.0)	3.0* (2.6-4.0)	(2.1-2.3), (2.6-4.0)*
Cholesterol (mg/dl)	136 (112-204)	282 (223-344)	328 (266-352)	155 (111-258)	211 (136-279)	211 (136-279)	(150-299), (136-279)*
Glucose (mg/dl)	88 (52-177)	129 (111-146)	109 (86-115)	145 (134-272)	adult range	–	(65-110)

*Data adapted from Harper et al: Age related variations in hematologic and biochemical test results in Beagles and Labrador Retrievers, *J Am Vet Med Assoc* 223:1436-1442, 2003; mean values. Kitten data from College of Veterinary Medicine, Cornell University and data adapted from Levy JK, Crawford PC, Werner LL: Effect of age on reference intervals of serum biochemical values in kittens, *J Am Vet Med Assoc* 228:1033-1037, 2006.

TABLE 37-1 Normal values for routine biochemical indicators of hepatobiliary disorders in young dogs and cats (median [unless otherwise stated] and range)—cont'd

Test	Kitten age					Normal adult reference range
	1-3 days (n = 55)	1 week (n = 55)	2 weeks (n = 79)	4 Weeks (n = 62)	8 weeks (n = 55)	
BSP% 30 min	N.D.	N.D.	N.D.	<3	<3	(0-3)
Total serum	<10	<10	<10	<10	<10	(0-10)
Bile Acids (βM/L)						
Total bilirubin (mg/dl)	0.1-1.1	0.1-1.6	0.0-0.7	0.0-0.2	0.0-0.6	(0.0-0.4)
ALT (U/L)	29-77	11-76	10-21	14-55	12-56	(28-91, 10-80)
AST (U/L)	21-126	15-45	14-23	15-31	14-40	(9-42, 5-55)
ALP (U/L)	1348-3715	126-363	116-306	97-274	60-161	(10-77, 10-80)
GGT (U/L)	0-5	0-5	0-4	0-1	0-2	(0-2)
Total protein (g/dl)	2.8-5.2	2.5-4.8	2.7-5.2	4.5-5.6	4.9-6.5	(5.4-8.1)
Albumin (g/dl)	1.9-3.1	2.0-2.5	2.1-2.6	2.4-2.9	2.4-3.0	(2.3-3.0, 2.4-4.1)
Cholesterol (mg/dl)	48-228	119-213	137-443	99-434	124-221	(150-270, 42-170)
Glucose (mg/dl)	52-163	105-145	76-158	99-152	94-143	(63-150)

symptomatic hypoglycemia is uncommon in neonatal cats and may reflect their carnivore-based metabolism. Neonatal dogs have overall poor glycemic regulation compared with adults, with slow recovery from either hypoglycemia or hyperglycemia. This is attributed to a relative insensitivity to endogenous insulin and suboptimal counterregulatory hormone responses (cortisol and epinephrine) in puppies. Consequently puppies can develop prolonged hyperglycemia after supplemental glucose administration.

Neonates have a relative deficiency of alternative energy sources (fat stores, gluconeogenic amino acids) to total body mass compared with adults. Only small amounts of fat are stored in the liver during the last trimester of gestation. Because lactate precedes use of alanine or glutamine for gluconeogenesis in puppies, and because lactate is preferentially used in the brain of hypoglycemic neonatal puppies, there may be an advantage in using lactate-containing fluids in symptomatic hypoglycemic puppies.

Maintaining euglycemia is important for the neonates' neurologic status because they have a brain-to-body mass carbohydrate requirement 2 to 4 times greater than adults. Unfortunately, even though the neonatal brain may preferentially accept lactate as an energy substrate, lactate availability may be insufficient. Ketones, an important alternative fuel during starvation, are insufficiently synthesized in neonates owing to their limited body fat, slow fatty acid mobilization, low ketogenic abilities, and their inability to survive the adaptation interval that precedes effective ketosis.

Although glucose regulation improves with age, puppies and kittens up to 4 months of age should be considered predisposed to hypoglycemia when anorexic or dehydrated. Conditions and clinical signs associated with neonatal/pediatric hypoglycemia are provided in Box 37-1. It is notable that severity of clinical signs increases with age such that hypoglycemia is more easily recognized in older animals. Thus maintaining a high index of suspicion for hypoglycemia is essential to achieve early diagnosis in a neonate. Treatment is aimed at achieving euglycemia, normalizing body temperature and hydration status, avoiding stress, and eliminating underlying causal factors.

Urea cycle function and blood ammonia concentrations

Function of the urea cycle matures at varying stages of fetal and neonatal development in different species. Urea cycle enzymes have not been directly quantified in fetal or neonatal dog or cat liver. Nevertheless, baseline ammonia values in clinically normal dogs and cats as young as 2 months are within the normal adult range, with the exception of some Irish Wolfhounds with apparent delayed closure of the ductus venosus.

Plasma ammonia concentrations can reflect portosystemic shunting caused either by congenital malformations of the portal circulation or secondary to portal hypertension (e.g., hepatic fibrosis, cirrhosis, portal vein thrombosis). Unfortunately because ammonia is labile in blood, immediate analysis is imperative. Samples must be transported from patient to equipment on melting ice, eliminating the routine transport to a commercial laboratory. It is well acknowledged that enzymatic methods for measuring blood ammonia concentrations lack precision. Ammonia is not routinely used in the author's clinical practice because of its unreliability and because there are better test alternatives: measurement of serum bile acids and detection of ammonium urate crystalluria.

Serum bile acids

Serum bile acids (SBAs) are well documented as a reliable method for estimating sufficiency of hepatic function and hepatoportal circulation. Bile acids are synthesized in hepatocytes from cholesterol, conjugated to an amino acid (taurine exclusively in cats; taurine or glycine in dogs), excreted into bile, and then undergo an efficient enterohepatic circulation. In adults, the enterohepatic circulation has 90% to 95% efficiency (each cycle). The utility of the endogenous meal-provoked bile acid challenge for assessment of liver function and perfusion has been fully investigated in neonatal, juvenile, and adult dogs and cats. In our laboratory, SBA concentrations in 1-day-old and 1-, 2-, and 4-week-old puppies and kittens are within the adult reference range. In older puppies and kittens, paired SBA samples (one before and one 2 hours after meal ingestion) concur with the adult reference range. The SBA test is reliable for detection of portal circulatory anomalies when paired samples (premeal and 2 hours postprandially) are evaluated. Random or fasted single samples are ill advised. Normal values may exist in animals with portosystemic vascular anomalies after a prolonged fast owing to circulatory delivery of arterial blood. Approximately 15% to 20% of dogs and 5% to 10% of cats have higher postprandial SBA concentrations relative to premeal values owing to delayed gastric emptying, intestinal transit, or perhaps gallbladder expulsion of bile (physiologic variation). Paired-sample (one before and one 2 hours after meal ingestion) SBA tests are recommended for vigorous routine assessments. Screening puppies for portosystemic vascular anomalies (PSVAs) using single random or fasted SBA concentrations is not recommended. Some animals with PSVA have normal fasting SBA values, and a few demonstrate the "backward" pattern described above. Physiologic variables influencing this test include (1) the gastric emptying rate, (2) the rate of gallbladder contraction and bile expulsion, (3) the rate of intestinal motility, (4) the

---

BOX 37-1   Signs of hypoglycemia

Weakness
Hypothermia
Dehydration
Inability to nurse
Persistent crying
Bradycardia or tachycardia
Irregular respiration
Apnea

functional status of the ileum where active bile acid transporters reside, and (5) the normalcy of the hepatobiliary structures and portal circulation.

Bilirubin metabolism

The fetal, neonate, and juvenile dog's capacity for hepatic uptake, conjugation, and excretion of bilirubin is remarkably mature compared with humans and several nonhuman primates. The fetal dog has substantial concentrations of bilirubin-conjugating enzymes. The capacity of the liver in the fetal, neonatal, and juvenile cat has not been similarly investigated. Some individual puppies have total bilirubin values mildly increased during the first 72 hours of birth, but this resolves within 2 weeks. Some kittens at birth and up to 14 days of age have total bilirubin values as high as 1.0 mg/dl (adult reference range, 0 to 0.2 mg/dl); values normalize by 4 weeks of age. The etiology of such high neonatal bilirubin concentrations remains unclarified.

Liver enzyme activity

Age-appropriate reference intervals for serum liver enzyme activity are essential for interpreting laboratory data in neonatal puppies and kittens. Differences in serum enzyme activities between neonates and adults reflect physiologic adaptations during the transition from fetal and neonatal life stages, trauma associated with birthing, colostrum ingestion, maturation of metabolic pathways, growth effects, differences in volume of distribution and body composition, and nutrition. Activity of serum alkaline phosphatase (ALP), aspartate aminotransferase (AST), creatine kinase (CK), and lactate dehydrogenase (LDH) usually increase greatly during the first 24 hours of life. In kittens, ALP, CK, and LDH activity exceeds adult values through 8 weeks of age, whereas AST increases only transiently after birth. The early increases in AST, CK, and LDH likely reflect muscle trauma associated with birthing, whereas ALP activity reflects bone isoenzyme associated with bone growth. Enteric absorption of colostral macromolecules during the first day of life causes a substantial increase in ALP in puppies and kittens, and of gamma-glutamyltransferase (GGT) in puppies (Figure 37-1, *A* and *B*). This phenomenon is not unique to dogs and cats as it has also been documented in neonatal calves, lambs, pigs, foals, and human infants. Studies also have confirmed significant differences in ALP activities develop between colostrum-deprived and suckling pups and kittens within 24 hours of birth, with a similar change in GGT also observed in puppies. These differences are short lived, resolving within the first 2 weeks, but can be used as a surrogate marker of effective colostrum ingestion. Studies have confirmed that colostrum contains substantially higher GGT and ALP activity than that resident in the serum of the respective dam or queen. For example, colostral or milk GGT in bitches is 100-fold and ALP is tenfold greater than sera until day 10. However, by day 30, GGT and ALP activity in milk is significantly lower than before suckling had commenced. Although a marked influence of colostrum on serum ALP activity in neonatal kittens also occurs, the effect on GGT

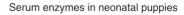
Serum enzymes in neonatal puppies

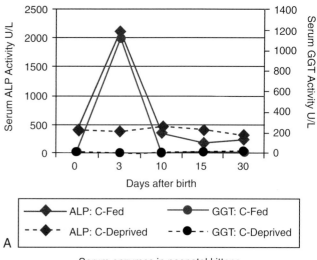

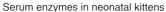

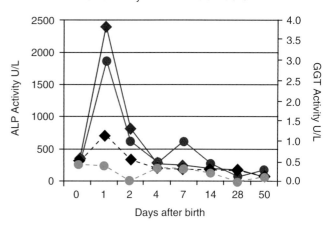

A

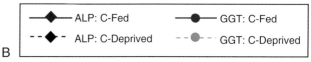
B

Figure 37-1 Liver enzyme activity in puppies **(A)** and kittens **(B)** immediately after birth showing the influence of colostrum ingestion on associated enzyme concentrations.

is modest compared with that in neonatal puppies. Sustained increases (first 6 to 12 months of life) in serum ALP activity in puppies and kittens (maximally threefold more than high normal adult reference values) reflect the bone ALP isoenzyme derived from osteoblast activity.

Albumin, globulins, coagulation factors, and protein C

Synthesis of albumin, many globulins, most coagulation, and many anticoagulant factors depends on the liver. Total protein and albumin concentrations in young dogs up to 4 weeks of age are below normal limits for adults, whereas protein concentrations in young cats are more variable (see Table 37-1). By 8 weeks of age, puppies have normal adult albumin concentrations, whereas total globulin values increase with age, reflecting cumulative antigenic challenge.

Although coagulation assessments are uncommonly completed in neonatal puppies and kittens, limited observations suggest that values fall within the normal adult ranges for prothrombin time (PT), activated partial thromboplastin time (APTT), and fibrinogen in animals as young as 8 weeks of age. Protein C, recently shown to discriminate normal puppies from puppies with PSVA, is influenced by adequacy of portal venous perfusion. Although liver failure and severe enteric protein loss also can compromise protein C activity, this anticoagulant factor is useful for differentiating PSVA from microvascular dysplasia (MVD) in young dogs.

Cholesterol

Serum cholesterol concentration can reflect hepatic functional and circulatory disturbances. Because cholesterol is synthesized in the liver, synthetic failure can cause marked hypocholesterolemia. Portosystemic shunting, either congenital or acquired, also causes mild to marked hypocholesterolemia. Because cholesterol is excreted into the biliary tree in bile, cholestasis can increase in cholesterol concentrations. A mild to moderate increase in cholesterol is apparent with acute obstructive jaundice and in some animals with acute severe hepatic inflammation (lacking synthetic failure). In 1- to 3-day-old puppies but not kittens, mild hypocholesterolemia is common (see Table 37-1). In puppies and kittens older than 2 to 4 weeks of age, serum cholesterol concentrations are within the adult normal range.

Hepatic hematopoiesis

Extramedullary hematopoiesis can develop in the liver of puppies or kittens through 4 months of age. However, in older juveniles, hematopoietic activity in the liver is usually restricted to disorders associated with a brisk regenerative anemia.

Hepatic mineral storage

Age-related variations in hepatic concentrations of iron, copper, zinc, and selenium (per gram of dry liver weight) have been reported for Beagle dogs from 8 to 193 days of age (Table 37-2). A decrease in hepatic iron concentrations during the first 20 days after birth likely reflects mobilization of iron for hemoglobin synthesis in bone marrow, the relative iron deficiency of a milk diet, and decrease in hepatic extramedullary hematopoiesis. In many species, hepatic copper concentrations are higher in pediatric individuals relative to adults. In dogs, hepatic copper concentrations change little with advancing age unless challenged with a copper-rich diet. In dogs with copper-associated hepatopathy (primary metabolic or copper transport disorder, dietary copper loading, cholestatic liver injury), hepatic copper concentrations significantly increase over time (see later discussion on Copper Storage Hepatopathy).

Hepatobiliary Disorders of the Young Dog and Cat

Survey of young dogs and cats (n = 444; puppies, n = 312 and kittens, n = 132) with liver tissue examined histologically

TABLE 37-2	Hepatic mineral concentrations in Beagles (mean ± standard deviation; μg/g dry weight)	
Mineral content	8 to 40 days of age (n = 10)	>40 days of age (n = 20)
Iron	1025 ± 882	585 ± 258
Copper	285 ± 75	304 ± 90
Zinc	225 ± 88	143 ± 30
Selenium	2.5 ± 0.4	1.9 ± 0.4

Summarized from Keen CL, Lonnerdal B, Fisher GL: Age-related variations in hepatic iron, copper, zinc, and selenium concentrations in beagles, *Am J Vet Res* 42:1884, 1981.

(biopsy or necropsy) over a 12-year interval in the author's hospital is detailed in Table 37-3. Various histologic and definitive diagnoses are represented. Hepatic necrosis, hepatic congestion, and hepatic lipidosis were the three most common histologic features. Hepatic congestion is of uncertain significance as this may represent a terminal or death-related change.

Congenital Anatomic Malformations
Gallbladder

Congenital malformations of the gallbladder are most common in the cat. Congenital division of the gallbladder is most common and is also referred to as an accessory, cleft, diverticular, or bilobed gallbladder (Figure 37-2). These malformations involve the initial subdivision of the primary cystic diverticulum or a bud from the neck of the embryonic gallbladder. Although such malformations do not cause clinical illness, they can cause confusion when recognized during abdominal ultrasonography as they may be mistaken for a cyst.

Common bile duct diverticulum

A cystic diverticular outpouching of the common bile duct near the sphincter of Oddi has been recognized in some cats. These may become a nidus of infection (rather like the human appendix), eventually leading to septic choledochitis and pancreatitis. Clinical signs are initially vague but may involve inappetence and vomiting. Thereafter, features cannot be differentiated from other causes of hepatobiliary jaundice until gross inspection during exploratory laparotomy. Resection of the cystic diverticulum, often combined with cholecystoenterostomy, and judicious antimicrobial therapy and supportive care are usually curative. Adequate hydration, ursodeoxycholate (7.5 mg/kg orally twice daily with meals) and S-adenosylmethionine (20 mg/kg orally daily 1 to 2 hours before feeding) are used to promote choleresis for several months postoperatively.

Biliary atresia

Congenital maldevelopment of the biliary tree is an unusual anomaly recognized in puppies and kittens. These patients are jaundiced and fail to thrive. There is no treatment.

TABLE 37-3 Hepatobiliary disorders in puppies and kittens less than 4 months of age: gross and histopathologic tissue evaluations		
Disorder	**Puppies** (n = 312)	**Kittens** (n = 132)
Infectious hepatopathies	68	18
Parvovirus	30	0
Herpesvirus	7	0
Canine distemper	11	–
Infectious canine hepatitis	4	–
Feline infectious peritonitis	–	17
Parasite migration	4	0
Hepatic abscessation	12	1
Severe hepatic necrosis	54	41
Hepatic congestion	63	25
Hepatic lipidosis	36	16
Extramedullary hematopoiesis	39	10
Cholangitis	9	10
Trauma (hematoma, laceration)	10	6
Nonspecific hepatitis	14	3
Portosystemic vascular anomaly	1	11
Hepatic atrophy	3	2
Vasculitis	1	0
Lymphosarcoma	1	0
Diaphragmatic hernia (liver involvement)	1	0

Cystic hepatobiliary lesions

Congenital and acquired hepatic cysts occur in both dogs and cats. Acquired cysts are uncommon in juvenile patients but may develop subsequent to trauma or inflammation and are usually solitary. Congenital or developmental cysts are commonly multiple and variable in size. Polycystic renal and liver lesions have been identified in Cairn Terriers and Persian cats during the first few months of life. Whereas cystic lesions may be parenchymal or ductal in origin, most hepatic cysts are ductal. These arise from primitive bile ducts and lack continuity with the normal biliary tree. If lining epithelium produces fluid, cysts transform into retention cysts. Cysts may be solitary or multiple in the polycystic disorder and vary in size from a few millimeters to several centimeters. Cats with polycystic liver malformations sometimes also have cystic lesions in the kidneys or pancreas. Although hepatic cysts are often asymptomatic, they may become symptomatic when they encroach on normal tissue or organs. Cysts adjacent to the gallbladder are most problematic. In polycystic feline liver disease, prolific production of extracellular matrix surrounding dysplastic ductal structures causes intrahepatic portal hypertension and subsequently development of acquired portosystemic shunts, abdominal effusion, and signs of hepatic encephalopathy.

Clinical illness associated with biliary cystic lesions in juvenile or young adult dogs and cats may be lacking or may remain vague (e.g., inappetence or vomiting caused by cyst

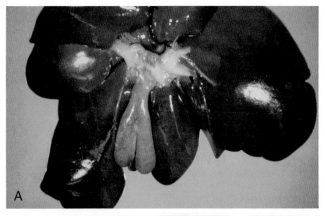

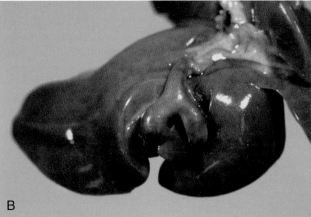

Figure 37-2 Bilobed gallbladders representing developmental anomalies in two cats. (From Hoskins J: *Veterinary pediatrics: dogs and cats from birth to 6 months*, ed 3, Philadelphia, 2001, Saunders, p 201.)

compression of the stomach). Diagnosis is accomplished with radiographic or ultrasonographic imaging. Ultrasonography discloses the cystic nature of lesions, as well as the extent of tissue involvement. When abdominal ultrasonography was used to phenotype Persian cats with the polycystic renal mutation, renal cysts were identified at 6 to 7 weeks of age in many cats. Cats lacking cystic lesions at 6 months were deemed unaffected. Although the diagnostic performance of abdominal ultrasonography in detecting the cystic renal lesions was exceptional (specificity, 100%; sensitivity, 75% at <16 weeks of age; and specificity, 100%; sensitivity, 91% at <36 weeks of age), this procedure has not been evaluated for detection of polycystic liver disease.

Cats with cystic liver lesions should be DNA tested for the renal polycystic gene mutation if they are intended for breeding. It remains unclarified if there are variants of this disorder associated with primary liver involvement. DNA testing is done using a cheek swab kit (available from felinegenome@ucdavis.edu). Treatment is usually not indicated for congenital cystic liver lesions unless a large cyst causes abdominal discomfort or fluid accumulation causes pressure effects on adjacent organs or tissues. Periodic aspiration of large problematic cysts has been used to manage some patients. Other alternatives include partial cyst wall resection, entire cyst excision, or removal of an involved liver lobe. In some Persian cats, the polycystic renal or hepatic involvement is recognized during the first few months of life. In some of these, polycystic kidney disease is rapidly lethal. In others, the disorder is mild, does not cause overt signs, and is recognized incidentally later in life.

Common Vascular Malformations Involving the Liver

Hepatoportal MVD and PSVA are related congenital inherited disorders of hepatic vasculogenesis or angiogenesis. An extensive genotyping project involving nine small dog breeds (in progress by the author) has confirmed the genetic relationship between these disorders with SBA concentrations designating affectation status. Each of these disorders is associated with SBA concentrations greater than 25 μmol/L. However, quantitative SBA values cannot reliably discriminate between these disorders. Current data support an autosomal dominant mode of inheritance with incomplete penetrance or a complicating regulatory element mutation and probable prenatal or perinatal lethality of the most severely affected dogs (PSVA). Pedigree studies suggest that up to 15% of dogs with PSVA remain asymptomatic to knowledgeable breeders and veterinarians. Unfortunately some of these dogs have been outstanding individuals and have been used as foundation stock, propagating the genetic defect. Because the historical, clinical, clinicopathologic, and histologic features of PSVA have saturated the veterinary literature during the past 30 years, most clinicians maintain a high index of suspicion for this disorder when presented with a vaguely ill young dog with high SBA values. However, it is important to acknowledge that the MVD phenotype is far more common than PSVA (10 to 30:1 depending on the breed and the pedigree structure). It is estimated that the frequency of PSVA ranges between 0.1% and 0.6% of the ill patient population in large specialty referral hospitals.

Portal hypoplasia versus portal hypoperfusion

Increased arteriole blood flow is a physiologic response to decreased portal venous perfusion and is a consistent histologic feature of any condition impairing hepatic portal venous perfusion (e.g., thrombi, venous obstruction). This adaptive response is associated with arteriolar tortuosity (coiling) and thickening of the arteriolar smooth muscle. Rather than portal hypoplasia, the functional terminology of *portal hypoperfusion* more accurately depicts the observed perfusion abnormality.

Hepatoportal microvascular dysplasia

MVD was originally well characterized in a family of Cairn Terriers with an increased incidence of PSVA. Extensive studies including organic anion dye clearance, colorectal scintigraphy, hepatic and portal ultrasonography, contrast radiographic portography, and liver biopsy (multiple liver lobes in each dog) confirmed MVD is associated with abnormal microscopic hepatic blood flow and a lack of macroscopic portosystemic shunting. In dogs with PSVA, hepatic

ultrasonography detected a subjectively small liver, abnormal portal to systemic vascular communications, and hypovascular intrahepatic portal perfusion. In dogs with MVD, intrahepatic portal vasculature was less well defined than in normal dogs; liver size was subjectively normal; and no large shunting vessels were identified. Radiographic portography confirmed macroscopic shunting only in dogs with PSVA but disclosed inconsistent portal venous perfusion among liver lobes in dogs with MVD. Dogs with only MVD demonstrated contrast retention in some liver lobes, consistent with differential perfusion among liver lobes, and a lack of well-distinguished tertiary portal branches. These findings correspond nicely with scintigraphic features described as portal streamlining in dogs scrutinized for PSVA that lacked a macroscopic shunt. Microscopic features in dogs with only MVD overlap with those observed in dogs with PSVA depending on the liver lobe sampled; lesions are inconsistent among different liver lobes. Cytologic imprints of liver biopsies in dogs with either MVD or PSVA usually demonstrate small binuclate hepatocytes.

Dogs with MVD are typically asymptomatic and do not develop hyperammonemia, ammonium biurate crystalluria, or uroliths. The MVD lesion is irreversible and often accompanies PSVA. Its presence explains why some dogs undergoing surgical PSVA ligation maintain increased SBA concentrations yet lack clinical signs. Definitive diagnosis of MVD from PSVA cannot be made based on the liver biopsy as lesions are similar. Because MVD lesions vary among liver lobes, a minimum of three biopsies from different liver lobes is recommended for definitive diagnosis. Needle biopsies are notoriously poor for ascertaining the presence of either MVD or PSVA because of small sample size and restricted lobe sampling.

The MVD phenotype explains why some dogs suspected of having PSVA based on abnormal liver function (SBA) and hepatic histology lack macroscopic shunting vasculature on contrast radiographic study, colorectal scintigraphy, and surgical inspection. It is important to realize the differences between MVD and PSVA. Dogs with MVD usually remain asymptomatic and do not require special liver diets or therapeutic interventions with lactulose, metronidazole, neomycin, antioxidants, or ursodeoxycholic acid. The typical liver affected with MVD has no necroinflammatory component. High bile acids in these dogs represent the circulatory flux of the enterohepatic bile acid circulation rather than injurious bile acids retained in tissues. Dogs with MVD followed long term (up to 15 years) maintained on a canine maintenance diet without additional therapies do not develop progressive liver injury. Because many small Terrier-type dog breeds have a 30% to 35% incidence of MVD, puppies should be tested using a paired SBA test at 4 months of age before adoption into a pet home. Knowing a dog's SBA status is important for future health care and assessments.

Portosystemic vascular anomaly

Several different types of PSVA have been described in dogs and cats, including but not limited to (1) persistent patent fetal ductus venosus (large breed dogs especially, inheritable in Irish Wolfhounds and Irish Deerhounds), (2) direct portal vein to caudal vena cava shunt, (3) direct portal vein to azygos vein shunt, (4) combination of portal vein with caudal vena cava into azygos vein shunt, (5) left gastric vein to vena cava shunt (common in cats and many small breed dogs), (6) portal vein hypoplasia or atresia with secondary multiple portosystemic shunts (comparatively rare), and (7) anomalous malformations of the caudal vena cava (rare). Additional subclassifications of PSVA are clinically useful to consider; these involve the different types of vascular malformations (extrahepatic and intrahepatic histologic lesions) in an individual.

Most animals with PSVA are diagnosed at a young age (4 weeks to 2 years), although some dogs have been 13 years of age at first diagnosis. There is no sex predilection. In dogs, Terrier breeds, especially Yorkshire Terriers, Maltese, Cairn Terriers, and several others, are commonly afflicted. Families of dogs have been studied in which a genetic predisposition is obvious (e.g., Yorkshire Terriers, Cairn Terriers, Tibetan Spaniels, Maltese, Havanese, Shih Tzu, Miniature Schnauzers, Irish Wolfhounds, and Scottish Deerhounds).

Although not commonly appreciated, not all dogs with PSVA are symptomatic. Most symptomatic dogs are "unthrifty" in appearance and often are the litter "runt." If not stunted early, most fail to keep up with growth expectations. Neurobehavioral signs (hepatic encephalopathy [HE]) may manifest early during the first few weeks of life owing to hypoglycemia (especially in toy breeds). Signs of HE also may manifest as the puppy or kitten is weaned onto growth-formulated diets from milk or when older animals are cutting teeth and swallowing blood. Failure to demonstrate overt signs of HE in the neonatal period relates to the protein and carbohydrate composition of the milk diet. Signs of HE are episodic and typically associated with meals. However, enteric parasitism can also provoke neurologic signs as a result of enteric inflammation and bleeding. Blood within the intestinal canal is highly encephalogenic in patients prone to HE. Neurobehavioral signs may involve propulsive circling, amaurosis (unexplained transient blindness), dementia (head pressing, staring, vocalizing), aggression (especially in cats), seizure, lethargy, or coma. Gastrointestinal signs may include anorexia, vomiting, constipation (worsens HE), diarrhea, or ptyalism (excessive salivation, in cats especially, often confused with upper respiratory tract infection). Urinary tract signs may include abnormally increased water consumption and increased urine production (polydipsia/polyuria) as a result of the effect of neurologic toxins or dysfunctional hepatic osmostats. Dogs with PSVA often have a markedly increased glomerular filtration rate (GFR) owing to their remarkable water flux. Ammonium biurate urolithiasis may cause stranguria or dysuria and hematuria. Rarely acute abdominal pain reflects ureteroliths. Fever (intermittent) may occur as a result of circulatory bypass of the hepatic reticuloendothelial system that normally provides immune surveillance against infectious material transported from the gut. Intolerance to certain drugs requiring hepatic biotransformation or first-pass elimination may be noted at the time of neutering (general anesthesia) or when anticonvulsant medications are needed to control seizure activity. Animals with PSVA become extraordinarily ill when challenged by infectious disorders (e.g., abscess, puncture wound, rickettsial infections).

Physical findings usually include a small body stature and unthrifty appearance. Abdominal palpation often discloses prominent kidneys. Large kidney size may relate to increased GFR, renal gluconeogenesis, and other designated metabolic functions not normally conducted by the kidney, as well as renal cell hypertrophy induced by high ammonia concentrations. Rarely cystic calculi are palpated. A unique copper-colored iris is observed in non–blue-eyed cats (Figure 37-3); this color is similar to the eye color in Persians and thus must not be interpreted out of context.

Major clinicopathologic features associated with PSVA include poikilocytes in cats (irregularly irregular erythrocytes); red blood cell microcytosis (small cells); low concentrations of blood urea nitrogen, creatinine, cholesterol, and glucose; variable liver enzyme activity and protein concentration; and ammonium urate crystalluria. However, some animals have few or none of these findings. Liver function assessments should include a provocative endogenous SBA challenge and use of the recently described protein C test. The protein C test involves measurement of an anticoagulant protease that depends on the liver and portal circulation for normal regulation. This test can help differentiate MVD from PSVA and thus assists in prioritizing expensive and invasive assessments.

Survey abdominal radiographs usually disclose a small liver and large or prominent kidneys. Urinary calculi usually are not radiodense. Abdominal ultrasonography usually discloses a small homogeneous liver. The anomalous shunting vessel may be identified, depending on operator skill. Color-flow Doppler allows detection of unusual turbulence in the vena cava cranial to the phrenicoabdominal vessels in most extrahepatic PSVAs. Intrahepatic PSVA is most easily visualized. The intrahepatic portal distribution often appears

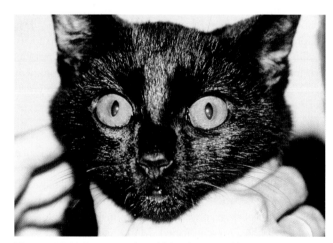

Figure 37-3 Copper-colored iris of a cat with a portosystemic vascular malformation.

hypovascular in animals with PSVA; however, some patients have partial hepatic perfusion, and these lobes may not appear hypovascular. Renal pelvic and cystic calculi, sand, or overt uroliths (rarely ureteral) may be identified.

Colorectal scintigraphy with a technetium pertechnetate-labeled enema is the least invasive method of documenting portovenous hepatofugal perfusion. A computer-linked gamma-camera records portal distribution of isotope either to the heart (shunt) or liver (no shunt present) within 3 minutes. This noninvasive technique usually confirms PSVA macroscopic shunting. Unfortunately it is unable to describe anatomic shunt location, to verify multiple (acquired shunts) versus single congenital shunts, and may miss shunts in very petite patients, splenic vein to azygos vein shunts, and shunts occluded by visceral compression while the patient is in lateral recumbency. Radiographic contrast portovenography is the "gold standard" for PSVA confirmation (Figure 37-4). Various methods have been described, including (1) mesenteric vein cannulation (requires surgery), (2) splenic vein cannulation (surgery or ultrasound guided), (3) splenic pulp

injection (percutaneous, ultrasound guided, or surgical; may cause infarcts/infection/hemorrhage), (4) arteriography via cannulation of the anterior mesenteric artery through the femoral artery (fluoroscopy directed, contrast dilution impairs strong shunt visualization), and (5) nonselective venography by rapid bolus jugular vein injection of contrast (useful only in very petite patients as contrast dilution is a problem). Mesenteric vein cannulation during exploratory laparotomy is most commonly used. Both right and left lateral recumbency portograms and a ventrodorsal porto-gram are used to verify that a PSVA has not been missed (Figure 37-5). Many extrahepatic PSVAs are better visual-ized on a single lateral projection; the side of best imaging is inconsistent. Left gastric vein shunts can resemble the

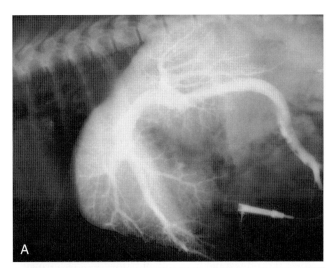
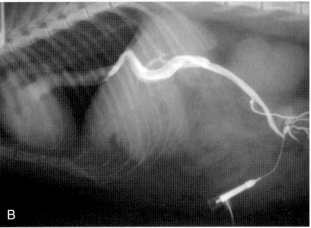

Figure 37-4 A, Portogram completed in a healthy dog with normal bile acid values. **B,** Mesenteric portogram in a cat with a left gastric vein shunt. Note the absence of contrast in the hepatic portal vasculature.

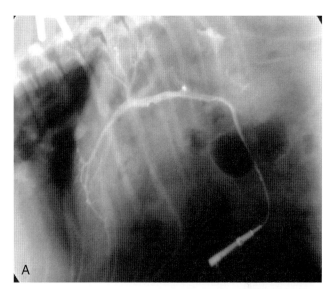
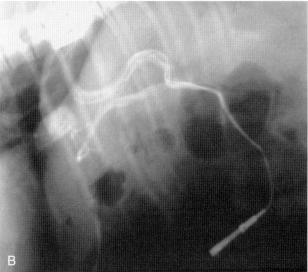

Figure 37-5 Positive contrast portograms of the same dog with a portosystemic vascular anomaly in right and left lateral recumbency. This study demonstrates how single-sided recumbency can fail to demonstrate shunting vasculature. So-called "portal streaming" or simply shunt compression by visceral structures explains these findings. **A,** Right side down. **B,** Left side down.

shape of a ductus venosus on lateral radiographs, each having an S or Z shape. A helpful but imperfect general rule is that intrahepatic PSVA can be differentiated from extrahepatic PSVA by location relative to the thoracolumbar spine. Most intrahepatic PSVAs have their caudal extent cranial to T13, whereas most extrahepatic PSVAs have their caudal extent caudal to T13.

Contrast multisector computed tomographic portograms provide the most informative studies for distinguishing aberrant portal vasculature. Equipment is costly and at present limited to large specialty facilities.

Generally these patients are referred for ligation of a PSVA, which is the definitive treatment for dogs demonstrating clinical signs. However, based on findings in the large genotyping study previously cited, clinical experience with dogs serendipitously discovered to have a PSVA at more than 9 years of age (asymptomatic dogs) and dogs managed medically long term (8 years), it is clear that not every dog with PSVA requires surgery. Furthermore, some dogs undergoing PSVA ligation cannot accommodate increased hepatic portal perfusion and develop multiple acquired shunts. A scheme explaining surgical outcomes relative to PSVA/MVD malformations is summarized in Table 37-4. Extrahepatic PSVAs are more amenable to surgical attenuation than many intrahepatic PSVAs (right divisional are more accessible than left divisional). Intravenous coils for occlusion of ductus venosus offer a new treatment option for intrahepatic PSVA. Success of PSVA surgical attenuation in cats is lower than in dogs. Placement of ameroid constrictors in cats is contraindicated because of the dismal response to full PSVA ligation. The general discussion that follows applies wholly to dogs.

Excellent outcome was found in 80%, good outcome in 14% (15/108;13 requiring a protein restricted diet, 1 requiring long term antimicrobials for HE, and 1 with grand mal seizures), and poor outcome in 7/108 dogs (6%, 6 dogs died of PSVA, 1 dog failed to improve clinical signs).

Medical management of PSVA is aimed at minimizing signs of HE and encompasses manipulation of dietary protein, modification of enteric flora, and avoidance of medications or substances augmenting or inducing encephalopathic signs. Careful regulation of dietary protein intake is critical. For dogs, a restricted protein diet (2.2 to 2.5 gm protein/kg body weight) derived chiefly from dairy and soy protein sources is best. Some dogs also tolerate chicken (white meat). Commercial diets formulated for dogs with hepatic insufficiency are convenient and function well in dogs with PSVA. Supplementation of such diets with additional cheese or cottage cheese to increase protein intake by 0.5 gm protein/kg body weight can be used to individually titrate protein intake to response. Diets can be modified with assistance from the free Nutritional Analysis Tools and System website (http://nat.crgq.com/mainnat.html). Meals should be frequent and small to maximize digestion and absorption. Minimizing colonic residue is helpful as colonic anaerobes degrade nitrogenous compounds to ammonia. Dogs with inoperable PSVA (severe MVD causing

intrahepatic portal atresia or extrahepatic portal atresia) have been managed for more than 3 years in the author's home without incident using commercial diets formulated for hepatic insufficiency. It is certain that dietary modification alone may be sufficient to abate clinical signs in dogs with PSVA. However, dogs with persistent ammonium biurate crystalluria or neuroencephalopathic signs should adjunctively receive lactulose dosed to achieve multiple soft stools per day (0.25 to 1 ml per 4.5 kg orally daily) and/or metronidazole (7.5 mg/kg body weight orally twice daily) or amoxicillin (especially cats, 2.5 mg/kg orally twice daily). Neomycin is the least desirable treatment for enteric flora modification. A small percentage of oral neomycin is absorbed and may result in renal injury or hearing loss with long-term administration. Milk can be used as an alternative for lactulose in some dogs and cats (lactose intolerance). Lactulose, a synthetic disaccharide indigestible by mammals, is fermented in the enteric canal to organic acids that acidify luminal contents. Colonic acidification promotes ammonium ion trapping, which reduces ammonia uptake into the portal circulation. Colonic acidification also inhibits enteric urease and protease activities. Organic acids promote bacterial nitrogen fixation and impose an osmotic catharsis (frequent soft stools) that promotes colonic evaluation of toxic substrates and products. If a commercial diet formulated for dogs or cats with hepatic insufficiency is used, additional vitamin supplements are not urgent. If a homemade diet is used, additional vitamins are recommended, taking care to avoid methionine supplements. Most dogs with PSVA have subnormal liver zinc concentrations, suggesting systemic zinc insufficiency. Zinc supplementation (1 to 2.5 mg elemental zinc/kg body weight/day) is recommended because zinc is essential for certain metalloenzymes (e.g., urea cycle). Zinc acetate is most commonly used (31% elemental zinc of formula weight) and can be compounded from Galzin (Gate Pharmaceuticals, North Wales, PA).

Medical and surgical management of minimally symptomatic patients is usually good. However, dogs with degenerative and nonsuppurative inflammatory lesions involving the hepatic venule may develop a progressive hepatopathy whether or not they undergo surgical treatment. Dogs with continued portosystemic shunting have increased susceptibility to systemic infections because of reduced function of hepatic macrophages. Thus prompt treatment must be provided for small wounds, cutaneous infections, and urinary tract infections. Attention also must be given to avoid conditions that can promote HE; these promiscuously expose patients to endogenous systemic or enteric toxins, nitrogen challenge, or promote dehydration and azotemia. Constipation must be avoided as colonic contents are an important toxin source contributing to HE. Management of acute severe HE requires mechanical cleansing of the colon with warm polyionic fluids until fecal debris is clear. Thereafter, instillation of a retention enema is used to modify enteric pH, flora, urease, and protease activities. Lactulose is the preferred retention enema solution. Dehydration, hypoglycemia, and electrolyte aberrations must be corrected.

TABLE 37-4   Malformations associated with extrahepatic and intrahepatic portosystemic vascular anomalies

	Single aberrant extrahepatic portosystemic communication	Two aberrant portosystemic shunts	MVD: attenuated intrahepatic portal tributaries (variably reduced flow to full atresia)	MVD: abnormal location and flow through hepatic venule: lobule outflow obstruction	Poorly developed extrahepatic portal vein (porta hepatis): extrahepatic portal hypoplasia	No extrahepatic portal vein in porta hepatis: portal atresia	Acquired portosystemic shunts	Ductus venosus, right or left divisional branch	Projected outcome: with successful surgical ligation*
Type 1	+	+/-	-	-	-	-	-	-	1
Type 2	+	+/-	+	-	-	-	- (possible with ligation)	-	2 or 3
Type 3	+	+/-	+	+	-	-	+/- (+ with ligation)	-	2, 3, or 4
Type 4	+	+/-	+	-	+	-	+/- (+ with ligation)	-	3, 4, 5
Type 5	+	+/-	+/-	-	-	+	+	-	4, 5
Type 6	-	-	-	-	-	-	-	+	1
Type 7	-	-	+	-	-	-	-	+	2 or 3
Type 8	-	-	+	-	-	-	+	+	4, 5

*"Cured" = 1; improved but retains high SBA = 2; requires medical Rx, retains high SBA = 3; no change = 4; worsened = 5.

Intrahepatic arteriovenous fistula

Congenital intrahepatic arterioportal fistulae unite a branch of the hepatic artery and portal vein and are uncommon malformations in the dog and cat. These vascular aberrations represent abnormal differentiation of the embryologic capillary plexus into arteries (sprouting) and veins (pruning). Arteriolarization of the portal venous system results in portal hypertension, development of multiple acquired portosystemic shunts, and commonly development of a transudative abdominal effusion. Nonhepatic systemic arteriovenous (AV) fistulae create a short circuit of arterial blood to the heart causing cardiac failure, effects analogous to the physiologic sequela of a chronic patent ductus arteriosus. However, when located in the liver, hepatic sinusoids impose hemodynamic resistance, blocking direct circulatory return of shunted arterial blood. Such patients do not develop cardiac sequela, but rather present with gastrointestinal signs (vomiting, diarrhea, melena) and HE. Age at initial diagnosis is usually within the first 2 years.

With the exception of abdominal effusion, historical, physical, and clinicopathologic findings resemble those affiliated with PSVA. All animals demonstrate high SBA concentrations and ammonium biurate crystalluria (examine three or more urine specimens). Abdominal ultrasonography equipped with color-flow Doppler rapidly identifies these malformations, AV admixture, and hepatofugal portal circulation. Liver lobes directly involved with the AV malformation are normal to large in size, and those distant to the malformation are atrophied. Contrast radiographic imaging of hepatic AV malformations requires injection into the anterior mesenteric or hepatic artery or into the jugular vein in very small patients. On inspection, affected liver lobes are prominent and may have numerous pulsating surface vessels. A continuous murmur accentuated during systole may be auscultated near the lesion. Palpation of the area may reveal a thrill.

Treatment of an intrahepatic AV fistula requires ligation of the nutrient artery and/or obliteration of the aberrant AV communication(s). Traditionally this has been accomplished by surgical resection of large malformations by hepatic lobectomy, ligating involved vessels, and/or establishing normal circulatory communications by vascular anastomosis. Caval banding, attempted in some dogs with intrahepatic AV fistula to rectify portosystemic shunting, provides no benefit and should not be done. Outcome to surgical interventions is poor, with many dogs dying during surgery or shortly thereafter; several dogs have developed portal venous or mesenteric thrombi. A small number of dogs have markedly improved with surgical procedure, which may reflect the nature of their AV malformations (location, distribution). It is common for survivors to manifest continued portosystemic shunting, recurrent abdominal effusion, and episodic HE. Medical management may require diuretics (furosemide combined with spironolactone) in conjunction with dietary sodium restriction to manage ascites and protein restriction (commercial diet for hepatic insufficiency) for episodic HE. Recent review of 22 dogs with hepatoportal AV fistula (treated surgically, with cyanoacrylate embolization, or both) had a dismal 25% good long-term outcome; 75% required continued diuretic therapy and/or dietary management for HE.

Neonatal Jaundice

There are no well-documented cases of inborn errors of bilirubin metabolism in dogs or cats causing neonatal jaundice. However, neonatal puppies have UDP-glucuronyl transferase activity (enzyme essential for bilirubin catabolism) lower than adult dogs. Activity of this enzyme matures within 28 to 42 days of age. Neonatal jaundice has been reported as a result of immunohemolytic anemia in puppies and kittens and in kittens with a hemolytic syndrome associated with neonatal isoerythrolysis. Neonatal isoerythrolysis may occur when kittens of type A or AB receive colostrally delivered anti-A alloantibodies from a type B dam.

Congenital Metabolic Abnormalities

Congenital disorders affecting the function or availability of lysosomal enzymes or effector proteins (activatory or protector proteins) necessary for catabolism of glycoproteins, glycolipids, glycosaminoglycans (mucopolysaccharides), gangliosides, and glycogen have been identified in humans and animal species, including the dog and cat. Such disorders cause tissue accumulation of undegraded storage products that impair organ or tissue structure and function with progressive clinical signs first emerging at a young age. Hepatomegaly is associated with some of these disorders when storage material accumulates in hepatocytes and/or Kupffer cells (fixed macrophages). A brief description of lysosomal storage disorders that may involve the liver, recognized in dogs and cats, is summarized here (Table 37-5).

Mannosidosis (deficiency in acid mannosidase) causes hepatomegaly, neurologic dysfunction (tremors, ataxia, hypermetria, and weakness), growth retardation, facial dysmorphia, and early death. Hepatic vacuolation is associated with membrane-bound mannose containing pentasaccharide. Demonstration of reduced intracellular alpha-mannosidase is diagnostic.

The mucopolysaccharidoses (MPS) are lysosomal enzyme defects impairing degradation of various glycosaminoglycans (connective tissue matrix components including dermatan sulfate, heparan sulfate, or keratan sulfate). Clinical features vary with the specific enzyme deficiency. Clinical features vary with different disorders and may include facial dysmorphia (rounded broad forehead, small ears, and dished face), corneal opacity, bone lesions (odontoid hypoplasia, vertebral exostoses, osteoporosis, coxofemoral luxation, lytic lesions in long bones and vertebrae), intervertebral disk degeneration, degenerative joint disease causing joint effusions and lameness, cardiac murmurs, growth retardation, neurologic abnormalities (i.e., cervical or thoracolumbar myelopathy, mental retardation), and early death. Metachromatic granules in leukocytes may also be recognized. Presumptive diagnosis of MPS is made based on a positive urine toluidine blue spot test, but definitive diagnosis is only confirmed on measurement of specific enzymes in fresh plasma, cultured

TABLE 37-5   Hepatic storage of glycosaminoglycans in feline and canine models of mucopolysaccharidoses I, VI, and VII

Disorder	Species	Deficiency	Hepatomegaly	Hepatocyte change	Other tissues affected
Mannosidosis	Cat	Alpha-mannosidase	Yes	Vacuolation of hepatocytes with mannose containing pentasaccharide storage material	Neurons; severe neurologic signs
Mucopoly-saccharidosis (MPS) I	Dog (Plott Hound, other single cases), DSH Cat	Alpha-L-iduronidase	Yes	Vacuolation of hepatocytes and Kupffer cells with MPS storage material	Facial dysmorphia, corneal opacity, osseous lesions, vertebral exostoses, intervertebral disk degeneration, degenerative joint disease, stunted growth, metachromatic granules in WBC, neurologic abnormalities, early death
MPS II: Hunter syndrome	Labrador Retriever	Iduronate sulfatase	Yes	Vacuolation of hepatocytes, biliary epithelium, sinusoidal lining cells, and hepatic macrophages with MPS storage material	Similar facial deformity but lack of bone effects as in MPSI; very slowly progressive neurologic syndrome (5 years)
MPS IIIa, San Filippo syndrome	Wirehair Dachshund, Huntaway Dog	Heparan N-sulfatase		Fine foamy vacuolation of hepatocytes with discrete membrane bound material, similar vacuolation in macrophages	Progressive neurologic syndrome
MPS IIIb	Schipperke	α-N-acetylglucos-aminidase	Yes	Vacuolation of hepatocytes and Kupffer cells and many other tissues with MPS storage	Lethargy, mental dullness, gradual onset neurologic signs (tremors, vestibular signs), lack of bone effects
MPS VI	Siamese, DSH cats, Miniature Pinscher, Welsh Corgi, Chesapeake Bay Retriever, Miniature Schnauzer	N-acetyl glucosamine 4-sulfatase (arylsulfatase B)		Vacuolation of hepatic macrophages	Facial dysmorphia, short stature, reduced bone growth, arthritis, corneal clouding, but variable clinical signs with different mutations
MPS VII	DSH Cat, German Shepherd Dog	B-Glucuronidase			
Glycogen storage disease (GSD) Ia (von Gierke disease)	Maltese	Glucose-6-phosphatase	Yes	Vacuolation of hepatocytes with glycogen and lipid	Early onset clinical signs with neuroglycopenia causing failure to thrive, collapse, and seizures
GSD II (Pompe disease)	Swedish Lapland dogs	Lysosomal alpha-glucosidase	No	None described	
GSD III, Cori disease	German Shepherd Dog, Curly-Coated Retriever	Glycogen debranching enzyme	Yes	Hepatocyte vacuolation due to glycogen accumulation	

Hepatic storage of glycosaminoglycans in feline and canine models of mucopolysaccharidoses I, VI, and VII, *Vet Pathol* 29(2):112-119, 1992.

dermal fibroblasts, or leukocytes. Practically, only symptomatic treatment for bone pain caused by skeletal deformities can be offered.

Gangliosidosis, caused by the lysosomal accumulation of incompletely catabolized gangliosides or glycolipids, has been documented in both dogs and cats. Affected animals develop neurologic signs as early as 2 to 3 months of age (progressive fine generalized muscle tremors, ataxia, and paresis) associated with ganglioside accumulation in the central nervous system. Visceral organs, including the liver, also accumulate membrane-bound cytoplasmic bodies microscopically characterized as multilamellar spherical cytoplasmic inclusions.

Glycogen storage disorders (GSDs) have been diagnosed in Maltese dogs (type Ia, defective glucose-6-phosphatase, von Gierke disease), Swedish Lapland dogs (lysosomal acid α-glucosidase deficiency, GSD II, Pompe disease), German Shepherd Dogs and Curly-Coated Retrievers (glycogen debranching enzyme, GSD III, Cori disease); and English Springer Spaniels (phosphofructokinase deficiency, GSD VII, Tarui disease). Only the GSD I and GSD III syndromes cause symptomatic hypoglycemia and profound hepatocyte engorgement with glycogen.

In Maltese dogs with GSD Ia (autosomal recessive trait), puppies have abdominal distention as a result of profound hepatomegaly at birth. Clinical signs attributable to symptomatic hypoglycemia develop within a few days (weakness, failure to nurse, mental dullness, and seizures). Puppies surviving beyond several weeks have poor growth rates, delayed development of neurological reflexes, and are difficult to wean to solid food. Abdominal ultrasonography reveals a diffuse hyperechoic hepatic parenchyma as a result of accumulation of glycogen and fat in hepatocytes. Clinicopathologic features include hypoglycemia, hyperlactacidemia, hypercholesterolemia, and hypertriglyceridemia. At death, the liver is grossly large and pale. Histologically, hepatocytes are markedly distended by vacuolar retention of glycogen and fat. A specific genetic defect has been characterized; carriers (heterozygotes) manifest no clinical effects.

Curly-Coated Retrievers with deficiency of glycogen debranching enzyme (GSD III, autosomal recessive trait) are identified at 6 to 9 months of age based on increased liver enzyme (alanine transaminase [ALT], AST, ALP) and inconsistently on CK activity. Fasting and postmeal serum bile acids, cholesterol, and triglyceride concentrations are normal. Clinical signs are mild in the first year of life but become overt with age and include lethargy, exercise intolerance, and episodic hypoglycemia (collapse and unresponsiveness). Grossly livers are friable, large, dark red, and have a finely irregular surface. Liver lesions include a diffuse vacuolar hepatopathy (hepatocyte glycogen retention). There are no fatty vacuoles nor necroinflammatory or fibrotic lesions. Carriers manifest no clinical effects. A specific genetic defect has been characterized, and a polymerase chain reaction (PCR)-based DNA test is available.

Canine GSD IIIa (glycogen debranching enzyme deficiency) reported in a family of German Shepherd Dogs was more severe than the disorder characterized in Curly-Coated Retrievers, with illness manifesting in puppies (lethargy, muscle weakness, hepatomegaly, and growth retardation). Disease severity limited survival to 15 months of age. Accumulated glycogen caused hepatomegaly and dysfunction in skeletal, cardiac muscle, smooth muscle, and the central nervous system (glia and neurons). Although the genetic defect has not been characterized, it is speculated to totally abrogate glycogen debranching enzyme function.

Copper Storage Hepatopathy

Bedlington Terriers have an autosomal recessive mutation causing an age-related accumulation of hepatic copper that causes a progressive hepatopathy and liver failure. A 13-kilobase pair deletion in the *COMMD1* gene (chromosome 10) has been verified in European dogs, and a PCR diagnostic test has been developed. Other *COMMD1* mutations exist in some affected Bedlington Terriers. Other chronic hepatopathies in dogs also may be associated with excess liver copper retention; these generally do not manifest in dogs less than 1 year of age, and it is not clear that copper retention in these dogs is an epiphenomenon of hepatocyte injury, relates to excessive dietary copper intake, or is a causal factor (West Highland White Terrier, Dalmatian, Labrador Retriever, Doberman Pinscher).

Copper, an essential component of certain metalloenzymes, is absorbed from food, circulates bound to plasma proteins, and is taken up into the liver. A complex hepatocellular copper transport system (chaperones, binding proteins, membrane transporters) disperses copper to essential storage sites and excretes excess copper into canalicular bile. In health, these mechanisms ensure a neutral copper balance with reasonable copper ingestion. Excess hepatic copper retention is easily identified in liver biopsies with copper-specific stains (e.g., rhodanine, rubeanic acid). However, hepatocellular copper excess must be verified by reconciliation of copper-specific stains and quantitative tissue copper measurements (expressed on a dry weight basis). Excessive hepatocellular copper leads to organelle and cell membrane oxidative injury and lysosomal degranulation causing cell necrosis, and a progressive hepatopathy. Initial injury occurs in zone 3 (centrilobular, periacinar). Dogs homozygous for the mutation develop a progressive hepatopathy that may become evident during the first year of life (high serum ALT activity). However, most affected dogs develop a progressive diffuse hepatopathy evident after several years of life. Homozygous normal and heterozygous carrier dogs usually have hepatic copper concentrations in the normal range (≤400 μg/g dry weight liver), whereas homozygous affected dogs develop increased hepatic copper concentrations during the first year. Hepatic copper concentrations greater than 2000 μg/g dry tissue are consistently associated with morphologic and functional evidence of a progressive hepatopathy that may proceed to cirrhosis without treatment. Older affected animals may develop hepatic copper concentrations greater than 10,000 μg/g dry tissue. Many affected dogs can be identified as early as 6 months of age based on hepatic biopsy (copper granule accumulation) and metal quantification before histologic evidence of hepatocellular injury. Some dogs require as long as 1 year before accumulating excessive hepatic copper. Although affected Bedlington Terriers may have evidence of increased hepatic copper as early as 8 to 12 weeks of age, biopsy at this age is unreliable for discriminating affectation status.

Copper-associated hepatopathy in Bedlington Terriers should be suspected in any individual with persistently high ALT activity. Although definitive diagnosis requires liver biopsy, genetic testing is useful in families with the characterized mutation. Measurement of serum or urine copper or ceruloplasmin (copper transport protein) concentrations does not have diagnostic value. In dogs with chronic copper-induced liver injury, hepatic mass replacement with fibrous tissue and regenerative nodules decreases the concentration of copper measured in sampled liver.

Life-long treatment with a copper chelator such as D-penicillamine or with zinc acetate that blocks enteric copper uptake is necessary for homozygous affected dogs. D-Penicillamine chelates copper within the circulation, promotes cupruresis, and provides antiinflammatory effects. A recommended dosage of D-penicillamine is 10 to 15 mg/kg body weight given orally every 12 hours 30 minutes before feeding. The most common adverse effects are vomiting and anorexia mitigated by initial dose reduction and gradual retitration and dose administration with food. If D-penicillamine is not tolerated, 2,2,2 tetramine may be used as an alternative chelator; 5 to 7 mg/kg is given orally every 12 hours 30 minutes before feeding. Vitamin C is contraindicated in liver disease associated with transition metal accumulation (copper, iron) because it may enhance oxidative injury. Pyridoxine supplementation (5 to 25 mg/day) is recommended with long-term D-penicillamine therapy. Vitamin E (10 IU/kg body weight/day) and S-adenosylmethionine (20 mg/kg body weight/day given orally on an empty stomach) are recommended antioxidants for dogs with excess hepatic copper storage. Prednisolone administration is not advised unless a dog is suffering a necrolytic or hemolytic copper crisis or an immune-mediated inflammatory process coexists. Dietary copper intake should be restricted to less than 5.0 ppm (dry matter basis) or no greater than 0.4 mg copper/day for a Bedlington Terrier. The amount of copper in commercial dog foods is variable, and the manufacturer should be contacted for specific information. Copper in the drinking water should not exceed 0.2 ppm (0.2 μg/L), especially if chelation therapy is the mainstay of therapy. It is prudent to avoid domestically softened water passing through copper pipes as this may contribute copper during initial flushing each day. Vitamin supplements should be investigated to determine their copper content before daily use. Nutritional support using home-cooked copper-restricted diets (e.g., avoiding organ meats, nuts, shrimp, and legumes) and commercial diets manufactured for dogs with liver disease have been successfully used in affected Bedlington Terriers. The reader is referred to the U.S. Department of Agriculture (USDA)

food tables to ascertain copper content in basic foods (http://www.nutritiondata.com/ or http://www.nal.usda.gov/fnic/foodcomp/Data/SR18/nutrlist/sr18w312.pdf). Dietary adjustments (energy, protein content) can be made using the NAT 2 freeware at the University of Illinois (also linked to the USDA food tables) at http://nat.crgq.com/mainnat.html.

Abnormal Urate Catabolism in Dalmatians

Dalmatians are predisposed to urate urolith formation as a breed-specific genetic disorder associated with hyperuricemia and hyperuricuria. Whereas normal dogs metabolize uric acid, a product of purine degradation, to water-soluble allantoin via hepatic uricase, all Dalmatians have an autosomal recessive defect in purine metabolism resulting in hyperuricosuria (ten- to twentyfold greater than other pure or cross-breed dogs). Defective membrane transport of urate compromises hepatocyte and renal tubular epithelium to uptake urate. The Dalmatian defect involves abnormal urate transport across cellular membranes. Although the molecular basis for the disorder is unresolved, the trait is linked (microsatellite linkage studies) to chromosome 3 (CFA03). The current hypothesis is that a promoter of urate membrane transport, made in the liver, is dysfunctional or absent.

Urinary excretion of uric acid in Dalmatians ranges between 400 and 600 mg/24 hours versus 10 to 60 mg/24 hours in non-Dalmatian dogs. Urinary uric acid/creatinine ratios range between 0.3 to 0.6 for normal puppies and 1.3 to 4.6 for Dalmatian puppies at 3 to 7 weeks of age and between 0.2 to 0.4 for normal dogs and 0.6 to 1.5 for adult Dalmatians. Although not all Dalmatians develop symptomatic urolithiasis, males have greater risk owing to their urogenital anatomy. Urate stones in Dalmatians often involve hundreds of very small stones that act as a conglomerate obstructing the penile urethra.

Treatment of dogs with symptomatic urate urolithiasis includes increasing their daily water intake (wet food), urinary alkalinization (increases urate solubility, goal pH between 6.5 and 7.0), dietary modification (reducing intake of urate precursors), titrated dosing with allopurinol (dosing based on uric acid urinary excretion), and scrotal urethrostomy (for males with recurrent obstruction despite medical strategies). Dietary modification involves selection of foodstuffs low in purines rather than focusing on protein restriction. Foods low in purines include bread and cereal (except whole grains), most vegetables excluding cauliflower, spinach, peas, mushrooms, and legumes (kidney beans, navy beans, lima beans, and lentils), fruit (avoid acidic citrus), nuts, pasta, eggs, cheese, milk, and butter. Foods with moderate purine content or risk include most poultry (chicken, turkey), fish and shellfish (except mussels and scallops), lamb, pork, and beef, oats and oatmeal, wheat germ and bran, and whole grain breads. Foods with high purine or risk include those noted above and organ meats (kidneys, liver, brains, hearts), game meats (venison, duck, goose), high purine seafoods such as sardines and mackerel, yeast (including brewer's yeast), and gravies made from organ meats. There are few prescription manufactured diets restrictive enough in purines to be appropriate for stone dissolution (Hills U/D); however, this diet is not an appropriate growth food for puppies. Thus affected puppies should have surgical removal of their stones as medical stone dissolution can take months (3 to 4 months is common). Allopurinol is used to inhibit xanthine oxidase, the enzyme transforming hypoxanthine to uric acid. Initial starting dose is 15 mg/kg body weight given orally every 12 hours. It is important to titrate the dose of allopurinol against the urinary uric acid concentration because inhibition of xanthine oxidase causes high urine concentrations of hypoxanthine and xanthine. Unfortunately excess urine xanthine concentrations can lead to xanthine urolithiasis. A 24-hour uric acid production test is used to titrate allopurinol dosing. All urine produced over a 12-hour interval is collected, mixed well, and an aliquot is submitted for measurement of uric acid. Optimal uric acid elimination approximates 300 mg/kg body weight/day. If output is much lower, the allopurinol dose is reduced; if output is much higher, the allopurinol dose is increased. However, scrutiny of dietary intake also is essential before recommending dose adjustments.

Hepatic Lipidosis

In a survey of histologically diagnosed liver disorders in puppies and kittens younger than 4 months of age ($n = 444$; see Table 37-1), hepatic lipidosis was diagnosed in 9.0%. Because most animals were evaluated for primary conditions in other organ systems or for infectious disorders, it is likely that hepatic lipidosis in this population represents a sequela of acquired nutritional inadequacies. A variety of metabolic disorders can disturb mobilization of triglycerides from the liver or enhance mobilization of peripheral fat stores to the liver. Whenever intrahepatic lipid synthesis or hepatocellular uptake of fat exceeds hepatic triglyceride dispersal, hepatic lipidosis ensues. It is well documented that the metabolic balance in juveniles is fragile. Studies have confirmed excess hepatic triglyceride accumulation in puppies born to undernourished bitches and in semistarved puppies fed only glucose at a rate of 60 kcal/kg body weight/day for 10 days. Two-month-old puppies completely starved for 24 hours also develop significantly greater hepatic triglyceride stores than normally fed control puppies. It is well established that cats have higher susceptibility to diffuse hepatic lipidosis compared with dogs. Any serious medical condition in the cat that induces anorexia can lead to diffuse severe hepatic lipid accumulation. Cytoplasmic hepatocellular vacuolation with triglycerides adversely influences hepatic function, leading to metabolic failure in affected cats. Nutritional support ensuring adequate intake of energy and protein, as well as providing essential amino acids, fatty acids, and water-soluble vitamins, is the major focus of treatment. Forced enteral feeding by gentle syringe alimentation, nasogastric intubation, or esophagostomy tube (especially cats) is necessary in most patients. Supplementation of cobalamin in B_{12}-deficient cats is essential. Oral supplementation with L-carnitine (250 mg/day, medical grade), taurine (250 to 500 mg/day), thiamine (50 to 100 mg/day), S-adenosylmethionine (190 mg/day on an empty stomach), and vitamin E (10 U/kg body weight/day) is recommended.

Selected Infectious Disorders Affecting the Hepatobiliary System

Hepatic Abscessation

Hepatic abscesses are more common in young puppies than in kittens. Hematogenous, omphalogenic, biliary, and peritoneal extension are reported sources of infecting organisms; postpartum umbilical infection is most common. After onset of clinical illness, health status deteriorates rapidly, culminating in death within 2 to 4 weeks. Occasionally seemingly healthy puppies die unexpectedly with the cause discovered on postmortem examination. Affected puppies usually range between 3 and 70 days of age and are from large litters. Although there is no evidence that individual bitches recurrently whelp litters with affected puppies, poor sanitation may be a predisposing factor. In kennels with recurrent puppy or kitten losses associated with omphalitis and liver abscessation, kennel sanitation may be the underlying cause. Isolated organisms include *Staphylococcus*, *Streptococcus*, *Salmonella*, and *Escherichia coli*. Affected neonates are usually stunted, emaciated, dehydrated, and may have abdominal distention as a result of hepatomegaly and peritonitis. Liver lobes may be adhered to one another and to adjacent viscera; there is no liver lobe predisposition. Unaffected lobes often have randomly distributed multiple foci of microabscesses and necrosis.

Liver Flukes

Hepatic trematode infection has been diagnosed in kittens as young as 4 months of age. The most common liver fluke in cats in North America is *Platynosomum concinnum*. Other species of flukes that may infect cats include *Amphimerus pseudofelineus*, *Opisthorchis tenuicollis*, *Metorchis albidus*, and *Metorchis conjunctus*. The life cycle of *P. concinnum* requires a tropical to semitropical climate and two intermediate hosts: a land snail (*Subulina octona*) and a lizard or marine toad. Cats acquire infection by ingestion of the second intermediate host. Once ingested, the parasite migrates up the common bile duct into the gallbladder, bile ducts, and pancreas. In 8 to 12 weeks, adult flukes produce embryonated eggs that are passed in feces. Recognition of fluke eggs in feces (fecal sedimentation) is the basis of definitive diagnosis. Clinical signs of liver injury are apparent by 7 to 16 weeks after infection and may include lethargy, inappetence, weight loss, emaciation, hepatomegaly, mucoid diarrhea, vomiting, and abdominal tenderness. The severity of clinical signs varies with the degree of the fluke infection; many naturally infected cats show no clinical signs. In experimentally infected cats, 62% returned to normal clinical health in 24 weeks without treatment. In heavily infected cats, clinical signs may develop before fecal shedding of ova. Circulating eosinophilia may develop and peak at 4 to 5 months after infection. Transient increases in serum AST and ALT activity develop during fluke migration through the liver. Serum ALP and GGT activities may remain normal or may increase depending on the numbers of developing flukes and the extent of invasion and obstruction of biliary structures. Cats with heavy fluke infection may become jaundiced, albeit some only transiently, as a result of biliary tree obstruction. Flukes within the gallbladder can be visualized ultrasonographically as hypoechoic foci. Histologic lesions in hepatic parenchyma and biliary structures include leukocyte infiltration, adenomatous hyperplasia of biliary structures, and periportal and periductal fibrosis. Chronic fluke infestation and bile duct obstruction may result in biliary cirrhosis. On postmortem examination, gross lesions may be absent; when apparent, enlargement of the gallbladder and bile ducts is found. Adult flukes and eggs are demonstrable in bile and within biliary structures. Treatment with praziquantel (20 to 40 mg/kg daily for 3 days) eradicates fluke infestation.

Canine Herpesvirus

Infection with canine herpesvirus causes an acute, rapidly fatal illness associated with hepatic necrosis. Puppies may have predisposition as a result of their poor thermoregulation and inability to mount a febrile response. Herpesvirus is not stable in the environment and must be acquired from a persistently infected carrier. Infection can be acquired in utero, during passage through the birth canal, by exposure to infected littermates, from oronasal secretions of the dam, or by fomite transmission. Abortions and stillbirths may follow in utero infections. Generalized, fatal infections develop in puppies exposed when less than 1 week of age. Puppies exposed when older than 2 weeks are comparatively resistant and often develop mild or inapparent infection. Diffuse necrotizing vasculitis and spread of virus into parenchymal organs, including the adrenal glands, kidneys, lungs, spleen, and liver, result in multifocal organ necrosis. Thrombocytopenia develops associated with disseminated intravascular coagulation as a result of the vasculitis and/or immune-mediated mechanisms. Meningoencephalitis is common, although puppies infected at less than 1 week of age usually die before neurologic signs develop. Survivors that had neurologic signs may have permanent neurologic deficits, most commonly cerebellar vestibular deficiencies. Ocular involvement may cause panuveitis, cataracts, keratitis, retinitis, and subsequent blindness.

Clinical signs of herpesvirus infection in puppies may include lethargy, decreased suckling, persistent crying, yellow-green diarrhea, rhinitis, abdominal pain, and incoordination. A distinct feature is the absence of fever. Petechial hemorrhages may be notable on mucous membranes and provide testimony to the thrombocytopenia and vasculitis associated with viremia. Death frequently occurs within 24 to 48 hours after onset of clinical signs in puppies less than 3 weeks of age. Puppies older than 3 to 5 weeks of age at exposure may develop only mild or inapparent infections. Passage of maternal protective antibodies or lymphocytes in colostrum can prevent illness in neonates.

Definitive diagnosis is made based on history, clinical signs, pathologic changes, and virus isolation. Hematologic and biochemical abnormalities are nonspecific and variable. Gross pathologic findings include disseminated multifocal 1- to 2-mm hemorrhages and areas of necrosis that are distinctly circumscribed in the liver, kidney, and lungs (Figure 37-6). Wedge-shaped renal infarcts develop subsequent to fibrinoid necrosis of interlobular arteries. Hepatomegaly, splenomegaly, and lymphadenopathy are common. Further information on systemic manifestations and treatment of herpesvirus infections can be found in Chapter 16.

Canine and Feline Parvovirus

Focal hepatitis and hepatic cord disorganization may develop in puppies and kittens infected with parvovirus. Twofold to fivefold increases in serum activity of ALT and AST may develop. In some cases, hepatic involvement is progressive, resulting in jaundice. Whether signs of hepatobiliary involvement are the result of parenchymal injury from viral infection, thromboembolic complications resulting from vascular lesions, or secondary to bacterial infection or endotoxemia (from breakdown of the gastrointestinal mucosal barrier) is unresolved. Seemingly, a poor prognosis is warranted when hepatic involvement becomes clinical (see Chapter 16).

Feline Infectious Peritonitis

Infection with feline coronavirus causing feline infectious peritonitis (FIP; herein referred to as FIPV) most often affects kittens and cats between 6 months and 5 years of age housed in a multiple-cat population. FIPV reflects a progressive and lethal coronavirus infection causing immune-mediated tissue injury. Tissue lesions are initiated by virus or viral antigen and host antiviral antibodies and complement. Humoral antibody responses increase virus pathogenicity, and cell-mediated immune responses play a decisive protective role. Effusive FIPV is thought to represent acute disease,

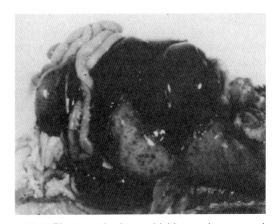

Figure 37-6 Photograph of petechial hemorrhages on visceral surfaces in a puppy with canine herpesvirus infection. Note hepatomegaly and diffusely mottled appearance of the liver associated with multifocal hepatic necrosis. (From Hoskins J: *Veterinary pediatrics: dogs and cats from birth to 6 months*, ed 3, Philadelphia, 2001, Saunders, p 217.)

occurring 4 to 8 weeks after infection or a stress-imposing event. The less common dry form of FIPV is considered to reflect a chronic form of infection. In dry FIPV, a 2- to 12-week interval of vague illness precedes initial presentation. Clinical signs include chronic undulant fever, inappetence, and weight loss. Plasma protein concentrations increase as a result of variable increases in globulins associated with an acute phase response. Coagulopathy reflects diffuse vascular injury and occurs in cats with severe inflammatory lesions or diffuse severe hepatic involvement. Coagulopathies and thrombocytopenia are more common in cats with effusive FIPV, and their presence portends a grave prognosis. Clinical signs of either syndrome ultimately depend on involved target organs. The clinical syndromes associated with FIPV are described in Chapter 16 on Viral Infections. Necrotizing hepatitis reflects immune complex–facilitated tissue injury, and lesions are associated with inflammatory perivascular cuffing. Animals with FIPV hepatitis may demonstrate anterior abdominal pain and hepatomegaly, with a subset becoming jaundiced. Serum ALT and AST activities are variably increased, ranging from twofold to tenfold normal values.

At present, diagnosis of FIPV is based on history, clinical signs, feline leukemia virus (FeLV) status, and, most importantly, histologic lesions and immunohistochemical demonstration of virus in tissue lesions or macrophages. Kittens with signs of hepatic involvement are poor candidates for immunosuppressive therapy.

Feline Leukemia Virus

Infection of kittens with FeLV may occur by vertical or horizontal transmission. By virtue of its oncogenic potential and ability to immunologically compromise its host, FeLV may be associated with neoplastic conditions and infectious disorders involving the liver of both pediatric and adult patients (e.g., see Toxoplasmosis below). Lymphosarcoma and myeloproliferative disease can develop in infected cats within weeks or months of virus exposure. Cats with hepatic neoplastic infiltrates often demonstrate nonpainful hepatomegaly. Jaundice indicates diffuse hepatic involvement or periportal infiltrates but less commonly signals impingement or infiltration of the common bile duct. Abdominal ultrasonography may or may not disclose mass lesions or foci of infiltrated regions involving hepatobiliary structures. Hematologic abnormalities may include a moderate to severe nonregenerative anemia and atypical cytology consistent with a myeloproliferative disorder or lymphosarcoma. Serum biochemical abnormalities are variable depending on the extent of hepatic involvement. Definitive diagnosis of FeLV infection is made by enzyme-linked immunosorbent assay for viral antigen or indirect fluorescent antibody labeling of infected cells. See Chapter 16 on Viral Infections.

Bordetella bronchiseptica

Accidental subcutaneous administration of attenuated live intranasal *Bordetella bronchiseptica* vaccine induces fever (within 2 days), a local inflammatory reaction at the injection site, and acute, nonseptic hepatocellular degeneration and necrosis. Chronic sustained liver injury has also been reported. Anecdotally, this accident has occurred several times in different veterinary facilities; in some cases dogs have succumbed to liver failure. Treatment with doxycycline for 3 weeks is advised. Some animals have required intravenous fluids and extended hospitalizations.

Virulent Systemic Calicivirus

Recently a highly infectious, vaccination-resistant, and virulent form of feline calicivirus (FCV) causing systemic disease and death has been described. Time from exposure to first clinical signs ranges from 1 to 12 days (median, 4 days). Affected cats show varying degrees of pyrexia, cutaneous edema, ulcerative mucositis and dermatitis, anorexia, facial and limb edema, lameness, upper respiratory signs, pulmonary edema and pleural effusion causing dyspnea, and jaundice. See Chapter 16 on Viral Infections. In one outbreak where biochemistry panels were available for 10 cats, 6 of 10 had hyperbilirubinemia (range, 0.6 to 3.9 mg/dl), and 5 of 10 had hypoalbuminemia (range, 1.1 to 2.1 g/dl). High serum enzyme activities included AST (3 of 10), ALT (2 of 10), and CK (5 of 10). Hepatic lesions include disruption of hepatic cords with hepatocyte individualization and zone 3 (centrilobular, periacinar) foci of necrosis associated with small accumulations of intrasinusoidal neutrophils and scattered intrasinusoidal fibrin deposits. Multifocal, peracute, pancreatic necrosis with adjacent fat saponification has been observed in some cats. Many clinical features and histologic lesions are associated with virus-induced vascular damage (e.g., edema, microthrombi, intrasinusoidal fibrin accumulation). Immunohistochemistry of liver tissue with anti-FCV antibody can confirm a definitive diagnosis. However, viral antigen was not discernable in hepatocytes in the initial report of virulent systemic FCV.

Strains of FCV causing virulent systemic FCV are genetically distinct from one another yet still cause similar clinical disease. Because these FCV strains are resistant to routine FCV vaccinations, cats with suspected infection should be handled with strict hygienic precautions.

Salmonellosis

Along with *Salmonella* spp., other enteric microorganisms such as *E. coli* also can be a source of hepatic parenchymal and biliary tract infection in young dogs that resembles the syndrome caused by *Salmonella*. *Salmonella* infection is associated with environmental or food or water contamination. Certain individuals are predisposed to infection by immunocompromising circumstances, such as malnutrition, parvoviral (vaccinal or field isolates) or FeLV infections, neoplasia, inherited immunoincompetence syndromes, glucocorticoid therapy, systemic or environmental stress, or neonatal life. Feeding of uncooked contaminated meat products (e.g., BARF diet), other forms of food contamination, and environmental transfer of bacteria by fomites are responsible for most infections. Puppies and kittens less than 1 year of age are more susceptible to infection and clinical illness than adults. Neonates may acquire infection from infected secretions from their dam (e.g., vaginal discharges, placentas, meconia). In utero infection may result in fetal death, abortion, or birth of weak "fading" puppies or kittens.

Salmonella spp. may exist in dogs and cats as a part of their normal enteric flora. Positive *Salmonella* fecal cultures occur in 1% to 36% of clinically healthy dogs and 0% to 18% of clinically healthy cats. Consequently isolation from feces does not confirm pathogenic infection without serotyping. Jaundice may reflect hepatic endotoxemia, hepatic infarction (development of disseminated intravascular coagulation), or bacterial colonization of hepatic parenchyma. Very young animals manifest the most severe clinical signs; puppies and kittens less than 7 weeks of age may not have a fever despite bacteremia and endotoxemia. Biochemical evidence of liver involvement includes increased serum activity of ALT, AST, and ALP and in some cases hyperbilirubinemia and hypoglycemia. Hypoglycemia also may reflect endotoxemia. Coagulopathy reflecting disseminated intravascular coagulation develops in animals with severe systemic or hepatic infection.

Hepatic necrosis has been documented in puppies with lethal infection. In these, multifocal foci of necrosis are the most common histologic lesion. Affected livers are grossly enlarged and have a mottled appearance. Bacterial organisms may be microscopically evident on routinely stained tissue sections. Hepatic colonization can follow either a clinical or subclinical infection. Suppurative meningitis also may develop in puppies or kittens. Definitive diagnosis of salmonellosis as the cause of illness relies on bacterial culture from involved tissues or body fluids that are normally sterile. Positive culture of fecal specimens cannot confirm a causal relationship with clinical disease.

Tyzzer's Disease

Clostridium piliforme (previously *Bacillus piliformis*) is a gram-negative spore-forming obligate intracellular bacterium that can cause enteric and hepatic infection in dogs and cats. Infection is precipitated by stress (e.g., crowding, unsanitary husbandry, weaning, or transportation), irradiation, and immunosuppression (e.g., glucocorticoid therapy). All species subject to infection develop necrotizing ileitis and colitis and multifocal hepatitis. Spontaneous infections in dogs and cats are believed to follow ingestion of bacterial spores passed in rodent feces. It is undetermined whether this organism also is an enteric commensal of the dog or cat. Most infections have been observed in laboratory-reared pediatric animals at the time of weaning. Infections are facilitated by stress or factors impairing immunocompetency. Clinical disease follows proliferation of organisms in enterocytes. Infected cells degenerate and slough, causing ulcer formation that permits mucosal translocation of bacteria into the portal circulation. Wide dispersal of organisms into the liver causes multifocal bacterial hepatitis. Presenting signs of natural infection in pediatric puppies and kittens include sudden onset of lethargy, anorexia, diarrhea (small amounts), abdominal tenderness, and rarely jaundice (cats). Within 24 to 48 hours of clinical illness, hepatomegaly and

abdominal distention are followed by hypothermia. Animals become nonresponsive and die shortly thereafter. Marked increases in serum ALT precede death.

Owing to the rapidly fatal course of infection, diagnosis is often made based on gross findings at necropsy. Inspection of the liver reveals many white-gray hemorrhagic 1- to 2-mm foci on the capsule and cut surfaces, with similar lesions on other viscera. The terminal ileum and proximal colon appear inflamed and thickened and contain foamy, dark-brown feces. Mesenteric lymphadenopathy is common. Definitive diagnosis is easily accomplished by histologic examination of liver sections. A multifocal periportal hepatic necrosis is associated with mononuclear cells and neutrophils at the margins of necrotic lesions. Clostridial organisms are easily identified within phagocytes in these areas in tissue sections with special stains (Giemsa, Warthin-Starry, or Gomori's methenamine-silver stains) or in fresh tissue imprints stained with methylene-blue or Diff-Quik. Organisms are not easily identified with routine hematoxylin and eosin staining of tissue sections. Treatment of Tyzzer's disease has not been successful owing to its rapid progression after realization that an animal is ill. Thus antibiotic efficacy is undetermined.

Toxoplasmosis

Toxoplasma gondii is a protozoal organism that can infect young dogs and cats, as well as many other young vertebrates. Cats can serve as either an intermediate or definitive host and are the only definitive host. Clinical signs associated with *Toxoplasma* infections vary depending on the chronicity of infection, host immune status, mode of infection, and target organs. *Toxoplasma* behaves as a pathogenic opportunist. Prenatal or lactationally acquired toxoplasmosis is generally more severe than postnatal infections. In utero infection can lead to stillbirths or acute severe neonatal illness or death from a fading puppy or kitten syndrome. Systemically infected puppies and kittens can appear normal at birth and continue to nurse but insidiously become lethargic, inappetent, and dyspneic and may demonstrate mucopurulent oculonasal discharge and develop progressive neurologic abnormalities with illness, culminating in death. Dissemination to multiple organs usually involves the liver and leads to jaundice, hepatomegaly, and abdominal effusion. Lesions may include multifocal necrotizing hepatitis or cholangiohepatitis.

Acute postnatal infection can develop in seemingly normal individuals following ingestion of large numbers of sporulated oocysts or bradyzoites. Again multiple organ dissemination is the rule, with clinical signs including inappetence, dyspnea, coughing, vomiting, diarrhea, hematemesis, enlarged tonsils and peripheral lymph nodes, splenomegaly, and hepatomegaly. Hepatic inflammation may be associated with anterior abdominal pain and peritoneal effusion and usually is associated with vomiting, diarrhea, and inappetence. Animals may become jaundiced as a result of diffuse hepatic necrosis or cholangiohepatitis. A survey of 100 cats with histologically confirmed toxoplasmosis confirmed clinical syndromes involving the liver in 93% of cats. Generalized systemic infections with toxoplasmosis are more common in dogs and cats less than 1 year of age.

Biochemical abnormalities indicating hepatic involvement include marked increases in serum ALT, AST, and ALP activities and hyperbilirubinemia. Diagnosis of toxoplasmosis is definitively confirmed by finding tachyzoites in histologic or cytologic specimens.

Clindamycin is the drug of choice for treating clinical toxoplasmosis in dogs and cats and also is recommended for pregnant animals. Oral and parenteral dosing is similar, 10 to 20 mg/kg body weight given orally or intramuscularly every 12 hours for 4 weeks. Clinical response is usually evident as early as 48 hours. Treatment response requires an adequately functioning immune system that can eliminate *Toxoplasma* organisms.

The zoonotic potential of fecal oocyst shedding must be considered when dealing with infected cats. Because cats only shed large numbers of oocysts during the first several weeks of infections, those with chronic infections (sustained IgG antibody titers) impose a smaller zoonotic risk.

Ascariasis

Hepatobiliary lesions produced by ascarid larval migration (*Toxocara* spp.) are commonly observed during necropsy of young dogs and cats. Most animals do not manifest clinical signs or laboratory abnormalities. However, severe hepatic and peritoneal migration, gallbladder rupture, and bile peritonitis have been observed in puppies.

Pregnant and lactating bitches reactivate larval forms encysted in tissues, leading to intestinal infection and the shedding of eggs into the newborn pups' environment. Therefore ascarid infection of neonates may occur by environmental contamination and egg ingestion or by transplacental or transmammary larval infection. After egg ingestion, larval forms of *Toxocara canis* and *Toxocara cati* penetrate the intestines and pass into the lymphatic system or portal circulation and travel to the liver. Larvae migrate through hepatic tissue and gain access to the lungs via the caudal vena cava, heart, and pulmonary arteries. Ascarids may also migrate from the gastrointestinal tract directly through the peritoneal cavity to the liver, causing transient abdominal discomfort and liver enzyme activity.

EXOCRINE PANCREAS

An important anatomic difference between the anatomy of the pancreas in the dog and cat is the fusion of the feline major pancreatic duct with the common bile duct. This difference may predispose the cat to intraductal pancreatic inflammation secondary to biliary obstruction or microbial infections. The pancreas possesses both exocrine (digestive) and endocrine (hormonal) functions. The islets of Langerhans (0.1- to 0.2-mm-sized islets comprise <1% of the adult pancreas, higher percentage at birth) and acini (approximately 80% of the pancreas) are derived from endoderm. Islet composition includes β cells (insulin producing, 68%),

α cells (glucagon producing, 20%), δ cells (somatostatin producing, suppress release of insulin and glucagon, 10%), and pancreatic polypeptide-secreting cells (2%). Rare cells include those producing vasoactive intestinal polypeptide (VIP; induces glycogenolysis and hyperglycemia, stimulates intestinal fluid secretion, can rarely cause secretory diarrhea) and enterochromaffin cells (synthesize serotonin, rarely can produce a "carcinoid syndrome"). Acinar cells are microscopically basophilic as a result of their prominent endoplasmic reticulum and Golgi structures and provide an apical oriented secretory complex transporting zymogen granules (inactivated digestive enzymes, periodic acid Schiff "+") to their apical plasma membrane. In health, the pancreas produces a bicarbonate-rich fluid containing digestive enzymes with secretions regulated by neural-humoral stimuli (vagus nerve, secretin, and cholecystokinin). Secretin, a peptide hormone produced in the duodenum in response to gastric acid and luminal fatty acids, stimulates water and bicarbonate release from pancreatic duct cells. Cholecystokinin, also a peptide hormone released from the duodenum in response to fatty acids, peptides, and amino acids, initiates discharge of digestive enzymes from acinar complexes. The repertoire of pancreatic enzymes includes trypsin, chymotrypsin, aminopeptidases, elastase, amylases, lipase, phospholipases, and nucleases. Trypsin, the major catalytic activator of the other enzymes, is initially activated by enterically produced enterokinase. Intrapancreatic control of enzyme activation is maintained by their storage in inactivated forms (zymogens) and colocalization with enzyme inhibitors. Certain systemic antiproteases also protect against inappropriate tissue enzyme activation (e.g., α1-antitrypsin, α1-macroglobulin).

Inflammatory disease of the pancreas primarily affects the exocrine portions and is uncommon in juvenile animals. However, pediatric pancreatitis has been associated with abdominal trauma, systemic infectious disease, and iatrogenic pancreatic injury during ovariohysterectomy (spearing with a spay hook or excessive manipulation of the pancreas). Infectious agents occasionally initiate pancreatic inflammation. In cats, pancreatitis has been associated with effusive FIP. Toxoplasmosis can directly invade pancreatic tissue. Ascarid migration (dogs, cats) and fluke migration in cats can damage pancreatic tissue or obstruct pancreatic ducts, leading to pancreatic inflammation. In cats, cystic duct malformations and development of choleliths also can compromise patency of the common bile duct, leading to pancreatic injury and inflammation.

Although seldom warranted in neonates or pediatric patients, laboratory confirmation of inflammatory pancreatic disease includes a complete blood cell count, serum chemistry profile, serum amylase and lipase, species-specific pancreatic lipase activity, survey abdominal radiographs, and abdominal ultrasonography. Definitive diagnosis of pancreatic inflammation requires reconciliation of test findings (particularly abdominal palpation, ultrasonography, and pancreatic lipase activity). Treatment of pancreatitis is supportive and managed similarly to that for an adult animal.

Pancreatic Exocrine Insufficiency

Exocrine pancreatic enzymes provide essential digestive functions such that loss of 90% of this capacity leads to maldigestion and exocrine pancreatic insufficiency (EPI) syndrome. Subclinical and clinical EPI syndromes have been characterized in dogs and are relatively rare in cats. Dogs with subclinical EPI have clinical signs masked by continued small-volume pancreatic enzyme secretion or digestion facilitated by alternative mechanisms (lingual or gastric lipases, gastric pepsins, intestinal mucosal esterases, and peptidases). Causes of canine EPI include pancreatic acinar atrophy (PAA; an apparent autoimmune lymphocytic inflammatory disorder), chronic pancreatitis, and pancreatic neoplasia. By far, PAA is most common and can affect dogs within the first year of life, although it usually becomes overt within the first 3 years. Long considered a hypoplastic pancreatic disorder, longitudinal studies have proven that PAA is the culmination of a lymphocytic immune-mediated inflammatory process.

Inherited PAA is not rare and has been intensively studied in German Shepherd Dogs and Rough-Coated Collie dogs in Finland, where 70% of dogs with EPI are German Shepherd Dogs and 20% are Rough-Coated Collies. A breed prevalence rate of 1% is reported. Although an autosomal recessive mode of inheritance has been proposed in German Shepherd Dogs, the trait may be polygenic or have incomplete penetrance. Accurate recognition of PAA as a syndrome requires acknowledgment that it also can represent the end result of pancreatic duct obstruction, ischemic tissue injury, toxicity, various nutritional deficiencies or imbalances, or defective secretory or trophic stimuli.

Clinical signs of PAA are variable but largely dominated by polyphagia, weight loss, excessive flatulence and borborygmi, and frequent, soft voluminous feces. However, some dogs vomit, some are inappetent, some are overweight, and rarely some dogs are hyperexcitable or aggressive. Progression of subclinical to clinical PAA varies widely; some dogs progress to full clinical disease within weeks, and others have slow progressive disease that never matures. At end-stage PAA, the pancreas is grossly diminished in size, thin, and transparent, with obvious ducts. Owing to the lymphocytic inflammatory lesion, the disorder has been more precisely labeled atrophic lymphocytic pancreatitis. Immunophenotyping has confirmed that CD3-positive T lymphocytes are involved with acinar destruction; histologic features mirror those associated with lymphocytic thyroiditis.

Routine clinical pathologic tests are not informative in most dogs with EPI. Serum ALT may be mild to moderately increased, reflecting uptake of noxious material from the small intestinal tract. Total lipid and cholesterol concentrations are usually low, whereas total protein, albumin, and globulin concentrations are usually normal. Serum activity of amylase and lipase is not informative. Serum canine trypsin-like immunoreactivity (cTLI) is the distinguishing test for EPI; the test is species- and pancreas-specific, measuring only pancreatic trypsin and trypsinogen that have entered the bloodstream directly from the pancreas. Healthy dogs have cTLI activity greater than 5.0 μg/L, whereas values less than 2.5 μg/L are diagnostic for EPI. Assessment of fasting cTLI values is recommended because even a transient postprandial increase of serum trypsinogen concentration can confuse test interpretation. Renal dysfunction also can obfuscate test interpretation because trypsinogen is eliminated by glomerular filtration. Low serum cTLI concentrations (<5.0 μg/L) on repeated tests can be used to detect subclinical PAA before overt EPI maldigestion can be recognized. Some dogs with minimal clinical signs have cTLI activity as low as others with end-stage PAA. Repeated cTLI measurements may be necessary to confirm subclinical PAA; the lower the cTLI value, the more certain the diagnosis. Notably, some dogs developing PAA have borderline low normal cTLI values. Although pancreatic biopsies can be safely collected, they are not recommended for early diagnosis of PAA because the pathologic process is unevenly distributed. Ultrasonographic diagnosis of PAA also is unreliable.

Treatment of clinical EPI requires pancreatic enzyme supplementation for the life of the patient. Most clinicians prefer powdered enzymes (pancrelipase) that are easily mixed with food: 3 g/meal for a 20- to 35-kg dog. Efficacy of enteric-coated enzyme tablets remains unsubstantiated; some studies suggest lower response rates and others no difference from powdered enzymes. However, tablet efficacy may be compromised by gastric retention. Rapid response to enzyme supplementation is usually evident during the first few weeks (weight gain, improved fecal consistency, and reduced flatulence and steatorrhea). Preincubation of digestive enzymes in food before feeding and supplementation with bile salts or antacids have no proven efficacy. Inhibition of gastric acid secretion with H_2 blockers remains controversial and is only recommended when response to enzyme therapy is suboptimal or inconsistent. Titrating the amount of supplemental enzymes mixed in food has been advocated by some clinicians but remains controversial. Too large a dose of powdered enzymes in food has been associated with oral bleeding that resolves on dose reduction.

Although diet modifications including low fat, high fiber, and low residue formulations have been recommended for dogs with EPI, studies have demonstrated wide variability in clinical responses among dogs. A highly digestible, low fiber, and moderate/low fat maintenance diet is recommended as the initial choice. Focus on individual patient needs and response to dietary changes and avoidance of radical dietary recommendations are prudent. The goal of diet modification coupled with responsible enzyme supplementation is reduced flatulence, borborygmi, fecal volume, and defecation frequency. Although a low fat diet may be useful during initial treatment, no long-term benefit has been demonstrated.

Dogs with subclinical PAA do not require treatment. However, dogs with partial PAA showing chronic intermittent gastrointestinal signs should receive a clinical trial of supplemental enzyme therapy. Patients with clinical PAA showing persistent signs despite enzyme replacement require a full diagnostic evaluation for inflammatory bowel disease or treatment for small intestinal bacterial overgrowth (SIBO). It is well acknowledged that EPI may be associated with secondary problems including SIBO, low cobalamin concentrations, and coexistent inflammatory bowel disease. Genesis of SIBO is attributed to loss of bacteriostatic factors normally supplied by pancreatic secretions and to greater availability of undigested enteric substrates that allow development of SIBO. Some evidence suggests that pancreatic enzyme replacement alone or administration of tylosin can abate SIBO. In SIBO, low cobalamin concentrations are proposed to reflect bacterial vitamin sequestration or failure to degrade nonintrinsic factor proteins (R proteins) that bind luminal cobalamin. Low cobalamin concentrations also may reflect deficient production of pancreatic intrinsic factor as a result of acinar atrophy. In one study of dogs with EPI, cobalamin concentrations were low in 82%; a smaller subset had severe hypocobalaminemia (<100 ng/L), which seemingly functioned as a negative prognostic indicator (i.e., shortened survival). Parenteral cobalamin administration is necessary in dogs with subnormal cobalamin concentrations; such treatment is inexpensive and safe, and a good response can be expected in 60% of treated dogs (one study). High folate concentrations, consistent with enteric microbial folate synthesis, have been documented in 37% of dogs with EPI (one study). Although SIBO has been anecdotally linked with EPI, this syndrome remains controversial, and neither high serum folate nor low serum cobalamin concentrations can accurately confirm its presence. Suspected SIBO does not predict favorable response to antibacterial therapy.

Testing for PAA using low serum trypsin–like immunoreactivity (sTLI) as a defining marker has permitted early diagnosis of dogs with subclinical disease. Nevertheless, immunomodulation during this stage cannot be advocated because of the slow onset of full PAA in some dogs and because some dogs with PAA remain asymptomatic for their lifetime. Because dietary sensitivities may complicate EPI, hypoallergenic diets may benefit some dogs during early treatment. Although some clinicians have used medium-chain triglycerides to increase the energy value of foods fed to undernourished EPI patients, benefit of this strategy remains unproven. The typical gastrointestinal signs of EPI are almost completely eliminated in nearly 50% of treated dogs. Poor responses are realized in approximately 20% of dogs (continued diarrhea, unthrifty appearance, and flatulence), and many of these are euthanized during the first year of diagnosis. Dogs failing to respond to treatment do not make good house pets. Unfortunately the high cost of enzyme supplements also has led to euthanasia of some dogs. At present, there is no evidence that combinations of antimicrobials, H_2 blockers, or powder versus tablet enzyme formulations improve response and/or survival in symptomatic dogs. Generally the long-term prognosis is good for dogs that survive the initial treatment interval. Although mesenteric torsion has been noted as a severe complication of EPI in German Shepherd Dogs, this complication has decreased in frequency with improved treatment regimens and enzyme preparations.

SUGGESTED READINGS

Center SA: Diseases of the gallbladder and biliary tree, *Vet Clin North Am Small Anim Pract* 39(3):543-598, 2009.

Center SA: Interpretation of liver enzymes, *Vet Clin North Am Small Anim Pract* 37(2):297-333, vii, 2007.

Center SA: Metabolic, antioxidant, nutraceutical, probiotic, and herbal therapies relating to the management of hepatobiliary disorders, *Vet Clin North Am Small Anim Pract* 34(1):67-172, vi, 2004.

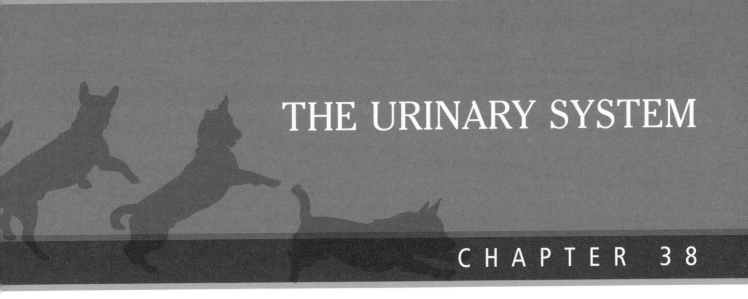

THE URINARY SYSTEM

CHAPTER 38

Jana M. Gordon, Michelle Anne Kutzler

The urinary tract of the dog and cat consists of the kidneys, ureters, urinary bladder, and urethra. The kidneys play an important role in the regulation of the body's water balance, electrolytes, and acid-base status. The kidneys are also involved in hormone metabolism and the elimination of toxins and wastes. Diseases of the urinary tract of puppies and kittens may be caused by congenital or acquired disorders. Congenital disorders are the result of abnormal development of the structures within the urinary tract, whereas acquired disorders may result secondary to congenital disorders or when the normally developed urinary tract becomes diseased. To further understand the congenital and acquired diseases of the urinary tract, a review of embryology and developmental physiology has been provided.

NORMAL DEVELOPMENT

The development of the kidney is complex. There are three stages of development: the pronephros, mesonephros, and metanephros (Table 38-1). A schematic diagram of this process is illustrated in Figure 38-1. Nephrogenesis continues for at least 2 weeks postnatally in the dog. In newborns, the inner glomeruli are larger than those in the outer cortex. However, all cells within the proximal convoluted tubules have a significantly smaller membrane area than the adult. These differences gradually disappear as the kidney grows.

In cats, normal renal development can be permanently altered by taurine deficiency. In addition to a decreased size, which is apparent by 8 weeks of age, kittens from dams with taurine deficiency have ureteral dilatation, large sclerosed glomeruli, proximal tubular flattening, epithelial atypia, reduced mitochondria at the apex of the tubule, and simplification of the tubule compared with age-matched controls.

The epithelial lining of the urinary bladder and urethra is endodermal in origin. The urinary bladder originates from the cloaca. The urorectal septum forms in the cloaca, which separates the rectum dorsally from the urogenital sinus ventrally. The cranial urogenital sinus becomes the vesicourethral canal and urinary bladder. The caudal urogenital sinus becomes the penile urethra in the male and urethra and vestibule in the female. The mesonephric ducts enter the dorsal aspect of the urogenital sinus in what becomes the trigone.

PHYSIOLOGY

Excretion and Reabsorption

During development, urine and wastes excreted by the fetal kidneys pass from the developing urinary bladder through the urachus into the allantoic cavity of the placenta. Waste products are then absorbed into maternal circulation. At birth, the neonatal puppy and kitten kidney is immature in both structure and function. Functionally the newborn has a lower glomerular filtration rate (GFR), renal plasma flow, and filtration fraction compared with the adult. The GFR increases with age postnatally. Glomerular capillary surface area and pore density increase between the first and sixth weeks after birth. Studies suggest that GFR and renal blood flow increase up to 11 weeks of age in the puppy and up to 9 weeks of age in the kitten before reaching adult levels.

There is limited evidence that puppies are capable of concentrating and diluting their urine at birth. When measuring urine-specific gravity, the urine may not be maximally concentrated, particularly in puppies less than 4 weeks of age, but this may be a reflection of the water content in their diet rather than an inability to concentrate their urine. Puppies also produce a higher daily urine volume and have an increased extracellular fluid volume compared with adult dogs. The urine and plasma osmolality in puppies and kittens increases with age and reaches adult values by 11 weeks of age in the puppy and 13 to 19 weeks of age in the kitten.

TABLE 38-1	Developmental embryology of the kidney
Stage	**Description**
Pronephros	• Cells of the intermediate mesoderm separate into an outer parietal and inner visceral layer forming the nephrocele. • Cords of cells extend from the parietal layer at the level of each somite and eventually become pronephric tubules. These tubules extend laterally and caudally until they join one another and form the pronephric duct. • Branches from the aorta form the glomeruli. Some glomeruli invaginate into the celom and become external glomeruli, and others invaginate into the pronephric tubules, becoming internal glomeruli.
Mesonephros	• The intermediate mesoderm in the thoracolumbar region proliferates and extends into the celomic cavity, forming the urogenital ridge. • The urogenital ridge will divide into the medial genital and lateral urinary ridge. Within the urinary ridge, the pronephric tubules stimulate the formation of the mesonephric tubules from invagination of the celom. • The medial aspect of the mesonephric tubule will invaginate and form Bowman's capsule. The lateral aspect of the mesonephric tubule joins the pronephric duct (now termed the mesonephric duct). As the mesonephric tubules and ducts develop, the pronephric ducts and tubules atrophy.
Metanephros	• The metanephric blastema develops within the sacral mesoderm. Ureteric buds develop from mesonephric ducts in the caudal embryo and extend cranially to the metanephric blastema. The ureteric bud becomes the collecting ducts and renal pelvis. • The previously described mesonephric ducts become metanephric ducts. A portion of the metanephric blastema, or tissue, becomes the rest of the tubular system (proximal convoluted tubule, loop of Henle, distal convoluted tubule) and joins the metanephric duct and Bowman's capsule to the collecting ducts formed by the ureteric buds. • The remainder of the surrounding metanephric blastema, or tissue, develops into the renal parenchyma.

Neonatal renal handling of water and electrolytes differs from adults. The fractional reabsorption of water in dogs is constant, whereas sodium excretion increases during the first 3 weeks. Increases in renal arterial blood pressure are associated with increases in both absolute and fractional sodium excretion by adult and newborn dogs. In puppies, the fractional excretion of potassium and phosphorus decreases between 9 and 27 weeks of age, whereas the fractional excretion of chloride and calcium increases in the developing puppy. Despite these findings, the fractional excretion of all electrolytes in the puppies in these studies was within the normal range established for adult dogs. When the fractional excretion of sodium, potassium, chloride, phosphorus, and calcium was evaluated in kittens from 4 to 30 weeks of age, the only significant change observed during the study period was an increase in fractional excretion of potassium, but all values were within adult reference ranges.

Postnatal excretion of uric acid decreases from 83% at birth to 51% by 90 days of age. Similar to human infants, the decrease in uric acid excretion with age appears to be unrelated to binding of uric acid to plasma proteins or to urine flow rate. The amount of protein in the urine is higher in newborn puppies but decreases within the first few months of life. Possible contributors to proteinuria include colostral proteins absorbed within the first few days of life, increased filtration by immature and fewer glomeruli, decreased renal tubular reabsorption, alkaline urine, urine concentration, and protein from cells in the urinary tract.

Micturition

Micturition in neonatal dogs and cats is mediated by a spinal somatovesical reflex that is initiated by perineal stimulation. The dam initiates urination by licking the perineum and consumes the excreted waste, which keeps the neonate and the environment clean and dry. The somatovesical reflex pathway disappears between 3 and 5 weeks of age and is replaced by a vesicovesical reflex, which is a supraspinal reflex pathway that is activated by bladder distention and is under voluntary control. This is also the age at which postural control develops, which enables the puppy or kitten to assume a proper stance for urination. Unanesthetized puppies and kittens less than 3 weeks of age do not evoke bladder contractions despite pressurized bladder distention. If the perineum is not stimulated, the bladder will continue to fill, causing abdominal distention.

EXAMINATION OF THE URINARY SYSTEM

Physical examination of the patient with urinary tract disorders may reveal urinary incontinence, lower urinary tract symptoms, or clinical signs of renal insufficiency or failure. Urinary incontinence may be intermittent and only noticed after the animal lies down for prolonged periods, or the incontinence may be more persistent, resulting in urine dribbling. When urine dribbling is noted, it is important to differentiate true incontinence from dribbling caused by overdistention, such as can be seen with urethral obstruction or neurologic bladder.

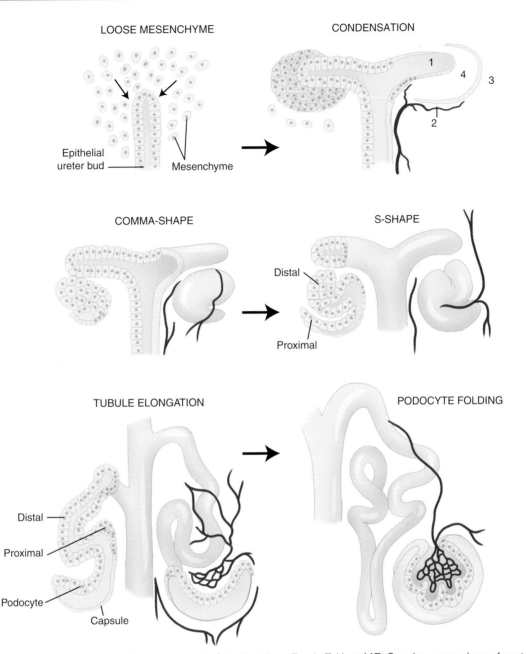

LOOSE MESENCHYME

Epithelial
ureter bud ——————— Mesenchyme

CONDENSATION

1
4
3
2

COMMA-SHAPE

S-SHAPE

Distal

Proximal

TUBULE ELONGATION

Distal

Proximal

Podocyte

Capsule

PODOCYTE FOLDING

Figure 38-1 Schematic representation of nephrogenesis. (Modified from Zoetis T, Hurtt ME: Species comparison of anatomical and functional renal development, *Birth Defects Research* 68(B):112, 2003.)

Lower urinary tract signs include pollakiuria, dysuria, stranguria, and hematuria. Lower urinary tract signs in young dogs and cats are seen most frequently with infections or calculi as a result of a congenital disease. Hematuria may be the only historic finding in diseases such as renal telangiectasia and idiopathic hematuria. If hemorrhage is severe, blood clots may form and lead to urinary tract obstruction. Anemia may also occur in dogs with idiopathic hematuria and renal telangiectasia.

Clinical signs of renal insufficiency include lethargy, poor growth, poor haircoat, weight loss, polydipsia, polyuria, and nocturia. With progression to renal failure, signs of uremia are seen, including anorexia, dehydration, pale mucous membranes, oral ulceration, halitosis, vomiting, hematemesis,

diarrhea, melena, and death. Kidneys may be palpably enlarged with polycystic kidney disease. In most dogs and cats with primary renal disease, kidneys may be normal or small in size. Signs related to renal secondary hyperparathyroidism are more common in young dogs because their bones are more metabolically active. These signs include enlargement of the maxilla and mandible, a pliable mandible, bone pain, and pathologic fracture.

Hematologic and biochemical abnormalities are most often seen in animals with renal failure and include azotemia, hyperkalemia, hyperphosphatemia, and metabolic acidosis. Regenerative anemia is occasionally found with renal failure as a result of gastrointestinal ulceration and hemorrhage. Regenerative anemia also occurs in cases of significant blood loss through the urinary tract as seen with idiopathic hematuria and renal telangiectasia. In cases of chronic renal failure, nonregenerative anemia may be present.

Examination of the urine may be normal or reveal isosthenuria, proteinuria, glucosuria, hematuria, crystalluria, pyuria, and/or bacteriuria. Urinary fractional excretion of electrolytes may be abnormal with some tubular disorders. Urine culture is indicated in cases of suspected infection of the upper or lower urinary tract.

Diagnostic imaging of the urinary system includes plain radiography, contrast radiography, ultrasonography, and cross-sectional imaging. Plain radiographs may be used to evaluate the size and position of the kidneys and urinary bladder. This may be difficult in emaciated animals or in the presence of peritoneal or retroperitoneal fluid. Soft tissue mineralization and certain types of calculi may also be visualized on plain radiographs.

Contrast studies of the urinary tract include excretory urography, antegrade pyelography, and retrograde contrast administration. Typically this is done with iodinated contrast agents. Excretory urography can be used as a crude measure of renal function because excretion of the contrast agent depends on renal blood flow, GFR, and tubular reabsorption of water. Most commonly, excretory urography is used to evaluate the kidneys and ureters for position and filling defects. With antegrade pyelography, iodinated contrast is injected directly into the renal pelvis in an attempt to identify lesions of the ureter.

Retrograde contrast studies involve placement of a balloon catheter distal to the area of interest, followed by administration of an iodinated contrast agent. This technique can be used to evaluate lesions in the vagina, urethra, urinary bladder, and distal ureters. With double-contrast cystography, iodinated contrast agent and air are administered through a urinary catheter. This is typically done to evaluate the wall of the urinary bladder for thickening or mass lesions, as well as its contents (e.g., calculi). However, care must be taken when placing any type of urinary catheter in a pediatric patient because of the possible risk of iatrogenic urethral perforation.

Transabdominal ultrasound is used primarily to evaluate the kidneys, urinary bladder, and proximal urethra. Ultrasound is a useful determinant of size and echotexture of the kidneys, as well as a means of identifying filling defects. The renal pelvis can be evaluated for dilation, calculi, and mineralization. Normal ureters are poorly visualized with ultrasound because of their small size, but if they are dilated, as can occur with an obstruction, they can usually be visualized with ultrasound. Occasionally the opening of the ureters into the urinary bladder can be seen as the expulsion of urine from the ureters into the urinary bladder. The urinary bladder wall can be assessed for abnormalities and the vesicular contents seen. Although transabdominal ultrasonography can be used for the proximal urethra in females and prostatic urethra in males, transrectal ultrasonography is necessary for the more distal portion of the female urethra and prostatic and pelvic portions of the male urethra in the dog.

Magnetic resonance imaging and computed tomography are occasionally used when developmental abnormalities are suspected. Computed tomography using intravenous urography is believed to be superior to traditional contrast radiography for the diagnosis of ectopic ureters.

Flexible and rigid endoscopy has both diagnostic and therapeutic implications in diseases of the urinary tract. Endoscopy allows visualization of the vagina, urethra, and urinary bladder of dogs and cats. Endoscopy can also be used to aid in obtaining biopsies, in performing urethral injections of collagen in cases of urinary sphincter incompetence, and in performing urethral and vesicular lithotripsy and stone removal.

Biopsy is necessary to definitively diagnose many primary renal disorders such as glomerulonephropathies, amyloidosis, and renal dysplasia. Biopsy is also indicated for definitive diagnosis of mass lesions within the urinary tract. In cases of recurrent urinary tract infections, biopsy of the urinary bladder wall may be indicated to identify deeper tissue infections.

CONGENITAL DISORDERS

Some congenital diseases are incompatible with life, and clinical signs of renal failure develop within the first few weeks of life. However, most of the diseases are not immediately life threatening, and clinical signs might not be apparent for several months or even years. The majority of congenital diseases manifest with urinary incontinence, lower urinary tract signs, renal insufficiency, or chronic renal failure.

Congenital disorders of the urinary tract may be caused by the presence of one or more abnormal genes. The end result may be production of an abnormal protein, failure to produce a normal protein, or production of excess amounts of a normal protein. In some instances, these mutations result in clinical syndromes that are sometimes identified in related animals. Familial or hereditary genetic diseases occur when a disease-causing gene is passed from one or both parents to offspring. The mode of inheritance is known for some of these diseases but not for others. Heritable diseases of the urinary tract have been identified in several breeds of dogs (Table 38-2) and cats (Table 38-3) and should be suspected when any of these breeds present with signs consistent with urinary tract disease. Newly affected breeds continue to be identified, and some of these conditions have been found in mixed-breed dogs and cats; therefore it is important that heritable diseases are not ruled out exclusively by signalment.

Ectopia

Ectopic kidneys are very rare in the dog and cat and occur as a result of failure of the metanephros to migrate from the sacral region of the embryo. They are typically located in the pelvis or inguinal region. One or both kidneys may be malpositioned and may be normal or small in size and are structurally and functionally normal. Diagnosis is made with radiography or ultrasonography.

TABLE 38-2	Canine familial or heritable urinary tract disorders	
Breed	**Disorder**	**Trait**
Alaskan Malamute	Renal dysplasia	
Basenji	Fanconi's syndrome	Familial
Bernese Mountain Dog	Membranoproliferative glomerulonephritis	Autosomal recessive
Beagle	Renal agenesis	Familial
	Membranoproliferative glomerulonephritis	Familial
Border Terrier	Renal dysplasia	
	Fanconi's syndrome	
Boxer	Renal dysplasia	Familial
Brie Sheepdog	Renal dysplasia	
Brittany Spaniel	Membranoproliferative glomerulonephritis	Autosomal recessive
Bull Terrier	Glomerulopathy	Autosomal dominant
	Polycystic kidney	Autosomal dominant
Bulldog	Renal dysplasia	
Bullmastiff	Glomerulonephropathy	Autosomal recessive
	Renal dysplasia	
Cavalier King Charles Spaniel	Renal agenesis	
	Xanthinuria	
	Renal dysplasia + agenesis	
Chinese Shar-Pei	Amyloidosis	
Chow Chow	Renal dysplasia	Familial
Cocker Spaniel	Renal dysplasia–related?	
Dachshund	Xanthinuria	
Dalmatian	Glomerulopathy	Autosomal dominant
	Uric aciduria	Recessive
Doberman Pinscher	Renal agenesis	Familial
	Glomerulopathy	Familial
Dutch Kooiker	Renal dysplasia	Familial
English Bulldog	Renal and ureteral duplication	
	Uric aciduria	
	Ectopic ureter	
	Urethrorectal fistula	
English Cocker Spaniel	Glomerulopathy	Autosomal recessive
English Foxhound	Amyloidosis	
Finnish Harrier	Renal dysplasia	Familial
Fox Terrier	Ectopic ureter	
German Shepherd Dog	Multifocal renal cystadenocarcinoma	Autosomal dominant
Golden Retriever	Renal dysplasia	Familial
	Ectopic ureter	
Great Dane	Renal dysplasia	
Labrador Retriever	Ectopic ureter	
Lhasa Apso	Renal dysplasia	Familial
Miniature Poodle	Urethrorectal fistula, urethroperineal fistula, urethral duplication	
Miniature Schnauzer	Renal dysplasia	Familial
	Fanconi's syndrome	
Newfoundland	Glomerulopathy	Familial
	Cystinuria	Autosomal recessive
	Ectopic ureter	
Norwegian Elkhound	Fanconi's syndrome	
Pekingese	Renal agenesis	
Pembroke Welsh Corgi	Ectopic ureter	
	Renal telangiectasia	
Poodle	Ectopic ureter	
Rhodesian Ridgeback	Renal dysplasia	
Rottweiler	Glomerulopathy	Unknown
Samoyed	Renal dysplasia	
	Glomerulopathy	X-linked
Scottish Terrier	Cystinuria	Autosomal recessive
Shetland Sheepdog	Renal agenesis	Familial
	Fanconi's syndrome	
Shih Tzu	Renal dysplasia	Familial
Siberian Husky	Ectopic ureter	
Skye Terrier	Ectopic ureter	
Standard Poodle	Renal dysplasia	Familial
West Highland White Terrier	Ectopic ureter	
Soft-Coated Wheaten Terrier	Renal dysplasia	Familial
	Membranoproliferative glomerulonephritis	Familial

Ectopic ureters occur in both puppies and kittens as a congenital abnormal termination of the ureters with the urinary bladder. Ectopic ureters are described as intramural or extramural. Intramural ectopic ureters enter the bladder wall and run transmurally but fail to empty at the trigone and instead continue transmurally and empty in the urethra or vagina vestibule. Extramural ectopic ureters bypass the urinary bladder completely and enter the urethra, vagina vestibule, or uterus. Females are affected more often than males. Ectopic ureters empty into the urethra of most females and prostatic urethra in males. Ectopic ureters may occur alone or with other developmental abnormalities of the urinary tract. Hydronephrosis may occur if the ureter ends in a blind pouch or forms a functional stenosis. An increased incidence has been found in English Bulldogs, Fox Terriers, Golden Retrievers, Labrador Retrievers, Newfoundlands, Poodles, Siberian Huskies, Skye Terriers, and Welsh Corgis. Clinical signs are related to variable degrees of urinary incontinence. Diagnosis is made with contrast radiography (excretory urogram with retrograde urethrogram or vaginogram), endoscopy, or cross-sectional imaging

TABLE 38-3 Feline familial or heritable urinary tract disorders

Breed	Disorder	Trait
Abyssinian	Amyloidosis	Autosomal dominant with variable penetrance?
Domestic Shorthair	Renal agenesis	
Oriental Shorthair	Amyloidosis	
Siamese	Amyloidosis	
Persian	Polycystic kidney	Autosomal dominant

(Figure 38-2). Surgery is the treatment of choice with transection and reimplantation or unilateral ureterectomy and nephrectomy. In some dogs incontinence persists, and pharmacologic management with diethylstilbestrol or phenylpropanolamine may be necessary.

Urethral ectopia occurs when the external urethral orifice is in an abnormal position. There is a report of an ectopic urethra terminating in the cranial vagina of a female English Bulldog and a report of a 2-month-old female cat with an ectopic urethra terminating in the rectum.

Duplication and Diverticula

There are sporadic reports in the literature of supernumerary kidneys. Fused kidneys may result in a variety of shapes, but horseshoe kidneys are the most common and result from fusion of the cranial or caudal poles of the kidneys within the pelvic canal. Kidney function is often normal. Diagnosis is made with radiography or ultrasonography. Fused kidneys are rare but have been reported in the dog and cat. Ureteral duplication has been reported in the dog associated with duplicated or supernumerary kidneys.

Complete or partial duplication of the urinary bladder with or without urethral duplication has been reported rarely in the dog. These dogs developed incontinence and dysuria. Surgery is the treatment of choice. Urethral duplication has been reported in male and female puppies. This anomaly is often associated with other developmental abnormalities, including renal hypoplasia, bilateral cryptorchidism, and duplication of the urinary bladder, vagina, vulva, penis (diphallia), scrotum (dipygus), descending colon, and rectum.

Urethral diverticula are tubular or saclike dilations opening into the urethral canal through an ostium at any point on its course. Congenital urethral diverticula are lined by urethral mucosa and contain a striated muscle layer. A Y-duplication is an incomplete urethral duplication in which the urethra splits to form an accessory channel opening to the perineum or anus. This type of duplication is rare but is

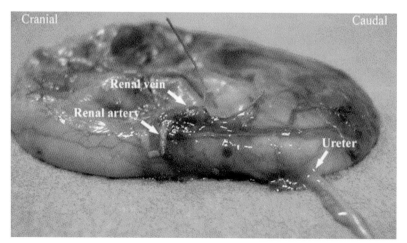

Figure 38-2 Gross appearance of left renal pelvis showing ureteral ectopia. The ureter arises from the caudal pole of the left pelvis. (From D'Ippolito P, Nicoli S, Zatelli A: Proximal ureteral ectopia causing hydronephrosis in a kitten, *J Fel Med Surg* 8:422, 2006, Figure 3.)

often associated with stenosis and hypoplasia of the normal penile urethra, a factor that could contribute to the complete stenosis of the urethral meatus. In these instances, the penile urethral meatus may not be patent. In some cases, a scrotal urethral fistula develops, and urine leaks from the fistula in the scrotum. A narrow-necked urethral diverticulum can be demonstrated with voiding using positive contrast cystourethrography.

Agenesis and Stenosis

Renal agenesis occurs as a result of failure of one or both kidneys to form. The failure could have occurred during any of the three stages of renal development in the fetus. Renal agenesis may be seen alone or with other developmental abnormalities in the urinary or reproductive tract of the dog and cat. There is a familial predisposition to renal agenesis in Beagles, Doberman Pinschers, Shetland Sheepdogs, and Cavalier King Charles Spaniels. The absence of one or both kidneys might be suspected on physical examination and confirmed with abdominal radiography, excretory urography, or transabdominal ultrasound. With unilateral agenesis, the other kidney may be hypertrophied. Bilateral renal agenesis is incompatible with life, but dogs and cats with unilateral renal agenesis may be clinically normal as long as the other kidney functions normally.

Ureteral agenesis has been reported in dogs and cats and is usually accompanied by ipsilateral renal agenesis. If disease is unilateral, animals are typically asymptomatic; however, bilateral disease results in death from uremia. In cases of bilateral ureteral agenesis, urine will not be present within the bladder and cannot be expressed from either kidney into its respective ureter. Ureteral stenosis is very rare in the dog and cat. Ureteral stenosis can occur at any location along the ureter but most commonly occurs at the ureteropelvic junction as the result of a developmental defect arising from abnormal differentiation of either the ureteric bud or the metanephros. The ipsilateral renal pelvis can be enlarged and filled with urine, indicative of hydronephrosis. Dilatation of the affected ureter is an ineffective treatment. Unilateral cases may be treated by nephrectomy. Unilateral ureteral obstruction may be relieved by segmental ureterectomy and anastomosis. However, it is important to mention that end-to-end ureteroureterostomy in the growing animal leads to severe anastomotic stricture, obstructive atrophy, and 100% ipsilateral renal loss at 1 year of age. Transureteroureterostomy in the immature nondilated ureter is safe and is followed by normally functioning upper urinary tracts at the end of 1 year of age, without evidence of damage to the recipient's ureter. The prognosis depends on the likelihood of successful treatment, and in cases of unilateral nephrectomy, on compensatory hypertrophy of the contralateral kidney.

Urinary bladder agenesis has been reported in a mixed-breed puppy with incontinence. Urethral agenesis has been reported in one 4-month-old female mixed-breed dog with urinary incontinence, which also had bilateral ectopic ureters that emptied into the vaginal floor.

Hypoplasia

Renal hypoplasia occurs when one or both kidneys are structurally normal but small in size with fewer nephrons, lobules, and calyces than a normal kidney. The decreased size is because of a reduced quantity of metanephric blastema or incomplete induction of nephron formation by the ureteral bud. If there is unilateral hypoplasia, the normal kidney may undergo compensatory hypertrophy, and there may be no clinical signs unless both kidneys are affected. One or both kidneys may be palpably small, but definitive diagnosis requires histology.

Urinary bladder hypoplasia has been reported in dogs and cats and is associated with ectopic ureters and may be a contributing factor to urinary incontinence seen postoperatively after surgical correction of ectopic ureters. The urinary bladder may gradually enlarge over time.

Urethral hypoplasia is uncommon but has been reported in the dog and in female cats with urinary incontinence resulting from congenital urethral sphincter mechanism incompetence. Episodes of dysuria and pollakiuria have also been described in patients with urethral hypoplasia with stenosis. In some instances, urethral hypoplasia occurs in conjunction with uterine hypoplasia and vaginal aplasia in females and stenosis of the urethral meatus in males. Diagnosis is made with urethral pressure profiling. Treatment options include collagen injections, diethylstilbestrol, and phenylpropanolamine (not effective in cats).

Renal Dysplasia

Renal dysplasia is defined as disorganized development of renal parenchyma caused by anomalous differentiation. Renal dysplasia occurs as a result of the persistence of fetal structures in focal areas within the kidney next to more normal structures. Most dysplastic kidneys also contain immature collecting ducts. Renal aplasia is an uncommon variant with more diffuse involvement. Abnormal primary structures include immature glomeruli, immature tubules, asynchronous differentiation of nephrons, persistent mesenchyme, persistent metanephric ducts, atypical tubular epithelium, and dysontogenic metaplasia. Secondary changes include compensatory hypertrophy and hyperplasia of normal nephrons, interstitial fibrosis, tubulointerstitial nephritis, pyelonephritis, dystrophic mineralization, cystic glomerular atrophy, microcystic tubules, retention cysts, and glomerular lipidosis.

Renal dysplasia is presumed to be familial in the Lhasa Apso, Shih-Tzu, Soft-Coated Wheaten Terrier, standard Poodle, Boxer, Chow Chow, Finnish Harrier, Malamute, Golden Retriever, Keeshond, Miniature Schnauzer, and Dutch Kooiker. There have been isolated reports of renal dysplasia in other breeds, including the Great Dane, Samoyed, Cocker Spaniel, Bulldog, Brie Sheepdog, Rhodesian Ridgeback, Border Terrier, and Bullmastiff.

The etiology of renal dysplasia and aplasia is unknown. Infection with the feline panleukopenia virus and canine herpesvirus has been associated with renal dysplasia in cats and dogs, respectively. Intrauterine taurine deficiency will also result in feline renal dysplasia. Clinical signs of renal dysplasia and aplasia may not develop for several months or years and are related to renal insufficiency or failure. Hematologic and urinary abnormalities may include anemia, azotemia, hypernatremia, hyperphosphatemia, hyperkalemia, isosthenuria, and proteinuria. Ultrasonographic examination may reveal kidneys with irregular margins and with parenchyma that is hyperechoic with poor corticomedullary definition (Figure 38-3). Histologic examination will demonstrate primitive underdeveloped glomeruli with dysplastic and disorganized arteriolar supply, abnormal Bowman's capsules, glomeruli, and abnormal, irregular, and orphaned tubules (Figure 38-4). However, concurrent pyelonephritis may complicate the diagnosis. This disease is progressive, and there is no cure. Treatment is supportive for clinical manifestations of renal failure.

Renal Amyloidosis

Amyloid is a protein produced as a result of increased production of serum amyloid A by the liver. Serum amyloid A is a protein typically released from the liver during inflammatory processes. Amyloid may be deposited in the glomerular capillary walls, mesangium, and medullary interstitium of the kidney. There is evidence that the disease is inherited in an autosomal recessive fashion in the Shar-Pei dog and autosomal dominant with variable penetrance in the Abyssinian cat. Renal amyloidosis is also familial in Beagles and Foxhounds, as well as Oriental Shorthair and Siamese cats. Shar-Pei dogs may have a history of intermittent fever and tarsal swelling. Oriental Shorthair and Siamese cats are more likely to have amyloid in their liver as well, resulting in hemoabdomen secondary to hepatic rupture. Proteinuria is commonly found in dogs and cats with renal amyloidosis with the exception of some Shar-Pei dogs and Abyssinian cats. In these breeds, amyloid may only be deposited in the medullary interstitium; thus proteinuria will not be seen in up to one third of affected animals. Regardless of where the amyloid is deposited, most dogs and cats develop clinical findings consistent with chronic renal failure by 1 to 6 years

of age. Nephrotic syndrome is more common with amyloidosis in the dog. Definitive diagnosis requires histopathology. Renal amyloidosis is progressive despite supportive care and carries a poor long-term prognosis.

Polycystic Kidneys

Polycystic kidney disease (PKD) is a condition in which multiple cysts replace areas of the renal cortex and medulla. Cysts in dogs and cats can occur as a result of obstruction of normal urine flow, abnormalities in the tubular basement membrane, or abnormal growth of the tubular epithelial cells. Cysts can range in size from 1 mm to more than 2 cm. The number of cysts can also be variable, and a single kidney may contain more than 200 cysts. In cats, Cairn Terriers, and West Highland White Terriers, cysts may also be present in the liver.

PKD is an autosomal dominant trait in Persian cats and Bull Terriers and is a suspected autosomal recessive trait in Cairn Terriers and West Highland White Terriers. In Persian cats, the mutation has been identified on the *PKD1* gene. Some dogs with PKD develop clinical findings consistent with chronic renal failure at an early age, whereas in other dogs and in cats, clinical signs may not develop for several years. Some cysts become large enough to cause abdominal distention or signs related to a space-occupying mass. PKD has also been identified concurrently with hereditary nephritis in the Bull Terrier.

There is a genetic test available for the *PKD1* mutation, which has good correlation with ultrasound detection of cysts at between 10 and 14 weeks of age. The exact mutation has not been identified in Bull Terriers; thus there is no genetic test available for these dogs. For breeds in which a DNA test is not available, ultrasonography is used to establish or eliminate a diagnosis of PKD by identification of anechoic, spherical structures that have smooth, sharply marginated walls. Cysts have been identified as early as 7 weeks of age. Ultrasonography was reported to have sensitivity of 75% when performed on cats 16 weeks of age or less and 91% when performed on cats 35 weeks of age or less.

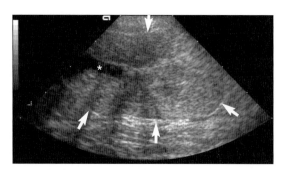

Figure 38-3 Sagittal ultrasound image of the caudal pole of the right kidney of a 15-week-old Bullmastiff presented with clinical signs compatible with chronic renal failure. (From Abraham LA, Beck C, Slocombe RF: Renal dysplasia and urinary tract infection in a Bull Mastiff puppy, *Aust Vet J* 81(6):337, 2003, Figure 1.)

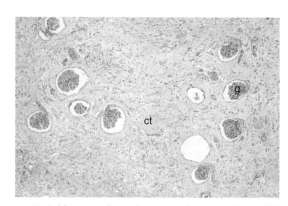

Figure 38-4 Hematoxylin and eosin-stained sections of kidney. Higher magnification (×100) illustrates atretic glomeruli (*g*) buried in dense connective tissue (*ct*). (From Abraham LA, Beck C, Slocombe RF: Renal dysplasia and urinary tract infection in a Bull Mastiff puppy, *Aust Vet J* 81(6):337, 2003, Figure 2B.)

PKD has not been described in cats less than 1 year of age without ultrasonographic evidence. The specificity of ultrasonography was reported to be 100% regardless of age. In animals with chronic renal failure, treatment is supportive. In cases of large cysts, marsupialization or ethanol ablation may be necessary as recurrence following drainage is common.

Perirenal Cysts

Perirenal cysts are sometimes referred to as capsulogenic renal cysts, capsular cysts, pararenal or perirenal pseudocysts, or capsular hydronephrosis. Perirenal cysts result in renomegaly caused by accumulation of fluid between renal parenchyma and the surrounding capsule so that it has no epithelial lining. Perirenal cysts can become very large, with the cyst lumen filled with yellow, urine-smelling fluid. Clinical signs associated with perirenal cysts include azotemia and a marked swollen abdomen. Congenital renal pelvis (pyelocaliceal) or ureteral diverticula may become cystic. Ureteral diverticula can arise from the distal ureter, midureter, and ureteropelvic junction. Also, blind-ending bifid ureter forms a ureteral diverticulum. A pyelocaliceal diverticulum is a cystic cavity lined by transitional epithelium, encased within the renal parenchyma, and connected to the pelvis by a narrow channel. Embryologically, the diverticulum formed as a result of a combination of the branching ureteric bud with the metanephric blastema.

Primary Glomerulopathies

A glomerulopathy is a disease restricted to the glomeruli without inflammation. This is in contrast to glomerulonephritis, in which tubulointerstitial and vascular disease occurs with glomerular disease. Primary glomerular diseases of the dog and cat should be suspected in any young purebred dog with persistent pathologic proteinuria. Certain breeds that develop familial glomerular diseases have been identified. Most progress to acute or chronic renal failure over months to years. Glomerulonephropathies have been described in many breeds, including the Beagle, Bullmastiff, Chow Chow, Miniature Schnauzer, Newfoundland, and Rottweiler. Additional inherited glomerulopathies are discussed below.

Samoyed Hereditary Glomerulopathy

Samoyed hereditary glomerulopathy is an inherited renal disease with an X-linked dominant mode of inheritance. The result is a mutation in the gene (COL4A5) encoding the α5 chain of type IV collagen molecules of the glomerular capillary basement membrane. Normally during development the α1/α2 heterodimer switches to the α3/α4/α5 heterotrimer. The α5 mutation results in the absence of the α3/α4/α5 heterotrimer necessary for normal type IV collagen formation in the glomerular basement membrane.

These dogs develop membranoproliferative glomerulonephropathy and glomerulosclerosis. There may also be thickening of the basement membrane of Bowman's capsule and renal tubules, periglomerular and interstitial fibrosis, and mononuclear interstitial inflammatory infiltrates. These light microscopic changes are nonspecific for this disease. Transmission electron microscopy is diagnostic of this hereditary glomerulonephropathy and reveals focal glomerular basement membrane splitting as early as 1 month of age that will progress to multilaminar splitting of the glomerular basement membrane.

Both males and females are affected, but males are affected more frequently (approximately 50% of male offspring from a carrier female) and develop a more severe, rapidly progressive form of the disease. Males develop proteinuria at 2 to 3 months of age, with chronic renal failure and death by 15 months of age. Affected females are often shorter in stature and develop a mild proteinuria that can last several years before renal failure occurs in the adult or older dog.

Bull Terrier Hereditary Glomerulopathy

Bull Terriers develop an autosomal dominant form of hereditary nephritis. The exact defect is unknown, but the α5 type IV collagen is unaffected in these dogs. Histologic features include thickening of the glomerular and tubular basement membranes and Bowman's capsule. Interstitial nephritis and fibrosis develop, as well as glomerulosclerosis and loss of nephrons. Electron microscopy is required for definitive diagnosis, and lamellation of the glomerular basement membrane is found as in other forms of hereditary nephritis.

Males and females are affected in equal numbers and with equal severity. Affected adult Bull Terriers have an elevated urinary protein/creatinine ratio. Urinary protein/creatinine ratio should be measured with caution in puppies less than 3 months of age because they often have incidental proteinuria. This disease has a variable course with reports of early proteinuria in affected dogs, but progression to renal failure may be anywhere from 11 months to 8 years of age.

English Cocker Spaniel Familial Glomerulopathy

There is an autosomal recessive form of hereditary nephropathy in the Cocker Spaniel. The mutation involves a gene (COL4A4) necessary for the formation of the α4 chain of the type IV collagen in the glomerular basement membrane. Histologic features include mesangial thickening, glomerular and periglomerular fibrosis, and interstitial inflammation. The glomerular basement membrane is thickened, with multilaminar splitting and fragmentation when evaluated with transmission electron microscopy. Males and females are affected in equal numbers and with equal severity. Proteinuria is commonly seen at 5 to 8 months of age, with occasional glucosuria and hematuria. Dogs develop chronic renal failure between 7 and 27 months of age.

Dalmatian Familial Glomerulopathy

An autosomal dominant form of hereditary nephritis has been reported in Dalmatians. The exact mutation is unknown, but the histologic findings on light and electron microscopy are similar to those found in other forms of hereditary nephritis. Dogs develop renal failure at 8 months to 7 years of age.

Doberman Pinscher Familial Glomerulopathy

A familial glomerulopathy has been found in Doberman Pinschers with an unknown mode of inheritance. Early in the course of disease, mesangial thickening is present, and as the disease progresses, glomerulosclerosis, interstitial inflammation, and interstitial fibrosis develop. Lamellation and excess matrix are found in the glomerular basement membrane when evaluated with electron microscopy. Males and females are affected equally, but a significant number of females had concurrent unilateral renal and ureteral agenesis. Proteinuria is common, but the time to development of renal failure is variable, with affected dogs developing acute or chronic renal failure and dying between 6 months and 8 years of age.

Soft-Coated Wheaten Terrier Familial Glomerulonephritis

Soft-Coated Wheaten Terriers develop familial glomerulonephritis. Females are affected more commonly than males, and dogs typically present with signs related to renal disease as adults. The mode of inheritance is unknown, but some of these dogs have a concurrent protein-losing enteropathy. There is some evidence that the protein-losing enteropathy precedes the development of glomerulonephritis and that a food hypersensitivity and impaired intestinal permeability predispose these dogs to immune complex formation and subsequent deposition in the glomeruli. Clinical signs are related to renal insufficiency and failure, including polyuria, polydipsia, anorexia, and vomiting. Laboratory abnormalities are consistent with renal failure and nephrotic syndrome, including anemia, azotemia, hyperphosphatemia, hypoalbuminemia, hypercholesterolemia, and proteinuria. The diagnosis is confirmed with renal biopsy, and histopathologic findings include membranous and membranoproliferative glomerulonephritis, glomerular sclerosis, and tubulointerstitial nephritis. Treatment is supportive for renal failure and protein-losing nephropathy.

Familial Glomerulonephritis in Bernese Mountain Dogs and Brittany Spaniels

Membranoproliferative glomerulonephritis with interstitial nephritis was diagnosed in 22 Bernese Mountain Dogs between 2 and 7 years of age. Eighteen of these dogs were female. The mode of inheritance is autosomal dominant with sex-linked dominance exchange. All the dogs developed proteinuria and azotemia. Most of the dogs also developed nephrotic syndrome. Brittany Spaniels also develop a membranoproliferative glomerulonephritis related to a deficiency in the third component of complement.

Tubulointerstitial Nephropathy of Norwegian Elkhounds

A noninflammatory tubulointerstitial nephropathy has been identified in a group of related Norwegian Elkhounds. The mode of inheritance is unknown, and it affects males and females with equal frequency. Azotemia, isosthenuria, proteinuria, and glucosuria may develop as early as 12 weeks of age.

Miscellaneous Congenital Disorders

Nephrogenic Diabetes Insipidus

Congenital diabetes insipidus is believed to be caused by a defect in the ability of the cells of the distal collecting tubules to respond to vasopressin released from the pituitary gland. This disease has been reported in puppies (especially Lhasa Apso) and kittens during the first month of life. Clinical signs include polyuria, polydipsia, nocturia, failure to grow, rough dry haircoat, gradual emaciation, occasional vomiting, and hyposthenuria. Urine-specific gravity ranges from 1.001 to 1.003. Prerenal azotemia with elevated blood urea nitrogen and creatinine may be present. The diagnosis is made by eliminating other causes of polyuria and polydipsia and a lack of response to water deprivation testing and exogenous vasopressin administration. Lhasa Apso puppies should be checked at 2 weeks of age to determine whether the kidney is effective in concentrating urine within the normal range of 1.006 to 1.017. If evidence exists of nephrogenic diabetes insipidus, then the administration of water by mouth (1 ml/oz of body weight once or twice daily) will prevent the occurrence of the acute dehydration syndrome. The decision to treat affected neonates must consider the possibility of future damage resulting from the plugging of the renal tubules with amorphous material of constituency similar to that observed in the first urine. Although initial treatment and rehydration may be successful, the plugged tubules will result in chronic nephritis and end-stage kidney disease by 4 to 10 months of age.

Congenital Interstitial Nephritis Secondary to Transplacental Infection

Oral inoculation with *Toxoplasma gondii* tissue cysts during pregnancy results in neonatal toxoplasmosis in cats. Under experimental conditions, interstitial nephritis occurs in 76% of kittens less than 4 weeks of age. Within the renal cortices, aggregates of macrophages, neutrophils, and fewer lymphocytes surrounded and replaced tubules. Tubular epithelial cells within these foci were often necrotic. Tachyzoites can be seen in tubular epithelium, interstitium, and within glomeruli. In dogs, experimental transplacental transmission of *Leishmania infantum* and canine herpesvirus results in interstitial nephritis (Figure 38-5). Canine herpesvirus is covered in detail in Chapter 16 on Viral Infections.

Ureteral Valves

Ureteral valve occurs as a result of persistence of mucosa and smooth muscle in the ureter. A semiannular ureteral valve was described in a 6-month-old female Collie resulting in hydronephrosis and incontinence.

Ureterocele

Ureterocele is a congenital cystic dilation of the ureter at the vesiculoureteral junction within the submucosa of the urinary

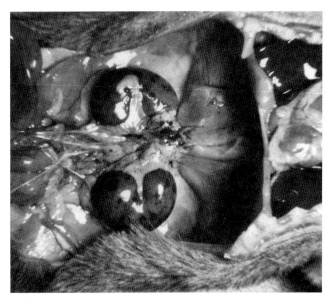

Figure 38-5 Interstitial nephritis caused by canine herpes infection. Petechial and ecchymotic hemorrhages can be visualized on the renal capsule. (From Mosier JE: The puppy from birth to six weeks, *Vet Clin North Am* 8(1):96, 1978, Figure 10.)

bladder wall. Ureteroceles may be unilateral or bilateral and simple (ureteral orifice in normal position) or ectopic (associated with an ectopic ureter). They are more frequently associated with ectopic ureters. Ureteroceles have not been reported in cats. Female puppies are more commonly affected than males. Urinary incontinence and clinical signs related to urinary tract infections are typically seen as a result of ureteral ectopia. Diagnosis can be made with contrast radiography and ultrasound.

Vesicoureteral Reflux

Vesicoureteral reflux results from reflux of urine from within the urinary bladder into the ureter. The reflux can occur from congenital malformation at the vesicoureteral junction or secondary from disease (e.g., interstitial nephritis) that interferes with normal function of the vesicoureteral junction. These animals may be at increased risk of developing urinary tract infections and pyelonephritis. Reflux is normal in puppies and occurs in a small number of normal adults. Diagnosis is made with contrast retrograde cystourethrography.

Vesicourethral Dysfunction in Manx Cats

Manx cats are predisposed to significant abnormalities of vesicourethral function because of spinal dysraphism (myelodysplasia) and other congenital spinal cord neuropathologic abnormalities. Manifestations of vesicourethral dysfunction include detrusor areflexia, autonomous pressure response to bladder filling, dysfunctional proximal urethra, and poor quality pelvic floor electromyographic activity. Histochemical studies of the bladder and urethra in patients with incontinence demonstrate a complete absence of adrenergic fibers, even in the trigone area.

Urachal Abnormalities

The urachus allows communication between the developing urinary bladder and the placenta. Normally the urachus would atrophy at birth. If this fails to occur, all or part of the urachus may remain. A patent urachus occurs when the entire urachus fails to close. Urachal cysts can occur with a focal failure to close anywhere along the length of the urachus. Vesicourachal diverticula form at the apex of the urinary bladder as a result of failure of urachal closure at the urinary bladder. Signs of patent urachus include omphalophlebitis, urine dripping from the umbilicus, and urinary tract infections. Urachal cysts are often found incidentally. Vesicourachal diverticula do not typically cause clinical signs but may become more apparent when underlying lower urinary tract disease is present. Diagnosis is made with contrast radiography (patent urachus, vesicourachal diverticula) and abdominal ultrasonography with cytology (urachal cyst).

Fistulae

Congenital communications between the urinary tract and other organ systems are rare in puppies and kittens. Communications between the urinary bladder and colon, the urinary bladder and uterine horns, and the urethra and rectum have all been reported.

CONGENITAL AND ACQUIRED URINE DISORDERS

Fanconi's Syndrome

Fanconi's syndrome is a complex tubular disorder involving impaired tubular resorption of amino acids, glucose, sodium, potassium, phosphorus, and uric acid. The disease has been described in many breeds, including Basenjis, Norwegian Elkhounds, Miniature Schnauzers, and Shetland Sheepdogs. In Basenjis the disease is familial, but the mode of inheritance is unknown. Fanconi's syndrome can also be acquired and has been reported in cases of nephrotoxicity. The most common clinical manifestations include polyuria, polydipsia, isosthenuria, proteinuria, and glucosuria. Metabolic acidosis and hypokalemia also occur. Glucosuria can lead to urinary tract infections. Renal failure may develop within weeks or several years after diagnosis. The diagnosis is often made using signalment and clinical findings. Treatment is variable and might include antibiotics for urinary tract infections, alkalinization therapy in cases of severe metabolic acidosis (pH < 7.0), potassium supplementation, and supportive care for chronic renal failure.

Renal Hematuria

Canine idiopathic renal hematuria or benign essential hematuria is a rare condition of severe and recurrent unilateral or bilateral renal bleeding in the absence of trauma, coagulopathy, or other obvious cases of hemorrhage. Renal hematuria has been reported in a Weimaraner, a Belgian Malinois, and a Catahoula Leopard Dog cross-breed. Reported clinical signs include stranguria, dysuria, and macroscopic blood and blood clots in the urine. Recurrent hematuria may be intermittent with urine color appearing grossly normal one day and grossly hematuric with large blood clots the following day. Complete ureteral obstruction (resulting in hydroureter and hydronephrosis) and urethral obstruction secondary to blood clots have also been reported. Large blood clots in the urinary bladder cannot be differentiated from other space-occupying masses by an excretory urogram or transabdominal ultrasonography (Figure 38-6). Renal hemorrhage can be diagnosed following visualization of macroscopic hemorrhage from the ureters during cystoscopy. If endoscopy is not available, cystotomy is performed and urine is obtained from catheterization of the individual ureters to determine whether blood is originating from one or both kidneys. Blood transfusions may be required in cases of severe anemia. Nephrectomy with ureterectomy is an effective treatment to remove the source of hemorrhage and to prevent the formation of blood clots in patients with unilateral renal hematuria.

Renal Telangiectasia

Renal telangiectasia has been reported in the Pembroke Welsh Corgi. These dogs develop hematuria and blood loss that may be significant enough to result in anemia. Histologically, blood-filled vascular structures are found within the kidneys and may be present in other organs.

Cystinuria

Cystine is an amino acid that is excreted in excess in the urine of some dogs and cats as a result of a proximal renal tubular transport defect. Males develop clinical signs more commonly than females, but this may be because of their narrower urethra. In Newfoundland dogs, the mode of inheritance is autosomal recessive and results in increased excretion and decreased reabsorption of cystine. There is also

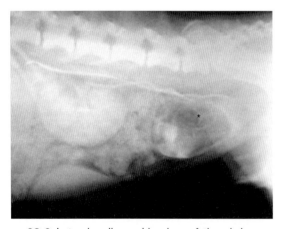

Figure 38-6 Lateral radiographic view of the abdomen of a 7-month-old, neutered male Catahoula Leopard Dog crossbreed following excretory urography. A filling defect is present within the bladder (*). The kidneys have a normal appearance. (From Hawthorne JC et al: Recurrent urethral obstruction secondary to idiopathic renal hematuria in a puppy, *J Am Anim Hosp Assoc* 34:512, 1998, Figure 1A.)

decreased reabsorption of the amino acids ornithine, lysine, and arginine in affected dogs. In Scottish Terriers, the mode of inheritance appears to be recessive. Clinical findings include cystinuria and cystine calculi. Not all cats and dogs with crystalluria develop calculi.

Hyperuricuria

Dalmatian dogs and English Bulldogs have increased quantities of uric acid in their serum. The Dalmatian dog has an autosomal inherited defect in its ability to transport insoluble uric acid into hepatic cells for conversion to its soluble form. Because of this defect, uric acid levels are increased in the blood, excreted in excess in the urine, and not reabsorbed adequately in the proximal tubules. Many Dalmatian dogs excrete uric acid in excess, but formation of urate uroliths is relatively rare. This supports a multifactorial etiopathogenesis to the formation of urate calculi in the Dalmatian dog. The cause of increased uric acid levels in the English Bulldog is unknown. Ammonium urate crystalluria and calculi also occur in dogs and cats with portovascular anomalies as a result of failure to solubilize uric acid. These animals most often present with signs related to hepatic encephalopathy, and calculi are found incidentally. The treatment of choice for calculi in the presence of a portovascular anomaly is surgical removal via cystotomy and correction of the vascular anomaly. Allopurinol is a xanthine oxidase inhibitor. Xanthine oxidase is a hepatic enzyme that converts hypoxanthine to xanthine and xanthine to uric acid. By inhibiting xanthine oxidase, uric acid production is decreased. Low protein diets are also used to decrease the amount of purines. A more neutral urine pH is also desirable to decrease the likelihood of ammonium urate calculi formation.

Xanthinuria

Xanthinuria is most common secondary to treatment with the xanthine oxidase inhibitor allopurinol. There have been a few reports of puppies (Dachshund and Cavalier King Charles Spaniel) and kittens with xanthinuria secondary to xanthine oxidase deficiency. Xanthine oxidase is a hepatic enzyme that converts hypoxanthine to xanthine and xanthine to uric acid. In its absence, there will be an accumulation of xanthine, and increased quantities will be excreted in the urine. Xanthine crystals cannot be differentiated from urate crystals; therefore diagnosis is typically made by evaluating calculi. Treatment for animals considered at risk for developing calculi consists of discontinuation of allopurinol, a low protein (purine) diet, and alkalinization of the urine.

Hyperoxaluria

Hereditary hyperoxaluria has been found in Domestic Shorthair cats and Tibetan Spaniels. Males are more frequently affected than females. These animals typically develop acute renal failure at 7 weeks to 1 year of age secondary to deposition of calcium oxalate crystals in the renal tubules. Neuromuscular function may also be compromised. Medical therapy should be formulated with the goal of reducing urine concentration of calculogenic substances.

Urolithiasis

Urolithiasis in male and female puppies and kittens (5 weeks to 5 months of age) is rare. Clinical signs may include dysuria, pollakiuria, stranguria, hematuria, and, in the event of a complete urethral obstruction, a firm, distended urinary bladder. Abdominal radiography will demonstrate the presence of a radiopaque mass(es) in the urethra and/or bladder. Some calculi are radiodense and some are radiolucent so contrast radiography may be required. Mineralization may also be seen in the kidneys as calculi can form there. Chronic inflammation caused by presence of uroliths may induce metaplastic transformation and ossification of the bladder wall or other segments of the urinary tract. Chemical analysis of pediatric uroliths reveals a composition positive for phosphates, carbonates, calcium, magnesium, and ammonia, and negative for urates and oxalates. General treatment principles are similar to those in adult animals and include diluting the urine, decreasing lithogenic substances, and manipulating urine pH to increase solubility.

ACQUIRED ANATOMIC DISORDERS

Hydronephrosis

Hydronephrosis is uncommon in the dog and cat. Females are most often affected. Hydronephrosis is defined as an abnormality of the kidney characterized by progressive dilatation of the renal pelvis and progressive atrophy of the renal parenchyma. It occurs as a result of obstruction to urine outflow owing to any cause and at any site from the renal pelvis to the urethral orifice. The pathologic changes are caused by pressure and ischemia within the kidney. Reported causes of unilateral hydronephrosis include uroliths or blood clots in the ureter or renal pelvis, unilateral ectopic ureter, accidental ligation of a ureter during ovariohysterectomy, ureteral stricture or stenosis, ureterocele, ureteral or renal pelvic neoplasia, and retroperitoneal tumor causing extraluminal ureteral compression. Permanent damage to the kidney may not occur if an obstruction is corrected within 1 week. Up to 25% of normal renal function can return if the obstruction is corrected within 4 weeks. However, ureteral obstruction lasting for more than 4 weeks may result in complete loss of renal function.

Clinical findings depend on the severity of the hydronephrosis. Physical examination findings include renomegaly. Bacterial infection of the hydronephrotic kidney can occur resulting in pyelonephritis, and associated clinical signs are lethargy, anorexia, pyrexia, leukocytosis with hematuria, pyuria, and bacteriuria. The diagnosis may be based on the history coupled with physical examination and laboratory findings consisting of uremia and confirmed by an enlarged kidney on transabdominal ultrasonography. Treatment is aimed at removing the underlying cause of the hydronephrosis if possible.

Neoplasia

Renal neoplasia is usually found in older dogs and cats, but nephroblastomas, carcinomas, lymphosarcoma, and undifferentiated sarcomas have been reported in young dogs and cats. Nephroblastomas occur in dogs younger than 6 months of age and are typically unilateral. Multifocal renal cystadenocarcinomas occur in German Shepherd Dogs with an autosomal dominant mode of inheritance. These dogs present much later in life (between 5 and 11 years of age) with signs involving the skin or genitourinary tract. In addition to bilateral renal cystadenocarcinomas, many develop nodular dermatofibrosis and uterine leiomyomas. Clinical findings might include a palpable abdominal mass or, in the case of renal lymphosarcoma, signs related to acute or chronic renal failure. Diagnosis of a renal mass is made with abdominal radiography or ultrasonography. Cytology and/or histopathology is required for a definitive diagnosis. Nephroblastomas, carcinomas, and sarcomas may remain local or invade surrounding tissues. Metastasis can occur to the regional lymph nodes, mesentery, liver, lungs, and bones. Unilateral nephrectomy and ureterectomy is the treatment of choice for tumors confined to the kidney. Unfortunately most tumors have spread locally or distantly at the time of diagnosis. Lymphoma is typically treated with multiagent chemotherapy but is associated with partial or complete remissions of only 1 to 3 months. Renal neoplasia carries a poor prognosis unless complete removal is possible.

Urinary bladder neoplasia is rare in puppies and kittens. Rhabdomyosarcomas have been reported in young dogs and are likely remnants of the urogenital ridge. These tumors are most commonly found in the area of the trigone. Signs are consistent with lower urinary tract disease and obstructive uropathy. Surgery has been used with limited success. A partial response with combination chemotherapy using doxorubicin, cyclophosphamide, and vincristine has been reported.

Malakoplakia of the Bladder

Malakoplakia is a chronic, granulomatous disease that is exceptionally rare in domestic animals. The pathogenesis of malakoplakia remains obscure, but it is currently proposed that defective assembly of macrophage microtubules compromises the structure and function of the phagolysosomes, which can affect many organs, including the bladder. Affected patients have a markedly enlarged bladder with a diffusely nodular mucosal surface that causes straining during urination (Figure 38-7). Urinalysis does not reveal

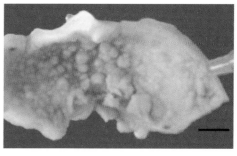

Figure 38-7 Urinary bladder of a 5-week-old kitten with malakoplakia. (From Bayley C, Slocombe R, Tatarczuch L: Malakoplakia in the urinary bladder of a kitten, *J Compar Pathol* 139(1):47, 2008, Figure 1, p 48.)

any abnormalities. Straining continues despite therapy, and euthanasia is the only humane option.

Urethral Prolapse

Urethral prolapse may result from trauma but is most often associated with genitourinary infection or excessive sexual excitement. Brachycephalic breeds (Boston Terrier and English Bulldog) have a higher reported incidence. The lesion is characterized by a granulating mass on the urethral orifice of the glans penis and the presence of chronic bloody preputial discharge. Amputation of the prolapsed urethra with suturing of the urethra to the glans penis has been successful. Surgical repair has been described using straight intestinal surgical needles or stay sutures placed perpendicularly to each other through the penile tissue and urethra posterior to the external orifice to prevent posterior retraction of the urethral mucosa.

SUGGESTED READINGS

DiBartola SP: Renal disease: clinical approach and laboratory evaluation. In Ettinger SJ, Feldman EC (eds): *Textbook of veterinary internal medicine*, ed 6, St Louis, 2005, Elsevier/Saunders, p 1719.

Feeney DA, Johnston GR: The kidneys and ureters. In Thrall DE (ed): *Textbook of veterinary diagnostic radiology*, ed 5, St Louis, 2007, Elsevier/Saunders, pp 693-707.

Kruger JM et al: The urinary system. In Hoskins JD (ed): *Veterinary pediatrics: dogs and cats from birth to six months*, ed 3, Philadelphia, 2001, Saunders, pp 371-401.

Lees GE: Juvenile and familial nephropathies. In *BSAVA manual of canine and feline nephrology and urology*, ed 2, Gloucester, 2007, BSAVA, pp 79-86.

Maxie MG, Newman SJ: Urinary system. In Maxie MG (ed): *Jubb, Kennedy, and Palmer's pathology of domestic animals*, vol 2, ed 5, St Louis, 2007, Saunders/Elsevier, pp 425-522.

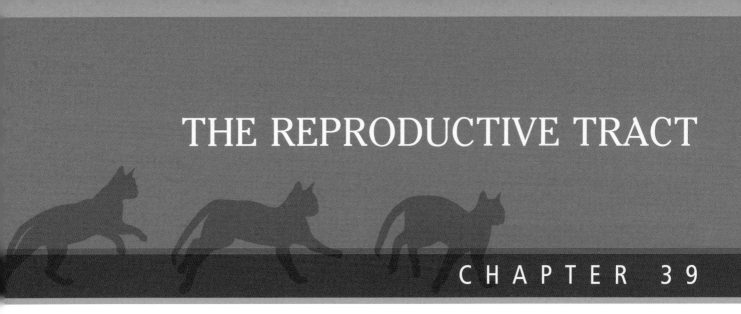

THE REPRODUCTIVE TRACT

CHAPTER 39

Michelle Anne Kutzler

SEXUAL DIFFERENTIATION

Normal sexual differentiation depends on the successful completion of three consecutive events: establishment of chromosomal sex, gonadal sex, and phenotypic sex. Chromosomal sex (normally XX or XY) is established at fertilization and maintained by mitotic division after that. Sexual differentiation is completed by 46 days of gestation (Table 39-1), where gestation lengths are 65 days for dogs and 64 days for cats.

In the early embryo, the gonads are undifferentiated (Figure 39-1). Gonadectomy of XX or XY embryos before gonadal differentiation results in the development of a female phenotype, leading to the conclusion that the basic embryonic plan is female. A gene located on the Y-chromosome (*Sry* gene) encodes a testis-determining protein that results in testis formation and establishes the male gonadal sex. *Sry* acts as a master switch turning on several genes that are located on other chromosomes, thus inducing a cascade of gene products that are necessary for testicular development. In the absence of the *Sry* gene, the default pathway to female gonadal sex is initiated, and an ovary develops.

Following gonadal differentiation, development of the internal and external genitalia occurs. In the early embryo, both sets of internal tubular structures (wolffian and müllerian) develop initially. Two testicular secretions (müllerian-inhibiting factor [MIF] and testosterone) are responsible for masculinizing the tubular reproductive tract (see Figure 39-1). MIF, a glycoprotein produced by Sertoli cells, causes the müllerian (female) duct system (uterine tubes, uterus, cervix, and cranial vagina) to regress. Testosterone, a steroid hormone produced by Leydig cells, promotes the formation of the vas deferens and epididymides from the wolffian ducts. Testosterone is metabolized to dihydrotestosterone (DHT) within the cells of the urogenital sinus, the genital tubercle, and the genital swellings to result in the formation of the prostate and urethra, the penis, and the scrotum, respectively. Androgen-dependent masculinization is mediated through the binding of testosterone or DHT to the androgen receptor protein, the product of a gene on the X-chromosome.

Canine and feline male external genitalia originate from an undifferentiated urogenital tubercle (which forms at the level of the embryonic cloacal membrane). As a direct result of the influence of DHT, the prepuce develops from a circular plate of ectoderm invaginating at the level of the distal tip of the penis, whereas the junction between the preputial and penile mucosa (balanopreputial fold) dissolves at a later stage, also as a direct result of the action of androgens. In the absence of DHT (as in the normal female), the caudal vagina, vestibule, and vulva develop. Determination of gender in newborn dogs and cats may be difficult because the difference at this age is a slightly longer anogenital distance in males (13 to 15 mm) versus females (7 to 8 mm) (Figure 39-2). A pseudohermaphrodite is an animal that has the gonads of one sex with the internal and/or external genitalia and/or the chromosomal complement of the opposite sex (Box 39-1).

TESTICULAR DESCENT

During fetal development, each testis moves to a position caudoventral to the inguinal canal from its original location near the caudal pole of the kidney. Testicular descent is coordinated by growth and regression of the gubernaculum. The gubernaculum extends from the caudal pole of the testis into the inguinal canal (Figure 39-3). Testicular descent occurs in three phases: intraabdominal, intrainguinal, and extrainguinal. During the intraabdominal migration, each testis moves toward its respective internal inguinal ring, and the caudal part of the gubernaculum enlarges enormously. The enlarging gubernaculum dilates the inguinal canal and extends the length of the scrotum, which facilitates the migration of the testis through the inguinal canal during the intrainguinal phase. In fact, the enlarged gubernaculum is present at birth and is frequently mistaken for descended testes in neonates. The extrainguinal phase is completed after birth in dogs and cats and involves regression of the gubernaculum, which guides/pulls the testis into the scrotum.

Gubernacular outgrowth and enlargement are mediated by MIF. Testosterone plays a role in the regression of the gubernaculum and the terminal differentiation into the proper ligament of the testis and the ligament of the tail of the epididymis.

The testes are in an abdominal or inguinal location at birth in puppies and kittens. The testes pass through the inguinal canal 3 to 4 days after birth but may move up and down within the inguinal canal until 10 to 14 weeks after birth. Therefore diagnosis for failure of testicular descent should not be made until the animal is at least 4 months of age. When palpating for the testes in young puppies and kittens, the clinician should place the index finger and middle finger on either side of the penis so that

TABLE 39-1	Timeline of sexual differentiation in canine fetuses*
Gestational age (Post-LH surge)	**Sexual differentiation**
32 days	Female and male gonads undifferentiated
36 days	Ovarian differentiation first detected in female embryos
36 days	Testicular differentiation first detected in male embryos
36 days	Müllerian duct regression in male embryos first observed
42 days	Wolffian duct regression in female embryos first observed
46 days	Müllerian duct regression in male embryos completed
46 days	Wolffian duct regression in female embryos completed

*Differentiation of fetal gonads and internal genitalia occurs between 32 and 46 days of gestation relative to the maternal preovulatory luteinizing hormone (LH) surge.

BOX 39-1   Pseudohermaphroditism

Pseudohermaphrodites are defined as male or female according to the presence of testes or ovaries, respectively. Female pseudohermaphrodites are rare in dogs and cats and result from iatrogenic prenatal exposure to either an exogenous androgen or progestogen. In humans, adrenogenital syndromes resulting in excess circulating androgens are a common cause of female pseudohermaphroditism. However, adrenogenital syndromes have not been described in small animals.

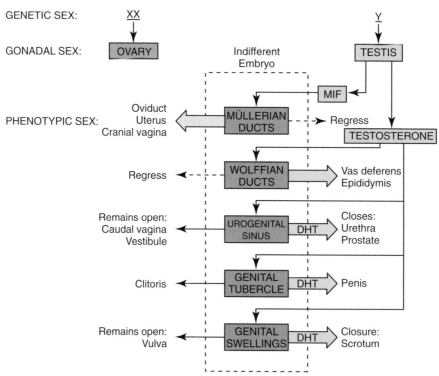

Figure 39-1 Differentiation of the internal and external genitalia after the gonad develops into a testicle or an ovary. *MIF*, Müllerian inhibiting factor; *DHT*, dihydrotestosterone. (Redrawn from Meyers-Wallen VN, Patterson DF: Disorders of sexual development in the dog. In Morrow D (ed): *Current therapy in theriogenology*, ed 2, Philadelphia, 1986, Saunders, pp 567-574.)

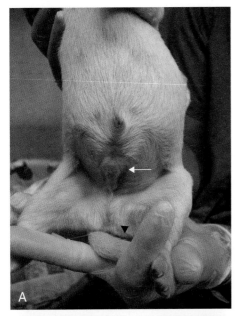

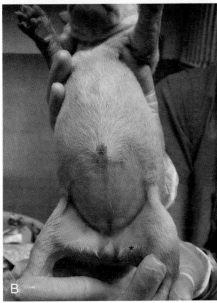

Figure 39-2 Anogenital distance in male **(A)** and female **(B)** 4-day-old Labrador Retriever pups. *Arrow* points to prepuce; *arrowhead* points toward scrotum; *asterisk* adjacent to vulva.

PUBERTY

Most puppies and kittens attain puberty between 8 and 19 months of age, with a range of 4 to 22 months for both males and females (Table 39-2). At 2 months after birth, the ovary measures 5 mm in diameter. Environmental factors can affect the onset of puberty. Most female cats born early in the season or exposed when young either to tomcats or cycling females or to increasing amounts of light show the first signs of estrus before similar individuals born later or not exposed to these factors.

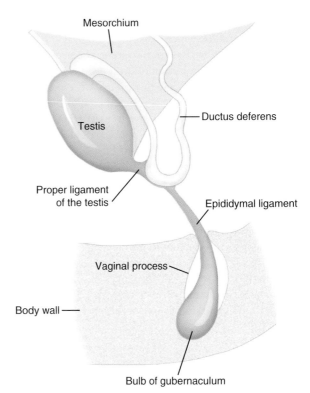

Figure 39-3 The normal relationship between the vaginal process, epididymal ligament, and gubernaculum. (Redrawn from Peter AT: The reproductive system. In Hoskins JD (ed): *Veterinary pediatrics: dogs and cats from birth to 6 months*, ed 3, Philadelphia, 2001, Saunders, pp 463-475.)

TABLE 39-2	Onset of puberty in the normal bitch and queen of reported breeds
Species/Breed	**Age at pubertal estrus**
Canine	
Beagle	7.2-23 months
Labrador Retriever	7.2-16.3 months
Mongrel	6.3-17.1 months
Feline	
Abyssinian	7-14 months
Birman	10-18 months
Burmese	4-19 months
Himalayan	4-16 months
Manx	9-18 months
Siamese	4-20 months
Domestic Shorthair	4.5-15 months
Domestic Longhair	6-18 months

Modified from Johnston SD: Premature gonadal failure in female dogs and cats, *J Reprod Fertil Suppl* 39:65-72, 1989.

the testes can be found by gentle traction in a front-to-back direction.

At birth, normal ovaries will have thousands of follicles. At the onset of puberty, a cohort of follicles is selected to begin development. Follicular development is promoted by the release of hypothalamic (gonadotropin-releasing hormone) and pituitary hormones (follicle-stimulating hormone and luteinizing hormone). As the follicles grow, they release estradiol, which causes the physical and behavioral signs of proestrus. Estradiol concentrations peak in mid proestrus and are near baseline during estrus in the bitch, whereas they remain elevated throughout estrus in the queen. Luteinizing hormone is released around the onset of estrus in dogs but only in response to external stimuli (e.g., mating) in cats. Puberty in both the female dog and cat is defined as the occurrence of the first estrus.

The testes contain spermatogonia, which divide to form spermatozoa near the time of puberty. Sperm development and testosterone secretion result from the release of the same hypothalamic and pituitary hormones as in the female. By 3.5 months after birth, there is sufficient testosterone to initiate the growth of penile spines in tomcats, which reach their full size when the cats are between 6 and 7 months of age. Growth or regression of the spines has been positively correlated with androgen-dependent mating activity. In male dogs, territorial marking behavior begins at the time of puberty.

REPRODUCTIVE DISORDERS IN MALE PEDIATRIC PATIENTS

Testicular Abnormalities

Congenital testicular abnormalities in cats and dogs include the congenital absence of one (monorchidism) or both (anorchidism) testes, testicular hypoplasia, and cryptorchidism. Puppies and kittens with XXY (Klinefelter's) syndrome are phenotypically male, have a normal penis and prepuce, and have reportedly normal sexual behavior. Epididymides and small testis are present within the scrotum. However, ejaculates do not contain spermatozoa, and histologic evaluation of testicular tissue reveals seminiferous tubular dysgenesis with no evidence of spermatogenesis. More than one X-chromosome is deleterious to normal spermatogenesis. The XXY syndrome can arise by meiotic nondisjunction of the sex chromosomes during male or female gametogenesis or by mitotic nondisjunction in the early zygote. Nondisjunctional events leading to abnormal sex chromosome constitutions occur randomly and are not the result of a heritable defect. This syndrome is particularly well known; domestic shorthaired tomcats with this condition often feature a calico or tortoiseshell coat. In cats, the genes for orange and black coat color are X-linked alleles. Males with this coat color may also be XX/XY chimeras or XY/XY chimeras. In these two karyotypes, normal testicular histology and spermatogenesis may be present. A sample karyotype form is shown in Figure 39-4.

Failure of the testis to descend into the scrotum (cryptorchidism) is a development defect. Unilateral cryptorchidism is 4 times more common than bilateral cryptorchidism. If only one scrotal testis is present, careful ultrasonographic or surgical exploration of the contralateral inguinal canal and abdomen may be necessary to determine whether the missing scrotal testis is retained, hypoplastic, or absent. Inguinal retention is 3 times more likely than abdominal retention. For abdominal retention, tracing the vas deferens retrograde from its insertion on the dorsal aspect of the prostate is a useful method to find the testis. Cases of bilateral cryptorchidism can be distinguished from anorchidism postpubertally using challenge testing (Box 39-2).

In puppies with undescended testes, the right testis is usually retained in the inguinal region. On the other hand, in kittens, abdominal retention is more common than inguinal retention. The presence of a strong cranial suspensory ligament that fails to break down and prevents gubernacular outgrowth and migration has been proposed in cryptorchid individuals. Although the production of testosterone by the interstitial (Leydig) cells continues in the cryptorchid testis, spermatogenesis does not occur because of the elevated intraabdominal temperature relative to the cooler temperature within the scrotum. As a result, the testicular germinal epithelium degenerates, and the cryptorchid testis becomes smaller and soft. In dogs, these changes may be responsible for the 5 times greater incidence of Sertoli cell tumors and 3 times greater incidence of seminomas in cryptorchid testes compared with scrotal testes.

The reported incidence of cryptorchidism ranges from less than 0.1% to 13% in dogs and 0.37% to 1.7% in cats. Occasionally this abnormality occurs in association with other congenital defects (e.g., hypospadias, inguinal and umbilical hernias). Dog breeds with a higher incidence of cryptorchidism include the toy, miniature, and standard Poodle, Pomeranian, Yorkshire Terrier, Miniature Dachshund, Cairn Terrier, Chihuahua, Maltese, Boxer, Pekingese, English Bulldog, Old English Sheepdog, Miniature Schnauzer, Siberian Husky, and Shetland Sheepdog. Dog breeds with a low incidence of cryptorchidism include the Beagle, Golden Retriever, Labrador Retriever, Saint Bernard, Great Dane, and English Setter. There are no data at present to support that cryptorchidism is a heritable defect in cats. However, Persian cats are overrepresented in feline surveys of cryptorchidism. Breeding trials in Boxers and Cocker Spaniels have confirmed that cryptorchidism is a heritable condition involving a sex-linked autosomal recessive trait.

BOX 39-2 **Two challenge tests used to differentiate between bilateral cryptorchidism and anorchidism**

Gonadotropin-releasing hormone (GnRH): 2 µg/kg intramuscularly (IM) for dogs and 25 µg IM for cats with a blood sample drawn 1 hour later for measurement of serum testosterone.
Human chorionic gonadotropin (hCG): 20 IU/kg IM for dogs and 250 IU IM for cats with a blood sample drawn 4 hours later for measurement of serum testosterone.
Serum testosterone concentrations exceeding 1 ng/ml following challenge testing support the diagnosis of cryptorchidism, and serum testosterone concentrations less than 1 ng/ml support a diagnosis of anorchidism.

KARYOTYPING FORM
Molecular Cytogenetics Laboratory, Room 314B Bldg. 1197,
Department of Veterinary Integrative BioSciences,
Texas A&M University, College Station, TX 77843
Voice: (979)862-2879; Fax (979)845-9972;
Contact e-mail: bchowdhary@cvm.tamu.edu or traudsepp@cvm.tamu.edu

Owner/agent name: _____

Address: _____

_____

Phone # _____

Date sample taken: _____

Signature of person taking sample: _____

SPECIES SAMPLED (*PLEASE PRINT*):

Name of the animal (Proband)	Registration number	Year of birth	Breed	Sex	Color

History of proband's father/sire:

History of proband's mother/dam:

Reasons for Karyotyping:

Fax/E-mail: (for sending results): _____

Invoice to (name/address): _____

(1) Blood samples **MUST be collected in 2 x 5 ml sodium heparin tubes** (e.g., Vacutainer) **AND 4 x 10 ml** EDTA tubes.
(2) Samples MUST be sent by overnight mail. Please wrap the tubes in paper towels and only then put them on ice to *avoid freezing*. Samples degraded during transit are sender's responsibility.
(3) PLEASE DO NOT send samples on a Friday. Also ensure that samples sent on a Thursday reach the lab by Friday noon. Normal turn-around time for results is 10 working days.
(4) **CHARGES (please make the checks payable to Texas AgriLife Research):**

1. $225 - basic chromosome analysis from blood (chromosome number count and assessment of the sex chromosomes). For species with available karyotype standard (cattle, horse, sheep, goat, pig, dog, cat).
2. $275 - basic chromosome analysis from blood (chromosome number count and assessment of the sex chromosomes). For species with NO karyotype standard (alpaca, llama, exotic species).
3. $350 - basic chromosome analysis from fibroblast cultures of any species.
4. $450 - basic chromosome analysis for insurance agencies and private companies.
Plus **additional $10** if we send the heparin tubes to you. Your veterinarian may charge an additional fee.
(5) **RESULTS:** The sender will be supplied with an image of a metaphase chromosome spread from a cell obtained from the sample. For detailed analysis (banded karyotype), there are extra charges.
(6) To ensure confidentiality, results will not be provided by phone, unless the requesting agency wants it.
(7) One copy of the results will be mailed or sent by fax or e-mail to owner/agent.

Figure 39-4 Sample karyotype form. (Reproduced with kind permission from Drs. B.P. Chowdhary (Director) and T. Raudsepp (Associate Director) of the Molecular Cytogenetics Laboratory at the College of Veterinary Medicine and Biomedical Sciences, Texas A&M University.)

Homozygous females appear to be phenotypically normal carriers that will transmit the gene to 50% of their offspring. Heterozygous males and heterozygous females will also be phenotypically normal carriers. Because of the heritable nature of this condition, professional organizations (e.g., British Veterinary Medical Association) recommend not breeding cryptorchid animals, their littermates, and their parents. Attempts to induce descent of the cryptorchid testis by hormonal treatments are relatively ineffective and do not correct the genetic flaw.

Internal Genital Tract Abnormalities

The excurrent tract includes the rete testis, efferent ducts, epididymis, vas deferens, and urethra. Cystic rete testis was observed in an 8-month-old cat during a routine castration. The cystic structure occupied approximately half of the right testis. Areas of active spermatogenesis alternated with areas of focal degeneration in the right testis, and no sperm were present in the right epididymis. A similar abnormality has not been reported in the dog. Unilateral epididymal aplasia has been reported in a fertile Siberian Husky and a 39,XXY male calico cat. Unilateral absence of the vas deferens, kidney, and ureter has also been reported in the dog and cat.

Both male dogs and cats possess a prostate gland, and cats also have paired bulbourethral glands. Congenital prostatic hypoplasia is rare in the dog and cat and usually associated with pseudohermaphroditism. Congenital bulbourethral gland abnormalities have never been reported in the cat. Several acquired diseases of the prostate have been reported in adult dogs (benign prostatic hyperplasia, chronic prostatitis, prostatic neoplasia) but do not occur in pediatric patients.

Persistent müllerian duct syndrome (PMDS) is an autosomal recessive trait in Miniature Schnauzers and Basset Hounds with expression limited to dogs with an XY-chromosome constitution that are also homozygous for the recessive genes. PMDS has also been reported in Persian cats, Domestic Shorthair (DSH) cats, and Domestic Longhair (DLH) cats. This syndrome results from the failure of müllerian-inhibiting activity (mutation in the gene for the MIF receptor) with normal synthesis of testosterone during development. As a result, müllerian-derived structures (uterine tubes, uterus, cervix, and cranial vagina) are retained. Approximately 50% of the animals affected with PMDS are either unilaterally or bilaterally cryptorchid but otherwise appear to be normal males externally. Affected males with scrotal testes are fertile. Male and female offspring, as well as parents and siblings of affected males, are carriers of the trait. Internally both testes are attached to the cranial ends of a normal uterus, with an epididymis associated with each testis (Figure 39-5). The vas deferens are present within the myometrium. The cranial portions of the vagina and prostate are often present. Externally normal male animals may go unnoticed until they develop pyometra or a urinary tract infection (or dysuria) or prostatic infection. Diagnosis is made by histologic examination of the internal genitalia and gonads, as well as cytogenetic determination of an XY karyotype. Squamous metaplasia of the prostate has been reported in animals affected with PMDS and concurrent Sertoli cell tumors. When removing the uterus, it is important to remove as much of the vagina as possible. Small-diameter communications between the cranial vagina and prostatic urethra are a source of ascending infection into the uterus.

External Genital Tract Abnormalities

Congenital abnormalities of the penis and prepuce in dogs and cats are duplication of the penis (diphallia), failure of

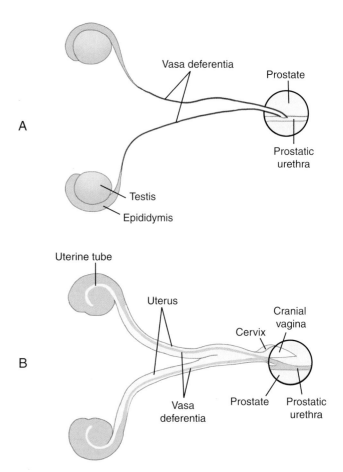

Figure 39-5 Schematic representation of genitalia in normal males **(A)** and affected males **(B)** with canine persistent müllerian duct syndrome. A narrow connection between the cranial vagina and the prostatic urethra, represented here by a dotted line, has been observed in at least one affected male. (Redrawn from Meyers-Wallen VN et al: Mullerian inhibiting substance is present in testes of dogs with persistent mullerian duct syndrome, *Biol Reprod* 41:881-888, 1989.)

the balanopreputial fold to separate (persistent penile frenulum), inability to protrude the penis from the prepuce (phimosis), preputial and penile hypoplasia from immaturity, and termination of the penile urethra at an abnormal location (hypospadias). Acquired abnormalities of the penis and prepuce in dogs seen during the first year include urethral prolapse and balanoposthitis.

A duplication of the cloacal membrane during embryonic development may lead to duplication of the urogenital tubercle, causing duplication of the penis and prepuce (diphallia). This rare defect has been reported in three 5- to 6-month-old dogs: one German Shorthaired Pointer and two unrelated Poodle cross-breed dogs. All three dogs presented with clinical signs of hematuria, pollakiuria, and inappropriate urination and also showed complete duplication of the urinary bladder. Diagnosis is made by visual inspection (Figure 39-6). One owner noticed two streams of urine during urination. Affected individuals may also be bilaterally cryptorchid with unilateral hydronephrosis and

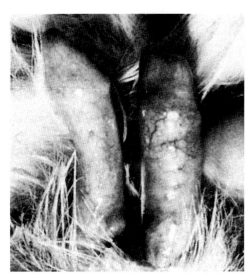

Figure 39-6 Diphallia in a 6-month-old Poodle cross-breed dog. (From Johnston SD, Bailie NC, Hayden DW, et al.: Diphallia in a mixed breed dog with multiple anomalies, *Theriogenology* 31:1253-1260, 1989.)

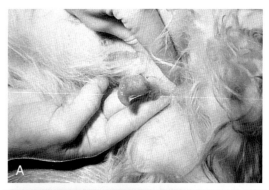

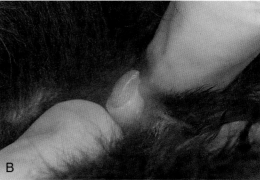

Figure 39-7 A persistent frenulum is demonstrated by complete retraction of the prepuce in this dog **(A)** and cat **(B)**. (**A,** From Johnston SD, Root Kustritz MV, Olson PN: *Canine and feline theriogenology*, Philadelphia, 2001, Saunders, pp 356-367. **B,** From Romagnoli S, Schlafer DH: Disorders of sexual differentiation in puppies and kittens: a diagnostic and clinical approach, *Vet Clin North Am Small Anim Pract* 36:573-606, 2006.)

unilateral renal agenesis, which may progress to renal failure secondary to pyelonephritis.

A persistent frenulum is a thin membrane of fibrous connective tissue joining the ventral aspect of the tip of the penis to the prepuce or the corpus of the penis, which may result in ventral or lateral deviation of the penile tips (phallocampsis) (Figure 39-7). Its presence is attributed to abnormal dissolution of the balanopreputial fold (an androgen-dependent process). This condition has been reported in several breeds of dogs, but Cocker Spaniels and Poodles are overrepresented. Persistent frenula also occur in cats. Animals affected with a persistent frenulum may be asymptomatic or may show discomfort during urination or copulation (erection). Additional clinical signs include excessive licking and dermatitis on the medial aspect of the hind legs secondary to urine scalding. Diagnosis is made by visual inspection. Treatment is made by transecting the frenulum with scissors, which can be accomplished with local anesthesia. Natural copulation by an affected dog has been reported after surgical correction.

The inability to protrude the penis from the prepuce (phimosis) is a defect that can be congenital in pseudohermaphrodites or in cases of congenital preputial stenosis. Congenital preputial stenosis has been reported in German Shepherd Dogs, Bouvier des Flandres, Labrador Retrievers, and Golden Retrievers and is likely heritable as it has been observed that several related litters and affected individuals have normal karyotypes. Severely affected neonates may develop balanoposthitis and septicemia resulting in death within the first 10 days after birth if not treated. Phimosis can also be an acquired condition secondary to inflammation, edema, neoplasia, or the presence of scar tissue as a consequence of wound healing after penile or preputial trauma. It has also been reported in an adult, intact DSH

tomcat presented for dysuria. If the preputial orifice is large enough to allow complete urination, patients may be asymptomatic except for an inability to protrude the penis during breeding. Diagnosis is made by visual inspection. Phimosis can be treated with preputial surgical enlargement by removing a V-shaped wedge of tissue at the level of the preputial orifice, which will prevent urine pooling and recurrent posthitis.

Dogs with preputial hypoplasia are generally presented for protrusion of the penis (owners may erroneously interpret this as a persistent erection problem) or urinary incontinence. Penile protrusion (paraphimosis) may lead to drying of the penile mucosa. Paraphimosis may also occur secondary to preputial stenosis or following castration. For preputial hypoplasia, surgical reconstruction of the prepuce (by creation of a pedicle extension flap) and, for less severe cases, phallopexy inside the prepuce have been successful in the dog.

Penile hypoplasia and penile immaturity indicate underdevelopment of the penis in absolute terms (hypoplasia) or in relation to body weight (immaturity). Penile immaturity (smaller diameter, decreased size, and radiodensity of the os penis) may be attributed to prepubertal gonadectomy. Penile hypoplasia has been reported in the Great Dane, Collie, Doberman Pinscher, and Cocker Spaniel. Penile hypoplasia has been reported in female pseudohermaphrodites (78,XX with ovaries and external genitalia that had been masculinized by prenatal androgen exposure; 78,XX [*Sry* +] with bilaterally cryptorchid testes and male external genitalia). Penile hypoplasia has also been reported in a male tortoiseshell cat with hypoplastic testis (38,XX in some cells and 57,XXY in others). Although affected animals may be asymptomatic, clinical signs may include dysuria, hematuria, and dripping of urine secondary to urine pooling and infection within the prepuce. Diagnosis is made by visual inspection. Histologic examination of gonadal tissue with karyotype evaluation is necessary to rule out an intersex condition. If indicated, penile hypoplasia can be treated by penile amputation and urethrostomy.

Hypospadias is a condition in which the prepuce and/or penile urethra does not close completely during development, resulting from incomplete closure of the urethral folds. An incidence of 0.003% has been reported for canine hypospadias, but it is important to note that the surveyed population did not include stillborn puppies, neonatal deaths of severely affected individuals, or dogs with undiagnosed, mild cases. Hypospadias occurs in conjunction with male pseudohermaphrodites and testicular feminization (see next paragraph). Hypospadias develops from inadequate fetal androgen production, insufficient fetal 5-α reductase activity, or ineffective fetal androgen receptors. 5-α Reductase is the enzyme that converts testosterone to DHT. Congenital deficiency of 5-α reductase, caused by an autosomal recessive trait, results in perineoscrotal hypoplasia, which resembles a vagina with a blind pouch. Individuals with this phenotype have wolffian duct structures (epididymis and vas deferens). Hypospadias can also be induced in genetically female dogs and cats following maternal administration of androgens or progestogens during pregnancy or by feeding the pregnant dam a diet deficient in vitamin A. In species other than the cat and dog, in utero exposure to estrogenic or antiandrogen endocrine-disrupting chemicals (e.g., phthalates, phytoestrogens) can also induce hypospadias. The urethral opening may be in the glans, the penile shaft, the prescrotal junction, or the perineum (Figure 39-8). Glandular hypospadias is milder, whereas perineal hypospadias is more severe. The condition may appear separately or in conjunction with other somatic defects, such as unilateral renal agenesis, cryptorchidism, bifid scrotum, and PMDS. Hypospadias is a familiar defect in certain breeds of dogs, such as the Boston Terrier. Affected animals may be asymptomatic, especially if only the glandular type is present, for which no treatment is necessary. The other forms are often characterized by urinary incontinence and inguinal dermatitis secondary to urine scalding and infection of regional mucocutaneous surfaces. Diagnosis is made by visual inspection and by catheterizing the urethra. To understand the etiology requires gonadal histology with karyotype evaluation. Treatment is made by surgical correction of the defect. Surgical repair depends on position and severity of the defect. Surgical

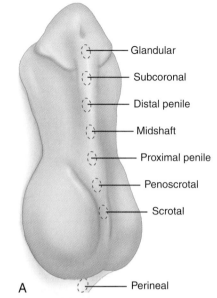

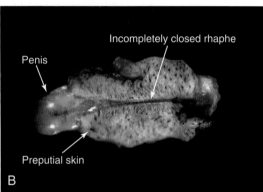

Figure 39-8 Failure of closure of the penile urethra and skin leads to a condition called hypospadias. **A,** Summary sketch of various locations of hypospadias. **B,** The incompletely closed rhaphe of the preputial skin extended caudally along the ventral midline. (**A,** From Symons J, Grady R: Disorders of the genitourinary system in the newborn. In Osborn LM, DeWitt TG, First LR, Zenel JA (eds): *Pediatrics*, Philadelphia, 2005, Mosby/Elsevier, pp 1352-1363. **B,** From Romagnoli S, Schlafer DH: Disorders of sexual differentiation in puppies and kittens: a diagnostic and clinical approach, *Vet Clin North Am Small Anim Pract* 36:573-606, 2006.)

repair of the defect generally requires separating the urethral mucosa from the skin at the mucocutaneous junction and suturing the incised edges of the urethral mucosa, taking care to avoid placing knots inside the urethral lumen (because this may cause calculus formation). Amputation of the penis and prepuce to the level of the urethral opening is generally performed in cases of penile hypoplasia, whereas complete penile amputation and scrotal or perineal urethrostomy are required in cases of scrotal or perineal hypospadias.

Testicular feminization is a recessive X-linked androgen receptor defect in male dogs and cats. Half (50%) of the male offspring from females carrying this defect will be affected with testicular feminization. Affected males have an XY karyotype, are bilateral cryptorchid, and have normal regression of müllerian structures with subnormal masculinization of internal and external androgen-responsive tissues. External genitalia vary from incompletely masculine (including hypospadias and persistent frenulum) to incompletely feminine (short, blind-ending vagina) (Figure 39-9). Affected males with female external genitalia are presumed by their owners to be females until puberty occurs, and clitoromegaly develops as a result of androgen stimulation from cryptorchid testes.

Prolapse of the distal penile urethra through the external urethral meatus is reported as a congenital idiopathic problem in young dogs and as a consequence of sexual excitement or urethral infection in adult dogs. This is a rare acquired disorder seen almost exclusively in English Bulldogs and Boston Terriers. The problem has not been reported in cats. Presenting complaints include penile bleeding and pollakiuria. Affected individuals may be presented for hemorrhage from the everted urethral mucosa. Recommended treatment is amputation of the everted tissue followed by suturing the urethral mucosa to the penile mucosa. Castration does not prevent recurrence, and some dogs that are left intact do not have recurrence.

Inflammation of the penile and preputial mucosa (balanoposthitis) is generally caused by normal bacteria flora but can also be caused by herpesvirus, blastomycosis infections, or transmissible venereal tumors. Affected individuals may be asymptomatic or may show irritation by licking of the affected area. Diagnosis is based on visual inspection, exfoliative cytology, and culture of the inflammatory lesions. In many cases, the best treatment for balanoposthitis in pediatric patients is benign neglect. Treatment of balanoposthitis from normal bacteria flora involves daily cleaning of the preputial orifice to remove exudate and irrigating the preputial cavity with saline or a dilute (10%) white vinegar solution. Treatment with systemic antibiotics may prolong the course of the infection and select from more pathogenic, resistant bacteria. Herpes viral infections tend to be self-limiting in neonates more than 3 weeks of age and require no specific treatment. Antifungal and chemotherapeutic therapies safe for pediatric patients should be instituted for blastomycosis infections and transmissible venereal tumors.

REPRODUCTIVE DISORDERS IN FEMALE PEDIATRIC PATIENTS

Ovarian Abnormalities

Congenital ovarian abnormalities are not typically diagnosed in pediatric patients in part because of sexual immaturity of most dogs and cats less than 12 months of age. Congenital ovarian abnormalities include presence of supernumerary ovaries, agenesis, hypoplasia, and atypical development (ovotestis). In the condition of supernumerary ovaries, two ovaries located ipsilaterally approximately 1 cm apart within the broad ligament were found on a cat. The two ipsilateral ovaries are each smaller than the contralateral ovary, but their total mass exceeds that of the contralateral ovary. Both unilateral and bilateral ovarian agenesis has been reported in dogs, whereas only unilateral ovarian agenesis has been reported in queens. Bilateral ovarian agenesis is a cause of pubertal failure (primary anestrus). Ovarian agenesis may be associated with other genital malformations or with uterus unicornis. Right unilateral ovarian agenesis was reported in association with the absence of the right uterine tube, right uterine horn, right half of the uterine body, right kidney, and right ureter. Ovarian hypoplasia in the bitch and queen results from an abnormal karyotype (XO, XXX, XO/XX, XO/XXOO, or X/XXX). Dogs and cats with X-chromosome monosomy (XO) are phenotypically female but have shortened statures compared with breed standards without other somatic abnormalities. Affected individuals fail to show pubertal estrus by 2 years of age (primary anestrus) as a result of bilateral ovarian dysgenesis. Diagnosis can be made from cytogenetic testing and/or histologic gonadal examination.

The triple-X syndrome reported in dogs is similar to humans. External and internal genitalia are phenotypically female but infantile because of the absence of estrogenic stimulation. Histologic examination of the ovaries reveals complete absence of follicles/oocytes (ovarian dysgenesis). This condition most likely results from chromosomal nondisjunction in meiosis.

True hermaphroditism is rare in the dog and cat population. True hermaphrodites have both ovarian and testicular

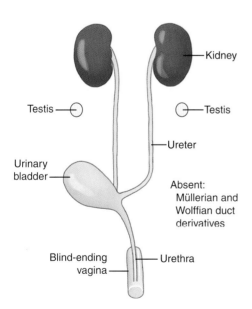

Figure 39-9 Schematic representation of the internal and external genitalia in a domestic cat with testicular feminization syndrome. (Redrawn from Meyers-Wallen VN et al: Testicular feminization in a cat, *J Am Vet Med Assoc* 195:631-634, 1989.)

Kidney

Testis

Testis

Ureter

Urinary bladder

Absent: Müllerian and Wolffian duct derivatives

Blind-ending vagina

Urethra

tissue. Ovotestes may represent one or both gonads, or one gonad may be an ovary and the other a testis. Several cases have been reported in the dog. True hermaphrodites can be either chimeras (XX/XY or XX/XYY) or possess an XX karyotype, with the latter being the most common in dogs. Only true hermaphrodite chimeras have been reported in queens. A chimera is an individual composed of two or more types of cells, each type arising from different sources and containing different chromosome constitutions. Fusion of two zygotes differing in sex chromosome constitutions accounts for some chimeras. The gonadal and phenotypic sex of chimeras depends on the sex chromosome constitution of the separate cell lines and their distribution in the gonadal primordium. If one cell line contains a Y-chromosome and the other does not, clearly demarcated ovarian and testicular tissue can develop within the same gonad.

True hermaphrodites with an XX-chromosome constitution (XX sex reversal) have abdominal unilateral or bilateral ovotestes and an enlarged clitoris (with an os clitoris) (Figure 39-10). Only rarely does the clitoris of normal bitches contain bone. Affected animals display primary anestrus, irregular estrous cycles, or normal fertility. This is an inherited defect in American and English Cocker Spaniels, Beagles, Chinese Pugs, Kerry Blue Terriers, Weimaraners, Soft Coated Wheaton Terriers, Doberman Pinschers, and German Short-haired Pointers. This defect involves a translocation of the *Sry* gene to the X-chromosome or to an autosome. The mode of inheritance is autosomal recessive. The parents of affected dogs are carriers, as are at least two thirds of the male and female siblings. Cases of XX sex reversal have also been reported in the Basset Hound, Vizsla, Soft Coated Wheaton Terrier, Pomeranian, Doberman Pinscher, American Pit Bull Terrier, Border Collie, Walker Hound, and Afghan Hound. In the Cocker Spaniel, affected dogs usually have persistent müllerian derivatives despite the presence of testicular tissue. Wolffian duct derivatives (vas deferens) can be found within the uterine myometrium. Diagnosis is made by visual inspection of clitoromegaly in an otherwise normal-appearing female. Histologic examination of the gonads reveals the presence of both ovarian and testicular tissue, and karyotype confirms an XX-chromosomal constitution.

Internal Genital Tract Abnormalities

The uterine body, cervix, and cranial vagina develop from paired müllerian ducts that fuse during embryonic life. Congenital anomalies in dogs and cats include segmental aplasia (uterus unicornis, segmental aplasia of the uterine horn, and aplasia of the caudal uterine body and/or cervix), uterine hypoplasia, partial fusion of the uterine horns, and duplication of a uterine horn. When one uterine horn is absent, the ovary and uterine tube are generally present on the affected side. This abnormality is usually an incidental finding during ovariohysterectomy (Figure 39-11). Heritability of uterine horn aplasia is unknown. Agenesis of the cervix has been reported in a bitch with the uterine body ending blindly. The uterus was separated from the vagina by a membranous

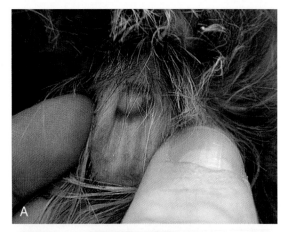
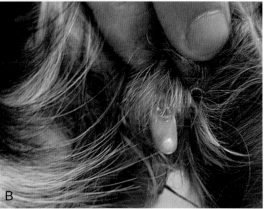
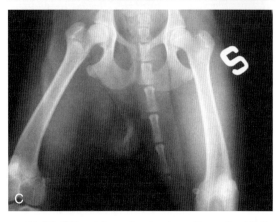

Figure 39-10 Clitoral hypertrophy in a 6-month-old English Cocker Spaniel. An enlarged clitoris can be noted dilating the vulvar lips **(A)** and can be fully appreciated following exteriorization by applying forward pressure against each vulvar lip **(B)**. On ventrodorsal radiography, ossification of the os clitoris can be observed **(C)**. (From Romagnoli S, Schlafer DH: Disorders of sexual differentiation in puppies and kittens: a diagnostic and clinical approach, *Vet Clin North Am Small Anim Pract* 36:573-606, 2006.)

tissue and became secondarily distended with fluid. Congenital cysts of the mesosalpinx that arise from wolffian duct remnants have also been reported. Surgical correction of segmental aplasia has not been described in these species, and the usual treatment is ovariohysterectomy.

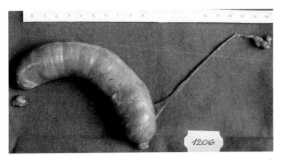

Figure 39-11 Unilateral uterine horn aplasia in a dog. (From Laznicka A, Jaresova H, Vitasek R, et al: Segmental aplasia of mullerian ducts in bitches—as case report, *Veterinarstvi* 47:410-412, 1997.)

External Genital Tract Abnormalities

A papillary projection of the caudal tip of each of these ducts pushes forward into the urogenital sinus to form the müllerian tubercle, which becomes canalized and fuses to the genital fold, forming the caudal vagina and vestibule. The vulvar lips develop from the genital swellings, and the clitoris originates from the genital tubercle. The hymen develops at the junction between the müllerian ducts and the urogenital sinus, and it is usually open at birth in dogs and cats. An incomplete fusion of each of these three embryonic structures within themselves and with each other causes developmental problems at specific sites of the reproductive system. Any ambiguity of the external genitalia should prompt clinicians to perform a thorough investigation of the urogenital system, including a contrast radiographic study of the urinary system. Congenital malformations of the reproductive system are often associated with congenital malformations of the urinary system (see Chapter 38).

Vulvovestibular anomalies can be observed by careful inspection of external genitalia in kittens and puppies and can often be corrected surgically. Congenital abnormalities of feline external genitalia include segmental aplasia of the cranial vagina, an impatent vagina and persistent hymen, presence of a common vulvovestibular-anal opening, and rectovaginal fistula. Vaginal septa, an imperforate hymen, vaginovestibular strictures, vestibulovulvar strictures, segmental aplasia of the vagina, and vulvar agenesis have been reported in the bitch. The most commonly reported vaginal anomalies of the dog are vaginal septa and circumferential vaginovestibular strictures. Although the reported incidence is low (0.03%), the true incidence could be higher because many cases probably go unnoticed if the bitch is not used for breeding. Dogs with congenital vaginal abnormalities may be asymptomatic. No breed predisposition has been identified, and heritability of vaginal anomalies is not well defined. Signs of vaginal septa or strictures in pediatric patients may be absent or may include vaginitis, urinary incontinence (most common), or urinary tract infections.

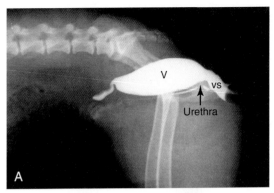

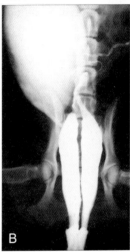

Figure 39-12 Lateral **(A)** and ventrodorsal **(B)** radiographic images of positive-contrast vaginograms from a dog with a vaginal septum (*V*, vagina; *vs*, vestibule). (**A** from Johnston SD, Root Kustritz MV, Olson PN: *Canine and feline theriogenology,* Philadelphia, 2001, Saunders, pp 225-242. **B** from Root MV, Johnston GR: Vaginal septa in dogs: 15 cases (1983-1992), *J Am Vet Med Assoc* 206:56-58, 1995.)

Most vaginal strictures and septa can be detected on vaginal digital examination just cranial to the urethral papilla. If nothing is palpable, the vagina should be examined with an otoscope, vaginoscope, or an endoscope. Contrast vaginography can also be performed (Figure 39-12). Briefly, the patient should be fasted for 12 to 24 hours, and an enema should be administered 2 to 3 hours before the procedure to improve the radiographic detail. The patient should then be anesthetized and placed in lateral recumbency. Iodinated contrast medium diluted with an equal volume of lactated Ringer's solution should be injected into the vagina through a Foley catheter, following inflation of the balloon at the level of the vestibule. The vulvar lips may also need to be held closed to prevent backflow of the contrast medium. Approximately 1 to 5 ml/kg of diluted contrast medium should be infused until back-pressure is felt on the syringe. Both lateral and ventrodorsal radiographic views should be obtained.

Vaginal stricture and septa can be treated with digital manipulation (manual dilation bougienage) in the case of membranous vaginal strictures or surgically via an episiotomy in cases of thicker vaginal strictures or vaginal septa. Vaginal strictures may be treated by performing vaginoplasty or vaginectomy. Vaginal septa must be excised. Surgical correction is also possible for the poor vulvar conformation.

It is not uncommon for female puppies with normal external genitalia to develop vaginitis between 3 and 6 months of age. Juvenile (puppy) vaginitis is vaginal inflammation and is associated with bitches that have not yet undergone puberty. No breed predisposition has been reported. Puppies younger than 6 months of age harbor significantly more coagulase-positive staphylococci than do older animals. The types of bacteria typically found in prepubertal vaginal cultures are listed in Table 39-3. Cranial vaginal culture specimens should be collected with a guarded swab through a vaginal speculum or otoscope cone.

Most dogs affected by juvenile vaginitis show minimal or no clinical signs. Scant mucoid discharge at the vulvar lips is the most common clinical sign described. However, some bitches may exude a large enough volume of discharge to be of concern to the owner, or some bitches may frequently lick their vulva. This condition is often self-limiting, and its resolution can be prolonged by systemic treatment with antibiotics. Conservative therapy including cleaning the perivulvar area with baby wipes or a non–alcohol-based otic cleanser will help to prevent moist dermatitis and allow vaginal inflammation and discharge to resolve spontaneously. If the clinical signs are severe and culture results reveal moderate to heavy growth of one or two bacterial species, the bitch can be treated with sensitive antibiotics. Adjunctive therapy may be considered with glucocorticoids (prednisone 0.5 to 1.0 mg/kg orally once or twice daily, then taper dose if effective) or estrogens (diethylstilbestrol 0.1 to 0.2 mg/kg orally once daily for 5 days, then taper to twice a week), remembering that estrogens used in prepubertal dogs will prematurely close physes. Prevention includes keeping the puppy's perineal area clean, especially for puppies with excess hair around the external genitalia and for puppies with poor external conformation (e.g., recessed vulva). A common question asked by veterinarians is whether dogs with juvenile vaginitis should be allowed to go through one estrous cycle before ovariohysterectomy. No studies have evaluated whether this would be beneficial. In a retrospective study describing seven dogs with juvenile vaginitis that were left intact, three improved after one estrous cycle, one improved after two estrous cycles, and three showed no improvement after

---

TABLE 39-3 Normal vaginal bacterial flora from puppies 1-11 weeks and 12-24 weeks of age*

Type of isolate	Age (1-11 weeks)	Age (12-24 weeks)
α-Hemolytic staphylococci	15%	19%
β-Hemolytic staphylococci	30%	14.3%
Bacillus spp.	15%	14.3%
Coagulase-negative staphylococci	30%	23.8%
Coagulase-positive staphylococci	65%	66.7%
Corynebacterium spp.	10%	9.5%
Escherichia coli	45%	38.1%
Klebsiella spp.	0%	4.8%
Micrococcus spp.	0%	14.3%
Neisseria spp.	0%	4.8%
Nonhemolytic staphylococci	20%	9.5%
Proteus spp.	15%	4.8%
Pseudomonas spp.	5%	0%

*In most cultures, more than one isolate was identified.
Modified from Olson PNS, Mather EC: Canine vaginal and uterine bacterial flora, *J Am Vet Med Assoc* 172:709, 1978.

BOX 39-3 Society for Theriogenology (SFT) and American College of Theriogenologists (ACT) position statement on mandatory spay/neuter procedures

The ACT and SFT believe that companion animals not intended for breeding should be spayed or neutered; however, both organizations believe that the decision to spay or neuter a pet must be made on a case-by-case basis, and this decision should be made between the pet's owner and its veterinarian, taking into consideration the pet's age, breed, sex, health status, intended use, household environment, and temperament. Although there are health benefits to spaying and neutering, these must be weighed against the health benefits of the sex steroids. In general, the advantages of spaying or neutering a pet include effective population control, decreased aggression, decreased wandering, decreased risk of being hit by a car, and decreased risk of mammary, testicular, and ovarian cancer. On the other hand, the disadvantages of spaying or neutering may include increased risk of obesity, diabetes, osteosarcoma, hemangiosarcoma, prostatic adenocarcinoma, transitional cell carcinoma, urinary tract infections, urinary incontinence, autoimmune thyroiditis, hypothyroidism, and hip dysplasia. Therefore the decision to spay or neuter a dog or cat should be made solely by the pet's owner with the direct input of its veterinarian and will depend on each particular animal's situation.

From Society for Theriogenology and American College of Theriogenologists: *Position Statement of Mandatory Spay-Neuter,* http://www.therio.org/displaycommon.cfm?an=1&subarticlenbr=213. Society for Theriogenology website; last Accessed Sept. 10, 2008.

multiple estrous cycles but had subsequent resolution by 3 years of age. This suggests that resolution may not be associated with hormonal changes but rather improved immunity with age. The decision when to perform the ovariohysterectomy should be made between the pet's owner and the owner's veterinarian, taking into consideration the pet's age, health status, intended use, household environment, and temperament (Box 39-3).

SUGGESTED READINGS

Johnston SD, Root Kustritz MV, Olson PN: *Canine and feline theriogenology,* Philadelphia, 2001, Saunders.

Peter AT: The reproduction system. In Hoskins JD (ed): *Veterinary pediatrics: dogs and cats from birth to six months,* ed 3, Philadelphia, 2001, Saunders, pp 463-475.

Romagnoli S, Schlafer DH: Disorders of sexual differentiation in puppies and kittens: a diagnostic and clinical approach, *Vet Clin North Am Small Anim Pract* 36:573, 2006.

THE NEUROLOGIC SYSTEM

CHAPTER 40

Linda Lou Blythe

The nervous system is a complicated collection of neurons, neuroglial cells, and blood vessels that function to acquire sensory input from the environment (afferent input), integrate it, and allow for a motor or glandular response (efferent output). The two major subdivisions are the central nervous system, which includes the brain and spinal cord, and the peripheral nervous system, which consists of peripheral nerves, lemmocytes, sensory receptors, and motor endplates. The autonomic nervous system (ANS) is composed of both central and peripheral nervous system components. The ANS is an involuntary system striving to maintain homeostasis of the body by activating smooth muscle, cardiac muscle, and glands.

NERVOUS SYSTEM DEVELOPMENT

Clinically, one needs to have an elementary understanding of how the nervous system is formed to appreciate anatomical problems that can arise in this development process and the clinical effects on neonatal and young dogs and cats. In an embryo, the nervous system develops from the ectodermal layer that lies dorsal to the notochord. A proliferation of these cells forms the neuroectoderm, which is also known as the neural plate. With differential rates of cellular proliferation, this neural plate invaginates to form first a neural groove and then, when the dorsal edges meet and fuse, a neural tube with an internal neural canal extending the length of the neural tube (Figure 40-1). A group of cells on the dorsal lateral aspect of the neural tube separate and become the neural crest cells. These cells will become the neurons that form the autonomic and spinal or dorsal root ganglia and the lemmocytes (Schwann cells) that will myelinate the peripheral nervous system.

The initial fusion of the neural groove in the neural tube takes place at what will be the caudal end of the brain, the rhombencephalon, and it progresses both rostrally and caudally (Figure 40-2). For reference, scientific and common names for the subdivisions of the brain are shown in Table 40-1. The rostral section develops into the brain, and the caudal section becomes the spinal cord. The brain initially forms into three distinct vesicles: the prosencephalon, the mesencephalon, and the caudal rhombencephalon. With differential grown of neurons in these three sections, the prosencephalon further subdivides into the telencephalon, the future paired cerebral hemispheres, and the internally located diencephalon (Figure 40-3). Likewise the rhombencephalon rostrally becomes the metencephalon (pons) and caudally the myelencephalon (medulla oblongata). The cerebellum arises from rapid outgrowth of the dorsal part of the metencephalon in a structure called the rhombic lip.

Inside the developing neural tube, the space of the neural canal also changes. In the caudal part of the developing brain, the canal changes into a dorsally flattened fourth ventricle shared by the metencephalon and myelencephalon. In the mesencephalon (the midbrain), the neural canal is the least changed, remaining a narrow passageway called the mesencephalic aqueduct (cerebral aqueduct) that is subject to blockage secondary to inflammation within the brain. In the diencephalon, the canal becomes a vertically arranged space, the third ventricle, extending from the top in the epithalamus to the bottom in the infundibulum of the diencephalon. It is in the telencephalon or cerebral hemispheres where the canal is most changed as it develops from a canal into two laterally and ventrally located paired lateral ventricles that follow the massive expansion of this subdivision, the cerebral hemispheres (see Figure 40-3). Each of these lateral ventricles connects with the third ventricle through an interventricular foramen, another narrow anatomical part of the ventricular system where inflammation can cause blockage of the cerebrospinal fluid (CSF) flow. Approximately 35% of the total CSF is produced in the lateral and third ventricle by a vascular-ependymal structure called the

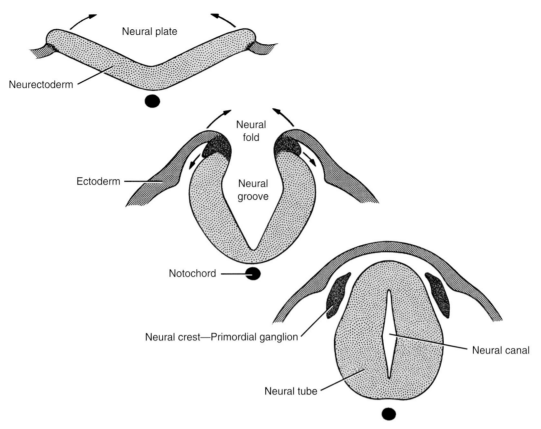

Figure 40-1 Development of the neural tube. (From de Lahunta A, Glass E: *Veterinary neuroanatomy and clinical neurology*, ed 3, St Louis, 2009, Saunders/Elsevier.)

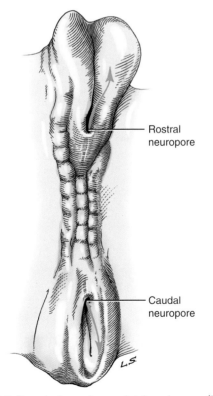

Figure 40-2 Dorsal view of neural tube closure. (From de Lahunta A, Glass E: *Veterinary neuroanatomy and clinical neurology*, ed 3, St Louis, 2009, Saunders/Elsevier.)

TABLE 40-1	Scientific and common names for the subdivisions of the brain
Scientific name	**Common name**
Diencephalon	No common name; contains thalamus, hypothalamus, and epithalamus
Mesencephalon	Midbrain
Metencephalon	Pons
Myelencephalon	Medulla oblongata
Telencephalon	Cerebral hemispheres; contains archicortex (hippocampus), pyriform lobe, and neocortex

choroid plexus. This CSF then flows caudally through the cerebral aqueduct to the fourth ventricle, where additional CSF is produced (approximately 23% of the total) and escapes from the interior of the brain through the lateral apertures in the metencephalon (pons) to flow into the subarachnoid space surrounding the brain and spinal cord. Absorption of CSF occurs primarily through one-way valves, the arachnoid granules (villi), into the venous sinuses. Malformation or inflammation that blocks the internal flow or the absorption of CSF will result in a clinical condition called hydrocephalus (see the next section).

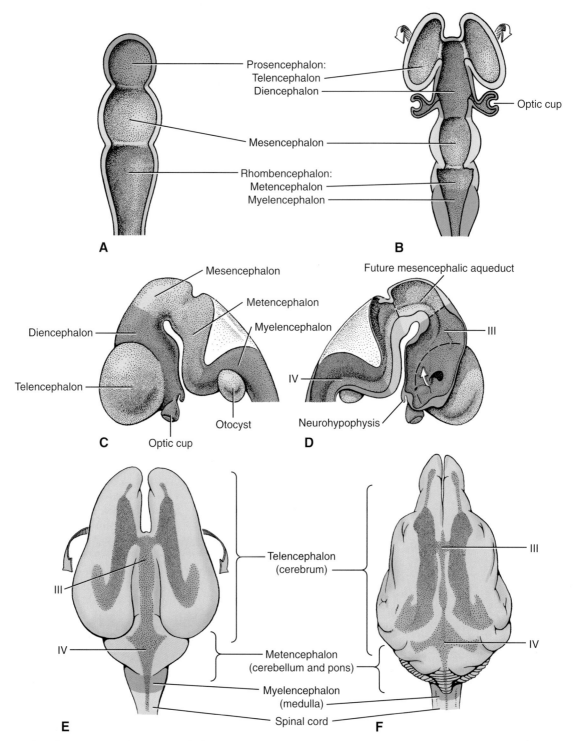

Figure 40-3 Development of brain vesicles. **A,** Three vesicle stages. **B** to **F,** Five vesicle stages, III, IV—ventricles. (From de Lahunta A, Glass E: *Veterinary neuroanatomy and clinical neurology,* ed 3, St Louis, 2009, Saunders/Elsevier.)

CONGENITAL OR ANOMALOUS BRAIN CONDITIONS WITH CLINICAL SIGNS FROM BIRTH TO 2 MONTHS OF AGE

As a reference, Table 40-2 provides definitions for the congenital neurologic conditions that are described more fully in the following paragraphs. In the developing embryo, failure of the rostral segment to properly fuse and develop results in several anomalous conditions collectively called cranial dysraphism. Anencephaly occurs when the cerebral hemispheres fail to develop. This is rare and most commonly causes the fetus to die in utero, but on occasion a puppy or kitten may live to be born and then die often within hours after birth. Encephaly is a condition in which the cerebral

TABLE 40-2 Definition of congenital neurologic conditions

Congenital neurologic condition	Definition
Cerebellar abiotrophy	A degenerative condition in which premature death of neurons in the cerebellum is caused by disruption of the metabolic processes necessary for cell vitality and function
Cerebellar hypoplasia	Failure of the cerebellar cortex to fully develop, often secondary to viral infection
Cerebral aplasia (anencephaly; prosencephalic hypoplasia)	Absence of cerebral hemispheres
Dandy-Walker syndrome	Malformation or absence of the cerebellar vermis
Hydranencephaly	Destruction or lack of development of the neocortex
Hydrocephaly	An enlargement of the cerebral ventricular system secondary to an increase in volume of CSF
Hydromyelia	Dilation of the central canal of the spinal cord
Lissencephaly	Absence of gyri and sulci in cerebral cortex
Meningocele	Protrusion of a fluid-filled sac of meninges through a defect in the calvaria
Meningoencephalocele (encephalocele)	Protrusion of brain tissue through a defect in the calvaria that is still covered by meninges and skin
Microencephaly	Overall reduction in the size of the brain
Porencephaly	Cystic cavities in the cerebral cortex usually secondary to infection
Syringomyelia	Cavitation of the spinal core parenchyma

hemispheres and meningeal coverings protrude from an opening in the calvaria. These puppies and kittens also die shortly after birth, if not before. Encephalocele is inherited in Burmese cats. In addition, pregnant queens exposed to griseofulvin may have their kittens in utero suffer these malformations and others, including agenesis of the corpus callosum and cyclopia. Reports of congenital anomalies in puppies born to bitches receiving griseofulvin during pregnancy have been reported. Meningocele, cranium bifidum,

and cyclopia are also a result of failure of the rostral segment to develop correctly.

Puppies and kittens with porencephaly have cysts inside the brain that are hypothesized to result from a fetal vascular malformation and may also occur with failure of the ventricular system to develop normally with concurrent hydrocephalus. It also may be a result of destruction of parts of the neocortex secondary to infection. Hydranencephaly is a condition in which the white matter of the neocortex is destroyed or fails to develop resulting in a fluid-filled meningeal sac in place of the brain tissue. In utero viral infection has been documented as one of the causes in large animals, dogs, and kittens. In the latter, the panleukopenia virus has been implicated, but these cases are rare compared with the cerebellar hypoplasia lesion of exposed prenatal and neonatal kittens. Vaccination of pregnant queens early in pregnancy is preventative for these conditions.

In almost all these anomalous conditions (cerebellar lesions being an exception), the newborn puppies and kitten die shortly after birth. In some, the abnormality is visible externally (e.g., hydrocephalus, encephalocele), whereas in others, such as hydranencephaly, the diagnosis is made during postmortem examination of the brain. Seizures may be seen before death.

Lissencephaly is a condition in all animals in which the gyri of the cerebral cortex are reduced in size or fail to develop. In Wire Fox Terriers, Irish Setters, and Lhasa Apsos, a genetic basis is suspected based on an increased incidence reported in these breeds. A report on a Korat breed of cats documented lissencephaly associated with microencephaly in which clinical signs of abnormal behavior, including self-mutilation, were evident. Common clinical signs of lissencephaly include visual deficits, lack of postural responses when testing conscious proprioception, varying depression (obtund) to hyperexcitability with aggression to owner, and seizures. Constant compulsive circling may also occur.

Hydrocephalus is a dilation of the ventricular system within the brain resulting in increased hydrostatic pressure from the CSF on the brain tissue, especially that adjacent to the lateral and third ventricles. This leads to either developmental failure (agenesis) or atrophy. Hydrocephalus can either be congenital or acquired after birth. Blockage of CSF flow within the brain is called internal hydrocephalus. Failure of the CSF to be absorbed, often secondary to meningitis and loss of the arachnoid granulations (arachnoid villi), is called external hydrocephalus. In either case, brain tissue fails to develop or atrophies as a result of increased CSF pressure within the skull. When this occurs in utero or shortly after birth before closure of the sutures of the skull, an enlargement of the skull occurs. The fetus may die in utero or shortly after birth. The enlarged head may cause a dystocia at the time of parturition because of the disproportionate size relative to the maternal birth canal. In less severe cases, a domed forehead may be present at birth or become evident to the owner between 2 and 3 months of age (Figure 40-4). The eyes may be malpositioned with ventral lateral deviation because of the prominent frontal areas mechanically

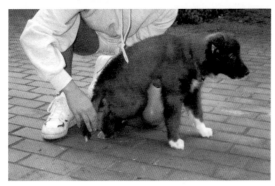

Figure 40-4 Mixed 3-month-old shepherd-breed puppy with domed head suggestive of hydrocephalus and loss of conscious proprioception postural responses.

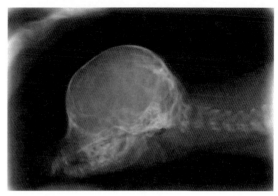

Figure 40-6 Lateral radiographic view of the skull from a dog with hydrocephalus showing enlargement, thinning of the bones of the calvaria, and a persisting open fontanelle.

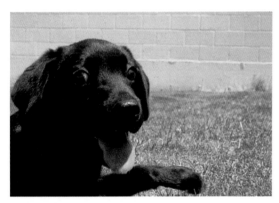

Figure 40-5 Ventrolateral deviation of the eyes in a 4-month-old Labrador Retriever puppy with congenital hydrocephalus.

affecting the orbits (Figure 40-5). Clinical signs of this age of puppy or kitten would include failure to thrive, seizures, behavioral signs ranging from aggression to depression, and possible absence of conscious proprioception responses and the menace response. If there are open fontanelles, ultrasound may be used to visualize the dilated ventricles. Radiographs of the skull may show an enlarged skull, thinning of the bones of the calvaria, and presence of a persisting open fontanelle (Figure 40-6). Previously the term "ground glass appearance of the calvaria" was used, which is not necessarily characteristic of hydrocephalus. Advanced imaging using computed tomography and magnetic resonance imaging (MRI) would also give a definitive diagnosis (Figure 40-7).

Hydrocephalus is most commonly a congenital condition of varying degrees of severity in both dogs and cats. Small breed dogs have been reported to be at increased risk. Examples include Maltese, Chihuahua, Pekingese, Lhasa Apso, toy Poodle, Pomeranian, Pug, English Bulldog, and the small Terrier breeds. Acquired hydrocephalus is more difficult to diagnose clinically because with all skull sutures closed, the skull does not change in size. It is most commonly caused by an infectious agent affecting the brain tissue. In these cases, the clinical signs are often more severe and rapidly progressive (Figure 40-8).

Increased CSF pressure in acquired cases may be measured, but this also puts the animal at risk for herniation of the brain under the tentorium cerebelli or through the foramen magnum. Increased cells and protein may indicate an active infection, and culture of the CSF may reveal the causative organism if it is bacterial. Detection of neutralizing antibodies from serum and CSF for viral causes of encephalitis (e.g., canine distemper, parainfluenza) may be useful in determining the causative agent. Sudden death may occur from both congenital and acquired hydrocephalus. Medical management with dexamethasone (0.25 mg/kg orally twice daily) or prednisone (0.25 to 0.50 mg/kg orally twice daily) may stop the progression and cause improvement in those animals whose neurologic deficits do not preclude them being a family pet. Corticosteroids reduce cerebral edema and often reverse clinical signs but should not be used if encephalitis is present as the result of an infectious agent. With improvement, the corticosteroid dose is reduced by one half for 1 week and then given every other day for several weeks. If signs are stable, the drugs may be discontinued and then given only as needed. In selected cases where medical management is not successful, a surgically placed CSF shunt may be elected. Under general anesthesia, a drainage tube with a one-way valve is placed from the lateral ventricle to the right atrium or the peritoneal cavity. In growing animals, the shunt may need to be replaced to accommodate the growth. Other complications of shunts include sepsis and occlusion of the tubing by fibrous tissue or clots.

Cerebellar disease is a common neurologic condition seen in young kittens and puppies. Cerebellar hypoplasia is common in kittens secondary to in utero or postnatal feline panleukopenia virus infections. The virus attacks the rapidly dividing granule cells and is cytotoxic to the Purkinje cell layer, both of which are located in the cerebellar cortex. In puppies, it is most likely an inherited condition, but canine herpesvirus and parvovirus may also be causative factors. Inherited congenital cerebellar disease is an autosomal recessive defect in Chow Chows, Bullmastiffs, Irish Setters, and some cats. It may be a primary cerebellar hypoplasia or malformation or a die-back process of a normally formed

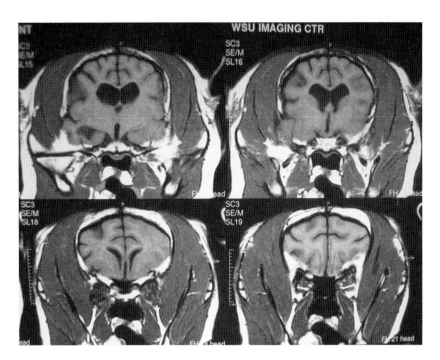

Figure 40-7 MRI of a dog with dilated ventricles that are diagnostic for hydrocephalus.

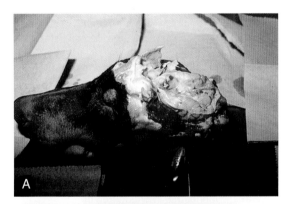

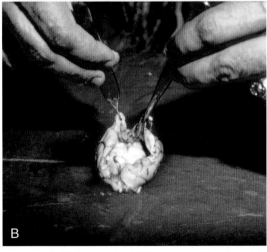

Figure 40-8 **A,** Eight-month-old Doberman Pinscher dog with sudden onset of clinical signs of seizures. Head size was normal, but on removal of the bone of the skull, the thinned cerebral cortices collapsed. **B,** Brain from the dog in **A** illustrating the markedly enlarged lateral ventricles and the thinning of the cerebral cortices.

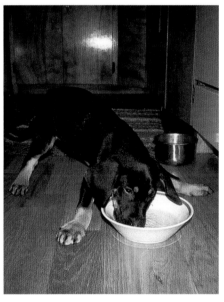

Figure 40-9 Eight-week-old mixed hound puppy with signs of cerebellar hypoplasia. Over time, this dog's clinical signs lessened, and only the hypermetria and loss of the menace response persisted. He lived to 10 years of age as a family pet.

cerebellum called cerebellar abiotrophy. Table 40-3 lists the breeds of dogs and cats most commonly affected by cerebellar abiotrophy. Postnatal cerebellar abiotrophy has been reported to be an autosomal recessive inheritance in Kerry Blue Terriers, Rough-Coated Collies, and Old English Sheepdogs and is suspected in Gordon Setters.

Regardless of the cause, clinical signs are similar in both puppies and kittens with head tremors, ataxia, and hypermetria (Figure 40-9). Postural responses of extensor postural

TABLE 40-3	Degenerative neurologic diseases of young cats and dogs		
Breed	**Disorder**	**Age at onset**	**Clinical signs**
Korat cat	GM$_1$ gangliosidosis	4-8 wk	Tremor, ataxia, blindness, seizures
Manx cat	Sacrocaudal malformation	Birth	Paraparesis, urinary-fecal incontinence
Siamese cat	GM$_1$, GM$_2$ gangliosidosis	3-6 mo	Ataxia, tremor, tetraparesis
	Mucopolysaccharidosis	6-8 wk	Stunted growth, broad face, corneal clouding, paraparesis may develop later
	Sphingomyelinosis	4-6 mo	Ataxia, tremor, hypermetria
	Congenital strabismus and nystagmus	Birth	Strabismus, nystagmus
	Cerebellar abiotrophy	<6 mo	Posterior/truncal ataxia, hypermetria, intention tremor
Afghan Hound	Hereditary myelopathy	3-8 mo	Paraparesis progressing to tetraparesis
Airedale Terrier	Cerebellar hypoplasia and abiotrophy	<6 mo	Ataxia, hypermetria, intention tremor
Akita	Cerebellar degeneration	<6 mo	Ataxia, hypermetria, intention tremor
	Congenital vestibular disease	Birth	Ataxia, rolling, head tilt
Beagle	Meningitis/vasculitis	<1 yr	Hyperesthesia, stilted gait, ataxia
	Cerebellar abiotrophy	<4 wk	Ataxia, hypermetria, intention tremor
Bernese Mountain Dog	Hypomyelination	<3 wk	Tremor
	Meningitis/vasculitis	<1 yr	Cervical hyperesthesia, stilted gait, pyrexia
	Cerebellar abiotrophy		Ataxia, hypermetria, intention tremor
Bluetick Coonhound	Globoid cell leukodystrophy	3-6 mo	Paraparesis progressing to tetraparesis, tremor
Border Collie	Cerebellar abiotrophy		Ataxia, hypermetria, intention tremor
Boston Terrier	Hemivertebrae	Variable	Often subclinical; may cause hyperesthesia, ataxia, paresis
	Hydrocephalus	<6 mo	Depression, blindness, circling, ventrolateral strabismus, enlarged calvaria
Bouvier des Flandres	Laryngeal hemiplegia	4-6 mo	Exercise intolerance, stridor, dyspnea
Boxer	Progressive axonopathy	3-6 mo	Paraparesis progressing to tetraparesis, hyporeflexia
Brittany Spaniel	Hereditary canine spinal muscular atrophy	4-6 mo	Crouching ataxic gait, proximal limb muscle atrophy, hyporeflexia
	Cerebellar abiotrophy		Ataxia, hypermetria, intention tremor
Bullmastiff	Cerebellar abiotrophy	6-9 wk	Ataxia, hypermetria, intention tremor
	Cervical spondylopathy	3-4 mo	Posterior ataxia, cervical hyperesthesia
Cairn Terrier	Globoid cell leukodystrophy	3-6 mo	Paraparesis progressing to tetraparesis, blindness, tremor
	Chromatolytic neuronal degeneration	4-7 mo	Paraparesis progressing to tetraparesis, hyporeflexia, head tremor; cataplexy
Chihuahua	Hydrocephalus	<6 mo	Depression, blindness, circling, ventrolateral strabismus, enlarged calvaria
	Neuronal ceroid lipofuscinosis	12-15 mo	Dementia, ataxia, seizures
	Neuroaxonal dystrophy	7 wk	Tremor, ataxia, hypermetria
Chow Chow	Dysmyelination	Birth-4 wk	Ataxia, tremor
	Cerebellar hypoplasia	Birth-4 wk	Ataxia, dysmetria, tremor
	Myotonia	2-4 wk	Muscle stiffness, myotonic dimple
Cocker Spaniel	Multisystem neuronal degeneration	6-10 mo	Seizures, tremor, ataxia, aggression
	Congenital vestibular disease	Birth	Ataxia, rolling, head tilt
Collie	Cerebellar degeneration	4-8 wk	Posterior/truncal ataxia, hypermetria, intention tremor
Dachshund	Sensory neuropathy	Birth-4 wk	Ataxia, decreased pain sensation, self-mutilation
	Narcolepsy-cataplexy	<6 mo	Excess sleep, postural collapse (cataplexy)

TABLE 40-3   Degenerative neurologic diseases of young cats and dogs—cont'd

Breed	Disorder	Age at onset	Clinical signs
Dalmatian	Congenital deafness	Birth	Deafness
	Cavitating leukodystrophy	3-6 mo	Paraparesis progressing to tetraparesis; behavioral abnormalities; visual loss
	Peripheral neuropathy	6-24 mo	Progressive weakness, distal limb muscle atrophy, laryngeal paresis
	Reflex myoclonus	2-6 wks	Muscular hypertonicity exacerbated by exercise
Doberman Pinscher	Narcolepsy-cataplexy	<6 mo	Excess sleep, postural collapse (cataplexy)
	Congenital vestibular disease	3-12 wk	Head tilt, ataxia, circling, nystagmus
English Bulldog	Hydrocephalus	6 mo	Depression, blindness, circling, ventrolateral strabismus, enlarged calvaria
	Sacrocaudal malformation	Birth	Paraparesis, urinary-fecal incontinence
	Hemivertebrae	Variable	Often subclinical; may cause hyperesthesia, ataxia, paresis
English Pointer	Sensory neuropathy	<6 mo	Distal limb anesthesia and self-mutilation
English Setter	Congenital deafness	Birth	Deafness
	Neuronal ceroid lipofuscinosis	12-15 mo	Dementia, ataxia, seizures
Finnish Harrier	Cerebellar abiotrophy	<6 mo	Posterior/truncal ataxia, hypermetria, intention tremor
German Shepherd Dog	Congenital vestibular disease	3-4 wk	Head tilt, ataxia
	Spinal muscular atrophy	<4 wk	Valgus deformity of thoracic limb(s) due to flexor contracture, tetraparesis
German Shorthaired Pointer	GM₁ gangliosidosis	6-12 mo	Dementia, blindness, seizures
Golden Retriever	Hypomyelinating polyneuropathy	<7 wk	Pelvic limb ataxia and weakness, hyporeflexia
	Cerebellar abiotrophy	<6 mo	Posterior/truncal ataxia, hypermetria, intention tremor
Gordon Setter	Hereditary cortical cerebellar abiotrophy	6-24 mo	Ataxia, dysmetria
Great Dane	Cervical spondylopathy	6-24 mo	Posterior ataxia progressing to tetraparesis
	Cerebellar abiotrophy	<6 mo	Posterior/truncal ataxia, hypermetria, intention tremor
Irish Setter	Hereditary quadriplegia and amblyopia	Birth-5 wk	Tetraplegia, tremor, nystagmus, seizures
	Cerebellar abiotrophy	<6 mo	Posterior/truncal ataxia, hypermetria, intention tremor
Jack Russell Terrier	Myasthenia gravis	6 wk	Episodic weakness
	Hereditary ataxia	2-6 mo	Paraparesis progressing to tetraparesis, ataxia, dysmetria
	Cerebellar abiotrophy	<6 mo	Posterior/truncal ataxia, hypermetria, intention tremor
Kerry Blue Terrier	Hereditary cerebellar cortical and extrapyramidal nuclear abiotrophy	9-16 wk	Ataxia, hypermetria, tremor, hypertonia
Labrador Retriever	Reflex myoclonus	2-4 wk	Muscle hypertonicity, extensor rigidity, opisthotonus increased with exercise
	Cerebellar abiotrophy	<6 mo	Posterior/truncal ataxia, hypermetria, intention tremor
	Spongiform encephalopathy	4-6 mo	Dysmetria, tremor, extensor rigidity
	Narcolepsy-cataplexy	<6 mo	Excess sleep, postural collapse (cataplexy)
	Cavitating leukodystrophy	4 mo-adult	Ataxia, blindness, depression
Lhasa Apso	Lissencephaly	<18 mo	Depression, poor housetraining, seizures
Maltese dog	Idiopathic tremor	6 mo-5 yr	Generalized tremor
	Hydrocephalus	<1 yr	Seizures, depression, poor housetraining
Miniature Poodle	Cerebellar abiotrophy	<6 mo	Posterior/truncal ataxia, hypermetria, intention tremor

Continued

TABLE 40-3	Degenerative neurologic diseases of young cats and dogs—cont'd		
Breed	Disorder	Age at onset	Clinical signs
Old English Sheepdog	Congenital deafness	Birth	Deafness
	Cerebellar abiotrophy	<6 mo	Posterior/truncal ataxia, hypermetria, intention tremor
Poodle	Atlantoaxial subluxation	6-18 mo	Hyperesthesia, ataxia, tetraparesis
	Sphingomyelinosis	4-6 mo	Ataxia, tremor, hypermetria
	Narcolepsy-cataplexy	<6 mo	Excess sleep, postural collapse (cataplexy)
Portuguese Water Dog	GM$_1$ gangliosidosis	<5 mo	Tremor, ataxia, dysmetria, nystagmus
Pug	Meningitis	<3 yr	Seizures, depression, circling, head pressing, blindness, cervical hyperesthesia
Rhodesian Ridgeback	Cerebellar abiotrophy	<6 mo	Posterior/truncal ataxia, hypermetria, intention tremor
Rottweiler	Neuroaxonal dystrophy	1-2 yr	Ataxia, hypermetria, head tremor
	Spinal muscular atrophy	<4 wk	Paraparesis progressing to tetraparesis, hyporeflexia, head tremor
Samoyed	Cerebellar abiotrophy	<6 mo	Posterior/truncal ataxia, hypermetria, intention tremor
	Hypomyelination	<3 wk	Tremor, inability to stand
Scottish Terrier	Scottie cramp	2-18 mo	Muscle hypertonicity following exercise
Siberian Husky	Laryngeal paralysis	<1 yr	Exercise intolerance, dyspnea, stridor
Silky Terrier	Glucocerebrosidosis	6-8 mo	Ataxia, tremor
Smooth-haired Fox Terrier	Hereditary ataxia	2-6 mo	Posterior ataxia, thoracic limb hypermetria
	Myasthenia gravis	4-8 wk	Episodic weakness
Springer Spaniel	Hypomyelination	Birth-4 wk	Ataxia, tremor
	Fucosidosis	6-18 mo	Behavioral changes, ataxia
	Myasthenia gravis	6 wk	Episodic weakness
Swedish Lapland	Hereditary neuronal abiotrophy	5-7 wk	Ataxia progressing to tetraplegia, atrophy of distal limb muscles, hyporeflexia
Tibetan Mastiff	Hypertrophic neuropathy	2-3 mo	Paraparesis progressing to tetraparesis, hyporeflexia
Weimaraner	Spinal dysraphism	Birth-4 wk	Simultaneous advancement of pelvic limbs
West Highland White Terrier	Globoid cell leukodystrophy	3-6 mo	Paraparesis progressing to tetraparesis, blindness, tremor
Yorkshire Terrier	Atlantoaxial subluxation	<1 yr	Tetraparesis, cervical hyperesthesia
	Hepatic encephalopathy	<1 yr	Ataxia, seizures, head pressing, circling, blindness

Modified from Hoskins JD, Shelton GD: The nervous and neuromuscular systems. In Hoskins JD (ed): *Veterinary pediatrics: dogs and cats from birth to six months*, ed 3, Philadelphia, 2001, Saunders, pp 427-430.

thrust, hopping, tactical placing, and knuckling are present as the affected animals know where their body is in space (proprioception), but when tested they appear incoordinated in their responses. This is in contrast to a cortical lesion where normal postural responses are commonly absent (see Figure 40-4). Failure to develop a menace response is also a clinical sign of cerebellar disease as normal blinking in response to a menacing gesture to the eyes requires coordination from the cerebellum. This condition is nontreatable and nonprogressive. Most juvenile and adult cats show the same clinical signs throughout life, whereas some affected dogs have reduced clinical signs as they age. Partial or complete absence of the vermis of the cerebellum has been reported in dogs (Figure 40-10). Moderate to severe signs of cerebellar dysfunction are present, and many of these animals have difficulty in righting themselves or standing.

Congenital peripheral vestibular disease has been reported in multiple breeds of dogs (German Shepherd Dogs, Doberman Pinschers, English Cocker Spaniels, Beagles, Akitas, Smooth Fox Terriers, and Shetland Sheepdogs) and cats (Siamese, Tonkinese, and Burmese cats). The etiopathogenesis is mostly unknown, but a lymphocytic labyrinthitis has been documented in two litters of Doberman Pinschers. Clinical signs include head tilt, circling, and rolling from birth or within a few weeks of age. There are no signs of central vestibular or brain involvement, and the clinical signs may spontaneously resolve or persist for life (Figure 40-11). Deafness may also be present in some cases. Diagnosis is based on clinical signs in young animals

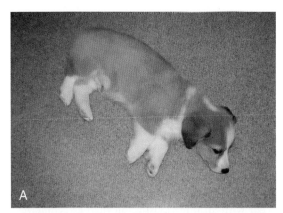

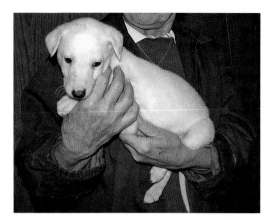

Figure 40-12 White 7-week-old Greyhound puppy with congenital deafness.

Figure 40-10 **A,** Clinical signs of congenital partial or complete absence of the vermis of the cerebellum include moderate to severe signs of cerebellar dysfunction with difficulty in righting themselves or standing. **B,** The vermis of the cerebellum is partially absent on the brain on the right. The brain on the left is normal for comparison.

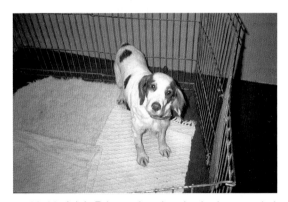

Figure 40-11 Adult Brittany female who had congenital vestibular dysfunction and circled constantly to the left. She was also deaf. This dog lived to 12 years of age as a family pet with no change in clinical signs.

as they begin to walk, and there is no known effective treatment.

Congenital and hereditary deafness is also seen in multiple breeds of white dogs and cats that have the white or merle color gene (Figure 40-12). In addition to the dominant white haircoat, iris coloring abnormalities (often blue eyes) are present. Deafness in these dogs is usually associated with developmental abnormalities of the peripheral cochlear

structure, including the organ of Corti, the spiral ganglion, and the cochlear nucleus. Six- to 8-week-old white puppies or kittens should be tested for their ability to hear and respond to sound on each side of their head. The condition may be unilateral or bilateral. There is no effective treatment for this condition.

Congenital spinal cord anomalies are not uncommon. The fusion of the neural plate in the embryo progresses caudally from behind the area that will develop into the rhombencephalon and may or may not completely fuse at the end of the spinal cord, the conus medullaris. In some cases, the neural canal is open at the end, and CSF can flow through the neural canal out into the subarachnoid space. In these cases, there is no clinical abnormality. The most common clinical abnormality relative to the failure of the neural tube to fuse normally in the caudal direction is spina bifida.

Neurologic form of spina bifida results when the caudal spinal cord and the dorsal aspect of the respective vertebrae fail to fuse during development, most commonly seen in the caudal lumbar, sacral, and caudal (coccygeal) segments. Cats bred to have short or no tails, such as the Manx cat, are most commonly affected. Many kittens are culled early in life because of gait deficits resulting from this condition. Selection of Manx cats with normal tails for breeding would markedly eliminate this genetic malformation. Sporadically, the English Bulldog, the Pug, and Boston Terriers have a similar condition with a presumptive inherited form in the English Bulldog.

When the spinal cord fails to develop, clinical lower motor neuron signs of flaccid paresis to paralysis, failure of pelvic limb musculature to develop, urinary and fecal incontinence, and flaccid anal sphincter and tail tone are evident. A "bunny hop" gait may also occur in animals that can walk. Other animals may have the classic vertebral lesions but no spinal cord abnormalities, and the animals are neurologically normal. In animals that are clinically affected, the skin over the dorsal spines of the affected vertebrae may have protrusion of the meninges and sometimes the spinal cord. There is no treatment for clinically affected animals to correct the deficits. Any exteriorized meninges and/or spinal cord should be surgically covered with skin to prevent infection.

Animals with minor clinical deficits should not be used for breeding.

CONGENITAL OR ANOMALOUS CONDITIONS WITH CLINICAL SIGNS FROM 2 TO 12 MONTHS OF AGE

Some congenital defects do not result in clinical signs at birth but are first seen after weaning. Less commonly seen are congenital defects such as spinal dysraphism and syringomyelia, which are also caused by failure or incomplete closure of the neural tube. Bony malformations such as block vertebrae, hemivertebrae, and transitional vertebrae may be present but not necessarily associated with neurologic clinical signs in the young dog or cat unless their growth causes misalignment and compression of the spinal cord.

Caudal occipital malformation syndrome is caused by occipital bone hypoplasia and a subsequent crowding of the caudal brainstem structures at the level of the foramen magnum. With this condition, there may be a concurrent syringohydromyelia in the cervical and/or thoracic spinal cord. Caudal occipital malformation syndrome has been reported to be hereditary in Cavalier King Charles Spaniels, but the mode of inheritance is not known. It has also been reported in toy breeds, including the Pomeranian, Yorkshire Terrier, and Maltese. In most cases, clinical signs of thoracic limb weakness, pelvic limb ataxia, and cervical scoliosis are localized to the cervical spinal cord segment with a neurologic examination. An additional clinical feature of persistent scratching at the affected region may be seen, especially when the dog is on a leash. Pain may be evident when the neck is touched or manipulated. Although the bony malformation is present in the neonate, clinical signs are usually not evident until after 6 months of age. The neurologic examination to localize the lesion, coupled with radiographs and MRI, is diagnostic. Surgery to decompress the nervous tissue has variable success rates depending on the initial severity of clinical signs and the time from onset to correction. Residual neurologic deficits may be present for life.

Atlantoaxial instability or subluxation is seen in small dog breeds, with clinical signs localized to the cranial cervical spinal cord and usually presenting in the first year. Clinical signs include cervical pain, tetraparesis and ataxia, and hyperreflexia with presence of the upper motor neuron sign of crossed extension reflex while in lateral recumbency. Diagnosis is made using plain radiography, and surgical approaches to stabilize this joint have reported success rates of 85% to 89%.

NEUROLOGIC EXAMINATION OF THE NEONATE AGED 0 TO 3 WEEKS

There are limitations to examining a neonate puppy or kitten because the nervous system is not fully developed at birth, and there are breed differences among dogs and even cats that complicate a precise interpretation of the neurologic examination. For example, a Greyhound puppy will develop the ability to stand before a smaller breed of dog such as a Maltese. In addition, the nervous system of the kitten develops more rapidly than the puppy. In the first 2 weeks, neonates spend time nursing or sleeping, most commonly lying close to littermates. They crawl around on the lower part of their thorax for the first 2 weeks and after that time are able to lift their heads and maintain an upright position. Vocalizations occur as they seek food or are disturbed, but continuous crying is abnormal (see Chapter 2). Continuous crying commonly indicates a cold or hungry pup but also may occur with an infectious lesion such as canine herpesvirus infection (see Chapter 16). In the latter case, clinical signs of depression, opisthotonus, and seizures may also be present.

Increased flexor tone of the limb muscles is seen the first 5 days followed by a shift to an increased extensor tone until 3 weeks of age. After this time, normal muscle tone is present. Deliberate postural responses tested in a standard neurologic examination vary as to when they appear, making neurologic examination of the neonate more difficult. They are all learned responses, but by 6 to 8 weeks they are fully developed. Evaluation of hopping, tactile placing, extensor postural thrust, and ability to hemiwalk may only be useful in the neonate when asymmetric lesions are present and differences are seen in response between right and left sides. Righting reflexes are present shortly after birth, which enables the neonate to nurse. Tendon tap reflexes (e.g., patellar reflex) may be hard to interpret in a puppy or kitten less than 3 weeks of age because of the increased extensor tone of the muscles. Flexor (pain or withdrawal) reflexes and a pain response to a noxious stimulus are present shortly after birth. A crossed extension reflex (pinching one foot and having the opposite limb extend) is present up to 3 weeks of age. After that time, the inhibition of the brain on the reflex develops. Presence of a crossed extensor reflex in a kitten after 17 days and in a puppy after 21 days indicates a brain or upper motor neuron lesion. The anogenital reflex is present at birth. It is elicited by stimulation of the perineal area resulting in urination and defecation. In nature, the dam elicits this reflex. Orphans will need manual stimulation to elicit this reflex by owner the first 2 weeks until voluntary control of these functions is developed (see Chapter 9). After 3 weeks of age, the anogenital reflex cannot be elicited. The panniculus or cutaneous trunci reflex is also present at birth.

Cranial nerve examination can be conducted in puppies and kittens after 2 to 3 weeks of age. The palpebral and corneal reflexes are present at birth but become more easily visualized after the eyelids open. Puppies' eyes open at 9 to 16 days, whereas in kittens, they open between 5 to 14 days (average of 8 days). The menace response in puppies may not appear until the third or fourth week because the retina is not yet fully developed before this time. For the kitten, there may not be a normal menace response until 21 days of age. It is important to remember that menace is a learned response, not a reflex.

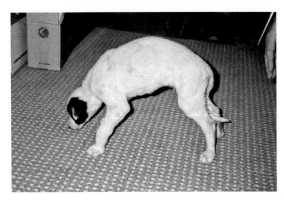

Figure 40-13 Seven-week-old Greyhound puppy with clinical signs of seizures, depression, pain on manipulation of head and neck, and loss of conscious proprioception postural responses. This puppy was reluctant to move and stood with his head down and back arched.

> **BOX 40-1**   **DAMNITT-V scheme of etiologies of neurologic disease**
>
> **D**egenerative
> **A**nomaly or congenital
> **M**etabolic
> **N**eoplastic or nutritional
> **I**nfectious or inflammatory
> **T**oxic
> **T**raumatic
> **V**ascular

Ear canals open in kittens between 6 and 14 days of age (average, 9 days) and have some testable hearing with response to sounds by 21 days. In puppies, ear canals open between 10 and 14 days of age, but hearing cannot be fully evaluated until after 3 weeks of age, when puppies have the motor control to look toward a sound. Disorders of the external ear can be found in Chapter 41. Evaluation of mental attitude is most important in neonates. Depression (Figure 40-13) or hyperexcitability with excessive vocalization would indicate brain disease. Seizures at this age may have a nutritional or metabolic etiology or be the result of an anomalous or infectious lesion in the brain. Causes of seizures can be divided into abnormalities within the brain (i.e., infection, brain tumor, trauma, or idiopathic epilepsy) or abnormalities outside of the brain in other organ systems, such as hypoglycemia, hypocalcemia, liver disease, or exposure to toxins. Ineffective nursing as a result of hypothermia may result in severe hypoglycemia and is a common cause of seizure activity in young puppies.

NEUROLOGIC EXAMINATION OF THE PUPPY OR KITTEN AFTER 3 WEEKS OF AGE

The purpose of this neurologic examination is to determine whether there is a neurologic lesion, and if so, where it is localized in the brain, spinal cord, or peripheral nerves. Once localized, the clinician can make a list of differential diagnoses and then determine the diagnostic tests to confirm or rule out a specific condition. The use of the DAMNITT-V scheme (Box 40-1) and the onset and progression of the clinical signs are good tools in the development of the list of differential diagnoses. An acute progressive disease might indicate an infectious lesion, whereas an acute nonprogressive set of clinical signs might suggest a traumatic or vascular etiology to the disease condition. Anomalous or congenital conditions have been covered in the previous section on the nervous system development.

After 3 weeks of age, the normal neurologic examination procedures can be performed with reliable results. It is beyond the scope of this chapter to fully describe the steps of the neurologic examination, and the clinician is referred to texts on general veterinary neurology. Briefly, evaluation of mental attitude, gait, cranial nerve function, postural responses, tendon and flexor (pain or withdrawal) reflexes, anal sphincter and panniculus (cutaneous trunci) reflexes, presence of sensation, muscle tone, and development needs to be done in a systematic way and the results recorded. Knowing the signalment of the animal, especially the breed of dog or cat, is useful as there are many degenerative conditions that are breed specific or predominant (see Table 40-3).

DEGENERATIVE DISEASES SEEN IN DOGS AND CATS BETWEEN 2 AND 12 MONTHS OF AGE

Many degenerative conditions have been reported in purebred dogs and cats. These conditions, as well as other neurologic conditions common to those breeds, are listed in Table 40-4. Cerebellar abiotrophy and cervical spondylopathy are two of the more common conditions. Cerebellar abiotrophy is a progressive degenerative condition of the cerebellum seen in multiple purebred dogs and cats (see Table 40-3), although sporadic cases have been seen in cross-breed dogs. Unlike cerebellar hypoplasia, for which clinical signs of ataxia, dysmetria, head tremors, and lack of menace response are evident shortly after birth, animals with cerebellar abiotrophy are normal for the first 6 to 8 weeks. Clinical signs consistent with cerebellar disease then become evident in the first year and become progressively worse. There is no treatment. Onset and progression of clinical signs vary depending on the breed. Progression may be limited to ataxia or may deteriorate to paraplegia or tetraplegia. A less severely affected animal may still be acceptable as a pet but should not be used as a breeding animal. The loss of the Purkinje cells in most breeds of dogs with this condition is believed to have a genetic autosomal recessive mode of inheritance.

Cervical spondylopathy is a common neurologic condition in fast-growing large and giant breeds of dogs. Most

TABLE 40-4	Neurologic storage diseases of young cats and dogs			
Breed	**Disorder**	**Enzyme deficient/ storage product**	**Age at onset**	**Clinical signs**
Balinese cat	Sphingomyelinosis (Niemann-Pick) (type C)	Sphingomyelinase (Sphingomyelin)	2-4 mo	Ataxia, incoordination, hypermetria
Domestic cat	Mucopolysaccharidosis II (Maroteaux-Lamy)	Arylsulfatase B	4-7 mo	Progressive paresis
	Globoid cell leukodystrophy (Krabbe)	β-Galactosidase (galactocerebrosidase)	5-6 wk	Ataxia, incoordination, tremor, paraparesis, hypermetria, visual impairment
	Metachromatic leukodystrophy	Arylsulfatase (sulfatide)	2 wk	Progressive motor dysfunction, seizures, opisthotonus
	Mucopolysaccharidosis I (Hurler)	α-L-Iduronidase	10 mo	Progressive motor dysfunction, seizures, opisthotonus; high incidence of meningioma in these cats
	Glycogenesis type II (Pompe)	α-Glucosidase		
	Ceroid lipofuscinosis (Batten)	Unknown	2-7 yr	Personality change, visual impairment, ataxia, incoordination, jaw champing, seizures
	Sphingomyelinosis (Niemann-Pick) (type C)	Sphingomyelinase (Sphingomyelin)	2-4 mo	Ataxia, incoordination, hypermetria
	Gangliosidosis GM$_1$, type 1 (Norman-Landing)	β-Galactosidase	2-3 mo	Tremors, incoordination, spastic paraplegia; visual impairment
	Gangliosidosis GM$_2$, type 2 (Sandhoff)	Hexosaminidase A and B	2 mo	Tremor, incoordination, spastic paraplegia
	Gangliosidosis GM$_2$, type 3 (Bernheimer-Seitelberger)	Hexosaminidase A	2 mo	Ataxia, incoordination, hypermetria
	Mannosidosis	α-Mannosidase (mannoside)	7 mo	Ataxia, incoordination, tremor, aggression
	Mucopolysaccharide VI Mucolipidosis II	Arylsulfatase B deficiency N-Acetylglucosamine-1-phosphotransferase deficiency		
	Gangliosidosis GM$_1$, type 2 (Derry)	β-Galactosidase	2-3 mo	Tremors, incoordination, spastic paraplegia
Korat cat	Gangliosidosis GM$_1$, type 2 (Derry)	β-Galactosidase	2-3 mo	Tremors, incoordination, spastic paraplegia
Norwegian Forest cat	Glycogenesis Type IV (Andersen)	α-Glucosidase		Seizures, hypoglycemia
Persian cat	Mannosidosis	α-Mannosidase (mannoside)	7 mo	Ataxia, incoordination, tremor, aggression
Siamese cat	Ceroid lipofuscinosis (Batten)	Unknown	2-7 yr	Personality change, visual impairment, ataxia, incoordination, jaw champing, seizures
	Mucopolysaccharidosis II (Maroteaux-Lamy)	Arylsulfatase B	4-7 mo	Progressive paresis
	Sphingomyelinosis (Niemann-Pick) (type C)	Sphingomyelinase (Sphingomyelin)	2-4 mo	Ataxia, incoordination, hypermetria
	Gangliosidosis GM$_1$, type 1 (Norman-Landing)	β-Galactosidase	2-3 mo	Tremors, incoordination, spastic paraplegia; visual impairment
	Gangliosidosis GM$_1$, type 2 (Derry)	β-Galactosidase	2-3 mo	Tremors, incoordination, spastic paraplegia

TABLE 40-4		Neurologic storage diseases of young cats and dogs—cont'd		
Breed	Disorder	Enzyme deficient/ storage product	Age at onset	Clinical signs
Australian Cattle Dog	Ceroid lipofuscinosis (Batten)	Unknown		Personality change, visual impairment, ataxia, incoordination, jaw champing, seizures
Basset Hound	Glycoproteinosis (Lafora)	(Glycoprotein?)	5 mo-9 yr	
	Globoid cell leukodystrophy (Krabbe)	β-Galactosidase (galactocerebrosidase)	1-2 yr	Ataxia, incoordination, tremor, paraparesis, hypermetria, visual impairment
Beagle	Glycoproteinosis (Lafora)	(Glycoprotein?)	5 mo-9 yr	Depression, seizures
	Globoid cell leukodystrophy (Krabbe)	β-Galactosidase (galactocerebrosidase)	4 mo	Ataxia, incoordination, tremor, paraparesis, hypermetria, visual impairment
Beagle-cross	Gangliosidosis GM₁, type 1 (Norman-Landing)	β-Galactosidase	3 mo	Tremors, incoordination, spastic paraplegia; visual impairment
Blue Heeler	Ceroid lipofuscinosis (Batten)	Unknown		Personality change, visual impairment, ataxia, incoordination, jaw champing, seizures
Bluetick Coonhound	Globoid cell leukodystrophy (Krabbe)	β-Galactosidase (galactocerebrosidase)	4 mo	Ataxia, incoordination, tremor, paraparesis, hypermetria, visual impairment
Border Collie	Ceroid lipofuscinosis (Batten)	Unknown		Personality change, visual impairment, ataxia, incoordination, jaw champing, seizures
Cairn Terrier	Globoid cell leukodystrophy (Krabbe)	β-Galactosidase (galactocerebrosidase)	2-5 mo	Ataxia, incoordination, tremor, paraparesis, hypermetria, visual impairment
Chihuahua	Ceroid lipofuscinosis (Batten)	Unknown	2 yr	Personality change, visual impairment, ataxia, incoordination, jaw champing, seizures
Cocker Spaniel	Ceroid lipofuscinosis (Batten)	Unknown	1.5 yr	Personality change, visual impairment, ataxia, incoordination, jaw champing, seizures
Dachshund	Ceroid lipofuscinosis (Batten)	Unknown	3.5-7 yr	Personality change, visual impairment, ataxia, incoordination, jaw champing, seizures
Dalmatian	Ceroid lipofuscinosis (Batten)	Unknown		Personality change, visual impairment, ataxia, incoordination, jaw champing, seizures
English Setter	Ceroid lipofuscinosis (Batten)	Unknown	1 yr	Personality change, visual impairment, ataxia, incoordination, jaw champing, seizures
English Springer	Gangliosidosis GM₁, type 1 (Norman-Landing)	β-Galactosidase	2-3 mo	Tremors, incoordination, spastic paraplegia; visual impairment
German Shorthaired Pointer	Gangliosidosis GM₂, type 1 (Tay-Sachs)	Hexosaminidase A	6-9 mo	Ataxia, incoordination, visual impairment, dementia
Japanese Spaniel	Gangliosidosis GM₂, type 1 (Tay-Sachs)	Hexosaminidase A	6-9 mo	Ataxia, incoordination, visual impairment, dementia
Lapland Dog	Glycogenesis type II (Pompe)	α-Glucosidase	1.5 yr	Incoordination, exercise intolerance
Miniature Pinscher	Mucopolysaccharidosis II (Maroteaux-Lamy)	Arylsulfatase B		Progressive paresis

Continued

TABLE 40-4	Neurologic storage diseases of young cats and dogs—cont'd			
Breed	Disorder	Enzyme deficient/ storage product	Age at onset	Clinical signs
Mixed-Breed Dog	Glycoproteinosis (Lafora)	(Glycoprotein?)	5 mo-9 yr	
	Mucopolysaccharidosis I (Hurler)	α-L-Iduronidase		Progressive motor dysfunction, seizures, opisthotonus
Mixed Poodle	Globoid cell leukodystrophy (Krabbe)	β-Galactosidase (galactocerebrosidase)	2 yr	Ataxia, incoordination, tremor, paraparesis, hypermetria, visual impairment
Plott Hound	Mucopolysaccharidosis I (Hurler)	α-L-Iduronidase		Progressive motor dysfunction, seizures, opisthotonus
Pomeranian	Globoid cell leukodystrophy (Krabbe)	β-Galactosidase (galactocerebrosidase)	1.5 yr	Ataxia, incoordination, tremor, paraparesis, hypermetria, visual impairment
Poodle	Glycoproteinosis (Lafora)	(Glycoprotein?)	5 mo-9 yr	
	Sphingomyelinosis (Niemann-Pick)	Sphingomyelinase (Sphingomyelin)	2-4 mo	Ataxia, incoordination, hypermetria
	Ceroid lipofuscinosis (Batten)	Unknown		Personality change, visual impairment, ataxia, incoordination, jaw champing, seizures
Portuguese Water Dog	Gangliosidosis GM$_1$, type 2 (Derry)	β-Galactosidase	5-6 mo	Tremors, incoordination, spastic paraplegia
Saluki	Ceroid lipofuscinosis (Batten)	Unknown	2 yr	Personality change, visual impairment, ataxia, incoordination, jaw champing, seizures
Springer Spaniel	Fucosidosis	α-L-Fucosidase	2 yr	Incoordination, behavioral changes, dysphonia
Sydney Silky Dog	Glucocerebrosidosis (Gaucher)	β-Galactosidase (glucocerebroside)	6-8 mo	Ataxia, incoordination, hypermetria
Terrier Mixed Breed	Ceroid lipofuscinosis (Batten)	Unknown		Personality change, visual impairment, ataxia, incoordination, jaw champing, seizures
Tibetan Terrier	Ceroid lipofuscinosis (Batten)	Unknown		Personality change, visual impairment, ataxia, incoordination, jaw champing, seizures
West Highland Terrier	Globoid cell leukodystrophy (Krabbe)	β-Galactosidase (galactocerebrosidase)	2-5 mo	Ataxia, incoordination, tremor, paraparesis, hypermetria, visual impairment
Yugoslavian Sheepdog	Ceroid lipofuscinosis (Batten)	Unknown		Personality change, visual impairment, ataxia, incoordination, jaw champing, seizures

Modified from Bagley RS: *Fundamentals of veterinary clinical neurology*, Ames, IA, 2005, Blackwell, p 124.

commonly affected are Great Danes and Doberman Pinschers. Genetic and nutritional factors have been implicated, but the exact etiopathology is unknown. Malformation of the mid to caudal cervical vertebrae and surrounding soft tissues compress the spinal cord. Compression results in the upper motor neuron signs of hypertonus, tetraparesis to tetraplegia, and ataxia of all four limbs, with the most prominent neurologic deficits seen in the pelvic limbs. In young Doberman Pinschers, instability causes more neurologic damage than vertebral malformation. Clinical signs may develop as early as 3 months of age. Contrast radiography with a myelogram or an MRI evaluation of the spine provides a diagnosis. Surgical stabilization and/or decompression has long been cited as the best treatment for long-term success, especially when done soon after recognition of the clinical signs. However, recent studies have provided evidence that medical therapy with corticosteroids may be equally beneficial in the long term.

METABOLIC AND NEOPLASTIC CONDITIONS THAT AFFECT THE NERVOUS SYSTEM

Most metabolic diseases occur in older animals with hepatic and renal diseases. Seizures are the most common clinical neurologic signs. An anomalous defect of a portacaval shunt in young dogs less than 1 year of age can result in clinical signs of seizures. In addition, there are a number of storage diseases that cause degeneration of the nervous system as a result of an enzyme deficiency or other inborn error of metabolism (see Table 40-4). Purebred cats and some breeds of dogs are most affected, although mongrel animals are not immune. Most commonly, the clinical signs of neurologic dysfunction are seen within the first year, often between 2 and 6 months of age. Clinical signs will depend on which part of the nervous system is most affected and vary from progressive ataxia to seizures (see Table 40-4). Currently there is no treatment to reverse these conditions.

Neoplasms of the central nervous system are almost nonexistent in neonates and rare in dogs and cats less than 1 year of age. A ganglioglioma has been reported in a 4-month-old Miniature Dachshund showing seizure-like neurologic signs. In all ages of dogs and cats, seizures are the most common clinical sign of neoplastic growths in the brain. However, seizures can have many causes as discussed above, including infections, trauma, idiopathic epilepsy, hypoglycemia, hypocalcemia, liver disease, or exposure to toxins. A complete physical and neurologic workup is needed to differentiate between these various causes. Brain tumors are best diagnosed by advanced radiographic techniques such as MRI.

NUTRITIONAL CONDITIONS THAT AFFECT THE NERVOUS SYSTEM

In neonates, hypoglycemia can be a result of inadequate nutrition and will result in seizures. Hypocalcemia is an electrolyte deficiency that can cause seizures in a young dog and cat. Thiamine deficiency occurs when growing kittens are fed an all-fish diet. Thiamine deficiency results in hemorrhages and malacia in the brainstem. Again, seizures are common, and cats have a characteristic ventroflexion of the head during the seizure. Other neurologic signs include changes in behavior, increased salivation, dilated pupils, incoordination, and progressive muscular weakness, with the disease progressing to death if supplementation with thiamine is not instituted. In a similar manner, young dogs that are fed cooked meat as a sole diet will develop paraparesis that can progress to convulsions and death. Improperly processed or stored dry food that has gone rancid has also been implicated in thiamine deficiency. To avoid problems, all dry food should be fed within 6 months of purchase. Additional information pertaining to nutritional diseases can be found in Chapter 44.

Use of commercial products specific for kittens and cats and not for dogs will help prevent taurine deficiency. Taurine is an essential amino acid requirement for felines but not for canines. Kittens of queens who were taurine deficient during pregnancy may be underweight at birth, grow slowly, have paresis, display a unique gait deficit with marked abduction of the pelvic limbs, and develop thoracic kyphosis. Early recognition and treatment of kittens with taurine can reverse the clinical signs. An irreversible blindness caused by retinal degeneration can occur in adult cats with chronic taurine deficiency.

INFECTIOUS AND INFLAMMATORY NEUROLOGIC LESIONS IN DOGS AND CATS

The bacterial, viral, and protozoal diseases of puppies and kittens and juveniles are covered in other chapters of this text (Chapters 15, 16, and 19, respectively). Infectious diseases causing inflammation of the brain or spinal cord are most common in puppies and kittens from 6 weeks to 6 months of age. Reduced maternal antibody protection, coupled with exposure to infected dogs before the establishment of the protective effects of the vaccines, is not an uncommon cause of viral encephalitis. Canine distemper virus and canine herpesvirus are the most common, but canine parvovirus type 2, adenovirus type 1, and parainfluenza virus all can cause meningoencephalitis in young dogs. The most common cause of viral infection of the brain in young cats is feline infectious peritonitis.

Bacterial encephalitis can occur in the neonate as a consequence of an ascending infection from the navel after birth, but this is not common. Clinical signs include fever, depression, reluctance to move, pain on manipulation of head and neck, loss of conscious proprioception postural responses, seizures, and possible cranial nerve deficits (see Figure 40-13). CSF analysis would confirm the inflammatory process by having a high neutrophil count coupled with a high CSF protein. Occasionally the causative bacteria can be isolated and identified from culture of the CSF. Treatment is with broad-spectrum antibiotics that cross the blood-brain barrier, such as potentiated sulfa drugs or chloramphenicol. Prognosis is guarded for recovery. Fungal, rickettsial, and protozoal organisms have also been reported to cause meningoencephalitis in young dogs and cats (see Chapters 17, 18, and 19, respectively).

TRAUMATIC NEUROLOGIC LESIONS OF YOUNG CATS AND DOGS

Trauma to the brain or spinal cord is also a consideration of etiology with any neurologic condition in a dog or cat of any age, although less so in the neonate. A "hit by car" etiology is very common in young animals exploring their environment. Onset is sudden with the worst clinical signs seen in the first 24 hours. Radiographs should be taken of the head or vertebral column, depending on neurologic localization of clinical signs. Therapy with antiinflammatory drugs and, in some spinal cord cases, corticosteroids often shows rapid improvement of clinical signs unless there is an unstable bony fracture that needs surgical repair.

TOXIN-INDUCED NEUROLOGIC DISEASES IN YOUNG CATS AND DOGS

Toxic lesions in neonates are not common. One litter of 4-week-old Border Collie puppies placed on wood chip bedding from South America had all puppies developing tremors of the body and the head within 24 hours, with some showing seizure activity. Retrospectively, no toxin was isolated, and pathology on two of the puppies did not demonstrate a morphologic lesion. One puppy raised to adulthood had spontaneously recovered by 4 months of age. History of exposure is most important as many toxins will affect the nervous system if young dogs or cats are exposed to them. Clinical signs often mimic diffuse cortical lesions, including seizures and muscle fasciculations.

Organophosphate toxicity will cause seizures and muscle fasciculation, as well as ANS signs of excessive salivation and lacrimation, and diarrhea. This may occur after improper exposure of puppies and especially kittens to some of the flea dips and flea collars used in adult animals.

Tetanus is caused by a tetanospasmin toxin produced by the bacterium *Clostridium tetani*. Dogs and cats are more resistant to the tetanus toxin than other species, but cases occur when there is a deep wound with contamination by these bacteria or even during shedding of deciduous teeth. Both localized and generalized tetanus are seen in dogs and cats. Figure 40-14 shows an 8-month-old Greyhound with tetanus with the classic generalized stiffness of limbs, prolapsed nictitating membrane, and contraction of the facial muscles in the lips and ears ("sardonic grin"). Excitement worsens the clinical signs. Treatment is aimed toward using antibiotics such as penicillin to kill the organism, antitoxin to neutralize any residual toxin, and supportive care.

A complete list of toxins that affect the nervous system, including pesticides, rodenticides, herbicides, fungicides, heavy metals, drugs, antifreeze, poisonous plants, detergents, and disinfectants, and toxins from animals and their primary effect on the nervous system can be found in Table 40-5. Additional information pertaining to toxin ingestion in pediatric patients can be found in Chapter 28.

VASCULAR ETIOLOGIES OF NEUROLOGIC DISEASE IN YOUNG ANIMALS

The most common vascular etiology of neurologic disease in young animals is from idiopathic fibrocartilaginous embolism. It occurs in both small and large breeds of dogs, cats, and other animals, including humans. This disease has an acute onset and can affect any part of the spinal cord. Unilateral lesions and asymmetric clinical signs are common. The clinical signs develop and progress rapidly within 1 to 2 hours from initial pain to unilateral or bilateral paralysis. After the initial onset of clinical signs, the condition is nonprogressive. Treatment is directed at reducing the swelling in the spinal cord using corticosteroids in the initial 24 hours of treatment and then supportive therapy until some level of recovery is achieved. Improvement is usually seen within the first few days with continued recovery over a period of 2 to 3 weeks. The prognosis is guarded and is relative to the ischemic damage sustained by the nervous tissue and the severity of clinical signs present.

IDIOPATHIC NEUROLOGIC DISEASE IN YOUNG ANIMALS

Idiopathic epilepsy is a recurrent seizure disorder with no known morphological lesions. Onset of clinical signs is seen in young dogs between 2 and 6 months of age, and the frequency and severity of seizures often increase over time. Extraneural and intraneural causes of seizure activity must be ruled out before diagnosing idiopathic epilepsy. Some breeds of dog, including the Beagle, Dachshund, German Shepherd Dog, Keeshond, and Belgian Tervuren are either proven or suspected to have a genetic factor that causes this disease. A high incidence of epilepsy has also been reported in Boxers, Cocker Spaniels, Collies, Golden Retrievers, Irish Setters, Labrador Retrievers, Miniature Schnauzers, Poodles, Saint Bernards, Siberian Huskies, and Wire Fox Terriers. Control is often possible with long-term treatment with phenobarbital or phenobarbital in combination with potassium bromide for recalcitrant cases. In large breeds of dogs, potassium bromide may be the first choice of an anticonvulsant.

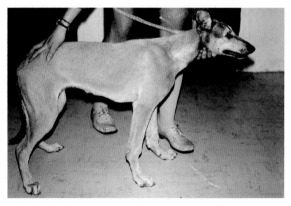

Figure 40-14 Eight-month-old Greyhound with sudden onset of stiffness of limbs, reluctance to move, lips pulled back ("sardonic grin"), and ears pulled dorsally. Excitement increased the clinical signs in the case of tetanus.

TABLE 40-5	List of common toxicants that affect the nervous system	
Use	**Toxicant**	**Primary Effect**
Pesticides	Chlorinated hydrocarbons	CNS stimulation
	Organophosphates	Binding of acetylcholinesterase
	Carbamates	Binding of acetylcholinesterase
	Pyrethrins	Blocking of nerve conduction and GABA inhibition
	Metaldehyde	CNS stimulation
	Arsenic	GI irritation
Rodenticides	Strychnine	Blocking of inhibitory interneurons
	Thallium	GI irritation, CNS stimulation, peripheral neuropathy, skin lesions
	α-Naphthyl thiourea (ANTU)	GI irritation, pulmonary edema, depression, coma
	Sodium fluoroacetate (1080)	CNS stimulation
	Warfarin	Anticoagulation
	Zinc phosphide	GI irritation, depression
	Phosphorus	GI irritation, CNS stimulation, coma
	Cholecalciferol	CNS depression, cardiac depression
	Bromethalin	Acute—CNS stimulation; chronic—CNS depression
Herbicides and fungicides	Numerous	GI irritation, CNS depression; some are stimulants
Heavy metals	Lead (see arsenic and thallium, above)	GI irritation, CNS stimulation or depression
Drugs	Narcotics	CNS depression
	Amphetamines	CNS depression
	Barbiturates	CNS depression
	Tranquilizers	CNS depression
	Aspirin	GI irritation, coma
	Marijuana	Abnormal behavior, depression
	Anthelmintics	GI irritation, CNS stimulation
	Ivermectin	Depression, tremors, ataxia, coma
Garbage	Staphylococcal toxin	GI irritation, CNS stimulation
	Botulinus toxin	LMN paralysis
Poisonous plants	Various	Various
Antifreeze	Ethylene glycol	GI irritation, CNS stimulation, renal failure
Detergents and disinfectants	Hexachlorophene	CNS stimulation or depression, tremors
	Phenols	GI irritation, CNS degeneration
Animal origin	Snake bite	Necrotizing wound, shock, CNS depression
	Toad (*Bufo* spp.)	Digitoxin-like action, CNS stimulation
	Lizards	GI irritation, CNS stimulation or depression
	Tick paralysis (*Dermacentor* spp., *Ixodes* in Australia)	LMN paralysis

CNS, Central nervous system; *GABA*, gamma-aminobutyric acid; *GI*, gastrointestinal; *LMN*, lower motor neuron.
From Lorenz MD, Kornegay JN: *Handbook of veterinary neurology*, ed 4, St Louis, 2004, Saunders, p 377.

SUGGESTED READINGS

Bagley RS: *Fundamentals of veterinary clinical neurology*, Ames, IA, 2005, Blackwell, pp 1-570.

Hoskins JD: Clinical evaluation of the kitten: from birth to eight weeks of age, *Compend Contin Educ Pract Vet* 12(9):1215, 1990.

Hoskins JD, Shelton GD: The nervous and neuromuscular systems. In Hoskins JD (ed): *Veterinary pediatrics: dogs and cats from birth to six months*, ed 3, Philadelphia, 2001, Saunders, pp 425-462.

Lavely JA: Pediatric neurology of the dog and cat, *Vet Clin North Am Small Anim Pract* 36:475, 2006.

Lorenz MD, Kornegay JN: *Handbook of veterinary neurology*, ed 4, Philadelphia, 2004, Saunders, pp 1-468.

THE SKIN AND EAR

Jon D. Plant

The normal pediatric integument of newborn dogs and cats undergoes significant change between birth and 6 months of age. The thicknesses of the epidermis and dermis increase twofold to threefold as the skin matures. During the same period, the integument as a percentage of body weight decreases from 24% to 12% in the dog. Meanwhile, there is a rapid replacement of reticulum fibers composed of type III collagen by mature type I collagen fibers in the dermis. These collagen fibers, as well as elastic fibers, increase in size and number during the first months of life.

The coat of kittens and puppies consists principally of fine hairs. At 12 to 16 weeks of age, hairs begin to thicken and decrease in curvature in a breed-specific manner, giving rise to the adult-type coat. Pigment of the skin and hair continues to develop into the adult phenotype until approximately 3 to 6 months of age.

GENODERMATOSES

Signs of congenital and hereditary skin disorders are most often observed during the first 2 to 3 months of age (Figure 41-1). In many cases, the genetic defect resulting in the disorder has not been fully characterized. Some of the described genodermatoses of dogs and cats are summarized in Table 41-1.

INFECTIOUS DISEASES

Young animals may be predisposed to infectious skin diseases as a result of either an immature immune system or a hereditary primary immunodeficiency. As the epidermal thickness increases and the protective function of the skin improves, puppies and kittens become less susceptible to viral, bacterial, and fungal infections.

Papillomas

Mucocutaneous viral papillomas are common in puppies. Smooth white lesions quickly progress to gray verrucous nodules that are often pedunculated (Figure 41-2). They are seen most often in the oral cavity and on the lips but may also occur on haired skin and conjunctiva. It is believed that various papilloma virus types have site predilections. The virus appears to be spread most often by direct contact but can survive for 2 months in the environment. There is a 1- to 2-month incubation period. Diagnosis can most often be made by clinical recognition in a puppy. Histopathology, if performed, reveals a hyperplastic and hyperkeratotic epidermis.

Papillomas typically regress in 2 to 3 months without therapy. In cases that fail to resolve or when treatment is otherwise warranted, cryotherapy is the treatment of choice. At least two freeze-thaw cycles are suggested. As long as the majority of lesions are frozen, all generally resolve, presumably by stimulating a host immune response.

Impetigo

Staphylococcus sp. impetigo is a nonpruritic superficial infection recognized commonly in puppies and rarely in kittens. Impetigo is characterized by nonfollicular pustules that occur most commonly in the nonhaired skin of the ventral abdomen. In contrast, in the adult dog, impetigo often results in larger pustules that span follicular units and is commonly associated with immunosuppression.

Cytology of the pustules will demonstrate neutrophils and intracellular cocci. Bathing every 3 to 7 days with a gentle shampoo containing an antibacterial ingredient such as chlorhexidine or triclosan is often sufficient to resolve impetigo. In severe cases that fail to respond to topical therapy, a 14-day course of a systemic antibiotic (amoxicillin-clavulanic acid or cephalexin) is indicated.

Dermatophytosis

Young animals carry an increased risk of developing dermatophytosis, reflecting their immature immune status and potential for exposure to carriers. *Microsporum canis* is the most frequent cause of ringworm in kittens and puppies.

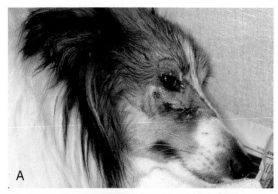

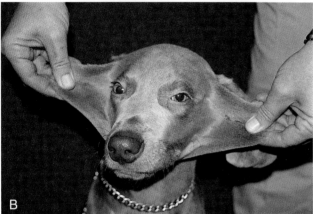

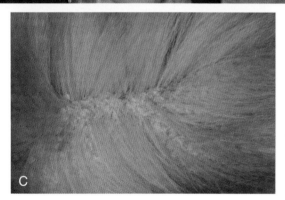

Figure 41-1 Examples of congenital and hereditary dermatoses. **A,** Canine familial dermatomyositis in a Shetland Sheepdog. **B,** Cutaneous asthenia (Ehlers-Danlos syndrome) in a 5-month-old Weimaraner. **C,** Ichthyosis in a Golden Retriever. (**B,** from Medleau L, Hnilica KA: *Small animal dermatology: a color atlas and therapeutic guide,* ed 2, St Louis, 2006, Saunders/Elsevier. **C,** courtesy Candace Sousa.)

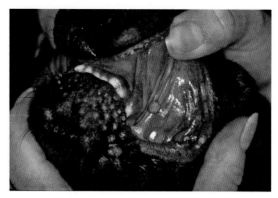

Figure 41-2 Multiple papillomas involving the lips and oral mucosa.

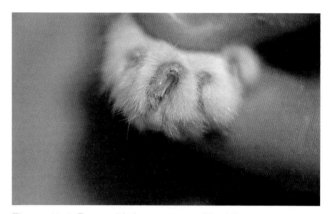

Figure 41-3 Paronychia in a cat caused by *Microsporum canis.* (From Medleau L, Hnilica KA: *Small animal dermatology: a color atlas and therapeutic guide,* ed 2, St Louis, 2006, Saunders/Elsevier.)

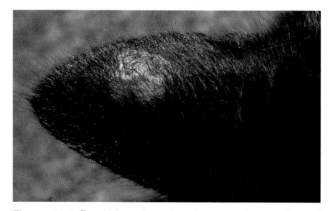

Figure 41-4 Focal alopecia and erythema on the ear pinna of a cat with dermatophytosis. (From Medleau L, Hnilica KA: *Small animal dermatology: a color atlas and therapeutic guide,* ed 2, St Louis, 2006, Saunders/Elsevier.)

Entire litters can develop lesions, typically multifocal alopecic, mildly erythematous patches that progressively develop papules, scales, and hyperpigmentation (Figures 41-3 and 41-4). Frequently affected areas of kittens and puppies include the head, muzzle, pinnae, and distal limbs.

Approximately 50% of *M. canis* infections will cause hairs to fluoresce with ultraviolet (Wood's) light examination. Microscopic examination of plucked hairs for ectothrix fungal spores also provides a rapid method of confirming the diagnosis. Incubating the hair for 15 to 30 minutes in KOH digests the keratin and may aid in visualization of the spherical spores. Fungal cultures should be performed to identify the species of ringworm.

In general, treatment of pediatric patients should be limited to topical products until they are approximately 16

TABLE 41-1	Genodermatoses of puppies and kittens			
Disease	Examples of affected breeds	Suspected mode of inheritance	Age of onset	Description
Acral mutilation syndrome	German Shorthair Pointer, English Pointer, English Springer Spaniel, French Spaniel	Autosomal recessive	2-12 mo	Self-mutilation of digits and feet (single or multiple), progressing to autoamputation; dogs are not lame despite severe lesions
Anhidrotic ectodermal dysplasia	Multiple dog breeds	X-linked recessive	Congenital	Hypotrichosis, alopecia, and thin dry skin accompany dental abnormalities (conical teeth, oligodontia)
Black hair follicular dysplasia	Papillon, Bearded Collie, Large Münsterländer, Saluki, Jack Russell Terrier, mongrel	Autosomal recessive	1-2 wk	Black areas of bicolor or tricolor pups develop dull coats, scales, hypotrichosis, and alopecia
Canine familial dermatomyositis	Collie, Shetland Sheepdog	Autosomal dominant	2-6 mo	Alopecia, erosions, and crusts develop over the face, pressure points, and tail tip (see Figure 41-1, *A*)
Color mutant alopecia	Doberman Pinscher, Irish Setter, Yorkshire Terrier, Dachshund, Great Dane	Autosomal recessive	6-24 mo	Individuals with color dilution, typified by blue Doberman Pinschers, lose hair over the trunk; normally colored areas are spared
Congenital hypotrichosis	Numerous breeds of dogs (e.g., American Cocker Spaniel, miniature Poodle) and cats (e.g., Birman, Siamese)	X-linked in dogs and autosomal recessive in cats	0-4 wk	Most are born with little or no hair; alopecia of the head, pinnae, ventrum, and caudal dorsum develops by 3-4 mo in those born with hair; skin may become scaled and hyperpigmented
Cutaneous asthenia (Ehlers-Danlos syndrome)	Numerous breeds of dogs (e.g., Beagle, Greyhound) and cats (Persian, Himalayan)	Autosomal dominant, autosomal recessive, and X-linked forms	Congenital	A group of diseases characterized by collagen disorders resulting in skin hyperextensibility and fragility; joint laxity, ocular abnormalities, and widening of the bridge of the nose may occur (see Figure 41-1, *B*)
Epidermolysis bullosa	Collie, Shetland Sheepdog, toy Poodle, German Shorthair Pointer, Persian, Domestic Shorthair	Autosomal recessive	0-12 mo	Vesicles, erosions, and ulcers of pressure points, areas subject to trauma, and oral cavity; onychomadesis may occur
Epitheliogenesis imperfecta	Numerous breeds of dogs and cats	Unknown	Congenital	Animals are born with variably sized, well-demarcated regions of ulcerated skin
Exfoliative cutaneous lupus erythematosus	German Shorthair Pointer	Autosomal recessive	6-48 mo	Severe scaling and alopecia develop on the head and progress over the dorsal trunk
Follicular parakeratosis	Rottweiler	X-linked	1 wk	Severe, nonpruritic scaling beginning on the muzzle and becoming generalized
Footpad hyperkeratosis	Irish Terriers, Dogue de Bordeaux	Autosomal recessive	<6 mo	Severe hyperkeratosis of the entire footpad surface
Hereditary nasal parakeratosis	Labrador Retriever	Autosomal recessive	6-12 mo	Hyperkeratotic crusts develop on the planum nasale
Ichthyosis	West Highland White Terrier, Norfolk Terrier, Jack Russell Terrier, Cavalier King Charles Spaniel	Autosomal recessive	Congenital	A group of diseases characterized by heavy scales, hyperpigmentation, and fissures (see Figure 41-1, *C*); specific findings vary depending on underlying epidermal defect

TABLE 41-1 Genodermatoses of Puppies and Kittens—cont'd

Disease	Examples of affected breeds	Suspected mode of inheritance	Age of onset	Description
Lethal acrodermatitis	Bull Terriers	Autosomal recessive	Congenital	Affected pups are lighter than littermates, growth is stunted, and they develop papular, pustular, and crusted dermatitis of the head and feet
Oculocutaneous albinism	Maltese, Doberman, Persian	Autosomal recessive	Congenital	Complete lack of ocular and skin pigment
Primary seborrhea	American Cocker Spaniel, West Highland White Terrier, Persian	Autosomal recessive	2 days-6 mo	Clinical syndromes vary with the breed affected; generally animals develop heavy scale, excessive sebum production, and lichenification

weeks of age. Topical application of 2% lime-sulfur dip every 5 to 7 days is suggested. A protective collar is applied until the patient is dry to prevent excessive ingestion through grooming. Care should be taken to ensure that body temperature is maintained after applying a full-body dip to a pediatric patient. Small, localized lesions can also be treated with topical clotrimazole or terbinafine creams applied daily. When possible, affected animals should be isolated and the patient's environment cleaned with 0.5% bleach. Caretakers should be educated regarding the zoonotic potential of dermatophytosis.

Treatment is continued until there is both a clinical resolution and a microbiological cure, as determined by follow-up fungal culture. Once the patient reaches 16 weeks of age, systemic therapy can be considered, following recommendations for adult dogs and cats. Oral itraconazole (5 to 10 mg/kg/day), terbinafine (30 to 40 mg/kg/day), or micro-sized griseofulvin (50 or 100 mg/kg/day) is commonly prescribed.

PARASITIC DISEASES

Demodicosis

Demodex canis, the common mite species causing demodicosis in dogs, is acquired by pups from their dams within the first days of life. As normal skin inhabitants, the mites reside in hair follicles without causing cutaneous changes in most dogs. Commonly young dogs develop localized demodicosis, defined by convention as five or fewer lesions. These are nonpruritic, alopecic lesions that often develop on the face or limbs, although other areas may be involved (Figure 41-5). Generalized demodicosis is diagnosed when more than five lesions are present. This is not a hard and fast rule, as fewer extensive lesions would also warrant a diagnosis of generalized demodicosis. Purebred dogs are at increased risk of generalized demodicosis. Breeds reportedly predisposed include the Shar Pei, English Bulldog, Alaskan Malamute, and a number of Terrier breeds.

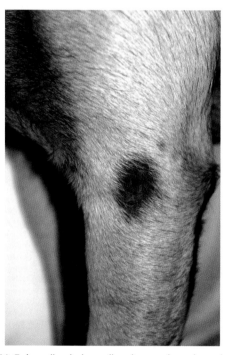

Figure 41-5 Localized demodicosis causing alopecia on the leg of a Pug. (Courtesy of Candace Sousa.)

Diagnosis is readily made with multiple deep skin scrapings. The skin is pinched to force mites to the surface, and the area is scraped with a mineral oil-coated scalpel blade or stainless steel spatula until capillary bleeding is observed. A 4× objective provides sufficient magnification to recognize mites easily and speeds scanning of the entire slide. Mites are more easily visualized with the condenser lowered into a position that increases contrast. Although occasional mites can be found on normal dogs, skin scrapings with multiple mites observed should be considered positive in the presence of characteristic lesions.

Treatment of juvenile-onset localized demodicosis is usually unnecessary as most cases respond without therapy.

Topical treatment with daily benzoyl peroxide gel or rotenone ointment (Goodwinol; Goodwinol Products Corporation, Pierce, CO) is of unproven efficacy but may provide some benefit while carrying little risk. Patients that do not resolve in 2 to 3 months require more aggressive therapy.

The safety of products used to treat generalized demodicosis has not been established in dogs less than 4 months of age. Weekly topical therapy with benzoyl peroxide-containing shampoo is recommended until the patient is older than 4 months of age and able to tolerate generalized therapy safely. Thereafter, treatment with amitraz dips (every 7 to 14 days), oral ivermectin (0.3 to 0.6 mg/kg/day), or oral milbemycin (1 to 2 mg/kg/day) follows the recommendations for adult dogs and is continued until clinical resolution and failure to demonstrate mites twice by skin scrapings performed 4 weeks apart.

Sarcoptic Mange

Because of the highly contagious nature of *Sarcoptes scabiei* var. *canis* infestation, entire litters of pups may be presented with typical lesions. These include a ventrally oriented papular rash, crusted and alopecic pinnal margins, and excoriations of the lateral elbows. Scratching usually is elicited by rubbing the ear margin (Figure 41-6). Pups are often exposed by an infested bitch. The mite has a 21-day life cycle. Once infested, pruritus usually begins within several days and steadily worsens over weeks. Superficial skin scrapings covering broad areas of affected skin may reveal the mites, characterized by unjointed pretarsi with terminal suckers. Looking for the mites' rapid movement on the slide helps identify them among the copious keratinaceous material, crusts, and hair often collected on the scrapings. However, negative skin scrapings are common, especially in early infestation, necessitating therapeutic trials when clinical suspicion warrants. A response to treatment confirms the tentative diagnosis.

Selamectin provides a convenient and effective treatment of sarcoptic mange for pups more than 6 weeks of age. Two doses 4 weeks apart are normally effective, although more frequent applications are often recommended in adults with severe infestations. Lime-sulfur dips applied every 5 to 7 days are a safe and effective alternative therapy for young puppies. If caretakers are affected, their lesions most often resolve with treatment of the patient.

Cheyletiellosis

Cheyletiella spp. mites may infest puppies, kittens, and rabbits. The three species of mites are not highly host specific. The mites complete their life cycle on the host, with eggs attached to hairs. These large mites are recognized by their hooked mouth parts. Pruritus varies from absent to moderate. Dog and cats may not display any lesions or may be heavily scaled and crusted, particularly over the dorsum. Mites may transiently infest humans, resulting in pruritic papules, often on the abdomen and forearms, similar to sarcoptic mange.

Superficial skin scrapings, trichograms (microscopic hair examination), and acetate tape preparations are used to demonstrate mites or eggs. All in-contact animals must be treated. Selamectin or fipronil is applied every 2 weeks 3 or 4 times. Alternatives, although less effective, include dips, powders, or sprays containing lime-sulfur, pyrethrin, carbaryl, or organophosphates. Lime-sulfur dips are the safest option when the age of the kitten or puppy precludes the use of other insecticides. In heavy infestations, the home environment should be treated with an insecticide to minimize zoonosis.

Pediculosis

Lice are host-specific, obligate parasites. Infestations of young dogs and cats are commonly associated with poor nutrition, overcrowding, and direct transmission from infested animals. Biting lice (*Trichodectes canis* and *Felicola subrostratus*) are recognized by their relatively broad heads compared with those of sucking lice (*Linognathus setosus*).

Infested pediatric patients display variable pruritus, progressive alopecia, and scale. Matting, erythematous papules, and anemia may develop in severe infestations. Lice and their eggs (nits) may be grossly visualized (Figure 41-7).

Treatment should be directed at all in-contact dogs or cats. Selamectin administered every 2 weeks for four treatments is safe, effective, and convenient. Alternatives include spot-on formulations, dips, powders, or sprays containing imidacloprid, fipronil, lime-sulfur, pyrethrin, carbaryl, or organophosphates, following manufacturer recommendations. The environment, bedding, and grooming tools of infested animals should be cleaned or replaced.

Fleas

Puppies and kittens are very susceptible to infestations with the cat flea, *Ctenocephalides felis*. Because of the flea's high reproductive potential, heavy infestations can develop rapidly. Litters of puppies and kittens can quickly become infested when the bitch or queen is not maintained on preventative

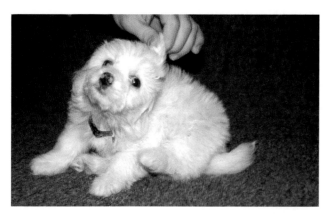

Figure 41-6 A positive pinnal-pedal reflex is highly suggestive of scabies. (From Medleau L, Hnilica KA: *Small animal dermatology: a color atlas and therapeutic guide,* ed 2, St Louis, 2006, Saunders/Elsevier.)

TABLE 41-2	Minimum approved age for use of selected flea products				
	Advantage	Frontline plus	Revolution	ProMeris	Capstar
Active Ingredient	Imidacloprid	Fipronil	Selamectin	Metaflumizone	Nitenpyram
Canine	7 wk	8 wk	6 wk	8 wk	4 wk and 2 lb
Feline	8 wk	8 wk	8 wk	8 wk	4 wk and 2 lb

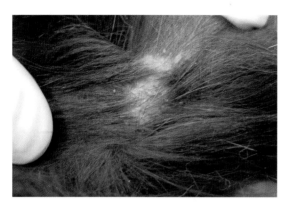

Figure 41-7 Lice nits visible in the coat of a kitten. (Courtesy Carmen Mendez.)

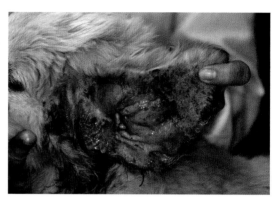

Figure 41-8 Acute, severe pinnal dermatitis caused by juvenile cellulitis in a Golden Retriever puppy.

flea control. Young animals may develop pruritus, erythematous papules, scales, alopecia, and excoriations. The severity of pruritus is often inversely related to age, as hypersensitivity to fleas develops over time. Areas that are commonly affected are the neck and ventral abdomen regions of cats and the ventral abdomen and dorsal lumbar regions of dogs.

Heavy infestations can lead to severe, life-threatening anemia, particularly in pediatric patients with relatively low blood volumes. Further, young kittens do not yet groom appreciably, a mechanism that helps reduce the flea burden of mature cats. Intensive care, including blood transfusions, may be required in severely anemic animals.

Flea products with excellent adulticidal activity are now available for use on puppies and kittens. Spot-on products are generally approved for kittens 8 weeks of age or older and for puppies 6 to 8 weeks of age or older (Table 41-2). Nitenpyram, available as an oral tablet, can be used in animals as young as 4 weeks of age and has a very rapid kill, appropriate for heavy infestations. For animals younger than the minimum approved age of these products, manual removal of fleas with a fine-toothed comb is recommended.

MISCELLANEOUS DISEASES

Juvenile Cellulitis

Also referred to as "puppy strangles," juvenile cellulitis is an idiopathic dermatitis and lymphadenitis, most commonly affecting puppies 3 to 16 weeks of age. Dachshund,

Golden Retriever, and Gordon Setter breeds are predisposed. Attempts to demonstrate organisms or transmit the disease have been unsuccessful. Erythematous papules and pustules develop on the lips, muzzle, eyelids, and ear canals. Submandibular lymphadenitis is profound. Pinnal edema, alopecia, and erythema may be the first lesions noticed (Figure 41-8).

Most pups respond well to 2.2 mg/kg prednisone daily. Within several days to 1 week, erythema, swelling, and lymphadenopathy improve substantially. However, to prevent relapse, the dose should be tapered slowly according to the response, over the course of 4 to 6 weeks. Refractory cases may respond to dexamethasone therapy in place of prednisone. Owners or breeders should be warned that some scarring can be expected because of the deep nature of the lesions.

Otitis Externa

In general, the ear canals of puppies and kittens are less prone to disease than those of adult animals, which more frequently suffer from chronic skin diseases that lead to otitis externa. Exceptions are otitis externa in puppies and kittens caused by infestation with the ear mite *Otodectes cynotis* and skin diseases occurring at a young age that can lead to ear disease. These include juvenile cellulitis, primary seborrhea, and ichthyosis. *Otodectes* sp. infestations are characterized by head shaking, pruritus, and crumbly brown to black aural exudate. Secondary excoriations of the pinnae, head, and neck are common.

Mites are most easily visualized by microscopic examination of aural exudate collected on a cotton-tipped swab. Occasionally ear mites are found on other regions of the skin with skin scrapings. The ears should be gently cleaned. Treatment options include systemic (selamectin, ivermectin, or moxidectin) and topical (ivermectin, moxidectin, or fipronil) protocols. All in-contact pets should be treated.

SUGGESTED READINGS

Medleau L, Hnilica KA: *Small animal dermatology: a color atlas and therapeutic guide,* ed 2, St Louis, 2006, Saunders/Elsevier.

Nagle T: Topics in pediatric dermatology, *Vet Clin Small Anim* 26:557, 2006.

THE MUSCULOSKELETAL SYSTEM

CHAPTER 42

Gert J. Breur, Sean P. McDonough, Rory J. Todhunter

Almost 20% of all dogs presenting with a musculoskeletal problem in a referral center are younger than 1 year of age. Of the diagnosed conditions, approximately 50% are related to bones, 35% to joints, and 15% to muscles and tendons. Similar epidemiologic data for kittens do not exist, but pediatric orthopedic conditions in cats appear to be less common than in dogs. Pediatric orthopedic conditions are often challenging for the clinician. Pediatric patients have a high activity level and are still in a phase of continuous growth and development. In addition, many pediatric orthopedic conditions caused by abnormal musculoskeletal development may bring further secondary abnormal musculoskeletal development, resulting in complicated clinical presentations. Indeed, to appreciate the intricacies of pathophysiology, diagnosis, and treatment of pediatric orthopedic conditions, a good understanding of musculoskeletal growth and development is required.

MUSCULOSKELETAL DEVELOPMENT

Canine and feline skeletal development follows a similar pattern and temporal sequence. During embryonic development, the first evidence of the developing skeleton, with the exception of the skull bones, is the so-called condensation of mesenchymal cells in the locations of future bones. The mesenchymal bone model transforms into cartilage and then into bone via endochondral and intramembranous ossification. Joints form between the developing bones by segmentation and cavitation, followed by the formation of the intraarticular structures. Muscles are derived from the mesenchyme immediately surrounding bones and joints. Tendon insertions form from the developing cartilaginous anlagen, and they connect secondarily to more proximally developed muscle masses during embryonic limb elongation. Later in prenatal development, the characteristic features of the fetus appear, and the size of the formed skeletal elements, joints, and muscle-tendon units increases.

Postnatal skeletal development is a continuation of the prenatal development and occurs via enlargement of the cartilaginous skeletal elements and mineralization through endochondral and intramembranous ossification. In both endochondral and intramembranous ossification, the mineralization process is initiated in matrix vesicles. Further mineralization is mainly regulated by the control of calcium and phosphorus metabolism via parathyroid hormone, calcitonin, and vitamin D. Longitudinal bone growth is the result of cartilage formation in epiphyses (where secondary ossification occurs) and growth (physeal) plates. In both locations, the mechanism by which bone enlarges is the same: new cartilage is formed, resulting in increased mass (length and width) that is then transformed into bone (endochondral ossification). In most long bones, growth plates contribute approximately 75% to 80% of the final bone length, whereas the epiphyseal growth centers contribute approximately 20% to 25%. Growth plates are also responsible for latitudinal bone growth (growth in width).

Most longitudinal bone growth takes place between 12 and 26 weeks of age. During this period, mineralization of all epiphyseal growth centers is completed at predetermined times, and growth plates have their most rapid rate of longitudinal bone growth and endochondral ossification. At the end of this period, epiphyseal bone growth is completed. Following this period, growth plate–associated bone length continues at a much slower rate until it ceases completely. At cessation of growth, growth plates fuse at predetermined times (Table 42-1). The rate of skeletal development and the final size of bones vary widely among canine and feline breeds. The optimal rate of skeletal development for a given breed is rarely known. An indicator for skeletal growth is body weight. Unfortunately puppy and kitten

443

TABLE 42-1   Age when ossification centers appear and growth plate fusion occurs in immature dogs

Anatomical site	Age when ossification center appears	Age when fusion occurs	Anatomical site	Age when ossification center appears	Age when fusion occurs
Scapula			**Pelvis**		
Body	Birth		Pubis	Birth	4-6 mo
Tuber scapulae	7 wk	4-7 mo	Ilium	Birth	4-6 mo
			Ischium	Birth	4-6 mo
Humerus			Os acetabulum	7 wk	5 mo
Diaphysis	Birth		Iliac crest	4 mo	1-2 yr
Proximal epiphysis	1-2 wk	10-13 mo	Tuber ischii	3 mo	8-10 mo
Distal epiphysis		6-8 mo to shaft	Ischial arch	6 mo	12 mo
Medial condyle	2-3 wk	6 wk to lateral condyle	Caudal symphysis pubis	7 mo	5 yr
Lateral condyle	2-3 wk		Symphysis pubis		5 yr
Medial epicondyle	6-8 wk	6 mo to condyle	**Femur**		
Radius			Diaphysis	Birth	
Diaphysis	Birth		Proximal epiphysis (head)	2 wk	7-11 mo
Proximal epiphysis	3-5 wk	6-11 mo	Trochanter major	8 wk	6-10 mo
Distal epiphysis	2-4 wk	8-12 mo	Trochanter minor	8 wk	8-13 mo
Ulna			Distal epiphysis		8-11 mo to shaft
Diaphysis	Birth		Trochlea	2 wk	3 mo condyle to trochlea
Olecranon	8 wk	6-10 mo	Medial condyle	3 wk	
Distal epiphysis	8 wk	8-12 mo	Lateral condyle	3 wk	
Carpus			**Patella**	9 wk	
Ulnar	4 wk		**Tibia**		
Radial	3-4 wk		Diaphysis	Birth	
Central	4-5 wk		Medial condyle	3 wk	6 wk to lateral
Intermediate	3-4 wk		Lateral condyle	3 wk	6-12 mo to shaft
Body	2 wk		Tuberosity	8 wk	6-8 mo to condyle
Epiphysis	7 wk	4 mo			6-12 mo to shaft
First	3 wk		Distal epiphysis	3 wk	8-11 mo
Second	4 wk		Medial malleolus	3 mo	5 mo
Third	4 wk		**Fibula**		
Fourth	3 wk		Diaphysis	Birth	
Sesamoid bone	4 mo		Proximal epiphysis	9 wk	8-12 mo
Metacarpus/Metatarsus			Distal epiphysis	2-7 wk	7-11 mo
Diaphysis	Birth		**Tarsus**		
Distal epiphysis (2-5)*	4 wk	6 mo	Talus	Birth-1 wk	
Proximal epiphysis (1)*	5 wk	6 mo	Fibular	Birth-1 wk	
Phalanges			Tuber calcis	6 wk	3-8 mo
First Phalanx			Central	3 wk	
Diaphysis (digits 1-5)	Birth		First	4 wk	
Distal epiphysis (digits 2-5)	4 wk	6 mo	Second	4 wk	
Distal epiphysis (digit 1)	6 wk	6 mo	Third	3 wk	
Second Phalanx			Fourth	2 wk	
Diaphysis (digits 2-5)	Birth		**Sesamoids**		
Proximal epiphysis (digits 2-5)*	5 wk	6 mo	Fabellar	3 mo	
Third Phalanx			Popliteal	3 mo	
Diaphysis	Birth		Plantar phalangeal	2 mo	
Volar sesamoids	2 mo		Dorsal phalangeal	5 mo	
Dorsal sesamoids	4 mo				

*Second phalanx absent or fused with first phalanx in first digit.

Modified from Owens JM: *Radiographic interpretation for the small animal clinician*, St. Louis, Ralston Purina Company, 1982, p 8; and Ticer JW: *Radiographic technique in small animal practice*, Philadelphia, 1975, Saunders, p 101.

growth (weight) curves have only been established for a few breeds.

ORTHOPEDIC EXAMINATION

The Young Dog with Hindlimb Lameness

Most clinicians start their orthopedic examination distally and proceed proximally. An overview of common causes for hindlimb lameness in pediatric dogs can be found in Box 42-1. Lameness isolated at the level of the foot may result from foreign bodies or lacerations of the digital pads or the tarsal pad, subluxated interdigital joints, paronychia, and sesamoiditis/fractured sesamoid bones. Lameness localized at the metatarsus includes fractures, ruptured flexor tendons (if the toes are off the ground), or some other soft tissue injury (like a failure of the flexor and retinacular support of the caudal distal hock joints or tarsal luxation). The latter condition will result in roundness of the caudal distal hock and proximal metatarsus with an overflexed hock. Tarsocrural luxation would result in non–weight-bearing lameness. All the normal bony protuberances around the hock should be palpable, and there should be no swelling or effusion of any joint. Hock swelling and effusion in a young dog could indicate talar osteochondrosis (OC) or infectious or inflammatory arthritis. Dogs with infectious arthritis will usually be extremely lame. Tibial distal metaphyseal bone pain and swelling, especially in a large or giant breed dog, could indicate hypertrophic osteodystrophy. Tibial diaphyseal bone pain on digital pressure could indicate panosteitis. German Shepherd Dogs are predisposed to panosteitis, but any large or giant breed dog can succumb. Lameness associated with stifle pain and effusion could be associated with rupture of the cranial (or caudal) cruciate ligament, patellar luxation (medial or lateral), infectious arthritis, patellar luxation, or OC of the femoral condyles. Femoral diaphyseal pain could

indicate panosteitis. The most common cause of lameness in the hindlimbs or hindlimb dysfunction in the young or growing dog is synovitis and osteoarthritis secondary to hip dysplasia. Pain on hip extension or a positive Ortolani test indicates hip dysplasia and secondary osteoarthritis. The Ortolani maneuver detects the palpable "click" of femoral head reduction into the acetabulum. Mild pain on hip extension also may be associated with iliopsoas muscle trauma. Severe pain during hip extension with simultaneous internal rotation of the hip joint is further indication of this condition. Infectious arthritis should always be on the list of differentials in an immature dog with marked lameness and joint pain or effusion. In small breeds, Legg-Calvé-Perthes disease or avascular necrosis of the femoral head will present as a mostly unilateral lameness that develops during growth and worsens with time. In cats with hip pain, slipped capital femoral epiphysis (SCFE) or hip dysplasia should be considered. Lumbosacral malformation or hemivertebra could also result in neurologic impingement and secondary hindlimb weakness or lameness. Neurologic conditions are discussed in greater detail in Chapter 40.

The Young Dog with Forelimb Lameness

Similar conditions of the digits and metacarpus occur in both the lower forelimbs and hindlimbs. An overview of common causes for forelimb lameness in pediatric patients can be found in Box 42-2. Angular limb deformities will be a cause of lameness more often in the forelimb than in the hindlimb. Angulation can be observed at the carpus in either a valgus or a varus direction, resulting in carpal pain on flexion from effusion and secondary osteoarthritis. Elbow subluxation as a result of premature closure of the distal ulnar physis is particularly debilitating and will be accompanied by effusion of the elbow joint, restricted range of motion, and sometimes crepitation. Distal metaphyseal bone pain and swelling indicate hypertrophic osteodystrophy in

---

BOX 42-1   **Hindlimb lameness**

Source of Lameness	Possible Etiologies	Diagnostic Tests
Isolated in the foot	Foreign bodies or lacerations of the digital pad and tarsal pad, subluxated interdigital joints, paronychia, sesamoiditis/fractured sesamoid bones	Palpation and radiography
Localized in the metatarsus	Fractures, ruptured flexor tendons (if the toes are off the ground) or some other soft tissue injury	Roundness of the caudal distal hock and proximal metatarsus with an overflexed hock
Hock swelling and effusion	Tarsal osteochondrosis or infectious or inflammatory arthritis	Radiography and synovial fluid analysis
Tibial distal metaphyseal bone pain and swelling	Hypertrophic osteodystrophy	Palpation and radiography
Tibial diaphyseal bone pain	Panosteitis	Digital pressure Radiography
Stifle pain and effusion	Rupture of the cranial (or caudal) cruciate ligament, patellar luxation	Palpation and radiography

BOX 42-2   Forelimb lameness

Source of Lameness	Possible Etiologies	Diagnostic Tests
Carpal pain on flexion	Effusion or secondary osteoarthritis	Angulation at the carpus in either valgus or varus direction
Elbow subluxation	Premature closure of the distal ulnar physis	Effusion of the elbow joint, restricted range of motion, and sometimes crepitation; radiography
Distal metaphyseal bone pain and swelling	Hypertrophic osteodystrophy in large and giant breeds	Palpation and radiography
Radial diaphyseal pain	Panosteitis	Palpation and radiography
Shoulder pain in young dogs	Osteochondrosis of the humeral head, shoulder instability, or biceps tendonitis	Palpation and radiography

large and giant breed dogs. Radial diaphyseal pain on pressure indicates panosteitis. Panosteitis can also occur in the proximal ulna and humerus, especially around the region of the nutrient foramen. Shoulder pain in young dogs could indicate OC of the humeral head, shoulder instability, or biceps tendonitis.

CONGENITAL MUSCULOSKELETAL DISEASES

Congenital diseases of bone, cartilage (joint deformity), and muscle (congenital myopathy) may be identifiable at birth or shortly thereafter and often have an inherited etiology. Congenital bone diseases can be further classified as dysostoses (malformation of individual bones, diseases of mesenchymal bone formation) and osteochondrodysplasias (developmental disorders of chondroosseous tissue, diseases of endochondral and/or intramembranous ossification).

Retarded Growth

Many patients presenting with a congenital musculoskeletal condition display retarded growth. Retarded growth of a puppy or kitten may be defined as reduced growth in terms of skeletal development or body weight when compared with normal littermates or a failure to attain the weight and/or height standards characteristic of a given breed. Selected puppy and kitten growth curves, as well as weight and/or height standards, can be found in Chapter 5 for some dog and cat breeds. Abnormal prenatal growth may affect the size of newborns and results in so-called "runts." Runts may not attain normal adult size because of inadequate compensatory growth after birth. Many diseases may result in retarded growth (Table 42-2).

A first step in the diagnosis of growth retardation is to determine the degree of retardation and the symmetry of the reduced body size (proportionate vs. disproportionate growth). Most endocrine, metabolic, or systemic diseases result in proportionally normal but reduced growth, whereas the osteochondrodysplasias and nutritional diseases usually result in disproportionate or abnormally reduced growth. A minimum database should include a family and nutrition

TABLE 42-2   Classification of growth retardation

Osteochondrodysplasia	Diseases of endochondral ossification
	Diseases of intramembranous ossification
Endocrinopathy	Growth hormone deficiency (German Shepherd Dog)
	Congenital hypothyroidism (Scottish Deerhound)
	Diabetes mellitus (Golden Retriever, Keeshond, Rottweiler)
Congenital disorders of cell metabolism	Lipid storage disease
	Glycogen storage disease
Nutritional deficiency	Major nutrients (essential amino acids, fats, carbohydrates)
	Minerals (calcium, phosphorus, zinc)
	Vitamins (A, D, E)
	Oxygen (heart and/or lung disease)
Chronic inflammation	Immunodeficiencies
	Intestinal parasite
Congenital or acquired major organ failure or insufficiency	Heart failure
	Hepatic failure (portosystemic shunts)
	Renal failure (progressive renal insufficiency, Fanconi's syndrome, polycystic renal disease)
	Digestive tract disease

Modified from Lorenz MD: Retarded growth. In Lorenz MD, Cornelius LM (eds): *Small animal medical diagnosis*, Philadelphia, 1993, JB Lippincott, pp 83-90.

history, complete blood count (CBC), serum chemistry, urine and fecal analysis (parasites), and radiographs of the radius and ulna. If an endocrinopathy is suspected, serum thyroxine, a thyroid-stimulating hormone test, growth hormone stimulation test, and/or determination of insulin-like growth factor-1 serum concentrations may be indicated.

Osteochondrodysplasia

Most patients with osteochondrodysplasias have reduced skeletal growth, characterized by abnormal endochondral and/or intramembranous ossification. The diagnosis of osteochondrodysplasias is based on the patient's signalment (breed), history (identifiable at birth or later in life, family, and nutrition history), clinical findings (proportionate or disproportionate, mentation), CBC, serum chemistry, urine analysis, endocrine evaluation as recommended for retarded growth, radiography (skull, appendicular and/or axial skeleton, epiphyseal growth centers, and/or growth plates), and growth plate histopathology (rib resection, percutaneous growth plate biopsy, or postmortem specimen) (Table 42-3). Chondrodystrophic dogs likely have an osteochondrodysplasia that can result in a tendency for relatively long trunks and short legs.

Dysostosis

Dysostoses may occur in the skull, axial, and/or appendicular skeleton. Diseases of mesenchymal bone formation in the appendicular skeleton are characterized by overrepresentation or a partial or complete absence of one or more bone elements. Patients usually present with a limb deformity and a severe, often non–weight-bearing lameness. The disease may be bilateral. Dysostoses can be diagnosed using radiography of the affected body region. Dysostoses of the appendicular skeleton may be subclassified as amelia, dimelia, hemimelia, ectrodactyly, polydactyly, and syndactyly (Table 42-4). The most commonly seen dysostosis is radial hemimelia. Treatment may be conservative (bandage or splint to prevent muscle contractures and bone deformities during rapid growth) or surgical (amputation, bone repair, or arthrodesis).

Joint Malformations

Severe joint malformations are rarely diagnosed and may range from complete absence of joints to bony fusion of skeletal elements. Abnormal epiphyseal development following trauma, congenital absence of ligaments (congenital elbow luxation), or asynchronous growth of adjacent paired bones (radial head subluxation) may also cause malformed joints. Joint malformations are diagnosed radiographically.

TABLE 42-3   Canine and feline osteochondrodysplasia

Breed	Trait	Mode of inheritance	Genetic test
Akita	Achondrogenesis	Unknown	No
Alaskan Malamute	Chondrodysplasia	Simple autosomal recessive	No
Beagle	Chondrodysplasia punctata	Unknown	No
	Multiple epiphyseal dysplasia	Simple autosomal recessive	No
	Osteogenesis imperfecta		No
Bulldog	Osteochondrodysplasia	Unknown	No
Bull Terrier	Osteochondrodysplasia	Unknown	No
Cocker Spaniel	Hypochondroplasia	Unknown	No
Great Pyrenees	Chondrodysplasia	Simple autosomal recessive	No
Irish Setter	Hypochondroplasia	Simple autosomal recessive	No
Labrador Retriever	Oculoskeletal dysplasia	Simple autosomal recessive	No
Miniature Poodle	Achondroplasia	Simple autosomal recessive	No
	Epiphyseal chondrodysplasia	Unknown	No
	Multiple epiphyseal dysplasia	Unknown	No
Mixed-breed dog	Mucopolysaccharidosis VII	Simple autosomal recessive	Yes*
Norwegian Elkhound	Chondrodysplasia	Simple autosomal recessive	No
Plott Hound	Mucopolysaccharidosis I	Simple autosomal recessive	Yes*
Samoyed	Oculoskeletal dysplasia without hematologic abnormalities	Simple autosomal recessive	No
	Oculoskeletal dysplasia with hematologic abnormalities	Unknown	No
Scottish Terrier	Achondroplasia	Unknown	No
	Idiopathic multifocal osteopathy	Unknown	No
Scottish Deerhound	Pseudoachondroplasia	Simple autosomal recessive	No
Domestic Shorthair cat	Mucopolysaccharidosis I	Unknown	Yes*
Siamese	Mucopolysaccharidosis VI	Simple autosomal recessive	Yes*
	Multiple cartilaginous exostoses	Unknown	No

*Clinical genetic testing available through PennGen (www.vet.upenn.edu/penngen).
Modified from Breur GJ, Lust G, Todhunter RJ: Genetics of canine hip dysplasia and other orthopaedic traits. In Ruvinsky A, Sampson J (eds): *The genetics of the dog*, New York, 2001, CABI Publishing, pp 267-298.

TABLE 42-4	Canine and feline appendicular dysostoses		
Disorder	Definition	Breeds with demonstrated heritable etiology	Mode of inheritance
Hemimelia	Complete or partial absence of one or more bones	Chihuahua	Unknown
		Domestic Shorthair cat	Autosomal recessive
		Siamese cat	Autosomal recessive
Ectrodactyly	Separation of metacarpal bones into a medial and lateral portion of the limb	Domestic Shorthair cat	Autosomal dominant
Polydactyly	Presence of one or more extra digits	Great Pyrenees	Autosomal dominant
		Collie	Autosomal recessive
		Saint Bernard	Autosomal recessive
		Australian Shepherd	X-linked lethal or sex-influenced autosomal
Syndactyly	Bony or soft tissue union between one or more digits	Domestic Shorthair cat	Unknown
		Australian Shepherd	X-linked lethal or sex-influenced autosomal

Modified from Towle HAM, Breur GJ: Dysostoses of the appendicular skeleton, *J Am Vet Med Assoc* 225:1685-1692, 2004.

Congenital Myopathies

Congenital myopathies are a group of primary, inherited diseases of skeletal muscle identified within the first weeks to months after birth. In most instances, the diagnosis of these diseases is based on breed, gender, history (age of onset, number of puppies affected in the litter), abnormal general physical exam (heart or diaphragm may be involved), abnormal neurologic examination (diffuse lower motor neuron signs with myotonia), elevated serum muscle enzymes, abnormal electromyography, and abnormal muscle histopathology. In selected disorders, the diagnosis can be confirmed with a molecular genetic test. A differential diagnosis for patients with lower motor neuron signs should include motor and sensory (viral), toxic, or autonomic neuropathies and polyneuropathies. Specific treatment for these congenital myopathies is not available, but supportive care may be beneficial.

ACQUIRED MUSCULOSKELETAL DISEASES

Acquired Bone Diseases

Acquired bone diseases do not have a primarily genetic etiology and are not identifiable at birth. They are classified as traumatic injuries, deformities, and nutritional, developmental, and miscellaneous disorders.

Traumatic Injuries (Fractures)

Approximately 40% to 50% of all dogs presented to referral centers with traumatic injuries are less than 1 year of age. Because of the continued growth and different mechanical properties of immature bone, treatment of musculoskeletal injuries of immature animals is often different and more challenging than treatment of such injuries in mature animals.

From a mechanical viewpoint, mature and immature bones are different. Compared with mature bone, immature bone is more resilient and elastic, resulting in different fracture types, like "greenstick" fractures in which the periosteal sleeve is left intact. The nutrient artery of immature long bones does not penetrate growth plates; therefore epiphyses rely solely on epiphyseal arteries for their blood supply. The periosteum of immature bone is thicker and more vascular than mature periosteum. It easily elevates from bone following trauma, and ensuing hematomas will facilitate rapid bone formation. Periosteum of immature animals, if intact, may also aid in the stabilization of fractures. It can be identified easily and sutured if needed. Immature animals also have more active periosteal, appositional bone formation and callus formation than mature animals. Compared with mature bone, screws and pins do not hold as well and strip easily and pull out of immature metaphyseal and epiphyseal bone because immature bone is more brittle than mature bone. Intramedullary pins have more anchorage in metaphyseal and epiphyseal bone because the medullary cavity of immature bone is relatively small compared with mature bone.

Fracture healing in young animals is more rapid (Table 42-5) and is characterized by abundant callus formation, active remodeling, more rapid clinical union, and a very low incidence of nonunions. Because of this rapid healing, fractures in immature animals should be treated as soon as possible. Immature animals have more compensatory mechanisms to correct for inadequate fracture reduction than mature animals. Inadequate reduction in craniocaudal and lateromedial direction is acceptable and will be corrected and remodeled. In contrast to mature animals, some bending at the fracture site may be acceptable and can be intrinsically corrected by young pups and kittens. Rotation following fracture reduction cannot be compensated for and may not

TABLE 42-5	Rate of fracture healing in dogs of different ages	
Age	IM Pin ESF (type I, some II)	Plate fixation ESF (type III, some II)
<3 mo	2-3 wk	4 wk
3-6 mo	4-6 wk	6-12 wk
6-12 mo	5-8 wk	12-16 wk
>1 yr	7-12 wk	16-30 wk

From Brinker WO, Piermattei DL, Flo GL: *Handbook of small animal orthopedics and fracture repair*, ed 3, Philadelphia, 1997, Saunders, p 155.
IM, Intramedullary; *ESF,* external skeletal fixation.

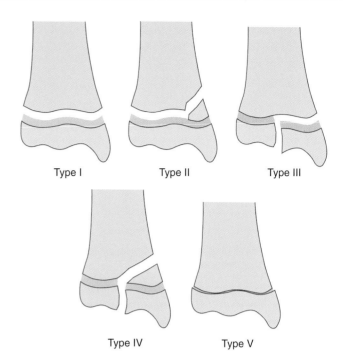

Type I   Type II   Type III

Type IV   Type V

Figure 42-1 Salter-Harris classification of growth plate separations. (From Fossum TW (ed): *Small animal surgery*, ed 3, St Louis, 2007, Mosby/Elsevier, p 951.)

be acceptable. Incomplete functional recovery following repair as a result of muscle contractures and adhesions (quadriceps contracture) is more common in immature animals than in mature animals. Therefore early physical therapy may be needed for complete return of function after fracture healing.

Because the growth plate is the weakest structure of immature long bones, the growth plate is a common site for injury. Traumatic growth plate injuries have been classified by Salter and Harris (Figure 42-1) in an effort to relate mechanisms, characteristics, and prognosis. A type I growth plate injury is characterized by a separation through the growth plate. A type II injury is a combined growth plate separation–metaphyseal fracture. A type III injury is a combined growth plate separation–epiphyseal fracture. A type IV injury is characterized by a combination of a growth plate separation with an epiphyseal and metaphyseal fracture. Type V injuries are caused by crushing of the growth plate, which results in premature closure and reduced bone length growth. Selected type I and II injuries may be amenable to casting. Growth plate separations are most commonly treated with K-wires or Rush pins, whereas epiphyseal and metaphyseal fractures may be stabilized with screws or K-wires.

Limb Deformities with Primary Skeletal Abnormalities

Limb deformities with abnormally shaped bones may be caused by dysostoses, osteochondrodysplasias, nutritional diseases, and growth plate injuries. Growth plate injuries are the most common cause of bone-induced limb deformity. Fractures involving the growth plates can involve either the complete growth plate or portions of it and may result in stunted or arrested growth (premature closure). Clinically this results in shortened bones or asymmetrical growth with subsequent angular deformity and/or rotational deformities of the affected bone in cases involving a partial growth plate closure. Because such complications are relatively common, owners should be advised about the possibility of deformity following skeletal injury in immature animals.

The choice between conservative and surgical treatment of deformities depends on many factors, including clinical

presentation. If the deformity is a cosmetic flaw only and not causing discomfort or lameness, treatment may not be necessary. If the deformity is associated with pain and lameness, surgical management is indicated. With surgical correction, the joint above and below the deformity is realigned to improve the mechanical function of the limb and to slow down the progression of osteoarthritis in the adjacent joints. If growth has been completed and there is no or minimal limb shortening, a corrective osteotomy (transverse, cuneiform, opening wedge, oblique, or dome) followed by stabilization of the osteotomy with either an external fixator or a bone plate is recommended. If growth has been completed and loss of bone length is part of the deformity, a corrective osteotomy followed by distraction osteogenesis may be considered. If continued growth is anticipated and there is already noticeable limb shortening, corrective osteotomy and distraction osteogenesis also may be indicated.

The effect of growth plate trauma may be amplified if the paired radius and ulna are involved. Trauma to the distal ulnar or the proximal or distal radial growth plate can cause asynchronous growth and unequal length of the radius and ulna. Asynchronous growth of the radius and ulna may be caused by other conditions as well. It may result in carpal valgus, elbow pain and incongruity, and/or cranial bowing of the radius (radius curvus) and is often associated with lameness. The first goal of treatment is reestablishment of elbow congruity to resolve elbow pain and facilitation of continued growth of radius and ulna with ulnar osteotomy (long radius) or ulnar ostectomy or radial lengthening (long ulna). If the deformity developed at a very young age, this procedure may have to be repeated if asynchronous growth continues and the elbow incongruity recurs. The second goal is correction of the angular deformity by a realignment of the elbow and radiocarpal joint, usually in a later separate surgery, with corrective osteotomy of the radius and ulna followed by stabilization of the radial osteotomy with an external fixator or bone plate.

If limb shortening is part of the deformity or continued impaired growth is a concern, distraction osteogenesis may be required (Figure 42-2). Treatment of deformities is often complex, and patients with deformity should be referred for further evaluation and possible surgical treatment as soon as the deformity is noticed.

Nutritional Diseases

Orthopedic diseases caused solely by nutritional deficiencies or oversupplementation have become rare. This group of diseases includes nutritional secondary hyperparathyroidism, hypovitaminosis D (rickets), hypervitaminosis D, hypovitaminosis A, hypervitaminosis A, and hypovitaminosis E. Additional information pertaining to nutritional diseases can be found in Chapter 44.

Developmental Orthopedic Bone Diseases

Craniomandibular osteopathy occurs in the Terrier breeds, especially the West Highland White Terrier (Table 42-6). The mode of inheritance is likely autosomal recessive. The

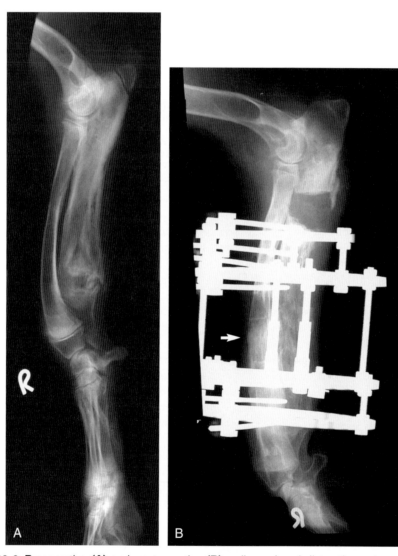

Figure 42-2 Preoperative **(A)** and postoperative **(B)** radiographs of distraction osteogenesis in a 17-week-old Great Dane with an angular limb deformity and a short limb caused by premature closure of the distal ulnar growth plate secondary to hematogenous osteomyelitis of the ulnar diaphysis and distal metaphysis. Note the mild elbow incongruity, radial bowing, radiolucency in the distal ulnar growth plate, and ulnar remodeling in the preoperative radiograph. The elbow incongruity was corrected using a proximal ulnar osteotomy. Distraction osteogenesis was chosen to lengthen the radius and ulna and to correct a mild carpal valgus. The arrow is pointing to the distraction zone in the radius.

TABLE 42-6	Breed predilections for selected developmental orthopedic diseases (DODs)	
DODs	**Breeds at increased risk**
Affected Bones	
Craniomandibular osteopathy	Cairn Terrier, Scottish Terrier, West Highland White Terrier
Hypertrophic osteodystrophy	Boxer, Chesapeake Bay Retriever, German Shepherd Dog, Golden Retriever, Great Dane, Irish Setter, Labrador Retriever, Weimaraner
Panosteitis	Afghan Hound, Akita, American Cocker Spaniel, American Staffordshire Terrier, Basset Hound, Bearded Collie, Bernese Mountain Dog, Boxer, Bull Terrier, Bulldog, Chesapeake Bay Retriever, Chow Chow, Dalmatian, Doberman Pinscher, English Setter, English Springer Spaniel, Giant Schnauzer, German Shepherd Dog, German Shorthaired Pointer, Golden Retriever, Great Dane, Great Pyrenees, Irish Wolfhound, Labrador Retriever, Mastiff, Neapolitan Mastiff, Newfoundland, Rhodesian Ridgeback, Rottweiler, Saint Bernard, Shar-Pei, Shih Tzu, Weimaraner, West Highland White Terrier
Affected Joints	
Shoulder joint osteochondrosis dissecans	Bernese Mountain Dog, Border Collie, Bouvier, Boxer, Bullmastiff, Chesapeake Bay Retriever, Dalmatian, English Setter, German Shorthaired Pointer, German Shepherd Dog, German Wirehaired Pointer, Golden Retriever, Great Dane, Great Pyrenees, Irish Wolfhound, Kuvasz, Labrador Retriever, Mastiff, Münsterländer, Newfoundland, Old English Sheepdog, Rottweiler, Saint Bernard, Standard Poodle
Distal humerus osteochondrosis dissecans	Chow Chow, German Shepherd Dog, Golden Retriever, Great Dane, Labrador Retriever, Newfoundland, Rottweiler
Fragmented medial coronoid process	Basset Hound, Bernese Mountain Dog, Bouvier, Bullmastiff, Chow Chow, German Shepherd Dog, Golden Retriever, Gordon Setter, Irish Wolfhound, Labrador Retriever, Mastiff, Newfoundland, Rottweiler, Saint Bernard
Ununited anconeal process	Basset Hound, Bernese Mountain Dog, Chow Chow, English Setter, German Shepherd Dog, Golden Retriever, Labrador Retriever, Mastiff, Newfoundland, Pomeranian, Rottweiler, Saint Bernard, Shar-Pei
Hip dysplasia	Airedale Terrier, Alaskan Malamute, Bearded Collie, Bernese Mountain Dog, Bloodhound, Border Collie, Bouvier, Briard, Brittany Spaniel, Bulldog, Bullmastiff, Chesapeake Bay Retriever, Chow Chow, English Springer Spaniel, German Shepherd Dog, German Wirehaired Pointer, Giant Schnauzer, Golden Retriever, Gordon Setter, Great Dane, Great Pyrenees, Keeshond, Kuvasz, Labrador Retriever, Mastiff, Neapolitan Mastiff, Newfoundland, Norwegian Elkhound, Old English Sheepdog, Pointer, Portuguese Water Dog, Rottweiler, Saint Bernard, Samoyed, Treeing Walker Coonhound
Legg-Calvé-Perthes disease	Australian Shepherd, Cairn Terrier, Chihuahua, Dachshund, Lhasa Apso, Manchester Terrier, Miniature Pinscher, Pug, Toy Poodle, West Highland White Terrier, Yorkshire Terrier
Distal femur osteochondrosis dissecans	Boxer, Bulldog, German Shepherd Dog, Golden Retriever, Great Dane, Irish Wolfhound, Labrador Retriever, Mastiff, Rottweiler
Patellar luxation (medial and lateral)	Akita, American Cocker Spaniel, Australian Terrier, Basset Hound, Bichon Frise, Boston Terrier, Bulldog, Cairn Terrier, Cavalier King Charles Spaniel, Chihuahua, Chow Chow, Flat-Coated Retriever, Great Pyrenees, Japanese Chin, Keeshond, Lhasa Apso, Maltese, Miniature Pinscher, miniature Poodle, Papillon, Pekingese, Pomeranian, Pug, Shar-Pei, Shih Tzu, Silky Terrier, Standard Poodle, Toy Fox Terrier, Toy Poodle, West Highland White Terrier, Wirehaired Fox Terrier, Yorkshire Terrier
Tarsocrural joint osteochondrosis dissecans	Labrador Retriever, Rottweiler, Bullmastiff

From LaFond E, Breur GJ, Austin CC: Breed susceptibility for developmental orthopedic diseases in dogs, *J Am Anim Hosp Assoc* 38:467-477, 2002.

bony formation along the mandible can be so severe that affected dogs may not be able to prehend and chew food (Figure 42-3). Treatment is supportive.

In young large or giant breed dogs, diaphyseal pain in one or multiple bones may be an indication of panosteitis.

Panosteitis is a self-limiting disease of unknown cause. One hypothesis revolves around decreased bone remodeling with intramedullary edema and excess bone formation. Additionally, excess calcium administered to young dogs drives down parathyroid hormone secretion, resulting in decreased bone remodeling around vessels as they traverse the cortex through the nutrient foramen. The diagnosis is made based on increased medullary opacity (Figure 42-4). Medullary enostosis of the diaphyseal and metaphyseal areas of long bones, especially the ulna, is observed histologically. German Shepherd Dogs are particularly vulnerable (see Table 42-6), which suggests a heritable component to this condition. Acute, intermittent, shifting (from leg to leg) lameness of variable severity is characteristic. Sensitivity to deep palpation along the long bones can be elicited with panosteitis. Because the condition is self-limiting, treatment is aimed at providing analgesia until the condition resolves.

Hypertrophic osteodystrophy is a developmental disease in immature, large, or giant breed dogs (see Table 42-6 for breed predispositions) in which the metaphyseal area of long bones becomes swollen and painful. The distal radius and ulna are most commonly affected, but the disease can affect the distal tibia. Failure or delay in cortical remodeling or progressive ossification of the metaphysis subjacent to the growth plate may be observed. Affected dogs may be febrile, toxic, and recumbent, requiring supportive therapy, although the cause of toxemia is still unclear. Because of the systemic nature of this condition, an infectious process and adverse reaction to distemper vaccination are proposed etiologies. Inflammation, hemorrhage, fractures, and extensive remodeling in metaphyseal trabeculae are hypothesized to result in bone abnormalities observed radiographically. Diagnosis is based on history, clinical signs, and variable lameness with swollen, warm, and painful distal metaphyses of long bones. The disease is often bilaterally symmetric. The diagnosis is confirmed radiographically with a metaphyseal lucent line parallel to the growth plate and periosteal proliferation (Figure 42-5). Periosteal mineralization may be observed on radiographs. Bridging of the growth plate as a result of periosteal proliferation or synostosis (which arrests growth) is likely in the most severely affected animals; therefore owners should be warned of the possibility of angular limb deformity.

Miscellaneous

Included in this group of diseases are incomplete bony fusion of the lateral and medial humeral condyle, retained cartilaginous core, slipped capital femoral epiphysis, and pes varus. Incomplete ossification of the humeral condyle is primarily seen in middle-aged spaniels. This condition may result in lameness or a pathologic medial, lateral, or Y condylar fracture in older animals. Lameness may be hard to diagnose, and the condition may be associated with bony proliferation along the lateral epicondylar crest. Fracture prevention and lameness treatment may consist of transcondylar screw placement. It has been suggested that this disease has a recessive mode of inheritance.

Retained cartilaginous cores are cones of growth plate cartilage projecting into the metaphysis and are commonly seen in immature dogs. They represent a failure of growth plate cartilage to convert into metaphyseal bone. They usually are a coincidental finding but may be associated with limb deformity. There is no treatment, and the cores will disappear spontaneously. Retained cartilaginous core may be caused by reduced metaphyseal blood supply.

SCFE (slipped capital femoral epiphysis) is a slow, progressive displacement of the proximal femoral metaphysis from the capital femoral epiphysis through the growth plate. This condition is nontraumatic and different from a Salter fracture-separation of the capital femoral growth plate. SCFE has been reported in both cats and dogs. Cats up to

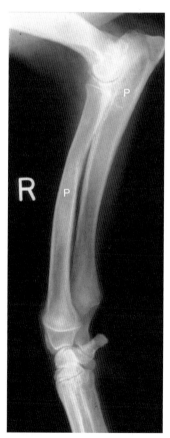

Figure 42-4 Left lateral radiograph of the radius and ulna of an 8-month-old Labrador Retriever with medullary enostosis in both ulnae. A periosteal reaction characteristic of panosteitis (P) is also present in the radial diaphysis.

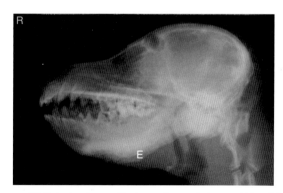

Figure 42-3 Lateral mandibular radiograph from a West Highland White Terrier with an exostosis (E) characteristic of craniomandibular osteopathy.

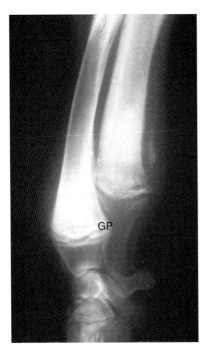

Figure 42-5 Radiograph of the distal radius and ulna from a 6-month-old Great Dane with hypertrophic osteodystrophy showing periosteal proliferation and development of two growth plates (GP) as a result of the metabolic interruption.

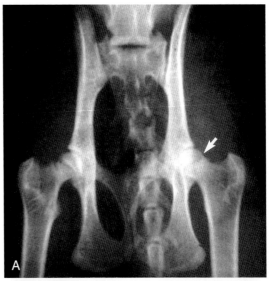

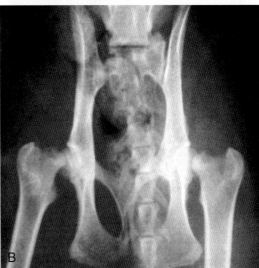

Figure 42-6 Ventrodorsal pelvic radiographs from a 20-month-old neutered male cat with bilateral slipped capital femoral epiphysis (SCFE) at 2 days **(A)** and 28 days **(B)** after the onset of lameness. At 2 days, a mild "slip" of the right femoral metaphysis and a wide radiolucent line in the left femoral head *(arrow)* indicating early SCFE is visible. By day 28, progression to bilateral complete physeal separation with bilateral osteolysis and sclerosis had occurred. (From McNicholas WT et al: Spontaneous capital femoral epiphyseal fractures in cats older than 1 year of age, *J Am Vet Med Assoc* 221:1731-1736, 2002.)

3.5 years of age may be presented with SCFE, and most are overweight neutered males with open growth plates. Affected patients present with a complaint of insidious hindlimb lameness and pain on manipulation of the hip joint. The diagnosis is based on radiographic changes (displacement of the proximal femoral metaphysis accompanied by resorption and sclerosis of the femoral neck) (Figure 42-6).

In early stages of the disease, ultrasound may aid in establishing the diagnosis. It has been suggested that the delayed growth plate closure is caused by hypotestosteronism following castration. Although surgical stabilization of the "slip" with K-wire may be possible, a femoral head and neck ostectomy is usually more appropriate because of the progressive resorption of the femoral neck. The prognosis with surgical excision is excellent. Slipped capital femoral epiphysis has been documented in dogs as well, but the etiology and pathophysiology are unknown. Treatment is as in cats, although a total hip replacement may be considered if the femoral neck is intact and the dog is large enough.

Pes varus is a varus deformity of the distal hindlimb in Dachshunds caused by nontraumatic premature closure of the medial distal tibial growth plate. Recommended treatment consists of an open-wedge osteotomy of the distal tibia followed by stabilization with a type II external fixator. The condition may be inherited.

Most osteomyelitis in puppies and kittens is bacterial in origin and may be hematogenous or posttraumatic. The chronic form, usually posttraumatic and associated with fractures, implants, bite wounds, or systemic illness, presents the same as in mature dogs and is treated similarly.

Hematogenous osteomyelitis is more often seen in immature than in mature animals. In the acute stage, patients present with localized pain, swelling, elevated temperature, and lameness. Radiographic signs include periosteal proliferation and sequestra but may be absent in early stages. In the acute phase, patients may have an elevated white blood count with a neutrophilic left shift. Samples for bacterial culture and antibiotic sensitivity may be obtained from the offending site via fine needle aspirates or medullary bone biopsy. Hematogenous infections usually are monomicrobial, and identified microorganisms include *Staphylococcus aureus*,

Staphylococcus intermedius, and *Escherichia coli*. Treatment should be based on clinical presentation and on the results of the antibiotic sensitivity of the causative microorganism. Referral to a specialist for further evaluation and treatment should be considered.

Joint Diseases

Approximately 35% of dogs younger than 1 year of age presented with a musculoskeletal problem are diagnosed with an arthropathy. These arthropathies may be classified as noninflammatory or inflammatory. About 95% of the arthropathies in growing dogs are noninflammatory.

Inflammatory Arthropathies
Infectious arthropathies

Bacterial infectious arthritis is uncommon in growing animals. It is caused either by penetrating wounds or hematogenous spread. Diagnosis is based on radiography and synovial fluid analysis. The synovial fluid analysis should include cytology, Gram's stain for identification of bacteria, and aerobic and anaerobic bacteriologic culture and sensitivity. Aggressive treatment is warranted and consists of evacuation of the exudate (aspiration or arthroscopy/arthrotomy) and local or systemic administration of antibiotics. *Borrelia burgdorferi* (Lyme disease), *Rickettsia*, and *Ehrlichia* organisms may also cause infectious polyarthritis in growing animals.

Noninfectious arthropathies

Occasionally rheumatoid arthritis may be diagnosed in growing dogs. Some polyarthropathies are unique to growing dogs. Semierosive polyarthritis in Greyhounds may be diagnosed in puppies as young as 3 months of age. Treatment may consist of prednisone with or without other immunosuppressive drugs (such as azathioprine). Suppurative arthritis has been described in association with canine juvenile cellulitis. Synovial fluid culture would be negative. Simultaneous treatment with antibiotics and prednisone may cure the disease.

Noninflammatory Arthropathies
Developmental orthopedic joint diseases

Developmental orthopedic diseases affecting joints are the most common arthropathies in growing animals and the most important cause for osteoarthritis or degenerative joint disease. Diseases in this group are usually breed-related, have a consistent age of onset, and a consistent clinical course (see Table 42-6). Most of these diseases are multifactorial or complex with genetic, nutritional, and environmental factors implicated in their etiopathogenesis. Alleles located at several quantitative trait loci influence the expression of complex phenotypes, like developmental orthopedic disease. Phenotypic expression of these alleles, most or all of which must be present for disease expression, is affected by environment such as diet, exercise, and litter effects. Signalment, history, and physical examination will usually localize the clinical problem to a region, joint, or portion of the long bones. Because many of these developmental orthopedic traits affect joints bilaterally, it is often wise to radiograph both sides even if only one side was found to be clinically affected at the time of examination. When growth is maximized, there is maximum opportunity for phenotypic expression if the dog carries the alleles that contribute to the trait. Offspring of Labrador Retrievers with hip dysplasia fed 75% of the ad libitum diet of age-matched control dogs had significantly less radiographic evidence of hip dysplasia and hip osteoarthritis than their ad libitum–fed counterparts.

Osteochondrosis

General OC is a systemic disease of endochondral ossification. It is characterized by interruption in conversion of cartilage to bone (endochondral ossification) in the epiphyses or the metaphyses. The terminal hypertrophic chondrocytes do not undergo apoptosis (programmed cell death), and vascular invasion is interrupted so the cartilage gets thicker until its nutrition by diffusion is compromised. Eventually the necrotic cartilage separates from the underlying subchondral bone (Figure 42-7, *A*). OC can present as either subchondral bone cysts or osteochondrosis(itis) dissecans (OCD). Dogs usually develop OCD (flaplike) lesions (Figure 42-7, *B*). A subchondral lucency or mineralized articular cartilage flap is seen on lateral radiographs of the shoulder in affected dogs. Various etiologies of OC have been proposed, including traumatic, vascular, genetic, endocrine/sex hormonal, conformational, and nutritional/environmental.

Shoulder
Shoulder osteochondrosis

Several breeds are predisposed for shoulder OC (see Table 42-6), and 50% to 70% heritability has been estimated in Labrador Retrievers. In Rottweilers and Bernese Mountain Dogs, heritability of OCD was 10% and 45%, respectively. Males outnumber females in incidence. The condition is bilateral in 20% to 85% of cases. Dogs usually present during the growth phase. The history may include mild to marked, intermittent forelimb lameness that was insidious in onset and may be more evident on one forelimb than the other.

The diagnosis is based on clinical signs, palpation, and radiography. Pain is palpated in full shoulder extension and sometimes when the humeral head is pushed against the glenoid in the flexed position. Effusion is not palpable in the shoulder area, and shoulder girdle muscular atrophy may be evident. Plain lateral shoulder radiographs may reveal evidence of an OCD flap, but some mineralized articular cartilage has to be present with the flap to see it radiographically. Sometimes intraarticular contrast is needed to highlight the flap, and air is effective as a contrast agent. A detached OCD lesion may detach and appear as a mineralized cartilage round body in the caudal cul-de-sac of the shoulder or cranially around the biceps tendon.

There are no long-term studies that report the results of surgical debridement compared with a conservative approach in a prospective manner. Surgical treatment of OCD of the

called elbow dysplasia. This syndrome includes ununited anconeal process, fragmented medial coronoid process, OC of the medial humeral condyle, ununited medial epicondyle, and asynchronous growth between the radius and ulna. In Labrador Retrievers, heritability of elbow osteoarthritis secondary to OCD or fragmented medial coronoid process was estimated at 27%. Bernese Mountain Dogs are at twelve-fold increased risk for elbow dysplasia. A heritable basis for elbow OC in Rottweilers and Golden Retrievers has been reported. Other breeds that are affected are the German Shepherd Dog, Saint Bernard, Great Dane, and Newfoundland (see Table 42-6). There is no gender predilection for elbow, stifle, or hock location of OC. The International Elbow Working Group in Europe and the Orthopedic Foundation for Animals (OFA) in the United States has an elbow registry similar to that for hip dysplasia. For evaluation, the OFA requires submission of a flexed lateral radiograph at 2 years of age or older.

The history of elbow dysplasia usually includes an insidious onset of forelimb lameness, exacerbated by exercise in growing large breed dogs. Examination of the dog shows a tendency to a stiff, choppy gait characterized by external rotation of the lower forelimb. Elbow dysplasia is bilateral in 20% to 50% of cases, but one elbow may be more clinically affected than the other; therefore lameness in one limb may predominate or lameness may shift from one forelimb to the other. Effusion may be bilateral and presents as an outpouching of the lateral elbow capsule underneath the anconeus muscle. Detection of elbow pain in young dogs by internal/external rotation with the elbow held at 90 degrees and detection of elbow pain in full extension should be followed up with radiography.

United anconeal process

Juvenile large dogs, especially the German Shepherd Dog, are the most commonly affected by ununited anconeal process (see Table 42-6). The ossification center of the anconeal process fails to undergo bony fusion to the ulnar metaphysis. Proposed etiologies include genetic, hormonal, metabolic, nutritional, traumatic, or OC. Not all dogs have a separate ossification center for the anconeal process. The usual time of anconeal process fusion to the ulna is 4 to 5 months of age or later in very large or giant breeds (e.g., Saint Bernard). The condition is bilateral in approximately one third of dogs. The flexed lateral radiographic view is helpful for diagnosis. Surgical excision was the traditional treatment of choice. However, lag screw fixation or dynamic ulnar osteotomy under appropriate circumstances are now advocated. The ulnar osteotomy is based on the concept that the lack of union to the ulna is caused by upward pressure from the radial head on the humeral condyle and secondary pressure on the anconeus by the humeral condyle. An ulnar osteotomy allows upward movement of the olecranon, thus relieving pressure on the anconeal process. The prognosis for function and slowing the progression of secondary osteoarthritis is fair to good. Union of the anconeal process following ulnar osteotomy may occur in younger dogs.

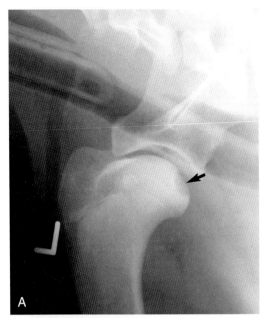
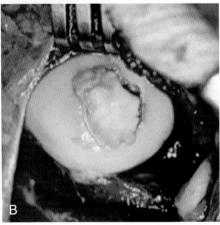

Figure 42-7 Radiographic **(A)** and intraoperative **(B)** images of osteochondrosis dissecans (OCD) lesions of the caudal aspect of the humeral head from a young dog. The subchondral defect *(arrow)* is visible on the caudal humeral head in **A**. The intraoperative image shows a large OCD lesion. (Courtesy Dr. Trotter, Cornell University.)

humeral head carries a good prognosis for functional recovery, whereas surgical intervention to treat OCD in other locations carries a guarded prognosis for recovery. Conservative management for shoulder osteoarthritis is no different from management of osteoarthritis of other joints—exercise modification, weight reduction if indicated, diet high in omega-3 polyunsaturated fatty acids, pain management with nonsteroidal antiinflammatory drugs and slow-acting, disease-modifying osteoarthritis agents like polysulfated glycosaminoglycans (PSGAGs) or glucosamine and chondroitin sulfate.

Elbow
Elbow dysplasia

Lameness localized to the elbow of young growing dogs with no history of trauma is usually caused by the syndrome

Fragmented medial coronoid process

Fragmented medial coronoid process is the most common developmental condition affecting elbows of growing dogs. Many dog breeds are predisposed, particularly Rottweilers and German Shepherd Dogs (see Table 42-6). Heritability is reported to be 28% and 40% for Labrador Retrievers and Rottweilers, respectively. Fragmented medial coronoid process is more common in male dogs and is often bilateral. Elbow incongruity from asynchronous growth between the radius, ulna, and humerus results in a shortened radius and relatively longer ulna, which may lead to a fragmented medial coronoid process.

Signs of elbow pain with no other radiographic changes consistent with ununited anconeal process or OC of the medial humeral condyle should raise suspicions of a fragmented medial coronoid process. The fragmented medial coronoid process can usually not be seen radiographically on standard views because of superimposition of the radial head and medial coronoid process. Elbow effusion, along with pain on internal and external rotation or full extension of the elbow, will be a tipoff. Pathognomonic radiographic signs of secondary osteoarthritis include sclerosis of the bone around the medial coronoid process, osteophytes on the medial coronoid and cranial radial head, and entheses along the dorsal olecranon toward the anconeus where the joint capsule attaches. The elbow is an unforgiving joint if it is affected by osteoarthritis. Early diagnosis is essential to treat the underlying developmental condition and slow progression of secondary osteoarthritis. If a diagnosis cannot be made by radiography, computed tomography, magnetic resonance imaging, arthroscopy, or exploratory arthrotomy should be used. Surgical excision of the fragmented medial coronoid process at the time of initial diagnosis before osteoarthritis is advanced is the recommended optimal treatment. Immature dogs have a better outcome than mature dogs because the regenerative power of the articular chondroepiphysis is higher than in younger dogs. Underlying conformational problems should be addressed (e.g., elbow incongruity), but mild cases can be difficult to diagnose radiographically.

Osteochondrosis of the medial humeral condyle

Many breeds are predisposed for this disease (see Table 42-6). OC of the medial humeral condyle occurs less frequently in Rottweilers compared with Labrador and Golden Retrievers. The clinical signs are similar to those of fragmented medial coronoid process, and sometimes the two conditions occur in the same joint. The diagnosis is made radiographically based on subchondral lucency of the medial humeral condyle, or occasionally an OCD-type flap can be seen. Treatment with surgical excision even in immature dogs carries a guarded prognosis for functional recovery. These lesions are on a weight-bearing surface of the elbow joint; thus the repair tissue and surrounding articular cartilage undergo mechanically induced degeneration, leading inevitably to secondary osteoarthritis. In one study, the outcome following medical and surgical treatment at 6 months revealed no difference in clinical signs.

Hip
Legg-Calvé-Perthes disease

Hip pain in immature toy and small breeds may be the result of Legg-Calvé-Perthes (LCP) disease. Synonyms include aseptic necrosis of the femoral head, coxa plana, and coxa magna. The clinical signs develop between 4 and 11 months of age. Many small breeds are predisposed (see Table 42-6), and a recessive mode of inheritance has been reported in Manchester Terriers. Unlike most other inherited orthopedic traits that are bilateral, this condition is often unilateral. Legg-Calvé-Perthes disease is diagnosed radiographically based on loss of femoral head integrity, subchondral lucency, and collapse (Figure 42-8). Histologic findings suggest that this disease results from infarction of epiphyseal and metaphyseal bone, including the epiphysis. Epiphyseal collapse is observed; thus articular cartilage and bone are both involved. However, the cause is still unknown. Although conservative management may be successful in early stages of the disease, conventional treatment is surgical excision of the femoral head and neck. This carries a good prognosis for a full functional recovery. Aggressive postoperative physical therapy is required to promote muscle development for the best long-term outcome.

Hip dysplasia

Canine hip dysplasia (CHD) is a developmental trait primarily affecting medium and large breed dogs. The trait develops during the period of rapid growth but is difficult to detect at a very young age with standard imaging (Figure 42-9).

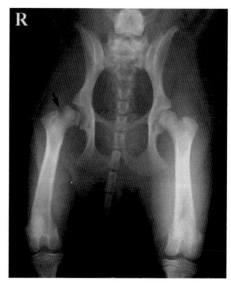

Figure 42-8 Ventrodorsal pelvic radiograph from a miniature Poodle with unilateral avascular necrosis of the femoral head (Legg-Calvé-Perthes disease) shown at *arrow*.

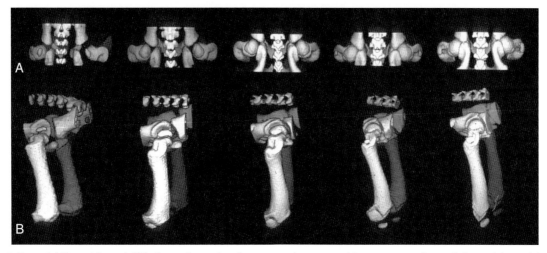

Figure 42-9 Dorsal **(A)** and lateral **(B)** three-dimensional computed tomographic reconstructions of the pelvis and femur from a Labrador Retriever beginning at 2 weeks of age and progressing to 10 weeks of age. The serial images illustrate the rapidity of bony maturation that occurs during the early growth period scaled to relative growth. (Courtesy Wendy Vanden Berg-Foels, Cornell University.)

CHD is characterized by faulty conformation and laxity of the hip joint that usually affects both hips. Clinically, early synovitis and capsulitis caused by subluxation is characterized by hindlimb lameness, reduced exercise tolerance, reluctance to jump, a "bunny hopping" gait when afflicted immature dogs run, poor hindlimb muscle mass, and laxity or pain in the hip joint. Radiographs reveal subluxation of the affected hip. Experimentally, Adequan (Luitpold Pharmaceuticals, Shirley, NY), a PSGAG, administered at 5 mg/kg subcutaneously or intramuscularly to dogs 6 weeks to 8 months of age significantly reduced the radiographic expression of CHD and also reduced the severity of secondary osteoarthritis.

Hip dysplasia affects dogs of all breeds, but it is more common as a clinical entity in large dogs. Many breeds are predisposed (see Table 42-6), and breed prevalence as estimated by the OFA varies from 1% to 75%. CHD has a heritable range between 0.25 and 0.7. Any medium to large breed dog (as well as small breeds and cats) and mixed breeds can express the trait. Pups with a genetic predisposition to CHD have hips that are grossly normal at birth. However, changes in the hip joint begin as early as the first few weeks of life. Coxofemoral subluxation may be palpable during weight bearing. A positive Ortolani sign indicates an abnormal hip.

The OFA will provide a provisional assessment of hip status at less than 2 years of age, and a definitive hip evaluation is given to dogs 2 years of age or older. According to the OFA, the sensitivity of the OFA radiograph at 12 months for later development of osteoarthritis in affected hips ranges from 77% to 99%, depending on the severity of the CHD at the earlier age. Ninety percent to 95% of dysplastic dogs have changes associated with CHD at 12 months of age. However, another study showed that of all dogs developing hip osteoarthritis over their lifespan, only 53% had radiographic evidence of a CHD at 2 years of age.

Hip status is graded on the OFA scale from excellent conformation to severe hip dysplasia; there are seven grades in all. The University of *Penn*sylvania *H*ip *I*mprovement *P*rogram (PennHIP) radiographic method measures the maximum amount of lateral distraction hip joint laxity (distraction index). There is a positive relationship between the distraction index and subsequent development of osteoarthritis. The best age for PennHIP screening is at early maturity. PennHIP also relies on the OFA-style radiograph to assess the degree of subluxation and secondary osteoarthritis. For the dorsolateral subluxation (DLS) score, the hips are imaged in a weight-bearing orientation under heavy sedation or general anesthesia with the dog positioned in ventral recumbency. The stifles are flexed and positioned under the hips so that the stifles are superimposed over the ischiatic table. The DLS score equates with the proportion of the femoral head covered by the dorsal acetabular rim.

For a single test under experimental conditions, the DLS score is the most accurate in detection of secondary hip osteoarthritis. A combination of the DLS score and Norberg angle provides a better estimate of a dog's likelihood of developing subsequent osteoarthritis than the DLS score alone. The Norberg angle is a measure of femoral head coverage on the OFA-style extended hip radiograph. The Norberg angle ranges from about 70 to 120 degrees, with the preferred angle more than 105 degrees.

Many hip-dysplastic dogs respond well to a combination of exercise modification, weight reduction if indicated, and antiinflammatory drugs. Food restriction during early growth to reduce weight gain and prevent obesity will limit the expression of CHD, as well as ease the pain associated with osteoarthritis. Juvenile pubic symphysiodesis at or before 3 months of age, triple pelvic osteotomy, femoral head and neck excision, and total hip replacement are all surgical treatment options for hip dysplasia.

Stifle

Femoral condylar osteochondrosis(itis) dissecans

Both the medial and lateral femoral condyles can be affected by OC. In a young growing large or giant breed dog (see Table 42-6 for breed predispositions) that has a lameness related to stifle effusion but a stable stifle joint, be suspicious of stifle OCD. Additionally, the stifle lameness that results from OC will have an insidious onset rather than the acute onset of lameness that results from cruciate ligament disruption, and dogs may be bilaterally affected. The treatment is the same as for OCs in other locations, but the prognosis is worse following surgical debridement of the condylar lesion than following debridement of a shoulder OCD lesion. Recently, osteochondral autografts have been used successfully to repair femoral OCD defects.

Patellar luxation

Medial patellar luxation occurs mainly in small or miniature dog breeds, but large breed dogs can also get medial patellar luxation. Lateral patellar luxation also occurs in large breed dogs but can occur in small or toy breeds. Many breeds are predisposed for this condition (see Table 42-6). Medial patellar luxation results in degeneration of the patellar articular surface and induces osteoarthritis in the femoropatellar joint, resulting in pain and lameness. Patellar luxation is classified as acquired or developmental. Developmental luxation is more common, and the patella can be displaced medially or laterally. Acquired traumatic patellar luxation is not common but can be seen in any breed subjected to trauma that tears the stifle retinaculum.

The degree of skeletal pathology associated with medial patellar luxation varies between mild and severe. In grade 1 luxation, the patella can be luxated manually, but spontaneous luxation of the patella during normal flexion does not occur. In grade 2 luxation, the patella may be manually displaced, or it may luxate with flexion of the stifle joint. The patella remains luxated until it is reduced by the examiner or by extension and derotation of the tibia by the patient. Clinically, the patella is in the correct location more than in the displaced location. In grade 3 luxation, the patella usually remains luxated medially but may be manually reduced when the stifle is in extension. However, after manual reduction, flexion and extension of the stifle results in spontaneous reluxation of the patella. Abnormalities of the supporting soft tissues of the stifle joint and deformities of the femur and tibia may be present. In grade 4 luxation, the proximal tibial plateau is typically rotated medially 80 to 90 degrees. The patella is permanently luxated and cannot be manually repositioned. The femoral trochlear groove is shallow or absent and can be associated with medial displacement of the quadriceps muscle, lateral torsion of the distal femur, lateral bowing of the distal one third of the femur, dysplasia of the femoral epiphysis, rotational instability of the stifle joint, and tibial deformity. Mirror image changes can occur with lateral luxation of the patella.

Patients with grade 1 luxations are not clinically affected. Patients with grade 2 luxations occasionally skip when walking or running. Lameness in patients with a grade 3 patellar luxation is constant. Patients with grade 4 luxations walk with the rear quarters in a crouched position because of inability to fully extend the stifle joints. Patellar luxations also occur in cats. Dogs with grade 2 to 4 luxation are candidates for surgical correction. Surgical techniques used to restrain the patella within the trochlear groove include tibial tuberosity transposition, soft tissue (joint capsule and fascia lata) release, soft tissue reinforcement, trochlear groove deepening, extracapsular suture restraint, and femoral and tibial osteotomies. Clinical signs and physical findings are similar to those seen with medial patellar luxations. Some patients with lateral patellar luxation concurrently have hip dysplasia. The treatment goals for lateral patellar luxation are similar to those for medial patellar luxation.

Cruciate ligament avulsion

Craniocaudal stifle instability is most commonly diagnosed in mature animals but also may occur in growing animals. In dogs younger than 4 to 5 months of age, the instability usually occurs because of avulsion of the cranial cruciate ligament from either the femoral or the tibial attachment site. Treatment may consist of reattachment of the avulsed fragment using diverging Kirschner wires or with tunneled cerclage wire. Alternatively, the avulsed ligament can be removed and the joint stabilized as with cranial cruciate ligament rupture. Alternatively, a tibial plateau leveling procedure or a proximal tibial epiphysiodesis may be performed. In dogs older than 4 to 5 months of age, craniocaudal stifle instability is usually caused by a mid-body rupture of the cranial cruciate ligament.

Tarsus

Tarsal osteochondrosis(itis) dissecans

Dogs with OCD of the talar ridges present with effusion of the affected tarsocrural joints at a young age. Labrador Retrievers, Rottweilers, and Bullmastiffs are predisposed (see Table 42-6). The lameness may be exacerbated by exercise. The diagnosis is made radiographically (Figure 42-10). Removal of the cartilage lesion may bring temporary relief, but the prognosis is guarded for good long-term function because of its weight-bearing location.

ACQUIRED MUSCULOTENDINOUS DISEASES

Acquired musculotendinous diseases do not have a primarily genetic etiology and are not identifiable at birth. They may be classified as infectious myopathies, traumatic myopathies, and traumatic tendinopathies. Myopathies and tendinopathies may be associated with limb deformities without primary skeletal changes, and tendon dislocations.

Infectious Myopathies

Infectious myopathies (myositis) in puppies or kittens may be bacterial or protozoal in origin. *Leptospira*

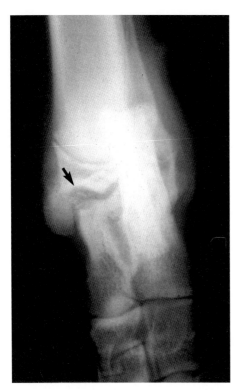

Figure 42-10 Photograph of a craniocaudal radiograph of a young dog with osteochondrosis dissecans of the medial trochlear ridge of the talus (*arrow*). Note the mineralization in the joint space.

icterohemorrhagica and *Clostridium* spp. have been identified as causes of bacterial myositis. In addition to systemic signs, patients have a stiff gait and painful muscles. The diagnosis is based on results of tissue culture and treatment consists of appropriate antibiotics and supportive care.

Protozoal myositis may be caused by *Neospora caninum* or *Toxoplasma gondii*. *N. caninum* is the most common. Puppies infected with *N. caninum* develop a progressive ascending paralysis and muscle atrophy. Puppies younger than 4 months of age often present with pelvic limb hyperextension that may not be reducible. Additional signs include mental depression, nystagmus, and seizures. The diagnosis is based on history (multiple littermates involved), clinical signs (progressive paralysis with pelvic limb hyperextension), increased serum creatinine kinase concentrations, serum indirect fluorescent antibody test, and muscle histology (electron microscopy, immunohistochemistry). Treatment may consist of trimethoprim-sulfadiazine, pyrimethamine, or clindamycin, but the prognosis is guarded. Because infections in puppies are most likely caused by transplacental transmission, retirement from breeding and treatment of the dam should be considered.

Traumatic Myopathies and Tendinopathies

Traumatic myopathies may be classified as direct and indirect muscle injuries. Direct trauma to muscles results in contusions (blunt, nonpenetrating trauma) or lacerations (penetrating trauma with a sharp object). The treatment of uncomplicated contusions consists of rest and may include cold compresses (only in acute stage to stop hemorrhage), bandages (to control edema), and nonsteroidal antiinflammatory medication. The patient should be free of major pain within 10 days. Recognized complications of contusions are compartment syndrome (increased pressure in a myofascial compartment followed by local neuromuscular ischemia and fibrosis) and myositis ossificans (dystrophic calcification within a muscle). Compartment syndrome is almost always a sequel of an automobile accident. Compartment syndrome of the quadriceps compartment is a commonly seen condition in puppies and kittens. If not treated properly, it may result in quadriceps contracture and fracture disease. Treatment consists of physical therapy or a fasciotomy to release the increased muscle compartment pressure. Myositis ossificans may be caused by intramuscular hematoma or laceration with subsequent fibrosis and dystrophic calcification and may adversely affect limb function. Physical therapy or surgical excision of the offending tissue has been recommended as treatment.

Partial lacerations may be treated conservatively with 2 to 3 weeks of rest and immobilization. A complete muscle laceration is an indication for surgical repair. Because most lacerations are associated with open wounds, the mode of surgical treatment depends on the condition of the wound. If the wound is clean with minimal tissue damage, primary repair is indicated. However, if the wound is contaminated, wound management with delayed repair is more appropriate. Return of function following treatment of lacerations in pups and kittens can be a major concern, and individualized treatment plans should include physical therapy.

Indirect muscle trauma is caused by stretching or a combination of activation and stretching of the affected muscle. In adult animals, this usually causes a muscle strain (synonyms: muscle pull, muscle tear). In pediatric patients, indirect muscle trauma also may result in an avulsion of the muscular or tendinous attachment of the affected muscle-tendon unit. For example, iliopsoas muscle trauma in puppies may result in a strain or an avulsion fracture of the lesser trochanter.

Like traumatic myopathies, traumatic tendon injuries can be classified as direct or indirect. Direct injuries, like contusions and lacerations, are treated as in adult animals. In young animals, indirect injuries of muscle-tendon units (MTU), caused by stretching or a combination of activation and stretching of the affected MTU, may result in avulsion fracture at an attachment site. Once the bone has become stronger, these injuries more commonly result in injuries at the myotendinous junction (muscle strain). Some examples of avulsions are avulsion fractures of the origin of the biceps brachii tendon, the triceps tendon, the popliteal tendon, and the long digital extensor tendon. Treatment consists of reattachment of the avulsed fragment. An uncommon avulsion is avulsion and subsequent mineralization of the flexor tendons originating from the medial humeral epicondyle. This condition is also called ununited medial epicondyle, and it has been suggested that this is a form of OC. The disease is seen in large breed dogs, and Labrador Retrievers seem overrepresented. Treatment may consist of surgical removal of the mineralized tissue.

Limb Deformities without Primary Skeletal Abnormalities

Several limb deformities caused by inadequate muscle function have been reported in the veterinary literature. Both decreased muscle tone (paresis or paralysis) and increased muscle tone (spasticity) can cause temporary and permanent limb deformity. Both decreased and increased muscle tone during skeletal growth may result in skeletal deformity, particularly at a very young age. In general, the etiology and pathophysiology of these diseases are poorly understood and treatment recommendations are sparse.

Two different carpal deformities have been described in puppies. Carpal hyperextension and carpal hypoextension (also called carpal flexural deformity) occur as soon as the pup stands, or soon after, and are probably both genetic and environmental in origin. It has been suggested that poor flexor muscle tone is responsible for radiocarpal joint hyperextension and that exercise may strengthen flexor muscles in young puppies. In older puppies, this condition may become irreversible, and pancarpal arthrodesis may be indicated. Radiocarpal joint hypoextension is most commonly seen in Doberman Pinschers, but other breeds may be affected as well. The etiology is unknown. Affected puppies usually present between 6 and 12 weeks of age. The disease is characterized by carpal hypoextension and varying degrees of tendon tautness of the flexor carpi ulnaris muscle. Treatment recommendations vary widely and may include exercise, rest, splinting, and change to an adult diet. In cases with mild flexor tendon tautness and a reducible radiocarpal joint, rest and change to an adult diet are sufficient to allow recovery within a couple of days. If the tendon is tight and the radial carpal joint is not completely extended, a couple of weeks of splinting should be included in the therapy. If the clinical signs do not resolve within a couple of days, tenotomy of the affected tendon(s) may be considered.

Hyperextension of the pelvic limb by extension of the stifle and tibiotarsal joints is another described deformity. Because flexion and extension of these two joints are interrelated, it may be difficult to determine whether the primary problem is related to the stifle or tibiotarsal joint. Three different types of pelvic limb hyperextension have been reported and are genetic or traumatic/mechanical in origin.

The first type is seen in young puppies and has been called hyperextension syndrome or genu recurvatum. The pelvic limb is kept in a hyperextended position, but the stifle and tibiotarsal joints can still be reduced. Mildly affected puppies may recover spontaneously, but more severely affected puppies require surgical intervention to maintain the affected leg in a flexed position. Successful use of external fixators and elastic bands to maintain the affected joint in a flexed position has been reported. If left untreated, the affected limb may become fixed (not reducible) in the hyperextended position (as in a quadriceps contracture), and surgical release of the contracted tissues and transarticular pinning of the stifle and tibiotarsal joints may be indicated.

A second type of pelvic limb hyperextension is seen in older puppies between 3 and 6 months of age. This condition is often seen in association with hip dysplasia, particularly in breeds with straight pelvic limbs like the Chow Chow and Saint Bernard. It also may occur following hip or stifle surgery. This condition does not convert into fixed hyperextension of the pelvic limb. The etiology of this condition is unclear. There is no specific treatment for this condition, although lengthening of the gastrocnemius tendon has been reported. If left untreated, tibiotarsal joint arthritis may develop.

The third type is a fixed (nonreducible) pelvic limb hyperextension. The most common cause for this condition is quadriceps contracture/tie down following fracture repair, which has been recognized in dogs and cats. Other conditions that may cause fixed pelvic limb hyperextension are severe muscle contusions, hyperextension syndrome, and *N. caninum* infections. Treatment depends on the genesis, severity, and maturity of the condition.

Dislocations

Dislocations of the biceps tendon, the proximal tendon of the long digital extensor muscle, and the superficial digital flexor tendon of the hindlimb have been reported. Luxation of the superficial digital flexor tendon may have a hereditary etiology. If tendon dislocations cause clinical problems, surgical treatment is indicated. Surgical treatment usually consists of reconstructing anatomical relationships.

SUGGESTED READINGS

Beale BS et al: *Small animal arthroscopy,* Philadelphia, 2003, Saunders/Elsevier.

Breur GJ, Lust G, Todhunter RJ: Genetics of canine hip dysplasia and other orthopaedic traits. In Ruvinsky A, Sampson J (eds): *The genetics of the dog,* New York, 2001, CABI Publishing, pp 267-298.

Houlton J, Collinson R: *British Small Animal Veterinary Association manual of small animal arthrology,* Ames, IA, 1994, Iowa State University Press.

Johnson AL, Schultz K: Orthopedics. In Fossum TW (ed): *Small animal surgery,* ed 3, St Louis, 2007, Mosby/Elsevier, pp 930-1356.

Piermattei D, Flo G, DeCamp C: *Handbook of small animal orthopedics and fracture repair,* Philadelphia, 2006, Saunders/Elsevier.

Shiers PK, Schulz KS: The skeletal system. In Hoskins JD (ed): *Veterinary pediatrics: dogs and cats from birth to six months of age,* ed 3, Philadelphia, 2001, Saunders.

THE EYE

Mary B. Glaze

THE OPHTHALMIC EXAMINATION

Examination of the neonate must take into account age-related variations in ocular appearance and response. Generally the eyelids open at 10 to 14 days of age, revealing a cloudy cornea that begins to clear within 24 hours. The patient should demonstrate a blink in response to a bright light when the lids open. Pupillary light reflexes are present within 24 hours of eyelid separation but remain sluggish for 3 weeks. Vision and menace responses are generally poor for the first 3 weeks and may not reach adult standards until 6 to 8 weeks of age. Reflex lacrimation begins when the eyelids open. Box 43-1 summarizes additional features of the neonatal eye.

THE GLOBE AND ORBIT

Congenital Abnormalities
Anophthalmos

Anophthalmos, or complete absence of the globe, is extremely rare. In most cases, careful examination of the orbital contents will reveal primitive ocular tissue.

Microphthalmia

Failure of the eye to develop to normal size is referred to as microphthalmia. The small globe is often associated with a correspondingly small palpebral fissure. Depending on the constellation of accompanying defects, vision may be normal, diminished, or absent. Microphthalmia with multiple colobomas is an autosomal recessive trait linked to merling in the Australian Shepherd (Figure 43-1).

In addition to small globes, dogs with *merle ocular dysgenesis* may have persistent pupillary membranes, cataract, equatorial staphylomas, choroidal hypoplasia, retinal dysplasia and detachment, and optic nerve hypoplasia. Vision is frequently impaired. Similarly affected breeds include the Great Dane, Collie, Shetland Sheepdog, Dachshund, and Catahoula Leopard Dog.

Microphthalmia is associated with inherited congenital cataracts in the Miniature Schnauzer, Old English Sheepdog, Akita, and Cavalier King Charles Spaniel, as well as with retinal dysplasia in the Bedlington and Sealyham Terriers, Beagle, and Labrador Retriever. In the Doberman Pinscher, microphthalmia, anterior segment dysgenesis, and retinal dysplasia are thought to be inherited as an autosomal recessive trait.

Microphthalmia, choroidal and optic disc colobomas, retinal dysplasia, and tapetal aplasia have been attributed to heredity and in utero viral infections in Domestic Shorthair kittens. Multiple anomalies, including colobomas, have also been described in Persian cats. Administration of griseofulvin to pregnant cats may cause microphthalmia in their offspring and has also resulted in anophthalmos, cyclopia, and optic nerve aplasia.

Atypical Eye Position

Strabismus refers to deviation of the eye from the visual axis. A lateral deviation or exotropia occurs in brachycephalic dog breeds, notably the Boston Terrier, Pug, Pekingese, and Shih Tzu. Convergent strabismus or esotropia is inherited in Siamese and Himalayan cats as an autosomal recessive trait, linked to pigment-defining genes that cause aberrant routing of optic nerve fibers. The strabismus is thought to be a compensatory mechanism for the abnormal visual input. Bilateral ventrolateral strabismus occurs with hydrocephalus because of enlargement of the calvaria and its effect on the globe-orbit relationship.

Atypical Eye Motion

A wandering movement of the eyes in puppies and kittens is associated with congenital blindness. Rapid, repetitive, involuntary movement of the eyes (nystagmus) commonly occurs in Siamese kittens and is likely related to the

461

BOX 43-1 Normal features of the immature canine and feline eye

Eyelids	Separate at 10-14 days
Globe position	Kittens demonstrate subtle divergent strabismus until 3-4 weeks
Tear film	Reflex tearing is present when eyelids separate
Cornea	Mild corneal edema begins to clear within 24 hours after eyelids open; corneal thickness continues to decrease until 6 weeks of age
Iris	Newborn blue-gray iris shows signs of adult coloration by 1 month of age; persistent pupillary membranes are seen until 6 weeks of age in puppies and 3 weeks of age in kittens
Lens	Vessels of the tunica vasculosa lentis are seen until 4 weeks of age
Fundus	The blue-gray tapetum gradually assumes adult coloration by 4 months of age; the optic disc appears smaller because of incomplete myelination, but caliber and distribution of retinal vessels are similar to adult
Vision/menace reflex	Visual reflexes are poor at 3 weeks of age, gradually improving until 6-8 weeks of age, as retina continues to differentiate
Pupillary light reflexes	Present within 24 hours of lid separation but sluggish until the retina matures during week 4
Dazzle reflex	Present when eyelids open

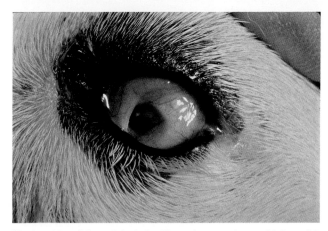

Figure 43-1 Microphthalmia. Note the prominent third eyelid, small cornea, and disproportionate amount of sclera visible in this merled Australian Shepherd.

objects and fight wounds are likely causes in young dogs and cats. Response to twice-daily warm compresses and a broad-spectrum systemic antimicrobial agent is generally rapid. If no response is seen within 24 hours, incise the oral mucosa behind the last maxillary molar with a blade, gently advance a closed hemostat through the pterygoid muscle, and partially open the hemostat within the orbit to establish drainage. In most instances, only a slight serosanguineous fluid appears. Damage to orbital structures occurs when the procedure is performed carelessly. Do not insert sharp instruments into the orbit that can damage the globe or its associated nerves and vessels. If exophthalmos is extreme, a bland ophthalmic ointment is applied to the corneal surface to prevent drying.

Orbital Neoplasia

Orbital neoplasia is extremely rare in animals younger than 1 year of age.

Traumatic Proptosis

Complete displacement of the eye from the orbit is most commonly seen in brachycephalic dogs, but any dog or cat may present with proptosis with sufficient cranial trauma (Figure 43-2). A completely displaced eye is a true ocular emergency. Prognosis for vision is always poor because of optic nerve injury, but the intact globe may be salvaged cosmetically.

A soft eye, indicating rupture of the fibrous tunic, or one with extensive avulsion of extraocular muscles or optic nerve should be enucleated. Those with severe intraocular hemorrhage usually shrink over time because of irreparable damage to the ciliary body.

General anesthesia is required to reposition the globe. After flushing the eye with sterile saline solution, a blunt probe, such as a spay hook, or preplaced sutures of 5-0 nylon are used to elevate the eyelid margins. Simultaneous gentle counterpressure is applied against the cornea with a moistened cotton ball or the flat surface of a scalpel handle to push the eye back into place. The eyelids are sutured closed

neuroanatomic abnormalities that produce strabismus. Vision is functionally normal. The nystagmus may lessen as the kitten matures.

Acquired Abnormalities
Orbital Cellulitis and Abscessation

Orbital inflammation is usually characterized by an acute unilateral exophthalmos, protrusion of the third eyelid, chemosis, pain on opening the mouth, and fever. Swelling or discoloration behind the last upper molar may occur. Foreign

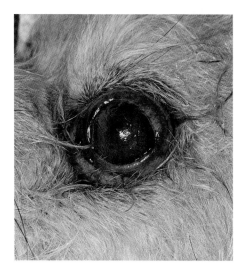

Figure 43-2 Proptosis. This mixed Terrier's globe is displaced in front of the eyelids and tightly positioned against the orbital rim, with minimal apparent anterior segment damage.

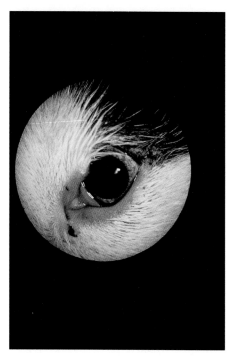

Figure 43-3 Eyelid agenesis. The superior temporal lid margin is absent in this 6-month-old Domestic Shorthair cat.

using horizontal mattress sutures of 5-0 nylon placed over stents. Sutures should enter the eyelid 3 to 5 mm from the margin and exit through the meibomian gland openings to prevent corneal damage.

A broad-spectrum systemic antibiotic and a tapering regimen of oral corticosteroids are recommended for 7 to 10 days. Injections should not be made into the orbital area. If the animal allows, topical antimicrobial ointment may be applied 3 or 4 times daily between the eyelid margins at the medial canthus. Warm compresses are recommended for 3 to 4 days after the replacement. One of the most frequent management errors is removing the tarsorrhaphy sutures prematurely. Sutures are left in place for 14 days or until the globe settles back into the orbit. Sequelae include lateral strabismus as a result of rupture of the medial rectus muscle, blindness, low tear production, and shrinkage of the eye (phthisis bulbi).

Enophthalmos

Enophthalmos describes an eye that has receded into the orbit. The Saint Bernard, Great Dane, Doberman Pinscher, Golden Retriever, and Irish Setter often appear enophthalmic owing to their large orbits and deeply set eyes. Congenital enophthalmos is most often associated with microphthalmia. Acquired causes include any painful ocular disorder, postinflammatory atrophy, loss of retrobulbar fat in debilitated or malnourished animals, phthisis bulbi, or Horner's syndrome with loss of sympathetic tone in the orbital fascia.

THE EYELIDS

Congenital Abnormalities

Premature or Delayed Eyelid Opening

A gradual increase in tear production triggers eyelid separation in the 10- to 14-day-old dog and cat. If the eyelids open prematurely, corneal drying and ulceration are likely to follow. Treatment consists of frequent application of a topical lubricating ophthalmic ointment to prevent corneal desiccation until tear production improves. A temporary tarsorrhaphy may be indicated in instances of progressive corneal ulceration.

Delayed eyelid opening may be associated with an accumulation of mucus or infectious exudate. If distended, the eyelids should be gently pried apart with firm digital pressure. The ocular surface is liberally flushed with sterile saline, and a fluorescein dye test is used to rule out corneal ulceration. Triple antibiotic ointment is recommended in the puppy, and erythromycin ointment is recommended in the kitten to treat *Staphylococcus* spp. and *Chlamydophila felis*, respectively.

Eyelid Agenesis

Eyelid agenesis occurs primarily in cats as a unilateral or bilateral anomaly. The condition is characterized by absence of the eyelid margin, almost always involving the lateral one third to two thirds of the upper eyelid (Figure 43-3).

Mild defects may be misinterpreted as entropion because of misdirection of adjacent hairs. Large defects lead to chronic irritation from direct contact of the cornea with facial hairs and from exposure secondary to imperfect lid closure. Small defects may be successfully managed with an ophthalmic lubricant ointment applied several times daily to reduce ocular irritation. Misdirected hairs can be cryoepilated or surgically everted using a modified Hotz-Celsus technique as for entropion. If one third or more of the eyelid is missing, pedicle grafts from the forehead or the temporal aspect of the lower eyelid are combined with rotational conjunctival grafts from the nictitans or inferior conjunctival cul-de-sac to repair the defect.

Entropion

Inversion of the eyelid margin occurs commonly in dogs but infrequently in the cat. The lower eyelid is more often affected. Accompanying clinical signs include increased tearing, squinting, corneal vascularization, and ulceration (Figure 43-4).

Several genes that define the eyelid structure, globe-orbit relationship, and facial skin are likely to influence the degree of entropion. The narrow palpebral fissure of the Chow Chow, the deeply set eye of the Golden Retriever, and the redundant facial folds of the Shar-Pei are examples of the variables that determine lid conformation. Painful ocular disorders also cause entropion secondary to spasm of the orbicularis oculi muscle. This mechanism is commonly implicated in cats with chronic herpesvirus infection.

Young animals with entropion but without corneal disease may be treated palliatively with an ophthalmic lubricant ointment to postpone surgery until the patient matures. Delaying surgery in the Shar-Pei may not be possible because of the severity of the breed's entropion and the risk of corneal ulceration. Temporary "tacking" is used to evert the lid margins and forestall corneal damage. The procedure is most effective when performed in the 3- to 4-week-old puppy. The older the animal is when tacking is first performed, the less likely it will be to correct the entropion without additional surgery. Local anesthetic blocks can be used in the very young animal, but masking the patient with isoflurane expedites the procedure. The first bite of a 5-0 nylon vertical

mattress suture enters 2 mm from the eyelid margin and engages about 4 mm of eyelid skin and subcutaneous tissue. Avoid suturing the eyelid margin directly because postsurgical notching can irritate the cornea. The needle is then reinserted into the skin and deeper tissue overlying the orbital rim, adjusting the tension to evert the eyelid margin in a slightly overcorrected position (Figure 43-5).

The number of required sutures varies with the individual patient. A topical lubricant ointment is applied twice daily. Ideally the sutures are left in place for weeks. Surgical staples may also be used, with the advantages of rapid placement and excellent retention.

As long as the cornea remains healthy, definitive surgery is ideally postponed until the patient is 6 months of age or older. The modified Hotz-Celsus technique is the classical procedure for entropion repair, everting the lid margin by removing an ellipse of eyelid skin equal to the amount of lid inversion. Preoperative assessment should be performed after application of a topical anesthetic to eliminate any spastic component that exaggerates the degree of entropion. It is also critical to establish a surgical plan before anesthesia, when enophthalmos and loss of eyelid tone alter eyelid position significantly. With the eyelid supported by a Jaeger lid plate inserted into the conjunctival cul-de-sac, the initial incision is made with a scalpel blade 2 to 3 mm from and parallel to the lid margin, along the line where the eyelid hair begins, extending at least 1 mm medially and laterally to the entropic section. The distal incision gently arcs, joining with the two ends of the primary incision and outlining the tissue that must be excised to successfully evert the margin. The incised ellipse of tissue is removed with scissors. The wound is closed with 4-0 to 6-0 simple interrupted braided nylon, silk, or polyglactin sutures, placing the first suture at the midpoint of the incision and continuing to bisect the remaining wound segments with sutures until the defect is perfectly apposed. Topical antibiotic ointment is applied to the eye twice daily until suture removal. A systemic nonsteroidal antiinflammatory drug (NSAID) provides satisfactory analgesia. The wound is protected with an Elizabethan collar.

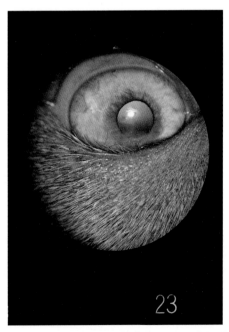

Figure 43-4 Entropion. The inferior temporal eyelid rolls inward, rubbing against the cornea and causing secondary vascularization in this young Chesapeake Bay Retriever.

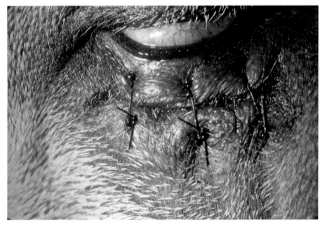

Figure 43-5 Eyelid tacking. Vertical mattress sutures are placed to temporarily evert the lid margin in this Shar-Pei puppy.

Sutures are removed in 10 days, although 6-0 polyglactin sutures are commonly left to resorb. A modification of the Hotz-Celsus procedure that excises an arrowhead-shaped area of skin around the lateral canthus can be used to correct the lateral canthal inversion in the Shar-Pei, Chow Chow, and Retriever breeds. A combination of techniques may be necessary in breeds with excessive facial folds or elongated lids, prompting referral of these patients to an ophthalmologist.

Ectropion

Ectropion refers to an everted eyelid margin, with secondary exposure of the bulbar conjunctiva. The conjunctival sac accumulates particulate debris and is often chronically inflamed. The condition is common in dogs with loose facial skin, including the Clumber Spaniel, Cocker Spaniel, Basset Hound, Bloodhound, and Saint Bernard. Some degree of ectropion is considered desirable in these breeds. Surgical correction is reserved for the most severely affected patients with secondary keratoconjunctivitis. The simplest method for correction shortens the lower eyelid by excising a wedge of tissue adequate to lift the eyelid into a more normal position. Patients with severe ectropion or those combined with entropion should be referred to an ophthalmologist for correction.

Distichiasis

Distichiasis refers to an extra row of cilia that protrude from the orifices of the meibomian glands along the eyelid margins. Congenital distichiasis occurs in the English Bulldog, Poodle, Cocker Spaniel, Golden Retriever, Shih Tzu, and Pekingese breeds and may be inherited as an autosomal dominant trait. The condition is rare in cats but is reported in the Abyssinian.

The mere presence of distichia does not justify their removal. Surgical treatment is reserved for those animals in which all other causes of tearing, conjunctivitis, and keratitis have been ruled out. Cryoepilation using liquid nitrogen or nitrous oxide and a 3-mm cryoprobe is a safe and effective method for managing numerous distichia. The eyelid is stabilized with a chalazion clamp, and the probe is positioned over the base of the affected meibomian glands, allowing the ice ball to extend just beyond the meibomian gland openings along the lid margin. The time necessary to reach this point varies with lid thickness and is likely to take longer in a Bulldog than a Poodle, for example. A double freeze-thaw technique is most effective. Eyelid swelling typically resolves in a matter of days, but marginal depigmentation can last for weeks to months.

Trichiasis

Trichiasis occurs when otherwise normal eyelashes or facial hairs deviate inward, contacting the surface of the eye. Secondary corneal changes include vascularization, pigmentation, or ulceration. Management of the trichiasis should begin with correction of any predisposing problem such as eyelid agenesis. Cryoepilation may be used to remove offending cilia, or a modified Hotz-Celsus procedure may be used to evert hairs away from the eye.

Ectopic Cilia

Occasionally cilia will penetrate through the conjunctiva lining the underside of the eyelid rather than emerge from the meibomian gland opening. The classical presentation is a young dog with a nonhealing superficial ulcer in the dorsal third of the cornea. Some dogs intermittently squint and tear but never ulcerate. The upper eyelid is more commonly affected. Magnification is required to demonstrate the small dark spot at the base of the meibomian gland that represents the tip of the emerging cilia (Figure 43-6).

En bloc resection of the palpebral conjunctiva and the affected meibomian gland is curative.

Acquired Abnormalities
Lacerations

Eyelid lacerations in dogs and cats are usually perpendicular to the lid margin. The lid's exceptional blood supply provides for excellent healing even when surgical correction is delayed. Minimal debridement and meticulous suturing are advised to preserve the lid margin and eyelid function. A two-layer closure will better control wound distraction by the orbicularis muscle. A deep layer of continuous 6-0 absorbable suture is used to reappose the conjunctiva and tarsus, taking care to bury knots that can damage the cornea. The lid margin is precisely apposed with 4-0 to 6-0 braided nylon, silk, or polyglactin in a figure-eight pattern, and a second

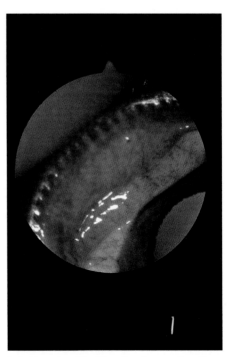

Figure 43-6 Ectopic cilia. The tip of ectopic cilia penetrates the conjunctiva at the base of a meibomian gland, appearing as a black dot just beneath the pinpoint central flash artifact.

layer of interrupted sutures is placed in the skin. Postoperative therapy includes topical broad-spectrum antibacterial ointment several times daily, oral antibiotic for 7 days, a systemic nonsteroidal for analgesia, and an Elizabethan collar to prevent trauma to the surgical site. Sutures of 4-0 and 5-0 material should be removed in 10 to 14 days, but 6-0 polyglactin resorbs without complication.

Allergic Reactions

Immediate hypersensitivity caused by insect stings, vaccines, or medication may initiate an IgE-mediated response that causes sudden and severe eyelid and conjunctival swelling. Clinical signs usually subside over 12 to 24 hours with warm compresses and oral antihistamines or corticosteroids. If the corneal surface cannot be visualized to rule out ulceration, a topical antibiotic or preservative-free artificial tear ointment is preferred over a topical corticosteroid to protect swollen and exposed conjunctiva.

Bacterial Infections

Acute eyelid swelling and pustule formation may precede facial pyoderma and lymphadenopathy in puppies with juvenile pyoderma. A hypersensitivity component to *Staphylococcus* spp. is thought to underlie the dramatic clinical signs. Topical antibacterial or corticosteroid medications are ineffective because insufficient drug levels are achieved in the eyelids. An oral antibiotic with efficacy against *Staphylococcus* spp. must be coupled with an oral corticosteroid for best response. Warm compresses of the eyelids may also help reduce secondary swelling. Complete resolution may take weeks.

Parasitic Infestations

Generalized or local infestation with a variety of ectoparasites causes alopecia, erythema, and pruritus of the eyelids. The more common parasites involved are *Demodex canis*, *Notoedres cati*, *Otodectes cyanotis*, and *Sarcoptes scabiei*.

Neoplasia

Eyelid tumors are rare in young dogs. Viral papillomas are usually pedunculated, with a cauliflower-like appearance. Oral papillomas may develop concurrently. The histiocytoma is smooth, tan to pink in color, and broad-based. One or several masses may arise quickly along the lid margin. Occasionally the eyelid mass accompanies systemic histiocytosis; thus careful systemic examination is advised. With either tumor, solitary masses may spontaneously regress in weeks to months. Surgical excision or cryotherapy is necessary only if the tumor is damaging the eye.

THE CONJUNCTIVA

Congenital Abnormalities

Dermoid

A dermoid is a congenital mass of tissue containing skin, hair follicles, and sebaceous glands (Figure 43-7). It most

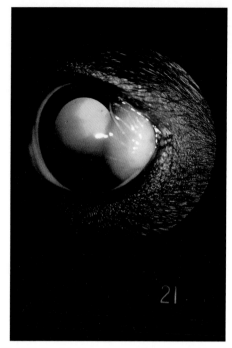

Figure 43-7 Dermoid. Aberrant nonpigmented skin with several surface hairs overlies the temporal conjunctiva and cornea in this Dachshund puppy.

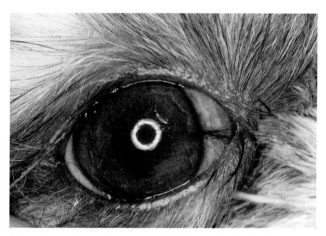

Figure 43-8 Medial canthal trichiasis. A tuft of hairs arising from the medial canthal caruncle can damage the cornea and misdirect tears in this young Shih Tzu.

commonly occurs in the temporal perilimbal conjunctiva and may also involve the adjacent eyelid and cornea.

Dermoids often cause ocular irritation and epiphora as a result of surface hairs contacting the ocular surface. Treatment involves careful dissection of the dermoid from the surrounding conjunctiva and underlying sclera. If the cornea is involved, a superficial keratectomy is also indicated.

Medial Canthal Trichiasis

Long hairs that arise from the medial canthal caruncle may wick tears over the lid margin, staining the periocular fur and predisposing to facial fold dermatitis (Figure 43-8).

Chronic contact also damages the corneal surface. The condition is most commonly seen in the Cavalier King Charles Spaniel, Lhasa Apso, Maltese, Shih Tzu, Pekingese, Poodle, and Pug. Cryoepilation is a simple, effective method of destroying the hair follicles within the caruncle. The caruncle may also be surgically excised, taking care to avoid damage to the adjacent nasolacrimal system.

Acquired Abnormalities
Allergic Conjunctivitis

Ocular allergy is rarely substantiated by other than response to topical antiinflammatory therapy or an association with systemic signs suggestive of atopy. Moderate conjunctival hyperemia, mild chemosis, serous ocular discharge, and pruritus are typical signs that occur bilaterally. Eosinophils and neutrophils are seen cytologically. Chronic antigenic stimulation may cause hyperplasia of lymphoid follicles in the conjunctival cul-de-sacs and on the bulbar surface of the third eyelids. A seasonal incidence is common. Symptomatic treatment with a topical corticosteroid is both beneficial and cost effective.

Bacterial Conjunctivitis

Bacterial conjunctivitis is characterized by conjunctival hyperemia, swelling, and mucopurulent discharge. In the dog, it is not a primary ocular disease but rather a consequence of a predisposing adnexal or lacrimal abnormality. Culture may reveal one or more types of bacteria, typically susceptible to a wide range of antibacterial drugs. Response to a topical antibacterial medication is usually rapid, but clinical signs recur once treatment is discontinued. A careful examination should be performed to rule out keratoconjunctivitis sicca (KCS), ectopic cilia, foreign bodies, entropion, ectropion, and nasolacrimal disease.

In contrast, the cat may exhibit a primary conjunctival infection by *C. felis*. Initial infection is characterized by a mild rhinitis and unilateral purulent conjunctivitis. Second eye involvement occurs 5 to 7 days later. Lack of corneal involvement may help differentiate the conjunctivitis from that caused by herpesvirus. Basophilic cytoplasmic inclusions in conjunctival scrapings performed during the first 2 to 9 days after onset of clinical signs are diagnostic, as are indirect fluorescent antibody (IFA) and polymerase chain reaction (PCR) testing in more chronic cases. Treatment consists of topical tetracycline or erythromycin ointment 4 times daily for 3 weeks or a 3-week course of oral doxycycline (5 mg/kg twice daily) or azithromycin (5 mg/kg daily).

Mycoplasma spp. are historically implicated in feline conjunctivitis. Controversy remains with respect to the organism's importance because infection cannot be established in the absence of other pathogens. Diagnosis is confirmed by demonstrating coccoid basophilic organisms in clusters on the epithelial cell membrane in the initial stages of infection or by PCR analysis of conjunctival swabs. Topical tetracycline is the medication of choice.

Viral Conjunctivitis

In the naive neonatal or adolescent cat, feline herpesvirus-1 (FHV-1) causes an acute conjunctival and respiratory infection. Clinical signs are directly related to the viral cytopathic effect on epithelial cells. The initial conjunctivitis is bilateral with pronounced hyperemia, accompanied by ocular discharge that changes from serous to mucopurulent. Pathognomonic dendritic corneal erosions may be overlooked if rose bengal is not used to stain the corneal surface. Kittens with viral conjunctivitis before eyelid separation will often have such severe conjunctival and corneal erosions that adjacent raw surfaces adhere together, creating symblepharon. These conjunctival adhesions can cause permanent prominence of the third eyelid, epiphora from obstruction of the nasolacrimal puncta, and corneal opacity.

Following recovery in 10 to 14 days from the initial herpesvirus infection, 80% of cats become latently infected carriers, and an estimated 45% of these will experience spontaneous viral shedding and/or recrudescence of clinical disease in the future. Subsequent episodes of conjunctivitis commonly occur without respiratory signs and affect only one eye. Diagnosis of herpetic conjunctivitis is more often based on history and clinical signs than on specific testing. Serology is predictably positive because of the widespread exposure of cats to herpesvirus. Viral detection using IFA or PCR testing fails to differentiate between wild and vaccinal virus.

Feline conjunctivitis should be considered infectious until proven otherwise. Topical corticosteroids may initially decrease hyperemia and swelling but are not recommended because they also prolong virus shedding and increase the risk of herpetic ulceration. Specific antiviral therapy is seldom used in the initial ocular-respiratory syndrome because of its self-limiting nature. If corneal ulceration is present, topical 0.1% idoxuridine may be compounded for topical use; its virostatic nature requires application 4 to 6 times daily. Topical 0.5% cidofovir requires only twice-daily application for 14 days but is much more expensive. Ocular signs improve in patients treated with oral famciclovir at a dose of 15 mg/kg every 12 hours for 14 days. Other oral antiviral medications are either ineffective or toxic to the cat. Lifelong oral L-lysine supplementation limits viral replication and may reduce the severity or frequency of relapses. The recommended dosage for kittens is 250 mg twice daily and for adult cats is 500 mg twice daily, usually supplied as a powder and mixed in food.

Dogs infected with canine distemper virus may exhibit conjunctivitis, ocular discharge, and reduced tear production. Conjunctival scrapings in the acutely infected patient may contain intracytoplasmic inclusion bodies.

THE LACRIMAL SYSTEM

Congenital Abnormalities
Lacrimal Punctal Atresia

The inferior and superior nasolacrimal puncta lie on the inner conjunctival surface of the eyelids, near the medial limit of the meibomian glands. In dogs, a congenitally imperforate inferior punctum is common, especially in the American Cocker Spaniel, Golden Retriever, miniature and toy Poodles, and the Samoyed. Epiphora is likely but may not be evident until several weeks of age. Diagnosis is made by examining the normal location of the opening, where the imperforate lumen is often identified by a cream-colored fluid beneath a thin layer of conjunctiva.

When the opposite punctum is cannulated and flushed, the conjunctiva overlying the imperforate punctum tents outward. It can then be grasped with fine forceps and incised with a 25-gauge needle or delicate scissors to create a punctal opening. Topical antibiotic-corticosteroid solution is applied twice daily for 7 to 10 days. Normal tear flow will usually maintain the opening, but some patients may require several daily flushings to ensure patency.

Lacrimal Punctal Scarring

In kittens, permanent scarring and blockage of the nasolacrimal puncta are common sequelae of herpetic conjunctivitis and secondary symblepharon.

Acquired Abnormalities
Keratoconjunctivitis Sicca

Inadequate aqueous tear production is a common disorder in dogs but one that seldom occurs in cats. Congenital acinar hypoplasia occurs in miniature breeds, including the Yorkshire Terrier, Pug, Chinese Crested, and Chihuahua. The congenital problem is commonly unilateral and characterized by extreme dryness and blepharospasm. Early lack of tears may cause delayed separation of the eyelids and early signs of corneal disease. Response to therapy is often negligible in these patients. Cats with eyelid agenesis may lack lacrimal glands or their ductules. Dogs with distemper and cats with acute or chronic upper respiratory tract infection secondary to herpesvirus may develop dry eye as a consequence of viral adenitis. Atropine administered as a preanesthetic agent or applied topically several times daily may transiently decrease tear production. Third eyelid gland removal increases the risk of KCS in predisposed dogs. Even a chronic uncorrected third eyelid gland prolapse may reduce its contribution to the aqueous tear film.

Breeds of dog with acquired KCS include the Cavalier King Charles Spaniel, English Bulldog, Lhasa Apso, Shih Tzu, West Highland White Terrier, Pug, Bloodhound, American Cocker Spaniel, Pekingese, Boston Terrier, Miniature Schnauzer, Samoyed, English Springer Spaniel, Poodle, and Yorkshire Terrier.

The early stages of the disorder are characterized by varying amounts of tenacious mucopurulent discharge, conjunctival hyperemia, and a dull, lusterless appearance to the corneal surface. As the lack of tears persists, gradual vascularization and pigmentation of the cornea occur, and corneal ulcers may develop. Eventually the canine cornea may pigment completely. Diagnosis is confirmed using a Schirmer tear test (STT). Values less than 10 mm in 1 minute are indicative of KCS. Values between 10 and 15 mm in 1 minute are highly suggestive of KCS, particularly in patients with typical clinical signs and in brachycephalic breeds of dog in general. Normal feline STT values are similar to those of dogs, although lower readings are often seen in anxious cats during the examination.

Patients with congenital sicca rarely respond well to therapy. Treatment of KCS consists of first cleansing the eye with sterile eyewash or saline. Topical cyclosporine A is used to stimulate natural tear production and to maintain mucin secretion by conjunctival goblet cells. If the patient fails to respond to twice-daily application of the 0.2% ointment (Optimmune; Schering-Plough, Kenilworth NJ) after 8 weeks, a 1% or 2% cyclosporine solution prepared by a licensed compounding pharmacy should be used in its place. If tear production still has not increased after several months, topical frequency can be increased or topical 0.03% tacrolimus solution can be added to the regimen along with the cyclosporine. If still no response is seen, a parotid duct transposition is indicated.

THIRD EYELID (NICTITATING MEMBRANE)

The third eyelid is supported internally by a T-shaped cartilage, encircled at its base by the gland of the third eyelid that produces 40% of the aqueous tear film. Lymphoid follicles are normally present on the posterior conjunctival surface. The only indications for third eyelid removal are severe, irreparable trauma and malignant neoplasia.

Congenital Abnormalities
Cartilage Eversion

Eversion of the cartilage is characterized by an outward curling of the nictitating membrane's leading edge (Figure 43-9).

Clinical signs include ocular discharge, conjunctival hyperemia, distortion of the lower eyelid, and infrequent keratitis. Eversion occurs in the Great Dane, Saint Bernard, Weimaraner, German Shorthaired Pointer, and Irish Setter. The Burmese cat may also be affected.

The deformed section of cartilage is surgically removed through an incision on the posterior surface of the third eyelid. The segment is carefully dissected from the surrounding conjunctiva and excised, rounding the edges to avoid sharp endpoints that could irritate the cornea. No sutures are required. Topical antibiotic ointment is applied twice daily for 1 week. The gland of the third eyelid may prolapse after cartilage resection.

Acquired Abnormalities
Follicular Hyperplasia

Lymphoid follicles are normally present on the posterior surface of the third eyelid. The semitransparent follicles enlarge in response to chronic antigenic stimulation and may become notably thickened and grossly visible near the

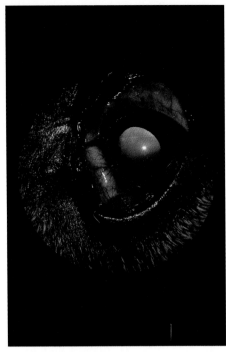

Figure 43-9 Everted cartilage. A bend in the third eyelid's T-shaped cartilage causes the leading edge to scroll outward, with secondary irritation in this Great Dane.

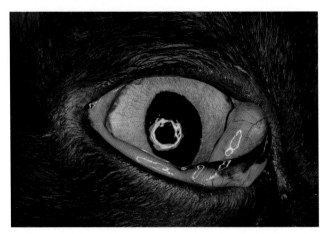

Figure 43-10 Nictitans gland prolapse. Commonly referred to as cherry eye, the gland of the third eyelid protrudes above the leading edge of the nictitans in this young Burmese cat.

leading edge. Symptomatic treatment with topical corticosteroid ointment is beneficial. Extremely hyperplastic follicles can be mechanically debrided with dry sterile gauze but should not be sharply excised or chemically cauterized.

Prolapse of the Nictitans Gland

Incomplete development of ventral soft tissue attachments causes the gland of the third eyelid to protrude, a condition commonly referred to as "cherry eye" (Figure 43-10).

Exposure of the gland often results in secondary conjunctival irritation, lymphoid hyperplasia, and ocular discharge. The Beagle, Boston Terrier, Cocker Spaniel, Lhasa Apso, English Bulldog, and Burmese cat are commonly affected.

A 30% to 57% decrease in tear production can be expected if the nictitans gland is removed, increasing the likelihood of KCS in susceptible patients. The abnormal gland position is also more than a cosmetic problem because tear production also decreases when the gland is chronically prolapsed.

Surgical repositioning of the gland is the treatment of choice. Repositioning techniques are divided into those that anchor the gland to adjacent tissue such as periorbital fascia, extraocular muscle, or sclera, and those that create a pocket for the gland by imbricating its overlying conjunctiva. Procedural details can be found in any veterinary ophthalmology textbook. Morgan's pocket technique works well in the majority of patients. Multiple techniques are combined in breeds such as the English Bulldog to improve results. Unfortunately retention of the gland does not always prevent KCS because breeds predisposed to glandular protrusion are also those with a generally higher incidence of dry eye.

Haws Syndrome

Bilateral third eyelid protrusion without other ocular abnormalities is fairly common in cats. The condition is often associated with vague gastrointestinal signs, including loose stools and diarrhea. The exact cause is unknown. A systemic autonomic imbalance has been theorized, but tapeworms and a rotavirus have also been implicated etiologically. The condition usually resolves in 4 to 6 weeks without treatment.

THE CORNEA

Congenital Abnormalities

Corneal Opacities

The cornea of the newborn puppy or kitten is transiently cloudy when the eyelids open at 10 to 14 days of age. Corneal thickness in the dog decreases over the first 6 weeks of life, presumably mirroring improved corneal endothelial function. It is not unusual to observe faint, irregular, maplike superficial opacities in the corneas of puppies younger than 10 weeks of age. These occur most often in the central cornea and gradually resolve without treatment by 12 to 16 weeks of age. Vision is unimpaired. Any breed of dog may be affected.

Cats with inherited lysosomal storage diseases may develop corneal opacities related to the accumulation of metabolic byproducts within corneal cells. Fine granular deposits within the stroma create a ground-glass appearance as early as 8 weeks of age, progressing over time to more obvious cloudiness in cats with GM_1 gangliosidosis, in cats of Siamese ancestry with mucopolysaccharidosis I and IV, and in Persian cats with α-mannosidosis.

Deep corneal opacities are usually associated with persistent pupillary membranes (PPMs), remnants of embryonic blood vessels that arise from the iris face. Attachment of residual strands to the inner corneal surface produces an opacity that is usually localized and nonprogressive, accompanied by thickening of Descemet's membrane (Figure 43-11).

There is no treatment. Heritable, clinically significant PPMs occur in the Basenji, Pembroke Welsh Corgi, Chow Chow, and Mastiff. Both minor and severe PPMs have been noted in a variety of other breeds.

Dermoid

Owners often notice this skinlike appendage soon after the animal's eyelids separate. The dermoid commonly affects the temporal cornea and conjunctiva in both puppies and kittens. Excessive tearing reflects corneal irritation by hairs on the dermoid surface. An increased incidence is recognized in the Saint Bernard, German Shepherd Dog, Dachshund, Dalmatian, and in the Burmese and Birman cat. Superficial keratectomy is curative and may be performed as early as 12 weeks of age.

Symblepharon

In the cat, adhesions of the conjunctiva to adjacent conjunctiva and/or cornea are common sequelae of infection that occurs before eyelid separation. The most likely pathogen is feline herpesvirus (FHV-1). The degree of opacification may be subtle, appearing as a thin vascularized membrane that obscures the limbus and overlies the cornea, or so severe that intraocular structures are obscured and vision is impaired (Figure 43-12).

Severe symblepharon is difficult to resolve surgically. Instead, prompt medical therapy of external eye disease and mechanical disruption of developing adhesions should be used to minimize symblepharon formation. Symblepharon is uncommon in dogs and more likely to follow chemical injury of the conjunctival and corneal surfaces.

Acquired Abnormalities
Corneal Dystrophy

Corneal dystrophies are familial, bilaterally symmetrical corneal opacities. Most corneal dystrophies in the dog are white in color, oval or circular in shape, refractile in nature, and located in the central or paracentral cornea. Histochemically the corneal deposits consist of cholesterol, phospholipids, and neutral fats that may affect any layer of the cornea.

The crystalline corneal dystrophy in the Siberian Husky is inherited as a recessive trait that may appear as early as 5 months of age. The affected corneas develop a central homogeneous gray haze. Although the corneal opacities seldom become dense enough to affect vision, breeding of affected dogs is not recommended. There is no treatment. A dense milky opacity occurs in the central cornea of Airedale Terriers as early as 6 months of age. Vision may be impaired as the dystrophy progresses. Pedigrees suggest a possible sex-linked, recessive pattern. A unique form of corneal dystrophy occurs in the Shetland Sheepdog, characterized by multifocal 1- to 3-mm circular or ring-shaped opacities that begin in the central cornea as early as 6 months of age (Figure 43-13).

Qualitative abnormalities of the tear film are implicated in the progression of the disorder as the dog ages. Treatment in the later stages consists of topical cyclosporine.

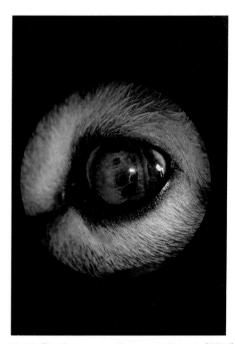

Figure 43-11 Persistent pupillary membrane (PPM)-related corneal opacity. Numerous PPMs extend from the iris face to the inner corneal surface, creating a permanent opacity in this Domestic Shorthair kitten.

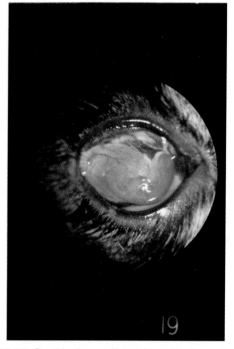

Figure 43-12 Symblepharon. Extensive adhesions of conjunctiva to the corneal surface limit vision in this Domestic Shorthair kitten following neonatal herpesvirus infection.

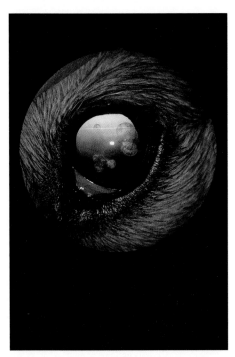

Figure 43-13 Corneal dystrophy. A unique bilateral dystrophy in the Shetland Sheepdog appears as multifocal circular white opacities across the corneal surface.

A rare progressive dystrophy occurs in the Manx cat, characterized by superficial edema in the central cornea as early as 4 months of age. The cornea progressively deteriorates, with accumulation of fluid-filled vesicles within the stroma. An autosomal recessive pattern of inheritance is suspected.

Corneal Edema

Ocular disease associated with canine adenovirus usually develops unilaterally from 1 to 3 weeks following infection or vaccination. The use of canine adenovirus type 2 vaccines was thought to have abolished the postvaccinal ocular response, but occasional reactions are still seen. Clinically, anterior uveitis is accompanied by complement-mediated injury to the corneal endothelium, producing severe corneal edema and the classical "blue eye." Treatment consists of topical corticosteroids and topical 5% sodium chloride ointment several times daily. Intraocular pressure (IOP) should be closely monitored. With or without treatment, the uveitis can lead to secondary glaucoma, especially in Afghan Hounds, Siberian Huskies, Samoyeds, and Norwegian Elkhounds. If endothelial damage is minimal, the edema resolves in 1 to 2 weeks. Partial or total corneal opacity persists in 20% of animals.

Pigmentation

Superficial corneal pigmentation is common in young brachycephalic dogs, notably the Pug, Shih Tzu, Lhasa Apso, and Pekingese. The pigmentation most often begins in the nasal corneal quadrant but may progress as a result of unresolved adnexal abnormalities and central exposure (Figure 43-14).

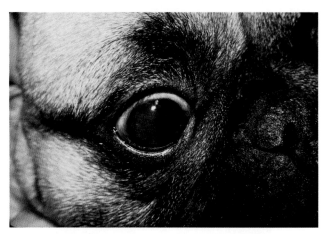

Figure 43-14 Pigmentary keratitis. Melanin discolors the medial and central cornea of this Pug with prominent eyes and corneal exposure.

Treatment is directed at correcting adnexal factors such as medial entropion, medial canthal and facial fold trichiasis, and lagophthalmos. Adequate tear production should be documented with an STT. The exposure secondary to lagophthalmos is addressed medically with topical lacrimogenics such as cyclosporine and/or surgically with a permanent partial tarsorrhaphy.

Corneal Sequestrum

A unique stromal necrosis occurs in the cat as a consequence of chronic corneal insult. Persian and Himalayan breeds are most commonly affected. Herpetic keratitis and adnexal disorders such as entropion, trichiasis, and lagophthalmos are implicated as etiologic factors. The problem is not common in patients younger than 6 months of age, but an iatrogenic sequestrum may develop following inappropriate use of a keratotomy for nonhealing corneal ulceration caused by herpesvirus infection in these young cats.

The corneal degeneration appears as a bronze discoloration of the stroma that often progresses to a dense black lesion of variable size and shape (Figure 43-15).

Vascularization and discomfort are variable. The abnormal tissue may slough spontaneously, but in some cats that process is protracted and painful. Definitive treatment requires superficial keratectomy.

Corneal Ulceration

A corneal ulcer is present when a break in the surface epithelium occurs, exposing the underlying stroma. Clinical signs include excessive tearing, squinting, conjunctival hyperemia, and varying degrees of corneal edema. Diagnosis is confirmed by fluorescein dye retention in the underlying stroma.

Although exogenous trauma by another animal or a foreign body is often implicated, most ulcers arise from inherent factors such as entropion, cilia disorders, exposure secondary to lagophthalmos, and inadequate tear production. A commonly overlooked etiology in young dogs is an

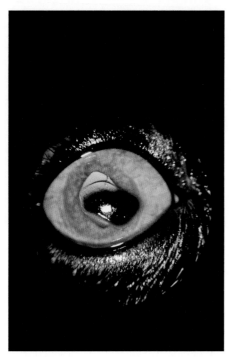

Figure 43-15 Sequestrum. A discolored area of necrotic corneal stroma developed in this young Persian cat with a chronic corneal ulcer.

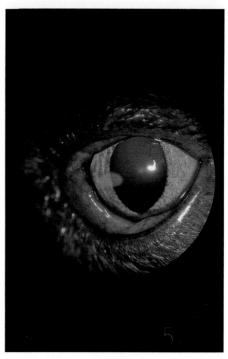

Figure 43-16 Ocular herpesvirus. Clinical signs of herpesvirus infection in this young Domestic Shorthair cat include conjunctival hyperemia, chemosis, and an elliptical fluorescein-positive superficial corneal ulcer.

ectopic hair that penetrates the conjunctival surface of the upper eyelid, classically producing a refractory ulcer in the upper third of the cornea. Refractory indolent ulcers caused by defective epithelial adherence to the underlying stroma do not occur in young dogs. In the cat, slow-healing corneal ulcers should be considered a consequence of herpesvirus infection until proven otherwise.

Management of an acute superficial corneal ulcer must first eliminate the ulcer's underlying cause. Initial therapy in the dog is directed at preventing bacterial infection, reducing the discomfort of secondary uveal spasm, and discouraging self-trauma. A broad-spectrum topical antibiotic solution is applied 4 times daily. If the pupil is miotic, topical 1% atropine is added to the regimen. Because of the long half-life of atropine's effects, a single application may be sufficient. Overzealous use of atropine reduces tear production and may compromise aqueous outflow in breeds predisposed to glaucoma. Brachycephalic patients will benefit from frequently applied topical lubricants. If corneal exposure is a significant factor, a partial temporary tarsorrhaphy should be considered to limit corneal drying. An Elizabethan collar is recommended to prevent ongoing trauma. Superficial ulcers treated in this manner should heal within 5 to 7 days. If not, the primary cause may still be present or secondary infection has occurred. Topical corticosteroids are contraindicated in ulcer management because they inhibit epithelial migration and mitosis, decrease stromal fibroblastic proliferation, limit inherent antimicrobial responses, and potentiate corneal enzymatic activity that can lead to rapid deepening of the ulcer. Topical NSAIDs can also slow corneal healing.

Corneal epithelial defects in the cat are most often the result of infection with FHV-1. Ulceration is dendritic or branching at first, but the viral cytopathic effect rapidly leads to more extensive geographic lesions (Figure 43-16).

Viral ulcers are superficial rather than deep. Ulceration can occur in young kittens after primary infection or in adult cats when stress or corticosteroid administration reactivates the latent virus. Antiviral therapy consists of lifelong nutritional supplementation with L-lysine to discourage viral replication; treating kittens with 250 mg twice daily and adults with 500 mg twice daily; compounded topical antiviral solutions such as 1% idoxuridine 4 to 6 times daily or 0.5% cidofovir twice daily for 14 days; and oral famciclovir at 15 mg/kg twice daily for 14 to 21 days. Herpetic ulcers are frequently resistant to treatment, and relapses are common.

Rapid deepening of an ulcer, a gelatinous ("melting") character to the stroma, and the appearance of a creamy, off-white cellular infiltrate are indications for a more aggressive medical regimen or referral to an ophthalmologist (Figure 43-17).

If an appropriate treatment plan is quickly implemented in response to these signs of enzymatic destruction and bacterial infection, complicated ulcers often resolve in the pediatric patient without difficult surgical procedures. A broad-spectrum topical fluoroquinolone such as ofloxacin is applied every 1 to 2 hours for the first 24 to 48 hours. The macroglobulins found in serum are used to counteract the destructive enzymes causing stromal melting. Serum is har-

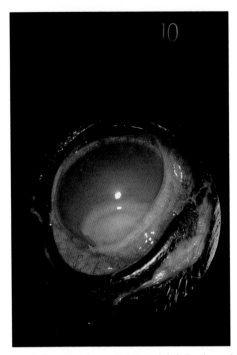

Figure 43-17 Septic ulcer. A bacterial infection should be ruled out in a deepening corneal ulcer, particularly when coupled with off-white to yellow cellular infiltrates at the ulcer site, progressive intraocular inflammation, and escalating pain.

vested aseptically from the patient or from a blood donor, refrigerated in a sterile dropper bottle, and applied topically as often as the antibacterial medication. A partial temporary tarsorrhaphy may be used to minimize corneal exposure in brachycephalic patients while still allowing assessment of therapeutic response. Frequency of therapy is decreased as the ulcer depth stabilizes, the corneal edema and infiltrates resolve, and the ulcer begins to epithelialize based on decreasing fluorescein retention. Oral antibiotics are not necessary in the face of such aggressive topical therapy.

Because secondary intraocular inflammation is likely to accompany a deep corneal ulcer, topical atropine is used judiciously to dilate the pupil and reduce ciliary spasm. Systemic corticosteroids or NSAIDs may be used to treat concurrent uveitis. Topical corticosteroids are contraindicated. Topical NSAIDs may also delay corneal healing and have been linked with ulcer progression in human patients with infected ulcers. An Elizabethan collar is essential. Topical ointments should not be used in ulcers that are nearing perforation or have already ruptured because entry of the ointment base into the anterior chamber will cause a significant inflammatory reaction.

Continued deepening of the ulcer despite aggressive medical therapy is indication for a conjunctival graft that provides mechanical support for the weakened cornea. A conjunctival graft performed by an experienced ophthalmic surgeon is highly successful. A third eyelid flap is much less effective at this stage of ulceration.

Traumatic Corneal Perforations

Perforating corneal wounds secondary to cat claw injuries are relatively common in puppies. The injured eye is painful, with corneal edema, aqueous flare, hyphema, iris congestion, and miosis. If the lens capsule is also perforated, lens antigens escape into the anterior chamber and stimulate a devastating immunologic reaction known as phacoclastic uveitis. The capsular wound may be difficult to visualize, but lens material may extrude into the anterior chamber or lens fibers can opacify within hours as a result of fluid absorption through the capsular defect.

Integrity of the corneal wound can be determined using the Seidel test, performed by touching a dry fluorescein dye strip to the wound surface. Focal dye retention is expected, but rivulets of apple-green color extending from the wound margin indicate aqueous leakage. A focal perforation may seal by means of stromal edema and fibrin plugs. Activity is restricted to minimize disruption of the seal. Broad-spectrum topical and systemic antibiotics are indicated to prevent secondary infection. Uveitis is treated conventionally with topical atropine and oral antiinflammatory medications (either corticosteroid or NSAID). Topical antiinflammatory drugs are not recommended because of the potential to slow healing of the corneal wound. Ophthalmic ointments should be avoided in a perforated eye; the oil base causes a severe reaction if introduced into the anterior chamber. Larger corneal perforations and lacerations require prompt surgical repair. An obvious tear in the anterior lens capsule is an indication for referral and possible lens extraction in addition to corneal repair.

Foreign Bodies

Corneal foreign bodies may adhere to the corneal surface or penetrate the cornea. After topical anesthesia with 1% proparacaine, a superficial foreign body can often be dislodged with a forceful stream of sterile saline. If unsuccessful, the tip of a 25-gauge needle may overcome the surface tension holding the foreign material in place. After removal, the underlying corneal defect is treated as a corneal ulcer. Deep or perforating foreign bodies should be referred for surgical extraction and subsequent repair of the corneal wound.

THE ANTERIOR UVEA

Congenital Abnormalities
Heterochromia

Heterochromia describes zones of different color in a single iris or refers to the iris of one eye being different in color from the other (Figure 43-18).

In most instances, heterochromia is of no clinical significance; however, an association between heterochromia and congenital deafness has been recognized in blue-eyed white cats and in a number of canine breeds, including the Australian Cattle Dog, Australian Shepherd, Boston Terrier, Dalmatian, English Bulldog, English Setter, and Old English Sheepdog.

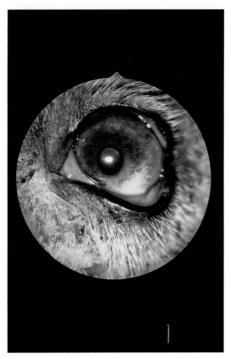

Figure 43-18 Heterochromia. There is no functional significance to the different colors seen within the iris of this Catahoula Leopard Dog, although some breed standards discriminate against the trait.

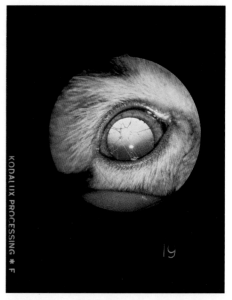

Figure 43-19 Persistent pupillary membranes. Remnants of an embryonic vascular network appear as interwoven strands, originating from the iris face and spanning the pupil of this 3-week-old Domestic Shorthair cat.

Pupillary Abnormalities

Abnormalities in pupil shape or location are rarely significant by themselves but may accompany other functional anomalies. Incomplete closure of the embryonic fissure creates a notch in the ventromedial pupillary margin known as a coloboma. The affected pupil assumes a teardrop shape. Colobomas are common findings in merled dogs, including the Australian Shepherd, Great Dane, Collie, and Dachshund.

Persistent Pupillary Membranes

PPMs are remnants of an embryonic vascular network that once spanned the pupil to supply nutrients to the developing lens. Pigmented strands persist on the anterior iris surface when the tissue fails to regress during late fetal or early neonatal development. Immediately after the lids separate, a network of fibers still may be seen over the pupillary space (Figure 43-19).

Individual PPMs may be confined to the iris surface or may extend to the cornea or lens, where they produce nonprogressive opacities at the attachment site. Treatment is not required. PPMs are inherited in the Basenji and occur with some frequency in the Pembroke Welsh Corgi, Chow Chow, and Mastiff. Severely affected dogs may be excluded from use in a breeding program. PPMs must be differentiated from postinflammatory adhesions that involve the pupillary margin.

Acquired Abnormalities
Anterior Uveitis

Inflammation is by far the most important abnormality of the iris and ciliary body. A variety of clinical signs characterize the inflamed eye, but the most sensitive indicators of uveitis are aqueous flare and a reduction in IOP. Nonspecific indicators of pain include tearing, blepharospasm, enophthalmos, and even lethargy. Conjunctival hyperemia results from vasodilation of conjunctival and episcleral vessels. Corneal edema develops when toxins, inflammatory mediators, and inflammatory cells damage the endothelium. Breakdown of the blood-aqueous barrier increases protein content within the aqueous (flare) and enables inflammatory cells and fibrin to enter the eye. The iris appears swollen and dull in color because of edema and cellular infiltrates (Figure 43-20). The pupil is classically constricted and sluggish in its reactions. An abnormal pupillary shape may result from adhesions of iris to lens known as posterior synechia. Ciliary body dysfunction reduces aqueous production and decreases IOP.

Anterior uveitis may result from disorders limited to the eye or may be secondary to systemic illness. Blunt contusion, perforating injury by a cat claw, rapidly developing cataracts, and corneal ulceration are common primary disorders in young animals. A growing number of infectious agents are implicated as causes of uveitis in dogs and cats. Even so, retrospective studies classified 60% of canine uveitis and 62% of feline uveitis as idiopathic.

As a general rule, therapy should be initially aggressive, tapering frequency of administration as clinical signs subside. In the absence of corneal ulceration, symptomatic treatment of anterior uveitis begins with topical 1% prednisolone

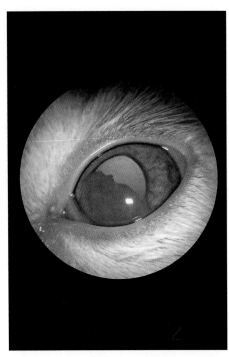

Figure 43-20 Anterior uveitis. A large fibrin clot and a prominently vascularized iris are seen in the normally blue eye of this 8-month-old Domestic Shorthair cat with intraocular inflammation secondary to feline infectious peritonitis.

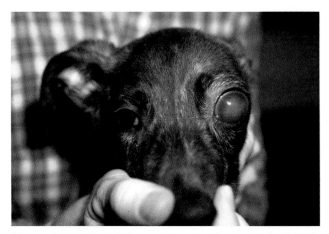

Figure 43-21 Buphthalmos. Exceptional scleral elasticity is responsible for the rapid and dramatic buphthalmos that accompanies glaucoma in puppies and kittens.

acetate at least 4 times daily. This particular corticosteroid penetrates the corneal barrier more effectively and provides higher intraocular drug levels than other antiinflammatory medications. Treatment should be continued for at least 2 weeks beyond resolution of clinical signs. Abrupt cessation of therapy may be followed by rebound inflammation. Cats often require long-term maintenance therapy to prevent relapses and secondary complications such as glaucoma.

Treatment also includes pupillary dilation with topical 1% atropine or 1% tropicamide. In addition to reducing the potential for adhesions between the iris and lens, these topical parasympatholytic agents relieve pain by reducing uveal muscle spasm and restore vascular permeability to normal. The inflamed iris does not dilate as readily as the normal iris; therefore several applications may be needed to achieve the desired pupil size. Once the pupil is dilated, reduce the frequency of application to the minimum effective dose. Keep in mind the potential for systemic absorption of atropine and its subsequent impact on tear production and gastrointestinal motility, particularly in these smaller patients. Atropine ointment reduces the likelihood that this bitter drug will traverse the nasolacrimal system and cause excessive salivation when licked from the nose.

GLAUCOMA

Glaucoma is simplistically defined as an increase in IOP beyond that compatible with normal vision and ocular physiology. Normal IOP ranges from 8 to 18 mm Hg. Congenital glaucoma is usually secondary to trauma or inflammation,

although rare instances of primary glaucoma have been reported in young animals. Elevations in IOP may occur at 3 to 6 months of age in puppies with developmental anomalies of the iridocorneal angle. Congenital open-angle glaucoma has been reported in 11 closely related Siamese cats, ranging in age from 3 weeks to 3 years, with moderate elevations in IOP. Atlases of feline ocular disease include examples of Persian and Domestic Shorthair kittens with congenital glaucoma.

The primary complaint in the young animal is often rapid and dramatic globe enlargement (Figure 43-21).

Additional clinical signs include ocular pain that appears to decrease over time, conjunctival and episcleral vascular congestion, and corneal edema. The pupil is classically dilated and nonresponsive. Within a matter of days, a sustained elevation in IOP causes irreversible optic nerve degeneration. In patients with secondary glaucoma, corneal opacities or posterior synechiae may implicate previous ulcerative disease and uveitis, respectively.

The goal of therapy is to return and prolong vision through control of IOP. To prevent ongoing damage to the optic nerve, IOP must be maintained below 20 mm Hg. IOP in patients with primary glaucoma may decrease within 1 hour of a single application of 0.005% latanoprost, a topical prostaglandin analogue that shunts aqueous through an alternative outflow pathway. Latanoprost is then continued once or twice daily until the patient can be evaluated by a specialist. Prostaglandin analogues should not be used in the treatment of glaucoma secondary to uveitis or anterior lens luxation. Intravenous mannitol, dosed at 1.0 g/kg, also reduces IOP rapidly by dehydrating the vitreous, but administration may be challenging in the very young patient. A topical carbonic anhydrase inhibitor (CAI) such as dorzolamide 2% (alone or in combination with timolol) or brinzolamide 1% is applied 2 to 3 times daily to reduce aqueous production. Side effects of hypokalemia, acidosis, or gastrointestinal upset are less likely to occur with a topical CAI than a systemic CAI such as methazolamide. Early referral to a veterinary ophthalmologist is advised once the diagnosis is made and emergency treatment is provided. Although the initial response to medical therapy may be dramatic, medication alone is generally ineffective in the long-term control of glaucoma in animals. Surgical procedures to maintain IOP in a potentially visual eye include cyclocryotherapy, laser cyclophotocoagulation, and gonioimplantation. Because elevated IOP should be considered painful even if the animal appears outwardly normal, procedures appropriate for the blind glaucomatous eye include evisceration with intraocular prosthesis placement or enucleation.

THE LENS

The normal lens often exhibits minor imperfections that can be easily detected with magnification in dogs and cats younger than 1 year of age. These include prominent anterior and posterior Y sutures and minute granules in the nucleus. Innocuous remnants of embryonic mesodermal tissue on the anterior lens capsule may appear as a mosaic of brown pigment spots identical in color to that of the iris.

Congenital Abnormalities

With the exception of cataracts, congenital anomalies of the lens are rarely seen in clinical practice. Aphakia, or absence of the lens, is extremely uncommon. A genetic basis has been proposed in the Saint Bernard. An abnormally small or microphakic lens is usually associated with other ocular malformations and has been reported in the Beagle, Doberman Pinscher, Miniature Schnauzer, and Siamese cat. A coloboma causes a segment of the normally curved equatorial lens to appear flattened. Lenticonus, a conelike protrusion of the posterior capsule and cortex into the vitreous body, often occurs in conjunction with other ocular anomalies in the Miniature Schnauzer, Doberman Pinscher, Cavalier King Charles Spaniel, Old English Sheepdog, Mastiff, Golden Retriever, Akita, Bouvier de Flandres, Bloodhound, Shih Tzu, and Persian cat.

Cataract

Cataract, or opacity of the lens, may be a congenital or acquired lens disorder. Congenital cataracts may not be recognized until the patient is 6 to 8 weeks of age when ocular examination is more easily performed (Figure 43-22).

These early-onset cataracts may be inherited or secondary to in utero or early neonatal influences; therefore it is important to question the owner or breeder regarding the presence of cataract in related animals or occurrence of any illness in the bitch or queen during gestation. Table 43-1 lists those canine breeds with heritable cataracts occurring before 1 year of age. A recessive mode of inheritance is implicated in Persian, British Shorthair, Himalayan, and Birman cats with early-onset cataract. Congenital cataracts are also common in animals with multiple ocular anomalies.

Attachment of a PPM may cause a focal anterior capsular cataract to develop. A focal posterior capsular/subcapsular cataract may accompany a patent or fibrotic remnant of the

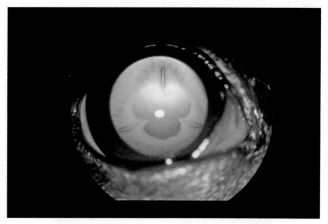

Figure 43-22 Congenital cataract. The prominent peripheral lens opacities highlighting the Y-suture in this 8-week-old Dachshund might be overlooked if the examination is performed without first dilating the pupil. (Courtesy Dr. David Ramsey.)

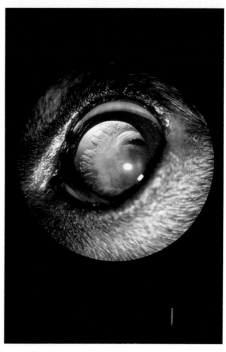

Figure 43-23 Persistent hyperplastic primary vitreous (PHPV). Progressive cataract formation with peripheral vacuolation accompanies frank hemorrhage within the lens of this young Dachshund with PHPV.

hyaloid artery. Persistent hyperplastic tunica vasculosa lentis and persistent hyperplastic primary vitreous (PHPV) are the most severe examples of persisting embryonic vasculature within the eye. Ocular lesions include fibrovascular proliferation with disruption of the posterior lens capsule, progressive cataract formation, and intralenticular hemorrhage (Figure 43-23).

These anomalies in the Doberman Pinscher and Staffordshire Bull Terrier are attributed to an incomplete autosomal dominant mode of inheritance. A breed predisposition is also recognized in the Bouvier des Flandres, Standard Schnauzer, and German Pinscher. Posterior capsular

TABLE 43-1	Features of inherited early-onset cataracts in the dog		
Breed	**Documented inheritance**	**Age of onset**	**Initial location**
Afghan Hound	Autosomal recessive	6-12 mo	Equatorial/posterior cortex
American Cocker Spaniel	Autosomal recessive	6+ mo	Anterior/posterior cortex
Boston Terrier	Autosomal recessive	Congenital	Posterior sutures/nuclear
German Shepherd Dog	Autosomal recessive	8+ wk	Posterior sutures/cortex
	Incomplete dominant	Congenital	Nuclear
Golden Retriever	Autosomal recessive	6+ mo	Posterior subcapsular
Labrador Retriever	Autosomal recessive	6+ mo	Posterior subcapsular
Miniature Schnauzer	Autosomal recessive	Congenital	Nuclear/posterior cortex
	Autosomal recessive	6+ mo	Posterior cortex
Norwegian Buhund	Autosomal recessive	Congenital	Fetal nucleus
Old English Sheepdog	Autosomal recessive	Congenital	Nuclear/cortex
Staffordshire Bull Terrier	Autosomal recessive	6+ mo	Posterior sutures/cortex
Welsh Springer Spaniel	Autosomal recessive	Congenital	Nuclear/posterior cortex
West Highland White Terrier	Autosomal recessive	Congenital	Posterior sutures

cataracts with intralenticular blood vessels have been noted in association with PHPV in two Domestic Shorthair cats, ages 6 and 9 months.

Acquired cataracts have been described in puppies and kittens fed only a commercial milk replacer in the first few weeks of life. Diffuse lens opacification and vacuolation near the posterior Y sutures appear in the third week of life. The cataracts are attributed to an arginine deficiency. The majority of the opacities fade to a perinuclear halo as the diet is corrected and the animals mature.

The mischievous behavior of puppies may predispose them to traumatic cataract formation. Trauma from cat claw wounds is suggested by a focal fibrinous exudate on the lens capsule in conjunction with a perforating corneal or scleral wound. Cataracts may also develop after electrical shock, as occurs from biting an appliance cord.

To date, surgical lens extraction is the only effective means of treating cataract in the dog. Recent claims that topical antioxidants or products containing carnosine may halt and reverse canine cataracts are contradicted by double-masked studies that show no improvement in lens opacity following treatment. Lens extraction by an experienced veterinary ophthalmic surgeon may be elected in patients with compromised vision. There is potential for cortical regrowth and recurring opacification when cataract surgery is performed in dogs less than 1 year of age. A second surgery may be required in these patients, accounting for the recommendation by some ophthalmologists to postpone surgery in the very young dog.

RETINA AND OPTIC NERVE

Examination of the fundus requires pupillary dilation with 1% tropicamide. Maximal mydriasis occurs in 15 minutes and lasts for 4 to 6 hours. Ophthalmoscopic examination of the fundus is challenging in a patient younger than 6 to 8

weeks of age. A monocular indirect ophthalmoscope (Pan-Optic; Welch Allyn Inc, Skaneateles Falls, NY) is a user-friendly tool that provides a wider field of view and penetrates cloudy ocular media more effectively than the direct ophthalmoscope.

The newborn fundus appears dark, with gradual changes in tapetal coloration from dark gray to lilac to blue by 4 to 6 weeks of age. The final brightly colored adult tapetal coloration may not be evident until 4 months of age. The amount of pigment in the ventral fundus varies. In the dog, the small, well-defined neonatal optic disc develops a fluffier white appearance as adult myelination occurs. In the cat, the adult optic nerve head remains round and darker than that of the dog.

Congenital Abnormalities
Collie Eye Anomaly

Collie eye anomaly (CEA) is a bilateral recessively inherited disorder found in the Collie, Shetland Sheepdog, Border Collie, and Australian Shepherd. Prevalence in the Collie may be as high as 60%. Diagnosis in the very young Collie is challenging because of its small, deeply set eyes, but examination at 6 to 8 weeks of age is advised to ensure that pigment does not mask lesions as the puppy matures. Lack of fundus pigmentation in merled animals also complicates the diagnosis because the lesions blend into the normal surroundings.

Choroidal hypoplasia is the fundamental defect, occurring alone or in combination with lesions of the optic nerve and sclera. A localized absence of tapetum and pigment temporal to the optic disc exposes large, irregularly spaced choroidal vessels against the scleral background. Vision is functionally normal (Figure 43-24).

A coloboma of the optic disc, found in up to 35% of affected animals, appears as a featureless pit in the disc

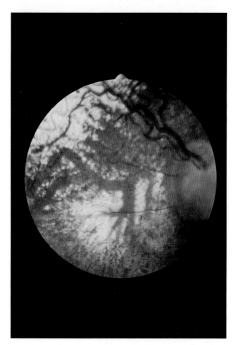

Figure 43-24 Collie eye anomaly. Choroidal hypoplasia occurs temporally to the optic disc in this young Sheltie, with anomalous choroidal vessels visualized against the scleral background. A retinal vessel at nine o'clock dips into a shallow defect (coloboma) in the optic disc.

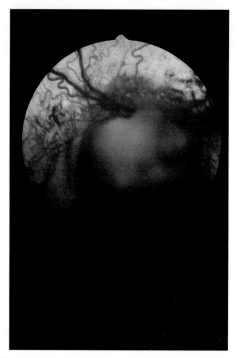

Figure 43-25 Scleral coloboma. Retinal vessels disappear at the margin of an extensive scleral deformity that surrounds and obscures the optic disc in this 9-month-old Boykin Spaniel.

surface with abrupt disappearance of retinal vessels at the defect margin. Similar defects can also occur in the sclera, often occurring adjacent to the optic disc (Figure 43-25).

Large colobomas likely produce visual field deficits ("blind spots"), but overall vision remains functional. Fewer than 10% of patients are born with blinding retinal detachments and associated hemorrhage. Although CEA is generally considered nonprogressive, an extensive coloboma may also predispose the affected dog to retinal detachment until 2 years of age.

Microphthalmia with Colobomas

Large equatorial colobomas occur in homozygously merled Australian Shepherds with a predominantly white haircoat. Retinal detachment occurs in an estimated 50% of affected animals. The disorder is inherited as an autosomal recessive trait with incomplete penetrance.

Retinal Folds

Pale linear folds are seen frequently in the nontapetal fundus of young Collies and occasionally in other breeds of dog. The folds probably represent a disparity in growth rates between the retina and fibrous tunic because the folds often disappear as the animal matures. These transient retinal folds are distinct from the retinal disorganization that occurs in retinal dysplasia.

Retinal Dysplasia

Retinal dysplasia is the result of faulty embryonic differentiation that creates linear folds and tubular rosettes within the sensory retina. Lesions may appear as striate or irregular areas of altered tapetal reflectivity, often in close proximity to the retinal vessels. Retinal detachment occurs secondary to concurrent vitreous abnormalities that result in giant peripheral retinal tears. Inherited forms of canine retinal dysplasia are most common, but maternal viral infections, trauma, and in utero toxicities can produce similar lesions.

The English Springer Spaniel inherits retinal dysplasia as an autosomal recessive trait. Lesions are bilateral, nonprogressive, and appear in the tapetal fundus as lightly colored round or linear lesions at 6 to 8 weeks of age, usually segregating along the retinal vasculature. As the tapetum matures, the folds appear darker against the tapetal background. Margins of the larger dysplastic foci appear hyperreflective, often with darkly pigmented centers. Focal or complete retinal detachments are sometimes seen. Vision is usually spared in the absence of retinal detachment.

Several types of retinal dysplasia are described in the Labrador Retriever. One form identified in field trial retrievers closely resembles that of the Springer Spaniel, with multifocal folds or irregularly shaped spots near the major blood vessels of the tapetal fundus. A dominant inheritance with incomplete penetrance is theorized. Geographic dysplasia appears as a more confluent irregular or U-shaped lesion within the tapetal fundus, with a darkly colored margin, scattered intralesional foci of hyperreflectivity, and central retinal elevation (Figure 43-26).

Visual impairment is likely. This geographic form is not always a congenital abnormality; thus a second examination

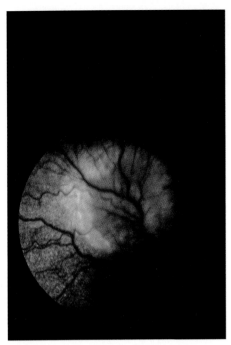

Figure 43-26 Geographic dysplasia. A roughly circular area of abnormal retina is characterized by a hyperreflective margin and a central retinal separation that obscures the underlying tapetum and bends the overlying vessels in this 6-month-old Labrador Retriever.

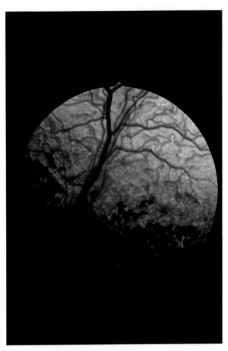

Figure 43-27 Dysplastic folds. Vision is clinically unaffected in this young Cocker Spaniel despite the widespread retinal dysplasia that appears as dark branching lines (folds) throughout the tapetal fundus.

is advised between 6 and 12 months of age. Generalized retinal dysplasia is characterized by retinal detachment and congenital blindness. Detachments also occur in conjunction with short-limbed dwarfism in Labrador Retrievers and Samoyeds. The causative gene has recessive effects on the skeleton and incomplete dominant effects on the eye.

Multifocal spots and branching folds occur in American Cocker Spaniels and Beagles without evidence of visual impairment or progression (Figure 43-27).

Mild forms of retinal dysplasia have also been seen in the Cavalier King Charles Spaniel, Golden Retriever, Rottweiler, and Yorkshire Terrier. Severe forms of retinal dysplasia with retinal detachment and blindness occur in Bedlington and Sealyham Terriers. Multiple ocular defects, including retinal dysplasia, occur in the Akita, Australian Shepherd, Chow Chow, Doberman Pinscher, Old English Sheepdog, and Saint Bernard. Generalized retinal dysplasia combined with PHPV occurs in the Miniature Schnauzer. A suspected hereditary multifocal dysplasia has been reported in related Somali cats.

Neonatal infection with canine herpesvirus, parvovirus, and adenovirus has been shown to cause retinal dysplasia. Radiation can also induce dysplasia in newborn pups. Intrauterine or early neonatal infections with feline panleukopenia and feline leukemia virus are documented causes of feline dysplasia. Retinal folds have been described in conjunction with retinal vessel tortuosity in cats with congenital cardiac and portacaval anomalies.

Congenital Stationary Night Blindness

Night blindness is evident in the Briard from birth as a result of a degenerative disorder of the neural retina and retinal pigment epithelium that includes a defect in retinal fatty acid metabolism. The resting pupil size is larger than normal. Most affected puppies also demonstrate a rapid horizontal nystagmus. Electroretinographic (ERG) rod responses are severely reduced to absent, but funduscopic changes are not evident until 2 to 3 years of age. Visual impairment does not progress. An autosomal recessive inheritance has been proposed. Subretinal injections of a corrective gene construct have improved vision and ERG amplitudes in affected puppies.

Tapetal Hypoplasia

Absence of the tapetum occurs sporadically in the Beagle as a simple recessive trait. With the choroidal pigment no longer obscured by the tapetum, the dorsal fundus appears dark in color rather than brightly reflective. Vision is unaffected.

Optic Nerve Hypoplasia

An abnormally small to absent optic nerve occurs as a recessively inherited disorder in the miniature Poodle. The defect is also seen on occasion in a variety of canine breeds, including the Beagle, Dachshund, Collie, Russian Wolfhound, German Shepherd Dog, Great Pyrenees, and Saint Bernard. Bilaterally affected animals are blind with dilated pupils. The affected optic disc is often less than half its normal size and

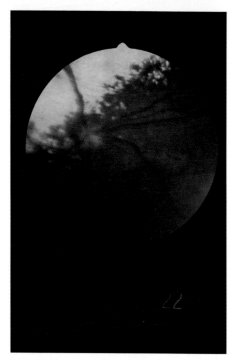

Figure 43-28 Optic nerve hypoplasia. Although retinal vessels and surrounding tissues appear normal, the optic disc is small, dark, and almost unrecognizable in this young Japanese Chin.

TABLE 43-2	Features of early-onset progressive retinal atrophy (PRA) in the dog		
Breed	Ocular signs	Behavioral signs	Mode of inheritance
Bullmastiff	6-12 mo	12-18 mo	AD
Collie	12-16 wk	6 wk	AR
Longhaired Dachshund	6-12 mo	6 mo	AR
Irish Setter	12-16 wk	6-8 wk	AR
Norwegian Elkhound	6-12 mo	6 wk	AR
English Mastiff	6-12 mo	12-18 mo	AD
Pit Bull Terrier	6 mo	6-12 mo	AR
Tibetan Terrier	10-18 mo	6-12 mo	AR
Cardigan Welsh Corgi	4 mo	8 wk	AR

AD, Autosomal dominant; *AR,* autosomal recessive.

dark in color, whereas the retinal vasculature is normal (Figure 43-28).

Unilateral hypoplasia may be a coincidental finding because the animal visually compensates with the unaffected eye. There is no treatment. Affected animals should not be bred. In the cat, hypoplasia of the optic nerve may result from in utero panleukopenia infection or administration of griseofulvin during the first half of gestation.

Optic Nerve Coloboma

Pits or notchlike defects in the optic disc are most often associated with CEA but occur occasionally in the American Cocker Spaniel, Brussels Griffon, Dachshund, English Springer Spaniel, and Golden Retriever. Colobomas also occur as one of a multitude of ocular anomalies in the Australian Shepherd and Basenji.

Acquired Abnormalities

Progressive Retinal Atrophy

Progressive retinal atrophy (PRA) is an inherited, bilateral, progressive disease of the retinal photoreceptors that ends in blindness. Early-onset PRA occurs in the Bullmastiff, Collie, Miniature Longhaired Dachshund, Irish Setter, Norwegian Elkhound, Old English Mastiff, Pit Bull Terrier, Tibetan Terrier, and Cardigan Welsh Corgi. Failure of the photoreceptor outer segments to develop normally, with subsequent degeneration of the photoreceptors linked to a deficiency in cyclic GMP phosphodiesterase, accounts for the early-onset disease in the Collie, Corgi, and Irish Setter. Early retinal degeneration in the Norwegian Elkhound is also linked to abnormal development of the photoreceptor outer segments. DNA-based tests have been developed that demonstrate the presence or absence of the actual gene mutation responsible for some of these inherited retinal degenerations (www.optigen.com). Table 43-2 summarizes the early-onset canine retinal degenerations.

Inherited retinal degenerations are relatively rare in the cat. An early-onset autosomal recessive degeneration has been identified in the Persian cat, with reduced pupillary reflexes at 2 to 3 weeks of age and complete retinal degeneration by 16 weeks of age. An autosomal dominant PRA has been described in the Abyssinian cat, with mydriasis occurring as early as 4 weeks of age, altered tapetal reflectivity developing by 8 to 12 weeks of age, and vision loss occurring by 1 year of age.

Patients with PRA first demonstrate their visual deficit in dim lighting. Progressive loss of day vision follows, culminating in total blindness. The pupils dilate as the disease progresses, but pupillary reflexes persist until late in the disorder. Ophthalmoscopically the tapetum appears increasingly hyperreflective as the retina thins and absorbs less light. Retinal vessels decrease in size and number. Focal depigmentation is commonly observed in the nontapetal fundus. Optic disc pallor and total absence of retinal vessels are signs of end-stage PRA.

Hemeralopia

Day blindness occurs in Alaskan Malamutes, with onset of behavioral changes as early as 8 to 20 weeks of age. The disorder also occurs in the miniature Poodle by 3 months of age. Dogs are visually impaired in daylight but function well at night and on overcast days. The fundus appears normal in affected animals. Diagnosis is confirmed by ERG.

Nonheritable Retinopathies

Retinal inflammation usually accompanies choroidal disease, with cellular infiltration, exudation, edema, or hemorrhage. The active inflammation is characterized by ill-defined areas of decreased tapetal reflectivity or nontapetal discoloration (Figure 43-29).

Choroidal exudates may also lead to retinal detachment. In contrast, inactive chorioretinitis lesions are well margin-ated, appearing hyperreflective within the tapetal region and depigmented in the nontapetal region. Pigment clumping may be seen at the center of the inactive inflammatory foci. Infectious causes of chorioretinitis in the young dog include canine distemper, toxoplasmosis, bacterial septicemia, and intraocular larval migrans by *Toxocara canis*. Causes in the young cat include feline infectious peritonitis, toxoplasmosis, histoplasmosis, and ophthalmomyiasis. Noninfectious causes range from toxins such as ethylene glycol to embryonic neu-roepithelial tumors such as medulloepithelioma. Treatment is generally directed at the underlying systemic disease, remembering that topical medication does not reach thera-peutic levels in the retina or choroid.

Posterior segment hemorrhage may occur as a nonspecific component of chorioretinitis or may accompany anemia or thrombocytopenia. Retinal vascular congestion occurs with congenital heart defects, such as atrioventricular septal defects and tetralogy of Fallot. Retinal hemorrhage and venous engorgement occur in cats with thiamine deficiency.

Feline nutritional retinopathy is relatively rare now that dietary levels of taurine have been increased in commercial cat foods, but an occasional domestic or exotic cat may demonstrate clinical signs when fed a vegetarian or home-made diet deficient in this essential amino acid. Lesions have been identified within 18 weeks of beginning a taurine-poor diet. A bilateral hyperreflective elliptical lesion develops temporal to the optic disc. This progresses to a horizontal hyperreflective band that extends across the tapetal fundus dorsal to the optic disc. Chronic taurine deficiency leads to generalized retinal atrophy and irreversible blindness.

Enrofloxacin has been linked with acute and severe retinal degeneration in cats. Affected cats present with dilated pupils, dramatic tapetal hyperreflectivity, and extreme retinal vessel attenuation within days of receiving enrofloxacin. In most, the blindness is permanent. Risk factors for fluoroqui-nolone toxicity include high dosage, prolonged treatment, intravenous administration, old age, and renal or hepatic disease. The dosage of enrofloxacin should never exceed the current manufacturer's recommended dose of 2.5 mg/kg every 12 hours, and even then enrofloxacin should be used with caution in the cat.

Retinal Detachment

Separation of the neural retina from the retinal pigment epithelium causes loss of function and secondary retinal degeneration. A focal detachment has little impact on vision, whereas a complete detachment is blinding. The displaced retina with its superficial vessels appears as a semilucent gray membrane that obscures underlying detail and decreases tapetal reflectivity (Figure 43-30).

Causes of retinal detachment in the young dog include congenital retinal disorders such as CEA or retinal dysplasia, PHPV, vitreous liquefaction leading to peripheral retinal tears in the Shih Tzu, trauma (including lens extraction), chorioretinitis, hypertension secondary to congenital renal or cardiac disease, and idiopathic disease.

The primary cause should be targeted. Retinal tears may be surgically repaired by an experienced veterinary

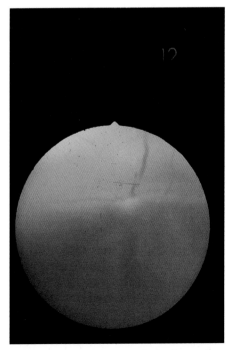

Figure 43-30 Retinal detachment. Retinal vessels are clearly visualized, but all other fundus detail is obscured beneath the complete retinal detachment in this young Labrador Retriever.

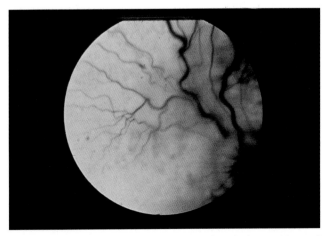

Figure 43-29 Chorioretinitis. Engorged retinal vessels and decreased tapetal reflectivity secondary to subretinal exudates characterize the active posterior segment inflammation in this young mixed-breed dog.

vitreoretinal surgeon. Once infectious disease has been ruled out, serous retinal detachments may respond to antiinflammatory doses of systemic corticosteroid, provided treatment is initiated before secondary retinal degeneration has occurred.

Optic Neuritis

Inflammation of the optic nerve results in vision loss of sudden onset. When bilateral, pupils will be fixed and dilated. If unilateral, the patient will exhibit anisocoria, with a partially dilated pupil on the affected side as a result of consensual input from the normal eye. The affected optic disc appears enlarged and hyperemic, with indistinct margins, peripapillary retinal elevation, and occasional hemorrhage. If the lesion is retrobulbar, the optic disc may appear normal. Causes of optic neuritis in the young dog and cat usually include infectious diseases that also affect other neurologic tissues, such as distemper and feline infectious peritonitis, and trauma, especially after proptosis of the globe.

The inflammation is treated symptomatically with high doses of systemic corticosteroids once infectious disease has been ruled out. Oral prednisone, starting at a daily divided dose of 2 to 4 mg/kg, is gradually decreased over a 3- to 4-week period. If the patient is going to respond, improvement usually occurs in the first 5 to 7 days. Optic atrophy and permanent blindness are common sequelae.

Papilledema

Passive edema of the optic nerve may be associated with increased cerebrospinal fluid pressure in congenital hydrocephalus or may be secondary to orbital inflammation. The treatment of papilledema is directed at the primary cause and in general it has a better prognosis than optic neuritis.

Optic Atrophy

Progressive degeneration of the optic nerve may follow optic neuritis, chronic papilledema, trauma, advanced retinal degeneration, glaucoma, or demyelinating disease. The optic disc appears shrunken and pale with decreased vasculature. The affected eye is irreversibly blind.

SUGGESTED READINGS

Cook CS: Ocular embryology and congenital malformations. In Gelatt KN (ed): *Veterinary ophthalmology*, Ames, IA, 2007, Blackwell Publishing, pp 3-36.

Gelatt KN, MacKay EO: Prevalence of primary breed-related cataracts in the dog in North America, *Vet Ophthalmol* 8(2):101-111, 2005.

Glaze MB: Congenital and hereditary ocular abnormalities in cats, *Clin Tech Small Anim Pract* 20(2):74-82, 2005.

Van der Woerdt A: Adnexal surgery in dogs and cats, *Vet Ophthalmol* 7(5):284-290, 2004.

Williams MM: Neonatal ophthalmic disorders. In Kirk RW, Bonagura JD (eds): *Current veterinary therapy X: small animal practice*. Philadelphia, 1989, Saunders, pp 658-673.

CLINICAL APPROACH TO PEDIATRIC NUTRITIONAL CONDITIONS

CHAPTER 44

Heather Prendergast

Neonates may not receive the appropriate nutrition for a number of factors, including insufficient milk production, the mother's death, an undeveloped gastrointestinal (GI) tract, or the inability to absorb nutrients. Neonates will not gain weight or may be unable to suckle normally as a result of a congenital defect or weakness.

Malnutrition can be caused by inadequate diet with poor quality ingredients, deficiencies, or excess supplementation. Inadequate protein and energy intake can lead to a decreased growth rate, inhibition of neural myelination and neurotransmission, decreased brain growth, and inhibited cognitive function. Patients with malnutrition may suffer from hypothermia, hypoglycemia, and dehydration.

Critically ill patients can receive nutritional support through a variety of routes, including enteral or parenteral feedings. Nutrition, both prenatal and postnatal, as well as during the first year of development, significantly influences the longevity and health of puppies and kittens.

At birth, the GI tract must transition from processing amniotic fluid to digesting milk. The release of hormones, digestive enzymes, activation of secretion, motility, and absorption are all adaptations that begin shortly after birth. These changes are critical to allow the GI tract to perform required functions.

Neonates have decreased pancreatic digestive enzymes, allowing the absorption of immunoglobulins from colostrum. Antibodies secreted in the mother's colostrum are only absorbed during the first 12 to 24 hours after birth. Pancreatic enzymes begin to be produced in response to ingestion of solid food; therefore consuming solid food is important to facilitate the development of normal GI tract function. GI motility is minimal the first month, a condition which must be taken into consideration whenever a neonate requires supplemental feeding.

PROPER NUTRITIONAL INTAKE

Excessive Nutrient Intake

Excess dietary energy and caloric intake may support a growth rate that is too fast for appropriate skeletal development and may result in a higher incidence of skeletal abnormalities. Excess calcium affects the skeletal system by increasing the severity of osteochondrosis. The absolute value of calcium appears to be more significant than the calcium/phosphorus ratio. Subsequently it is contraindicated to supplement large breed puppies with calcium when they are fed a complete and balanced commercial diet.

Osteochondrosis dissecans (OCD) is a disruption in endochondral ossification that results in focal lesions. OCD occurs in the physis and/or epiphysis of the growth cartilage. Factors affecting OCD include age, gender, breed, rapid growth rate, and excess nutrients. Great Danes, Labrador Retrievers, Newfoundlands, and Rottweilers are at an increased risk. Overnutrition and/or excess caloric intake results in abnormal weight gain relative to skeletal structure and disruption of chondrocytes, leading to OCD. See Chapter 42 for more information about OCD.

Canine hip dysplasia (CHD) is a genetic disorder of large and giant breeds but can also be influenced by nutrition. Evidence suggests that rapid growth and weight gain in early development increase the risk for CHD. See Chapter 42 for more information about CHD.

Hypervitaminosis D

Excess vitamin D is usually caused by inappropriate supplementation or rodenticide poisoning, and can be fatal. Increased levels of vitamin D can cause hypercalcemia and hyperphosphatemia, resulting in metastatic calcification. Symptoms may include vomiting, diarrhea, limb stiffness,

483

increased respiratory rate, anorexia, muscle weakness, and polyuria/polydipsia. Diagnosis is generally made by questioning the history of the diet. Tests can be submitted to a laboratory to verify vitamin D toxicity and should include parathyroid-related hormone protein, phosphorus, and 25-OH-cholecalciferol. Treatment can be initiated by removing the excess vitamin D source. The prognosis can be guarded, depending on the severity of the condition. Dissolution of calcifications can be slow and generally incomplete.

Nutritional Secondary Hyperparathyroidism

Nutritional secondary hyperparathyroidism is a common skeletal disorder that occurs as a result of hypervitaminosis D and/or a mineral imbalance caused by an inadequate diet. Diets that are composed mostly of meat are deficient in calcium and/or have an inverse Ca/P ratio. Because of the deficient calcium in the diet, the parathyroid glands enlarge and release large amounts of parathormone. The elevated levels increase osteoclastic resorption, therefore increasing calcium release into the bloodstream. Puppies and kittens develop severe bony lesions that can be seen radiographically. Bones may appear "moth eaten" and have poor density. The cortex will appear thinned, and the medullary cavity is widened. Because of the increased calcium release, blood levels will appear low normal. However, serum alkaline phosphatase levels, as well as parathyroid hormone (PTH) levels, will increase.

Symptoms of nutritional secondary hyperparathyroidism may include lameness, fractures, inability to walk, incoordination, muscle twitching, and seizures. Fractured vertebrae are common in severe cases. Treatment consists of changing the patient to an Association of American Feed Control Officials (AAFCO)-approved diet, fracture support, and strict confinement for 4 to 8 weeks. Serial radiographs can be taken to monitor improvement. Calcium and vitamin D supplementation are not advised because the complete and balanced AAFCO diet will have appropriate levels. If blood samples are to be taken to check the PTH levels, samples must be taken before switching diets because the PTH levels can rapidly equilibrate. Once the diet has been changed and the fractures have healed, the patient can completely recover from the imbalanced diet.

Deficient Nutrient Intake

Nutritional deficiencies appear when the patients' nutritional requirements exceed the maintenance requirements. This can include periods during gestation, lactation, and growth. Deficiencies in protein, essential fatty acids, and zinc result in keratinization defects and are most commonly caused by generic foods that are low in fat and have excessive mineral supplementation. Low quality protein decreases the digestibility of the food. Essential fatty acids are generally deficient in low quality foods and can be damaged when overheated for a lengthy period. Deficiencies in vitamin A can lead to retinal, visual, and digestive problems.

Vitamin E deficiency is rare because the use of vitamin E (a natural preservative) to maintain fats that are poorly stabilized is common. Vitamin B deficiency is also rare and usually manifests as a dermatologic condition.

Deficiency in zinc is generally caused by foods that are high in phylates, which chelate zinc. These foods include those high in bran and are often oversupplemented with calcium. Copper deficiency is common in homemade diets that are not correctly supplemented and often also contain excess calcium, zinc, or iron. Calcium competes with the absorption of zinc, copper, and iodine. The percentage of absorption is often less than 30% but greatly improves when the trace elements are provided in inorganic form with chelated amino acids.

Thiamine Deficiency

Thiamine deficiency is generally seen in cats that eat diets high in nonprocessed fish. The energy metabolism of the cat is compromised, resulting in weakness, blindness, head drop, and other neurologic disturbances. Cats may act interested in food but will not eat. Laboratory testing can determine thiamine deficiency; however, it generally takes an extended period to get results. Diagnosis can be made from history of diet, symptoms, and by the response to therapy. Response is generally observed after 1 to 2 days of treatment. Thiamine should be diluted 100 to 250 mg into 100 ml of NaCl fluids, which can then be administered subcutaneously daily. The pH of thiamine is approximately 5, necessitating diluting the product to increase the comfort level of the patient. The course of treatment continues until symptoms regress.

Hypokalemia

Hypokalemia is usually secondary to the depletion of potassium stores, either from loss through the GI tract or renal compromise. Symptoms include weakness and persistent ventroflexion of the neck, crouched posture, and muscular pain. Most symptoms resolve after the supplementation of potassium either orally or intravenously. Intravenous fluids with potassium supplementation should be mixed well before administration because sudden death can result from high levels of infused KCl. Oral supplementation is generally regarded as the safest method of administration. Patients should be monitored closely because potassium levels tend to rebound within 2 to 3 days of treatment. Supplementation may be lifelong as those who have experienced hypokalemia are at high risk of reoccurrence. Potassium gluconate can be administered orally to both puppies and kittens at 2 mEq/4.5 kg twice daily. The dosage can be adjusted as needed to maintain proper potassium levels.

Taurine Deficiency

Deficiency in taurine can be caused by an inadequate diet. AAFCO has minimum requirements for both dry and canned cat food as taurine bioavailability is decreased in canned food. Taurine is an essential amino acid for cats and is required for proper cardiac function and conjugating bile acids. Taurine is also lost in feces as a result of bacterial degradation in the intestinal tract. There is no evidence that suggests taurine is an essential amino acid in dogs; however, research shows that it may be conditional. Taurine is also necessary for bile acid conjugation in dogs, and dilated cardiomyopathy in Cocker Spaniels and Golden Retrievers has been associated with plasma taurine deficiency. Some lamb meal and rice diets have been suspected to have taurine deficiencies, but this suspicion has not been confirmed. Plasma or whole blood taurine levels can determine deficiencies. Dogs may be supplemented with taurine at 500 mg orally twice daily; cats can be supplemented with 250 mg orally twice daily.

Hypoglycemia

Proper nutritional intake is key for neonates because they lack sufficient glycogen storage, fat reserves, and reduced precursors for gluconeogenesis. They are unable to maintain glucose levels for extended periods. Maintenance of glucose requires several interrelated factors, some of which neonates have marginal abilities, including digestive absorption, liver and muscle glycogenolysis, and liver gluconeogenesis.

Hypoglycemia can be caused by vomiting, diarrhea, intestinal parasites, sepsis, hypothermia, or inadequate nutritional intake. Hypoglycemia can also be secondary to a variety of conditions, including endotoxemia, septicemia, portosystemic shunts, and glycogen storage abnormalities.

Hypoglycemic symptoms can include lethargy, anorexia, depression, incoordination, muscle tremors, and seizures. Normal glucose levels are 80 to 140 mg/dl. Patients are considered hypoglycemic with glucose levels less than 50 mg/dl. Hypoglycemia most commonly occurs in toy breed puppies but can occur with any neonate.

Hypoglycemic patients should be treated with 10% to 25% dextrose intravenously at 1 to 2 ml/kg. Dextrose given orally rarely reverses a hypoglycemic crisis. Once the patient responds, a 5% to 10% dextrose drip can be initiated until the patient is eating normally. Neonates have an immature metabolic regulatory mechanism; therefore glucose levels should be carefully monitored, and dextrose administration should be adjusted accordingly. Any fluids that are administered should be warmed to 100° F (38° C) to prevent hypothermia.

Traditionally owners have been advised to keep some syrup on hand, and should hypoglycemic symptoms occur (or reoccur) they can apply a small amount to the neonate's gum line while in transport to the veterinary clinic. This technique probably does no harm, but its effectiveness has been questioned recently. Often 50% dextrose solution is sent home for oral application if necessary. L-Carnitine increases the liver's ability to convert fat to glucose and can be given to prevent hypoglycemic episodes from reoccurring. L-Carnitine can be administered at 50 mg/kg by mouth twice daily.

Hypothermic patients should not be fed until their temperature is 97° F (36.1° C) because hypothermia decreases GI motility and digestion. Decreased motility can cause curdling of milk in the stomach.

NUTRITIONAL SUPPORT

The purpose of dietary support either by enteral nutrition (EN) or parenteral nutrition (PN) is to provide adequate nutrition, promote health, and to prevent and treat deficiencies. Proper nutritional support can prevent deterioration of the immune system and improve wound healing. Many animals presented for veterinary care are in poor medical condition secondary to metabolic, infectious, or traumatic insults and are already suffering from decreased nutritional intake. This nutritional deficit could increase the adverse affects of previous and current underlying diseases. Administration of appropriate EN or PN to critically ill patients is an important part of their therapy. Each patient should be evaluated to determine which type of nutritional support would be appropriate. What is the physiologic state of the patient? What nutrients does the patient need? What formulas are available to meet those needs? How will the formula be administered?

Patients that are younger than 2 weeks and have lost weight or have not eaten for 3 or more days, have excessive losses through vomiting and diarrhea, or have an increased nutritional need as a result of trauma, surgery, or infection are candidates for nutritional support (Box 44-1). Parenteral support should be limited to paralyzed or comatose patients with severe GI dysfunction. When an adequate catheter is placed, either total PN or partial PN support can be administered.

Some patients may still have an appetite or regain an appetite while EN or PN is being administered. Always offer fresh food and water to help stimulate oral intake. Once caloric intake meets/exceeds nutritional requirements, nutritional feedings can be decreased gradually to allow endocrine equilibration and to prevent rebound hypoglycemia.

Enteral Nutrition

Increased or decreased nutritional needs should be considered when addressing illnesses associated with nutrition. A puppy's or kitten's nutritional state may vary as a result of decreased intake, increased losses, increased nutritional requirements, or altered absorption.

When determining the dietary requirements of the patient, age, breed, and species should be taken into consideration. The goal is to maintain body weight and condition. Resting energy requirement (RER) can be calculated as:

$$RER\,(kcal/day) = 30\,(weight\ in\ kg) + 70$$

This equation gives an estimated maintenance requirement (Box 44-2). Energy requirements can be estimated by multiplying the RER × 1.5.

Adequate protein is required to help facilitate recovery and optimize immune function. Canines require 4 g/kg, whereas felines require 6 g/kg. Those with hypoalbuminemia or protein loss through the GI tract should have higher protein content, whereas those with preexisting liver or kidney conditions should have restricted protein content.

BOX 44-1   **Possible indications for nutritional support**

Patients Known to Be Protein-Energy Malnourished

Any patient in critical care unit
Recent weight loss of ≥5% to 10% of body weight
Decreased food intake or anorexia for ≥3 to 5 days
Generalized weakness and lethargy for ≥5 days
Hypoalbuminemia
Lymphopenia unassociated with severe stress or drug therapy
Presence of a nonhealing wound, delayed wound healing, or a decubital ulcer
Presence of a chronic, unrelenting fever or other signs of infection or sepsis
Poor body condition characterized by easily epilated hair and cracked nails

Patients with Conditions Known to Cause Protein-Calorie Malnutrition

Recent severe trauma or major surgery
Resection of ≥70% of the small intestine
Chronic vomiting or diarrhea
Protein-losing nephropathies
Increased nutrient needs with neoplasia
Peritonitis, pleuritis, or chylous effusion with effective, progressive drainage
Large wounds or burns, with persistent exudative losses
Use of drugs that promote catabolism
Chronic or massive hemorrhage
Cachexia

Patients with Conditions Associated with Poor Food Intake

Fractures of the mandible or maxilla
Congenital hard- or soft-palate clefts
Recovery from major oral or nasal surgery
Severe generalized stomatitis, glossitis, pharyngitis, and esophagitis
Severe periodontal disease
Neurologic conditions associated with coma or seizures requiring sedation
Tetraplegia that prevents patient from eating
Bilateral cranial nerve V or XII palsies
Severe oropharyngeal or cricopharyngeal dysphagia
Megaesophagus
Esophageal stricture or foreign body
Following esophageal resection
Following extensive stomach disease, surgery, or resection
Following extensive intestinal surgery or resection
Anorexia with refusal to eat because of various metabolic diseases (e.g., renal failure, pancreatitis, hepatic failure)
Severe persistent vomiting
Withholding food for ≥3 to 5 days because of therapeutic or diagnostic procedures

From Tams TR: *Handbook of small animal gastroenterology*, ed 2, St Louis, 2003, Saunders/Elsevier.

BOX 44-2   **Enteral feeding worksheet for dogs and cats**

1. Calculate resting energy requirement (RER):
   Body weight 2 to 45 kg: $RER \text{ (kcal)} = 30 \, Wt_{kg} + 70$
   Body weight <2 or >45 kg: $RER = 70 \, (Wt_{kg}^{0.75})$
   Body weight = _____ kg
   RER = _____ kcal
2. Calculate illness energy requirement (IER)*:
   Illness factor = 1.2 to 1.4 for dogs
   Illness factor = 1.1 to 1.2 for cats
   $IER = RER \times \text{illness factor}$
   IER = _____ kcal
3. Calculate amount of diet to feed:
   Daily volume to feed: IER ÷ energy density (kcal/ml)
   Daily volume = _____ ml
4. Evaluate responses and modify as needed:
   Weight changes often reflect fluid dynamics in the early period after injury. Caloric requirement may need to be increased or decreased depending on animal's metabolic rate and response to nutritional support.

Modified from Marks SL: The principles and practical application of enteral nutrition, *Vet Clin North Am Small Anim Pract* 28:677, 1998.
*Animals should be fed their RER initially, and have their body weights, physical examination findings, and ongoing losses carefully evaluated before gradually increasing their caloric intake based on the IER formula.

Arginine is an essential amino acid that is important for wound healing and promotes positive nitrogen balance and immune function. Glutamine is the principal nutrient for enterocytes and is important for nitrogen balance. The branched chain amino acids valine, leucine, and isoleucine decrease trauma- and sepsis-induced muscle catabolism and improve nitrogen retention. Taurine is an essential amino acid in cats and is required for cardiac function.

Fluid maintenance is approximately 50 to 100 ml/kg/day and may need to be increased if vomiting, diarrhea, or polyuria exists. Many canned diets contain a sufficient amount of fluids possibly meeting requirements. Body weight increases or decreases with hydration or dehydration; adjusting fluid intake can be assessed by measuring changes in body weight daily.

Vitamin and mineral content has rarely been studied and is difficult to monitor in critically ill patients; therefore using a complete and balanced diet is essential. However, over-supplementing can be detrimental, can easily occur, and usually increases the risk of compromising the patient.

The macronutrient composition of a variety of veterinary diets is provided in Table 44-1.

Enteral dietary therapy is practical, safe, easy, and economical. Enteral nutritional support can be delivered by a variety of methods, including eating, orogastric tube, nasogastric tube, esophageal tube, gastrostomy tube, or enterostomy tube (Table 44-2). Enteral nutritional support may be contraindicated in patients that have a bowel obstruction, severe malabsorption conditions, inflammatory bowel disease, or an adynamic ileus.

TABLE 44-1	Macronutrient composition of selected veterinary liquid enteral formulations					
		Caloric density (kcal/ml)	Nutrients (% of total kcal)			
Product	Protein type		Protein	Fat	Carbohydrate	Formula characteristics
Prescription diet Canine & Feline a/d (Hill's)	Liver Chicken Corn flour Casein	1.3	34	55	4	Isotonic, lactose free, fiber 1.3% DM, adequate taurine, fatty acid ratio (n6:n3 = 2.2:1)
Eukanuba Maximum-Calorie Canine & Feline (Iams)	Chicken Chicken by-product meal	2.1	29	66	5	Isotonic, lactose free, fiber 1.6% DM, adequate taurine, fatty acid ratio (n6:n3 = 8.3:11)
CliniCare Canine (Abbott)	80% casein 20% whey	1.0	20	55	25	Isotonic (230 mOsm/kg), lactose free, fiber free, fatty acid ratio (n6:n3 = 6.4:1)
CliniCare Feline (Abbott)	60% casein 40% whey	1.0	30	45	25	Isotonic (235 mOsm/kg), lactose free, fiber free, adequate taurine, fatty acid ratio (n6:n3 = 6.4:1)
CliniCare RF Specialized Feline (Abbott)	80% casein 20% whey	1.0	22	57	21	Isotonic (165 mOsm/kg), lactose free, fiber free, adequate taurine, fatty acid ratio (n6:n3 = 6.4:1)

From Ettinger SJ, Feldman EC: *Textbook of veterinary internal medicine*, ed 7, St Louis, 2010, Saunders/Elsevier.

TABLE 44-2	Advantages and disadvantages of enteral feeding devices	
Enteral feeding device	Advantages	Disadvantages
NE or NG tube	Ease of placement No general anesthesia NG tube allows for gastric decompression	Limited to liquid diets Short term (<14 days) Can be irritating; requires E-collar Can dislodge if patient sneezes or vomits Contradicted in facial trauma or respiratory disease Increased risk of vomiting with NG vs NE tube
Esophagostomy tube	Blenderized pet foods or liquid diets can be used Well tolerated by patient Ease of placement Can feed as soon as patient awakens from anesthesia Can be removed at any time Good long-term option	Requires general anesthesia Risk of cellulitis or infection at site Can dislodge if patient vomits Can cause esophageal irritation or reflux if malpositioned
Gastrostomy tubes	Blenderized pet foods or liquid diets can be used Well tolerated by patient Good long-term option	Requires general anesthesia Risk of cellulitis or infection at site Risk of peritonitis Must wait 24 hours after placement before feeding Must wait 10 to 14 days before removing
Jejunostomy tube	Requires liquid diet Able to feed distal to pylorus and pancreatic duct	Requires general anesthesia Technically more difficult to place Risk of cellulitis or infection at site Risk of peritonitis Risk of tube migration with secondary GI obstruction Must wait 24 hours after placement before feeding Requires CRI feeding Requires very close monitoring Short-term option

From Silverstein DC, Hopper K: *Small animal critical care medicine*, St Louis, 2009, Saunders/Elsevier.
CRI, Constant rate infusion; *GI*, gastrointestinal; *NE*, nasoesophageal; *NG*, nasogastric.

Liquid diets should only be administered in tubes 5 French (Fr) or smaller. Eight-French tubes can be used for a convalescent diet, whereas tubes 12 Fr and larger can be used to administer a blended canned diet.

The volume to be administered per feeding should be determined by the caloric density of the food; the calculated required daily caloric intake should then be divided into the proper number of feedings per day. For patients more than 3 months of age, six to eight feedings should be administered on day 1, decreasing to four to six feedings on day 2 and three feedings on day 3. Neonates should have a higher number of feedings per day.

Some clinicians advise to feed one third of the total caloric intake on day 1, increasing to two thirds of the caloric intake on day 2, and feeding the full caloric recommendations on day 3. Others advise to feed the entire caloric requirements starting on day 1.

Should any questions arise regarding the correct placement of a feeding tube, a radiopaque material can be injected into the tube and radiographed. This will help view the placement of the tube and confirm whether any materials are leaking into the abdominal cavity. The area of tube placement should be cleaned daily to prevent site infection.

It is important to prevent premature tube removal by the patient. Elizabethan collars are highly recommended, as well as bandages, sweaters, or T shirts. If a patient will receive care at home, clients should be educated that other pets can also remove the tube.

Tubes can become occluded with food, which can be prevented by feeding a commercially prepared diet rather than a blended canned diet. The tube should be flushed with water every time feeding is complete. Should the tube become occluded, a carbonated beverage can be useful. Infusing a small amount of sparkling water or cola can break down the occlusion.

Complications can include vomiting, diarrhea, and abdominal cramping. Vomiting can be caused by rapid and overadministration of diet. Abdominal cramping may be the result of rapid administration or the food not warmed to body temperature. Diarrhea may be caused by stress, nutrient composition, and/or rapid administration.

Oral

Every attempt should be made to encourage pets to eat before placing a tube. Many patients do not want to eat in the hospital. If it is possible, sending patients home may encourage eating as they are in a familiar, stable environment. Using highly palatable foods and encouraging patients to eat by hand-feeding can stimulate them. Heating the patient's food increases the aroma and palatability of the diet. A syringe may be used to force feed, but this may increase the stress of the pet, and nutritional requirements may not be met on larger patients. Drugs can be used to help stimulate appetite but should be used with caution in patients with preexisting medical conditions. Table 44-3 lists drugs currently available to help stimulate appetite.

BOX 44-3	Appropriate tube size, French (Fr)

Kittens: 3 Fr
Puppies <350 g: 5 Fr
Puppies 350-500 g: 10 Fr
Puppies >500 g: 14 Fr

Orogastric Tubes

Placement of orogastric tubes can be stressful to pediatric patients, and if long-term feeding will be necessary, it may be more beneficial to place another type of feeding tube. A red rubber feeding tube should be used. Appropriate tube sizes are listed in Box 44-3.

Before placing the tube, measure from the tip of the patient's nose to the last rib and mark the measurement on the tube to help ensure that the tip of the tube will be in the stomach. It is important to remeasure and remark weekly as the patient grows. Place the puppy or kitten in sternal recumbency with the head forward but not fully elevated (full extension of the head closes the esophagus and fully opens the larynx, increasing the risk of tube placement into the lungs). The tube should pass easily down the left side of the mouth into the esophagus. Advance to the mark that is measured on the tube. If an obstruction is felt before reaching the mark on the tube, then the tube is in the trachea. Remove the tube and start over. Tube placement can also be checked by placing a stethoscope on the stomach, infusing a small amount of air into the tube, and listening for air in the stomach. Some clinicians feel that the orogastric tube should be filled with milk before placement into the stomach. This will then prevent air from filling the stomach. A stethoscope can still be used to listen for the sounds associated with filling the stomach. Once the tube is confirmed in the stomach, infuse the formula over a 2-minute period. When finished, kink the tube and remove quickly, helping to prevent any formula from dripping out of the tube while removing.

Prevent overfeeding or feeding too rapidly. Gastric overdistention can cause delayed gastric emptying, bloat, and diarrhea. Regurgitation can occur through the nose. Excess air intake can also cause bloat and make the puppy uncomfortable. It is strongly advised to ensure proper body temperature because hypothermia can also cause delayed gastric emptying. The maximum stomach capacity for a puppy is approximately 50 ml/kg of body weight. The maximum stomach capacity for a neonate kitten is approximately 4 ml/100 g of body weight. Additional information about placing orogastric tubes in neonates can be found in Chapter 2.

Nasoesophageal/Nasogastric Tube

Nasoesophageal or nasogastric tubes may be an excellent choice for animals that are malnourished and/or not candidates for surgical placement of a gastrostomy tube. A polyvinyl chloride feeding tube can be placed with local anesthesia (Box 44-4). The tube should be gently passed through the

TABLE 44-3	Appetite stimulants that can be used in cats (C) and dogs (D)			
Agent	**Dose**	**Route**	**Frequency**	**Species**
Diazepam	0.5-1 mg/lb	PO	As needed	C
	0.05-0.1 mg/lb	PO	As needed	D
	0.025-0.05 mg/lb	IV	As needed	C, D
	0.5-2.0 mg	IV	As needed	C
Oxazepam	0.15-0.2 mg/lb	PO	As needed	C, D
	2-2.5 mg	PO	As needed	C
Flurazepam	0.05-0.1 mg/lb	PO	As needed	C
	0.05-0.25 mg/lb	PO	As needed	D
Chlordiazepoxide	2 mg	PO	As needed	C
Cyproheptadine	2 mg	PO	q8-12h	C
Prednisone	0.125-0.25 mg/lb	PO	q48h	C, D
Boldenone undecylenate	5 mg	IM/SQ	q7d	C
Nandrolone decanoate	10 mg	IM	q7d	C
	2.5 mg/lb (maximum 200 mg)	IM	q7d	D
Stanozolol	1-2 mg	PO	q12h	C, D
	25-50 mg	IM	q7d	C, D
Megestrol acetate	0.5 mg/lb	PO	q24h	D
B vitamins	1 ml/L fluids	IV	CRI	C, D
Cobalamin	0.25 mg/lb	SQ	q24h	C
	0.5 mg/lb	SQ	q24h	D
Elemental zinc	0.5 mg/lb	PO	q24h	C, D
Potassium	0.25-0.5 mEq KCl/lb	PO	q12h	C, D
	3 mEq K gluconate	PO	q6-8h	C, D
Interferon alfa-2b	3-30 IU	PO	q12h	C

From Tams TR: *Handbook of small animal gastroenterology*, ed 2, St Louis, 2003, Saunders/Elsevier.
PO, Orally; *IV*, intravenously; *IM*, intramuscularly; *SQ*, subcutaneously; *CRI*, constant rate infusion.

BOX 44-4	Appropriate nasoesophageal tube sizes

Kittens: 3.5 Fr
Puppies <22 lb: 5 Fr
Puppies >22 lb: 8 Fr

nares and down the esophagus to the desired premeasured location. Confirmation of tube placement can be made by administering 3 to 5 ml of sterile saline into the tube. If the patient coughs, it is in the trachea and should be removed. Remember very young neonates have a poor cough reflex. The tube is simply secured by placing a suture at the nose and on the head (Figure 44-1). An Elizabethan collar should be applied to prevent tube removal by the patient.

Water should be placed in the tube and capped when finished, preventing intake of air, reflux of esophageal contents, and occlusion of the tube by diet. Patients can eat and drink around the tube. The nasogastric tube can remain in place for several weeks, until adequate nutritional requirements have been met by the patient, and can be removed at anytime.

Complications associated with a nasogastric tube include rhinitis, dacryocystitis, esophageal reflux, vomiting, aspiration pneumonia, and obstruction of the tube. The tube should be removed should any of the above occur.

Pharyngostomy Tube

Pharyngostomy tubes are generally not recommended but may be needed to provide nutritional support to anorexic patients that are suffering from protein-calorie malnutrition, as well as those that will not ingest food and water orally. One advantage that the pharyngostomy tube has over the nasogastric tube is the diameter of the feeding tube. Pharyngostomy tubes are generally 12 to 24 Fr, therefore accommodating a larger variety of diets. The esophagostomy tube is preferred over the pharyngostomy tube because of ease of placement and fewer complications. If the pharyngostomy tube is improperly placed, coughing, gagging, and partial airway obstruction may occur.

Patients should be placed under general anesthesia and intubated with an endotracheal tube. Proper and aseptic techniques should be used when placing a pharyngostomy tube. Once placed, water should be instilled in the tube and it should be capped, preventing the intake of air, reflux of esophageal contents, and occlusion of the tube by diet. When the tube is no longer required, the suture used to stabilize the tube can be cut, the tube removed, and the wound will heal by contraction and epithelialization.

Esophagostomy Tube

Esophagostomy tube feeding is advised for patients that have disorders to the oral cavity or pharynx. It is contraindicated in patients with esophageal stricture, upcoming

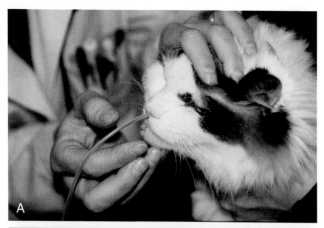

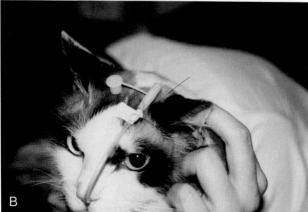

Figure 44-1 A, The tip of the nasoesophageal tube has been lubricated and passed into the ventral meatus by positioning the animal's head in a normal angle of articulation. **B,** The naso-esophageal tube can be secured to the skin on the dorsal midline between the eyes with tape "butterflies." A second tape tab should be secured as close to the nostril as possible using either suture material or glue. (From Ettinger SJ, Feldman EC: *Textbook of veterinary internal medicine*, ed 7, St Louis, 2010, Saunders/Elsevier.)

oral surgery, esophagitis, or megaesophagus. Tubes greater than 12 Fr can be used, allowing a variety of blended diets to be used. Once placed, water should be instilled in the tube and it should be capped, preventing the intake of air, reflux of esophageal contents, and occlusion of the tube by diet. When the tube is no longer required, the suture used to stabilize the tube can be cut, the tube removed, and the wound will heal by contraction and epithelialization.

Patients generally tolerate the tubes well, and maintenance of the tube is simple; owners can feed easily and maintain the tube at home. Patients can eat and drink around the tube, and once adequate nutritional intake is accomplished, the tube can be easily removed. Esophageal tube placement eliminates coughing, laryngospasm, or aspiration (Figure 44-2).

Gastrostomy Tube

A gastrostomy tube placement is indicated for anorexic patients with a functional GI tract distal to the esophagus,

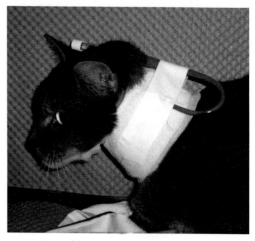

Figure 44-2 Cat with esophagostomy tube. (From Silverstein DC, Hopper K: *Small animal critical care medicine*, St Louis, 2009, Saunders/Elsevier.)

as well as in patients undergoing surgery to the oral cavity. Tube placement is contraindicated in patients with severe gastric disease or uncontrolled vomiting and in comatose patients. Advantages of the tube include ease of feeding and maintenance, patient tolerance, and larger tubes to accommodate blended diets.

General anesthesia must be used, and feeding cannot be initiated for 12 hours postoperatively. Tubes must remain in place for at least 7 to 14 days before removal to encourage adhesion between the stomach and abdominal wall. If the tube is removed early, there is an increased risk of gastric contents leaking into the abdominal cavity. Vomiting can be caused by several factors, including too rapid instillation of food, administering food that is not near body temperature, or a preexisting condition.

Once the tube is placed, water should be instilled in the tube and it should be capped to prevent the intake of air and occlusion of the tube by diet.

Enterostomy Tube (Jejunostomy)

Patients that undergo oral, pharyngeal, esophageal, gastric, pancreatic, duodenal, or biliary tract surgery may be candidates for an enterostomy feeding tube. Immediate feedings of a highly digestible, low bulk diet can be accomplished. Advantages of enterostomy feedings include bypassing the upper GI tract while still providing enteral support, decreased stimulation of the pancreatic enzymes, and fewer metabolic complications. Disadvantages include feeding an all-liquid diet, maintaining a constant rate infusion, and an increased potential for peritonitis.

When administering an all-liquid diet, the rate and volume must be regulated to prevent overdistention. A constant rate infusion must be given over an 8- to 10-hour period. Feeding cycles are divided into two 12-hour periods. During the first cycle, one quarter of the daily caloric intake is administered over 8 to 10 hours, with a 2- to 4-hour period of rest for the GI tract. If the patient tolerates the administration well, the second cycle is started with half of the daily caloric intake, administered over 8 to 10 hours, followed by a 2- to 4-hour rest period. A third cycle can then be administered with the full caloric intake, administered over 8 to 10 hours.

Parenteral Nutrition

Parenteral support may be indicated when a patient is unable to receive sufficient calories by an enteral route. Central parenteral nutrition (CPN) places a catheter directly into the right atrium or cranial or caudal vena cava. A nutrient mixture is administered via this central line. Peripheral parenteral nutrition (PPN) places a catheter in a peripheral vein and is indicated when a central line cannot be placed. In neonates and small pediatric patients, the intramedullary route can be used for parenteral nutrition.

When developing a nutritional protocol for parenteral support, the following should be considered: calories required; ingredients needed for specific metabolic conditions; protein, fat, and carbohydrate requirements or restrictions; and desired electrolyte levels. Human formulations are available but do not meet the requirements of animals. Desired formulas can be requested and made from a veterinary nutritionist. Compounded formulas must be made in a sterile environment and following the rules and regulations of the U.S. Pharmacopeia. Increased rates of sepsis have been reported with substandard compounding of formulas.

Phlebitis is a common side effect of catheters placed for CPN and PPN. Factors affecting phlebitis include catheter type, solution pH, blood vessel size, rate of infusion, blood flow rate, and medical condition.

A central line is hard to place but has the advantages of decreased phlebitis and a greater variability of solution to be administered over longer periods.

Metabolic complications associated with parenteral feeding include anemia, thrombocytopenia, hyperglycemia, hyperlipidemia, hyperuremia, hyperbilirubinemia, hyponatremia, and hypokalemia. By calculating the correct formula, the above-mentioned metabolic conditions can be avoided.

Mechanical complications may include catheter dysfunction, displacement, thrombophlebitis, leaking administration lines, line occlusion, and/or equipment failure.

SUGGESTED READINGS

Hand M et al: *Small animal clinical nutrition*, ed 4, Marceline, MO, 2000, Mark Morris Institute.

Hoskins JD: *Veterinary pediatrics: dogs and cats from birth to six months*, ed 3, Philadelphia, 2001, Saunders.

Kirk R: *Current veterinary therapy XIII: small animal practice*, Philadelphia, 2000, Saunders.

Tams TR: *Handbook of small animal gastroenterology*, ed 2, St Louis, 2003, Saunders/Elsevier.

THE ENDOCRINE SYSTEM

CHAPTER 45

Deborah S. Greco*

Endocrine and metabolic disorders affecting puppies and kittens from birth until 6 months of age may manifest as clinical problems related to growth or water metabolism (polydipsia and polyuria). Most commonly, endocrine and metabolic disorders affect growth of the animal; in particular, puppies are often presented to the veterinarian for assessment of delayed or aberrant growth. Other endocrine disorders of small animals, such as juvenile-onset diabetes insipidus (DI) or diabetes mellitus, affect water metabolism resulting in excessive thirst and/or urination, which can cause difficulty during house-breaking.

PITUITARY DISORDERS

Central Diabetes Insipidus

DI is a disorder of water metabolism characterized by polyuria, urine of low specific gravity or osmolality, and polydipsia. It is caused by defective secretion of antidiuretic hormone (ADH; central DI) or by the inability of the renal tubule to respond to ADH (nephrogenic DI). Deficiency of ADH (or vasopressin) can be partial or complete. Central DI is characterized by an absolute or relative lack of circulating ADH and is classified as primary (idiopathic and congenital) or secondary. Secondary central DI usually results from head trauma or neoplasia. Both central DI and nephrogenic DI are rare disorders.

Central DI may appear at any age, in any breed, and in either gender; however, young adults (6 months of age) are most commonly affected. The major clinical signs of DI are profound polyuria and polydipsia (>100 ml/kg/day; normal, 40 to 70 ml/kg/day), nocturia, and incontinence usually of

several months' duration. The severity of the clinical signs varies because DI may result from a partial or complete defect in ADH secretion or action. Other less consistent signs include weight loss because these animals are constantly seeking water, as well as dehydration.

Routine complete blood count, serum biochemical, and electrolyte profiles are usually normal in animals with DI. Plasma osmolality will often be high (>310 mOsm/L) in those with central or nephrogenic DI as a result of *dehydration*. Puppies with primary (psychogenic?) polydipsia will often exhibit low plasma osmolality (<290 mOsm/L) as a result of *overhydration*. When abnormalities such as a slightly increased hematocrit or hypernatremia are present on initial evaluation, they are usually secondary to dehydration from water restriction by the pet owner. In DI, the urinalysis is unremarkable except for the finding of persistently dilute urine (urine specific gravity, 1.004 to 1.012).

Diagnostic tests to confirm and differentiate central DI, nephrogenic DI, and psychogenic polydipsia include the modified water deprivation test or response to ADH supplementation. The modified water deprivation test is designed to determine whether endogenous ADH is released in response to dehydration and whether the kidneys can respond to ADH. The more common causes of polyuria and polydipsia should be ruled out before this procedure. Failure to recognize renal failure before water deprivation may lead to an incorrect or inconclusive diagnosis or cause significant patient morbidity. Normal renal concentrating abilities are not present in a puppy until 4 to 6 months of age. Congenital renal dysplasia can cause early signs of renal failure. A simpler way to differentiate between primary or psychogenic polydipsia and DI is to compare water consumption before and 3 to 5 days after desmopressin acetate administration (2 to 3 drops nasally twice daily); a 50% reduction in water consumption is consistent with a diagnosis of central DI.

*Adapted from Greco DS: Pediatric endocrinology, *Vet Clin Small Anim* 36(3):549-556, 2006.

Treatment consists of replacement of the deficient hormone (ADH) in the form of desmopressin acetate. Desmopressin, used to treat bedwetting in children, is available as a nasal spray; however, the nasal delivery apparatus should be removed before administration to a dog or cat as it can be uncomfortable for them. Two to 3 drops of desmopressin acetate nasally or onto the conjunctival sac twice daily is recommended to control polydipsia and polyuria in most animals with DI. It is important to counsel clients about the fact that water deprivation in the untreated central DI patient can be problematic.

Abnormalities of Statural Growth

Many pediatric endocrine disorders are manifested as abnormalities of statural growth. Causes of inadequate growth can be divided into two broad categories: intrinsic defects of growing tissues (skeletal dysplasias, chromosomal abnormalities, and dysmorphic dwarfism) and abnormalities in the environment of growing tissues (nutritional, metabolic, environmental, and endocrine). Intrinsic defects of growing tissues include most of the genetic and chromosomal abnormalities that result in growth failure. Genetic disorders may be suspected based on clustering of disease in certain breeds or lines of dogs and cats (e.g., chondrodystrophy of Alaskan Malamutes). Diagnosis may require pursuing pedigree analysis, genetic testing, or both.

Abnormalities of the environment of growing tissues are the most common and easily identified disorders. A thorough dietary history will reveal inadequate quantity and/or quality of feeding. Metabolic disorders, such as portosystemic shunting, pancreatic insufficiency, congenital heart disease, and congenital renal failure, may be identified by characteristic clinical signs and laboratory data. Endocrine causes of growth retardation include juvenile hypothyroidism, juvenile type I diabetes mellitus, juvenile hyperadrenocorticism, and hypopituitarism.

Endocrine growth abnormalities can be divided into two groups based on the type of dwarfism present. A proportionate dwarf exhibits small stature but precisely the same dimensions as the adult animal; proportionate dwarfism is characteristic of isolated growth hormone (GH) deficiency. In contrast, a disproportionate dwarf has a normal-sized head and trunk with short legs; disproportionate dwarfism is characteristic of hypothyroid- and hyperadrenocorticism-mediated dwarfism (Figure 45-1). Other endocrine causes of abnormal growth (e.g., juvenile diabetes mellitus) result in subnormal stature (not true dwarfism) and a normally proportioned, emaciated animal.

Pituitary Dwarfism

Pituitary dwarfism results from destruction of the pituitary gland via a neoplastic, degenerative, or anomalous process. It may be associated with decreased production of other pituitary hormones, including thyroid-stimulating hormone (TSH), adrenocorticotropic hormone (ACTH), luteinizing hormone (LH), follicle-stimulating hormone (FSH), and GH. Pituitary dwarfism is most common in German

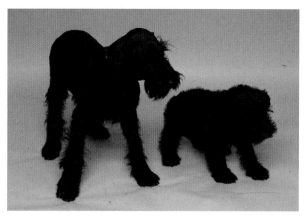

Figure 45-1 Disproportionate dwarfism in an 8-month-old hypothyroid Giant Schnauzer puppy compared with a normal littermate. (From Greco DS: Pediatric endocrinology, *Vet Clin Small Anim* 36(3):549-556, 2006.)

Shepherd Dogs 2 to 6 months of age. Other affected breeds include Carnelian Bear Dogs, Spitz, Miniature Pinschers, and Weimaraners. The disease is inherited as a simple autosomal recessive trait in German Shepherd Dogs and occurs as a result of cystic Rathke's pouch. The first observable clinical signs of pituitary dwarfism are slow growth noticed in the first 2 to 3 months of life and mental retardation usually manifested as difficulty in house-training. Physical examination findings may include proportionate dwarfism, retained puppy haircoat, hypotonic skin, truncal alopecia, cutaneous hyperpigmentation, infantile genitalia, and delayed dental eruption. Clinicopathologic features include eosinophilia, lymphocytosis, mild normocytic normochromic anemia, hypophosphatemia, and occasionally hypoglycemia resulting from secondary adrenal insufficiency. Differential diagnoses include other causes of stunted growth, such as hypothyroid dwarfism, portosystemic shunt, diabetes mellitus, hyperadrenocorticism, malnutrition, and parasitism. Diagnosis is made by measuring serum GH concentrations (no longer commercially available) or serum somatomedin C (insulin-like growth factor 1 [IGF-1]). The advantage of IGF-1 is that it is not species specific. There is usually a subnormal response to exogenous TSH and ACTH stimulation tests; furthermore, endogenous TSH and ACTH are decreased in affected dogs as a result of panhypopituitarism. A thyrotropin-releasing hormone (TRH) stimulation test would be abnormal as well.

THYROID DISORDERS

Congenital Hypothyroidism

Congenital hypothyroidism is a relatively common endocrine disorder of human infants, resulting in mandatory testing of neonates. In contrast, reports of congenital hypothyroidism in dogs and cats are relatively few. Only 3.6% of the cases of canine hypothyroidism occur in dogs younger than 1 year of age. Congenital hypothyroidism may be caused by aplasia or hypoplasia of the thyroid gland, thyroid ectopia, dyshormonogenesis, maternal goitrogen ingestion, maternal radioactive iodine treatment, iodine deficiency (endemic goiter), autoimmune thyroiditis, hypopituitarism, isolated thyrotropin deficiency, hypothalamic disease, or isolated TRH deficiency.

Because thyroid hormone secretion is essential for normal postnatal development of the nervous and skeletal systems, congenital hypothyroidism is characterized by disproportionate dwarfism, central and peripheral nervous system abnormalities, and mental deficiency. In addition, many of the signs of adult-onset hypothyroidism, such as lethargy, inappetence, constipation, dermatopathy, and hypothermia, may be observed.

Congenital hypothyroidism, regardless of cause, results in characteristic historical and physical examination features. Both dogs and infants have a history of large birth weight (in babies this is the result of prolonged gestation), followed by aberrant and delayed growth. In puppies, the first signs of abnormal growth occur as early as 3 weeks after birth, and abnormal body proportions are evident by 8 weeks of age. This is similar to human infants who are normal at birth but, if undiagnosed, exhibit characteristic signs by 6 to 8 weeks of age. Historical findings in hypothyroid puppies, such as lethargy, mental dullness, weak nursing, delayed dental eruption, and abdominal distention, are also observed in hypothyroid children.

Physical features of hypothyroid dwarfism in children include hypotonia, umbilical hernia, skin mottling, large anterior and posterior fontanelles, macroglossia, hoarse cry, distended abdomen, dry skin, jaundice, pallor, slow deep tendon reflex, delayed dental eruption, and hypothermia. In dogs with congenital hypothyroidism, hypotonia, macroglossia, distended abdomen, dry skin, delayed dental eruption, and hypothermia have been described (see Figure 45-1; Figure 45-2). In addition, because dogs develop more rapidly and become weight bearing sooner than human infants, gait abnormalities and disproportionate dwarfism are prominent features of canine congenital hypothyroidism. Midface hypoplasia, broad nose, and a large protruding tongue are some of the sequelae of untreated hypothyroidism in humans. Similar facial features, such as broad maxillae and macroglossia, were observed in affected puppies. In humans, delayed eruption of permanent teeth is observed in untreated congenitally hypothyroid individuals; delayed dental eruption is characteristic of hypothyroid puppies treated after 4 months of age. In humans and in dogs, both macroglossia and effusions of the body cavities are the result of myxedematous fluid accumulation. Hypothyroid puppies often exhibit haircoat abnormalities, including retention of the puppy haircoat and thinning of the haircoat.

Thyroid hormone is crucial for proper postnatal development of the nervous system. As a result, a significant number of properly treated and all untreated hypothyroid infants exhibit poor coordination and speech impediments later in life. Delayed treatment often results in low perceptual-motor, visual-spatial, and language scores in children with

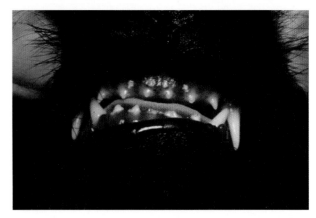

Figure 45-2 Delayed dental eruption in an 8-month-old hypothyroid dwarf Schnauzer puppy. (From Greco DS: Pediatric endocrinology, *Vet Clin Small Anim* 36(3):549-556, 2006.)

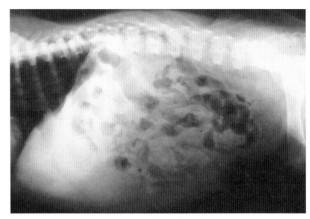

Figure 45-3 Epiphyseal dysgenesis in an 8-month-old hypothyroid puppy. (From Greco DS: Pediatric endocrinology, *Vet Clin Small Anim* 36(3):549-556, 2006.)

congenital hypothyroidism. If treatment is delayed beyond 4 to 6 months in human babies, intelligence is irreversibly affected, and mental retardation may ensue. Mental retardation is also likely in hypothyroid puppies; however, no objective evidence of delayed or aberrant intelligence is available to assess affected pups. Because the bulk of cerebellar development occurs postnatally, Purkinje cell growth is also significantly affected by congenital hypothyroidism. In humans and puppies, if treatment is delayed, signs of cerebellar dysfunction, such as ataxia, are observed.

Skeletal abnormalities, such as delayed maturation and epiphyseal dysgenesis, are the hallmark of congenital hypothyroidism. Delayed epiphyseal maturation is observed in the vertebral bodies and long bones of affected puppies. Epiphyseal dysgenesis, which is characterized by a ragged epiphysis with scattered foci of calcification, is observed in both humans and dogs with untreated congenital hypothyroidism (Figure 45-3). Normal epiphyseal development proceeds from a single center; however, in hypothyroidism, thyroid deficiency leads to the development of multiple epiphyseal centers, each with its own calcification progression. Disorderly epiphyseal calcification leads to secondary arthropathies in children suffering from untreated congenital hypothyroidism.

Clinicopathologic features of congenital hypothyroidism include hypercholesterolemia, hypercalcemia, and mild anemia. Hypercholesterolemia develops in both congenital and adult-onset hypothyroidism because of decreased hepatic metabolism and decreased fecal excretion of cholesterol. Hypercalcemia secondary to congenital hypothyroidism is the result of decreased renal clearance and increased gastrointestinal absorption of calcium. Decreased thyroid hormone stimulation of erythropoietic precursors results in a mild normocytic, normochromic anemia in some puppies suffering from hypothyroidism.

It has been well established that thyroxine is essential for the proper transcription, translation, and secretion of GH by pituitary somatotrophs. In humans (and most likely dogs), circulating GH concentrations are very high during the first few days after birth but rapidly decrease during the subsequent few weeks to levels just slightly above those in adults. In a previously reported case of congenital hypothyroidism, the dog exhibited a blunted GH response to xylazine but had a normal GH response to provocative stimulation following treatment of the hypothyroid state.

Diagnosis of congenital hypothyroidism is based on clinical signs, supporting clinicopathology, and thyroid function testing. It is vital to remember that normal puppies 5 to 6 weeks of age have serum total thyroxine (TT_4) concentrations 2 to 3 times higher than normal adult dogs. Therefore a serum TT_4 of 2.0 μg/dl, which is normal for an adult dog, would be low in a 6-week-old puppy and indicative of thyroid dysfunction. Serum free thyroxine (FT_4) would also be expected to be higher in normal neonatal dogs. A recent report of TT_4, FT_4, total triiodothyronine (TT_3), free triiodothyronine (FT_3), and reverse T_3 (rT_3) in puppies from birth to 12 weeks of age confirmed the suspicion that TT_4 and FT_4 are high in neonates. At birth, TT_4 was within the normal range, but by 1 week of age and until 5 weeks of age, the serum TT_4 was 2 to 3 times the normal adult range. Surprisingly, TT_3 and FT_3 were much lower in these neonatal puppies, suggesting an inability of neonatal animals to convert T_4 to T_3 peripherally. The advent of the endogenous canine TSH assay should allow discrimination of primary congenital hypothyroidism from secondary hypothyroidism (TSH deficiency). Puppies with primary hypothyroidism (e.g., thyroid dysgenesis, dyshormonogenesis) would be expected to have elevated endogenous TSH concentrations, whereas puppies with TSH deficiency should have subnormal endogenous TSH concentrations. Specific studies on endogenous TSH in neonatal canines have yet to be performed.

Treatment of congenital hypothyroidism in puppies and kittens is similar to treatment in the adult animal (22 to 44 mg/kg in the dog and 11 mg/kg brand-name L-thyroxine once daily in the cat). Some authors have suggested that hypothyroidism may be a cause of neonatal mortality in puppies; therefore 1- to 3-week-old pups in high-risk breeds may be screened.

PANCREATIC DISORDERS

Juvenile Diabetes Mellitus

Diabetes mellitus, a common endocrinopathy of adult dogs and cats, is rarely observed in puppies and kittens. All reported cases of diabetes mellitus in juvenile dogs and cats have been type I or insulin-dependent diabetes mellitus. Many canine juvenile diabetes mellitus cases, as in humans, are thought to have a viral etiology. Dogs suffering from juvenile diabetes mellitus usually present between 3 and 6 months of age. A genetic basis for diabetes mellitus is suspected in the Keeshonden and Samoyeds. Predisposed breeds for diabetes mellitus include Pulik, Cairn Terriers, Miniature Pinschers, Miniature Poodles, Miniature Schnauzers, Dachshunds, and Beagles.

In young dogs and cats, stunted growth is often associated with diabetes mellitus as a result of calorie deprivation. In dogs, progressive polyuria, polydipsia, and weight loss develop relatively rapidly, usually over several weeks. Another presenting complaint of diabetes mellitus in puppies is acute onset of blindness caused by cataract formation. Diabetic cataracts can develop rapidly, and the owner may notice that the puppy is suddenly bumping into furniture and other obstacles. The most common physical examination findings are dehydration and muscle wasting or thin body condition. Emaciated diabetic animals may have concurrent underlying disorders, such as exocrine pancreatic insufficiency, particularly those with juvenile-onset diabetes. A diagnosis of diabetes mellitus should be based on the presence of clinical signs compatible with diabetes mellitus and evidence of fasting hyperglycemia and glycosuria.

Treatment of juvenile diabetes mellitus may be challenging. Because these animals grow rapidly, insulin requirements may change drastically daily or weekly. The author has had success in treating 12-week-old Greyhound puppies with an initial dosage of 0.5 U/kg Lente insulin subcutaneously twice daily. Pork Lente insulin (Vetsulin; Intervet International B.V., Boxmeer, The Netherlands) is recommended. The puppies must be fed 3 to 4 times daily; additionally, regular insulin is administered at a dosage of 0.1 to 0.2 U/kg subcutaneously with meals. A growth formulation, rather than high-fiber foods, should be fed to growing puppies and kittens. Caloric requirements should be calculated for a growing animal. Management of concurrent exocrine pancreatic insufficiency will require the use of oral pancreatic extract and antibiotics for bacterial overgrowth.

SUGGESTED READINGS

Campbell KL: Growth hormone-related disorders in dogs, *Compend Cont Educ Pract* 10(4):477-482, 1988.

Feldman EC, Nelson RW: *Canine and feline endocrinology and reproduction*, Philadelphia, 1987, Saunders, pp 55-90.

Greco DS, Chastain CB: Endocrine and metabolic systems. In Hoskins JD (ed): *Veterinary pediatrics: dogs and cats from birth to six months*, ed 3, Philadelphia, 2001, Saunders, pp 353-355.

Greco DS, Peterson ME, Cho DY: Juvenile-onset hypothyroidism in a dog, *J Am Vet Med Assoc* 187:948-950, 1985.

SELECTED ZOONOTIC DISEASES: PUPPIES AND KITTENS

CHAPTER 46

Emilio DeBess

Puppies and kittens in their first year of life may become significant carriers of zoonotic diseases, which they acquire through various routes. Zoonosis is a communicable disease that humans may acquire from insect vectors, food, and direct and indirect contact with animals. Historically, more than 200 zoonotic viruses, rickettsiae, bacteria, fungi, and parasites have been identified throughout the world. Zoonotic infections are often acquired orally either by food or fecal-oral transmission. Children are at a higher risk of contracting zoonotic diseases because of their curious nature than adults or elderly persons. Therefore it is important for veterinarians to be aware of zoonoses, especially those that are related to direct pet contact, since 63% of households in the United States have at least one pet.

Because of the breadth of this topic, this chapter will discuss a limited number of zoonotic diseases (Table 46-1) to provide the reader with an understanding of the disease process.

RINGWORM (DERMATOPHYTOSIS)

Ringworm (see Chapter 17) is the most common zoonotic disease in the United States. Ringworm (dermatophytosis) is a fungal disease of cats, dogs, sheep, rabbits, cattle, and horses that invades keratinized structures (e.g., hair, horn, nails, feathers, and skin). Although it is self-limiting, clearing without treatment may take several months. Cats, especially young cats, can harbor the fungus without any noticeable clinical signs, thereby serving as an unsuspecting reservoir of infection.

Ringworm is readily transmitted to people by direct contact with infected animals, fomites (e.g., bedding), or contaminated environment such as the soil. The infections are spread mainly by spores, which are very long lived and can persist in the environment for years in blankets, clothing, bedding, combs, and other grooming tools.

Species that cause ringworm belong to the genera *Microsporum* and *Trichophyton*. These genera of fungi are somewhat unusual in that they produce asexual spores; sexual spores are produced so infrequently that they have not been observed. The most common source of ringworm in people is *Microsporum canis*, a species most often found on cats and dogs. When diagnosed, ringworm should be treated to limit the transmission of the fungus to humans.

The classic lesion is a circular patch characterized by broken stubby hair, scaling or crusting, and redness. The lesion will appear to spread outward, often with a central area of healing. Animals may have just a single lesion or many.

Diagnosis is usually made by microscopic examination of hairs from the site of the lesion for the characteristic spores lining the outside of the follicles. For a definitive diagnosis of ringworm, a fungal culture should be done as this is the most reliable diagnostic test for ringworm; however, it may take up to 3 weeks before any growth is seen. Single lesions (mild infection) can be spot treated with topical antifungal creams. Oral medications are available for more severe infections.

Because of its zoonotic potential, the best ringworm prevention is treating infected animals as soon as possible to avoid its spread to other animals or humans and to improve the likelihood of recovery without reinfection. Pet owners (particularly those with young children or immune-compromised individuals in the home) should be advised of the human heath risk and referred to their physician if lesions appear on any humans in the household. Because ringworm spreads easily, it is best to keep infected animals away from others until the infection has cleared.

ENTERIC INFECTIONS

Although a more comprehensive discussion of enteric infections may be beyond the scope of this review, several points related to animal-associated infections are relevant. Household pets may become ill with *Campylobacter* and *Salmonella*, but transmission from pets to humans is not common

TABLE 46-1	Top zoonotic threats from dogs and cats in the United States		
Disease	**Pathogen/vector**	**Incubation period**	**Syndrome (clinical/laboratory)**
Ringworm	*Microsporum* and *Trichophyton*	10-14 days	Circular patch characterized by broken stubby hair, scaling or crusting, and redness
Salmonellosis	Numerous serotypes of *Salmonella* are pathogenic for both animals and people	12-36 h, with a range 6-72 h	Acute enterocolitis, with sudden onset of headache, abdominal pain, diarrhea, nausea, and sometimes vomiting
Campylobacteriosis	*Campylobacter jejuni* and less commonly *Campylobacter coli*	2-5 days, with a range of 1-10 days	Acute bacterial enteric disease of variable severity characterized by diarrhea, abdominal pain, malaise, fever, nausea, and vomiting
Giardiasis	*Giardia duodenalis*, a flagellate protozoan	7-10 days, with a range of 3-25 days	Clinical symptoms include chronic diarrhea, steatorrhea, abdominal cramps, bloating, frequent loose and pale greasy stools, fatigue, and weight loss
Toxoplasmosis	*Toxoplasma gondii,* an intracellular coccidian protozoan of cats	10-23 days	Frequently asymptomatic or present as an acute disease with only lymphadenopathy, or one resembling infectious mononucleosis, with fever, lymphadenopathy, and lymphocytosis persisting for days or weeks
Toxocariasis	*Toxocara canis* and *Toxocara cati*, predominantly the former	In children, weeks or months	Usually mild disease, predominantly of young children, characterized by eosinophilia of variable duration, hepatomegaly, hyperglobulinemia, pulmonary symptoms, and fever
Cryptosporidiosis	*Cryptosporidium parvum*, a coccidian protozoan	1-12 days, with a range of 3-7 days	The major symptom in human patients is diarrhea, which may be profuse and watery, preceded by anorexia and vomiting in children
Cat scratch disease (CSD)	*Bartonella henselae*, also *Bartonella quintana*, may also produce illnesses among immunocompromised hosts, but does not cause CSD	Usually 3-14 days from inoculation to primary lesion and 5-50 days from inoculation to lymphadenopathy	Characterized by malaise, granulomatous lymphadenitis, and variable patterns of fever
Rabies	Rabies virus, a rhabdovirus of the genus *Lyssavirus*	Usually 3-8 wk, rarely as short as 9 days or as long as 7 yr	Acute viral encephalomyelitis; onset is often heralded by a sense of apprehension, headache, fever, malaise, and indefinite sensory changes often referred to the site of a preceding animal-bite wound
Animal bites	*Pasteurella* sp., streptococci, staphylococci, *Moraxella*, and *Neisseria, Fusobacterium, Bacteroides, Porphyromonas,* and *Prevotella*	12-72 h	Infected bite wounds are characterized by swelling, erythema, and warmth at the site of injury; purulent drainage, abscess formation, fever, regional adenitis, and elevated white blood cell count may be seen

compared with person-to-person and food-borne spread. The majority of *Giardia* infections in children are spread from person to person, especially in daycare settings; however, animal reservoirs of *Giardia* and other parasites may also contaminate surface water and may cause human disease.

Larval Migrans

Visceral larval migrans can occur in humans after infection by *Baylisascaris procyonis, Toxocara canis, or Toxocara cati* eggs. Following ingestion of infectious eggs, larvae penetrate the intestinal wall and migrate through the tissues, leading to eosinophilic granulomatous reactions involving the skin, lungs, central nervous system (CNS), and eyes. Ocular larval migrans most commonly involves the retina and can cause reduced vision, strabismus, uveitis, and endophthalmitis. Because the disease is transmitted by the fecal-oral route, human cases of *Baylisascaris* infection typically occur in younger age groups, mainly infants, who often engage in oral exploration of their environment and therefore are more likely to ingest *Baylisascaris* eggs. No effective therapy exists for the visceral form of *B. procyonis* larval infection. Adult *T. cati* has also been detected in some infected children.

The prevalence of *B. procyonis* in raccoons living in Portland, Oregon was assessed in 69 raccoons collected from wildlife control agencies. Infection with *B. procyonis* was assessed through the harvesting of adult worms from the intestines of raccoons. Fifty-eight percent of sampled raccoons were found to be infected with *B. procyonis*. Juveniles had the highest prevalence (70%) and heavier adult worm burdens (mean = 35 worms). The data suggest that juvenile raccoons are the major potential source of *B. procyonis* in Oregon.

Cutaneous larval migrans can be induced with infection by three species of hookworms infecting dogs and cats in the United States: *Ancylostoma caninum, Ancylostoma braziliense*, and *Uncinaria stenocephala*. Larvae are released from eggs passed into the environment in feces; infectious larvae infect humans by skin penetration. Larval migration results in the development of an erythematous, pruritic cutaneous tunnel. Occasionally larvae will reach the lungs and cornea. *A. caninum* has also been linked with eosinophilic enteritis in humans.

Prevention revolves around controlling animal excrement in human environments. Because hookworm and roundworm infections are sometimes occult, anthelmintics such as pyrantel pamoate should be routinely administered to all puppies and kittens at least twice, 14 to 21 days apart. In puppies, pyrantel could be given every 2 weeks between 2 and 8 weeks of age. Pyrantel could be given to high-risk kittens at 6, 8, and 10 weeks of age. Fecal centrifugation and flotation and direct fecal examination should be performed twice yearly on all dogs and cats to check for other parasites, particularly if they go outdoors.

Parasitic Infections

The molecular characterization of *Giardia* and *Cryptosporidium* has given rise to a more epidemiologically meaningful taxonomy. More important, molecular tools are now available for further typing of isolates of the parasites directly from clinical and environmental samples. As a consequence, information on zoonotic potential has been obtained, although the frequency of zoonotic transmission is still not completely understood.

Giardiasis

Giardia, a flagellate with worldwide distribution, may cause significant gastrointestinal disease in dogs, cats, and people. The organism has a wide host range; mammalian isolates are all currently classified as *Giardia duodenalis*. Using DNA sequences from a number of different genes, there appear to be two or three genotypes of *Giardia* in people, as well as two distinct genetic groups isolated exclusively from dogs. However, whether these genotypes vary in biologic activity, including their zoonotic potential, is for the most part unknown. There have been varying results concerning cross-infection potential of *Giardia* spp. isolates. In one study, *Giardia* spp. from humans were inoculated into cats; the cats were relatively resistant to infection. In contrast, evaluation of human and feline *Giardia* spp. isolates by isoenzyme electrophoresis suggests that cats could serve as a reservoir for human infections.

Because it is impossible to determine zoonotic strains of *Giardia* spp. by microscopic examination, it seems prudent to assume feces from all dogs and cats infected with *Giardia* spp. to be a potential human health risk.

Fecal examination should be performed on all dogs and cats at least yearly, and treatment with anti-*Giardia* drugs like praziquantel-pyrantel-febantel, fenbendazole, or metronidazole should be administered if indicated. Albendazole is also effective for the treatment of giardiasis but has been associated with neutropenia. Vaccination against *Giardia* could be considered in animals with recurrent infection; this practice is being evaluated as a possible therapeutic approach.

Cryptosporidiosis

People infected with the coccidian parasite *Cryptosporidium parvum* suffer severe gastrointestinal tract disease, including diarrhea and vomiting. Many infected individuals require hospitalization for the administration of intravenous fluid therapy. Infection of immunosuppressed individuals may be life threatening; people with AIDS may never be cured. Cryptosporidiosis has been documented in people and cats or dogs in the same environment, suggesting the potential for zoonotic transfer. *C. parvum* oocysts have been documented in feces of many domestic dogs and cats in the United States, Japan, Scotland, Australia, and Spain.

Until recently, no specific treatment was available. Although nitazoxanide is approved for treating cryptosporidiosis in immunocompetent patients 1 to 11 years of age, a review of (uncontrolled) data on nitazoxanide in treating cryptosporidiosis in patients with HIV argued that it might also be useful in this population.

Toxoplasmosis

Toxoplasma gondii is a protozoan parasitic disease and perhaps one of the most common small animal zoonoses; approximately 30% to 40% of adult humans in the world are seropositive, suggesting previous or current infection by *T. gondii*. The overall prevalence in the United States reported by the National Health and Nutritional Examination Survey (NHANES) between 1999 and 2004 was found to be 10.8%. In addition, seroprevalence among women of childbearing age (15 to 44 years) was 11%. People are most commonly infected by *T. gondii* after ingesting sporulated oocysts or tissue cysts.

In cats *T. gondii* multiplies in the wall of the small intestine and produces oocysts during what is known as the intraintestinal infection cycle and then excreted in great numbers in the cats' feces. Cats previously unexposed to *T. gondii* will usually begin shedding oocysts 10 days after ingestion of infected rodent tissue and continue shedding for around 10 to 14 days, during which time many millions of oocysts may be produced. Oocysts are hardy and may survive in the environment for well over 1 year. The oocysts must be in the environment 1 to 5 days before they sporulate and become infective. Therefore cat feces in litter boxes that are not cleaned daily can be potentially hazardous. The life cycle starts with a *Toxoplasma* parasite in the brain of a mouse or a rat. Since the parasite can only multiply in the cat's intestines, research has shown that *Toxoplasma* migrates up to the brain of the mouse or rat. As a result, the behavior of the mouse or rat changes, so when it smells a cat or cat urine, it subsequently loses the fear for cats. Cats then consume the infected mouse or rat, and at that point *Toxoplasma* enters the intestines of cats to multiply and continue its life cycle.

Toxoplasma gondii oocysts are not infectious when passed by cats. Most cats are fastidious about cleaning and do not leave feces on their fur. Bioassay failed to detect oocysts on the fur of cats 7 days after they were shedding millions of oocysts in their feces. These findings, supported by epidemiologic studies, suggest that touching individual cats is an unlikely way to acquire toxoplasmosis. In general, veterinary health care providers are no more likely than the general population to be seropositive for *T. gondii* infection. Because oocysts are passed unsporulated and noninfectious, working with fresh feline feces (<1 day old) is not a risk for veterinary health care personnel.

There is no serologic assay that accurately predicts when a cat may have shed *T. gondii* oocysts in the past. Most cats that are shedding oocysts are seronegative and would shed the organism if infected. Most seropositive cats have completed the oocyst-shedding period and are unlikely to repeat shedding. But because humans are not probably, nor commonly, infected with *T. gondii* from contact with individual cats, and because serologic test results cannot accurately predict the oocyst shedding status of seropositive cats, testing healthy cats for toxoplasmosis is of little clinical use. Fecal examination is an adequate procedure to determine when cats are actively shedding oocysts but cannot predict when a cat has shed oocysts in the past.

Fortunately clinical disease is generally mild following primary infection of immunocompetent people. Self-limiting fever, malaise, and lymphadenopathy are the most common clinical abnormalities, and the majority never realize when their first *T. gondii* infection occurred. The disease is potentially confused with infectious mononucleosis.

About 80% of women of child-bearing age in the United States are susceptible to acute infection with *T. gondii*. Transmission of the parasite to the fetus can result in mental retardation, seizures, blindness, and death. Some health problems may not become apparent until the second or third decade of life. An estimated 400 to 4000 cases of congenital toxoplasmosis occur in the United States each year.

The importance of *T. gondii* as a zoonotic disease should not be underestimated. However, it is very difficult to acquire toxoplasmosis from an individual cat. Once passed into the environment, sporulated oocysts survive for months to years. Most people are infected by ingesting sporulated oocysts from the environment, such as in gardening, and acquire toxoplasmosis by ingesting tissue cysts in undercooked meat, working with soil, or drinking contaminated water. For example, clinical toxoplasmosis developed in a group of people following a common drinking water exposure in a riding stable and in a group of people drinking contaminated water in British Columbia and Panama.

Ingestion of *T. gondii* in tissues can result in human toxoplasmosis, and eating undercooked meat, working with soil, and drinking contaminated water are probably the most common means by which the infection is acquired in the United States. Fortunately, *Toxoplasma* in meat is easily killed by proper cooking, freezing, or irradiation. *T. gondii* is considered nonviable by heating to internal temperatures of 152° F (67° C). *Toxoplasma* cysts are killed at 10° F (−12° C); freezing meat in domestic freezers for 24 hours usually renders *T. gondii* nonviable. Other suggestions to reduce the likelihood of contracting toxoplasmosis include boiling or filtering all water collected from the environment, wearing gloves or carefully washing hands after working with soil or raw meats, and thoroughly washing produce from the garden before ingestion. Ingestion of raw goat's milk can also result in human toxoplasmosis.

To prevent infection from cats, cover the children's sandbox when it is not being used. If cats are owned, a litter box liner should be used, and the litter box should be cleaned daily. Immunosuppressed persons including pregnant women should not clean litter boxes. Sporulated oocysts are extremely resistant to most disinfectants, and their inactivation requires exposure to 10% ammonia for 10 minutes; cleaning with scalding water or steam is most practical.

Bacterial Infections

Salmonella spp., *Campylobacter jejuni*, *Escherichia coli*, and *Yersinia enterocolitica* infect dogs and cats and can cause disease in humans. Gastroenteritis can occur in both dogs and cats following infection by these agents; *Y. enterocolitica* is probably a commensal agent in animals but induces fever, abdominal pain, and bacteremia following infection of humans. Puppies and kittens less than 6 months of age with campylobacteriosis can present with subclinical symptoms as well as with signs of ileocolitis. The chief clinical presentation is diarrhea due to the action of cholera-like enterotoxins and cytotoxins. Other symptoms include vomiting and anorexia. *Campylobacter* is commonly isolated from the feces of asymptomatic kittens. In fact, 49% of puppies and 45% of kittens, particularly strays or those living in kennels, may harbor *Campylobacter.*

Helicobacter pylori causes ulcers in people and has been isolated from a colony of cats; however, the zoonotic risks are currently undetermined. Infected pets and people in the same family have been found to be infected with *Helicobacter* spp. However, it is possible the human led to the infection of the animal.

Salmonella infection in cats and dogs is often subclinical. Approximately 50% of clinically affected cats have gastroenteritis, and many are presented with abortion, stillbirth, neonatal death, or signs of bacteremia. If neutrophils are noted on rectal cytology, culture for *Salmonella* and *Campylobacter* is indicated. Infection occurs after fecal-oral or fomite exposure, and prevention is based on sanitation and control of exposure to feces.

Recent studies evaluating raw food diets found that 80% of food samples contained *Salmonella* bacteria and that 30% of the dogs in the study were shedding *Salmonella* bacteria in their stool. Several studies have concluded that cats and dogs fed raw meat contaminated with *Salmonella* are at risk for development of salmonellosis and may pose a disease risk to their owners and handlers. Feeding of raw meat contaminated by *Salmonella* and recovery of *Salmonella* from the feces of sled dogs and Greyhounds has been documented, suggesting a risk of human infection from contact with infected dogs and cats. Adult dogs are often asymptomatic, but any infected animal or person will shed the organism for at least 6 weeks, thus acting as a source of exposure to other animals or people. *Salmonella* organisms are very difficult to remove from the environment and easily survive 3 months in soil.

Prevention is based on sanitation and control of exposure to feces. Antibiotic therapy can control clinical signs of disease but should not be administered to subclinical *Salmonella* carriers because of risk of antibiotic resistance. In bacteremic animals, parenterally administered quinolones are usually effective at controlling clinical signs of disease.

CAT SCRATCH DISEASE

Cat scratch disease (CSD) is caused by a *Rickettsia*-like organism known as *Bartonella henselae*. Although approximately 90% of CSD patients have a history of cat contact, there are anecdotal cases of CSD associated with dog, rabbit, and monkey contact. The United States has 57 million pet cats (one third of American households have them); thus there is a large reservoir from which *B. henselae* can be acquired by humans.

Although frequently seen in humans, CSD is not reportable and disease burden is not available. In 1992 to 1993,

Connecticut found the overall incidence of the disease to be 3.7 cases/100,000/year, with a peak incidence in children less than 10 years of age (9.3/100,000/year) and a median age of 14 years. In this survey, 52% of patients were female; 11% required hospitalization; and no deaths were reported.

In an uncomplicated case of CSD, a nontender papule develops at the site of inoculation followed by regional adenopathy, which develops 1 to 2 weeks later. Regional nodules enlarge for 2 to 3 weeks and then recede over the next 1 to 2 months. Nodes may be small and asymptomatic or massively enlarged and last several months. Most of the commonly enlarged nodes are axillary (45%), cervical/submandibular (26%), and groin (18%). Nodes may suppurate late in their course and require needle aspiration for relief. Fever occurs in approximately one half of symptomatic patients; systemic symptoms such as malaise, anorexia, and headache can also be present.

Prevalence of *B. henselae* among cat populations varies worldwide. The genotype Houston I is more prevalent in the Far East, and the genotype Marseille is dominant in western Europe, Australia, and the western United States. Cats are usually asymptomatic, but uveitis, endocarditis, neurologic signs, fever, necrotic lesions at the inoculation site, lymphadenopathy, and reproductive disorders have been reported in naturally or experimentally infected cats.

Cat contact is usually required for transmission of CSD. Because most cases have a benign course, avoiding cats is unwarranted. Exposure to kittens or young cats—especially kittens with fleas—is associated with the development of CSD in immunocompetent hosts. Fleas spread the bacteria between cats, although currently there is no evidence that fleas can transmit the disease to humans. Once a cat is infected, the bacteria live in the animal's saliva. Immunocompromised patients will want to control cat fleas. They may also wish to limit their exposure to both kittens (preventing bites, keeping the kitten's nails trimmed) and stray cats, which tend to carry *B. henselae* more frequently than older domestic cats.

ANIMAL BITES

Animal bites are a significant public health problem in the United States, and the number of bites appears to be increasing. There are substantially more dog bites than cat bites, and dog bites account for most animal bite wounds encountered in the emergency departments. Ninety percent of animal bites are from dogs and cats; of these, up to 18% of dog bites and up to 80% of cat bites eventually become infected, with occasional sequelae of meningitis, endocarditis, septic arthritis, and septic shock.

An estimated 77.5 million dogs lived in the United States in 2009, accounting for approximately 5 million dog bites per year. Of these bites, 800,000 required medical attention, 10,000 needed hospitalizations, and 20 people, mostly young children, died; 368,245 were seen in emergency departments.

On average in the United States each year, 18 people lose their lives to a dog bite.

Children less than 14 years of age accounted for 42.0% of the dog bite–related injuries in the United States; the rate was significantly higher for boys than for girls. Dogs were more likely to bite on the arm or hand (45.3%), bite someone they knew, and bite during the summer months. Cat bites appear to become infected more frequently.

A recent microbiologic study of dog and cat bites revealed that most infected bite wounds harbor multiple organisms, especially *Pasteurella* spp. Isolated aerobic organisms such as streptococci, staphylococci, and *Neisseria* are found in both dogs and cats. *Moraxella* spp., a common aerobic, is commonly found in cats. The most common anaerobes were *Fusobacterium*, *Bacteroides*, *Porphyromonas*, and *Prevotella*.

Bite wounds should be cleansed thoroughly and promptly. Bites by cats and humans are those most likely to be infected. When bite wounds are suspected to be infected, empiric antibiotics that treat *Pasteurella*, staphylococci, streptococci, and anaerobes should be administered. Common choices include amoxicillin/clavulanate or clindamycin plus trimethoprim/sulfamethoxazole. Tetanus prophylaxis should be considered. Treatment with a β-lactam antibiotic and a β-lactamase inhibitor is appropriate.

All patients should be evaluated and treated for any life-threatening problems; subsequently wounds should be carefully explored to ensure that the depth and extent of the wound are documented. Irrigation of wounds under pressure and debridement help to decrease the chance of infection developing. The decision to close lacerations from bites must be made on a case-by-case basis, taking into account the location of the bite, the time since the bite, and any evidence that may suggest infection.

Infected bite wounds are characterized by swelling, erythema, and warmth at the site of injury. Purulent drainage, abscess formation, fever, regional adenitis, and elevated white blood cell count can be seen. Infections in which *Pasteurella* spp. play a role often become symptomatic within 1 day and may spread rapidly. If fever is present in an immunocompromised patient after a dog or cat bite, systemic infection with *Capnocytophaga canimorsus* is possible.

Rabies should be formally considered in all animal bites, and local health department officials should be contacted if necessary for advice on animal disposition and the need for postexposure prophylaxis.

As our human population changes and grows, so does the dog population. Dogs are working less and moving inside and closer to families. More than half the national dog bite injuries (58.0%) occurred in the dog or victim's home, with the family dog listed as the primary source of the bite. As the interaction between dogs and humans increases, so does the physical and financial impact of dog behavior on human life. Teach children basic safety around dogs and cats, such as remaining motionless when approached by an unfamiliar animal or not approaching unfamiliar animals, playing with a dog only when supervised by an adult, and not disturbing a dog who is sleeping, eating, or caring for puppies.

METHICILLIN-RESISTANT *STAPHYLOCOCCUS AUREUS* IN PETS

Methicillin-resistant *Staphylococcus aureus* (MRSA) was named in 1961 to describe isolates of *S. aureus* in which resistance to methicillin (and, more broadly, to the entire class of β-lactam antibiotics) had been detected. Until the late 1990s, MRSA infections were problematic primarily in the hospital setting, as the disease was limited to those with "established health care risk factors" (frequent contact with health care system, previous infection or colonization, or a history of invasive devices or procedures).

The jump of MRSA to animals was expected because of the close relationship between animals and humans. In the late 1990s, reports of MRSA infection and colonization in pets were reported, and the number of isolates has increased dramatically in the past few years. Although this increase may be partially the result of increased testing and reporting, MRSA is definitely emerging in pet populations throughout the world. The role of pets in transmission of MRSA is still unclear; however, recent evidence suggests that MRSA can be transmitted between humans and their pets in both directions. Reports of MRSA infection and colonization in pets indicated that pets tend to be infected with strains that are predominant in the human population in their area.

Accordingly, the "USA100" hospital-associated MRSA strain accounted for the initial MRSA isolations from pets in North America. Not surprisingly, the "USA300" community-associated MRSA strain has now emerged as a cause of disease in pets. MRSA is emerging as an important veterinary and zoonotic pathogen, and the epidemiology of MRSA in household pets may take a parallel course to that in humans.

Until 2005, there were relatively few case reports of MRSA in animals. MRSA has now been identified in cats, dogs, horses, and pigs. *Staphylococcus intermedius* is the most common skin flora isolated from dogs and cats. However, even now the resistance gene associated with MRSA is detected in multidrug-resistant *S. intermedius* isolates.

Between October 2003 and December 2006, we documented 14 MRSA infections in companion animals at the University of Minnesota Veterinary Medical Center. The animals often present with nonhealing skin lesions or postoperative infections. Interestingly, the pets' owners were human health care providers, had been recently hospitalized, or were caring for a recently hospitalized family member. Most of the isolates from animals have been indistinguishable from the strains associated with human health care facilities (clonal group USA100).

Not all MRSA cases in animals have been related to humans. A recent outbreak in horses occurred at the Ontario Veterinary College in 2002 following several cases of postoperative or catheter-site infections. The investigation identified 27 infected horses seen at the veterinary college and 17 infected personnel. Most of the human patients reported direct contact with an MRSA-positive horse. Widespread environmental contamination was observed, with 62% of horse stalls previously housing an MRSA-positive horse testing positive. Equipment, such as stethoscopes, muzzles, and twitches, was also found to be contaminated with MRSA. This outbreak was attributed to the emergence of a novel MRSA strain in horses and subsequent spillover to their human caretakers. As a result, several infection-control measures, including routine equine surveillance and periodic human and environmental sampling, were instituted to control the outbreak and prevent further spread. Glove use was required for people handling any horse, and full barrier precautions and isolation were applied to all MRSA-positive horses.

Humans and pets can share both affection and infection. Veterinarians can be helpful in the diagnosis of zoonotic ailments. A 1987 study estimated that approximately 4 million pet-derived infections occur annually in the United States, with direct medical costs exceeding $300 million. Most pet-associated infections are preventable with simple measures like adequate hand washing, proper disposal of animal waste, and ensuring that infected animals are diagnosed and treated. Increased communication between primary care physicians and veterinarians could improve treatment and prevention of these conditions.

SUGGESTED READINGS

Bass JW, Vincent JM, Person DA: The expanding spectrum of *Bartonella* infections: II. Cat-scratch disease, *Pediatr Infect Dis J* 16:163, 1997.

Boyer K, McLoeod R, Marcinak J: *Toxoplasma gondii* (Toxoplasmosis). In Long SS, Pickering LK, Prober CG (eds): *Principles and practice of pediatric infectious diseases,* New York, 2009, Churchill Livingstone, pp 1267-1287.

Glaser C, Lewis P, Wong S: Pet-, animal-, and vector-borne infections, *Pediatr Rev* 21:219, 2000.

Heymann DL: *Control of communicable diseases manual,* ed 19, Washington DC, 2008, American Public Health Association.

Noah DL et al: Epidemiology of human rabies in the United States, 1980-1996, *Ann Intern Med* 128:922, 1998.

Talan DA et al: Bacteriologic analysis of infected dog and cat bites, *N Engl J Med* 340:85, 1999.

Zangwill KM: *Bartonella* infections, *Semin Pediatr Infect Dis* 8(1):57, 1997.

Page numbers followed by *f* refer to figures; *t* to tables; *b* to boxes.

503